Central Regulation of Autonomic Functions

Central Regulation
of Autonomic Functions

Edited by

ARTHUR D. LOEWY

K. MICHAEL SPYER

NEW YORK   OXFORD
OXFORD UNIVERSITY PRESS   1990

Oxford University Press

Oxford   New York   Toronto
Delhi   Bombay   Calcutta   Madras   Karachi
Petaling Jaya   Singapore   Hong Kong   Tokyo
Nairobi   Dar es Salaam   Cape Town
Melbourne   Auckland

and associated companies in
Berlin   Ibadan

Library of Congress Cataloging-in-Publication Data
Central regulation of autonomic functions
edited by Arthur D. Loewy, K. Michael Spyer.
p.   cm.   Includes bibliographical references.
ISBN 0-19-505106-8
1. Nervous system, Autonomic—Physiology.   I. Loewy, Arthur D.
II. Spyer, K. Michael. [DNLM: 1. Autonomic Nervous System—physiology.
WL 600 C397] QP368.C45   1990   612.8′9—dc20   DNLM/DLC
for Library of Congress   89-22825   CIP

Printing 9 8 7 6 5 4 3 2 1

Printed in the United States of America
on acid-free paper

PREFACE

The importance of the autonomic nervous system in regulating body functions has been appreciated for many years. The anatomy and, to a lesser extent, the physiology of the system were cogently described in Langley's monograph entitled *The Autonomic Nervous System* (Heffer & Sons, Cambridge), which was published in 1921. His book had an immense impact on the field.

With the development and application of a wide range of new experimental techniques in anatomy, physiology, and pharmacology, many traditionally held beliefs about autonomic function have changed or are in the process of being revised. Several excellent discussions of such advances have been published. The textbook by D. Purves and J. W. Lichtman (1985), *Principles of Neural Development* (Sinauer, Sunderland, MA), summarizes current knowledge of the development of the autonomic nervous system, and the 1987 monograph by J. B. Furness and M. Costa, *The Enteric Nervous System* (Churchill Livingstone, Edinburgh), surveys what is now known about the anatomical and neurochemical organization of the enteric nervous system. In addition, the issue of chemical cotransmission in the autonomic nervous system has been recognized through the outstanding contributions of a number of scientists, and these have been reviewed by G. Burnstock (1986) in his article "The Changing Face of Autonomic Neurotransmission," published in *Acta Physiologica Scandinavica* 126, 67–91, and by J. M. Lundberg and T. Hökfelt (1986) in a review article, "Multiple Coexistence of Peptides and Classical Transmitters in Peripheral Autonomic and Sensory Neuron-Functional and Pharmacological Implications," published in *Progress in Brain Research* 68, 241–262.

The idea that a wide spectrum of chemical transmitters operates at the level of the neuroeffector, the autonomic ganglia, and the central nervous system (CNS) has been clearly established. At many of these sites, the physiological actions of the various neurotransmitters and modulators have been studied at the cellular level. At the other end of the spectrum, the physiological description of autonomic reflexes has established that visceral afferents function not solely in transmitting nociceptive sensations but also as an integral part of the control mechanisms for homeostatic regulation of virtually all visceral functions.

In light of these exciting developments, it is perhaps surprising that so little appears to have changed over the last 20 or so years in the general appreciation within the medical and scientific communities of the role of the CNS in regulating autonomic functions. In many ways the prejudices and misconceptions that have grown out of this ignorance seem to have been perpetuated in typical textbook accounts of the autonomic nervous system. This is un-

fortunate in view of the dramatic advances in neuroanatomical techniques involving immunohistochemistry and axoplasmic transport tracing that have provided abundant new information on regions of the brain and the spinal cord that control the autonomic nervous system.
Neurophysiological studies at the single cell level have also contributed significantly to a
greater understanding of the role of the CNS in aspects of autonomic nervous system control.

The purpose of this volume is to redress this imbalance. Our initial intention was to be
comprehensive, but we concluded that it was better to concentrate on the areas in which
enough new ideas had developed to justify a revision of classical concepts. In doing so, we
were convinced that a mildly didactic approach was required rather than a traditional schol-
arly review as presented in volumes such as the *Handbook of Physiology* (American Physiological Society, Oxford University Press). Clearly, certain features of autonomic control are
underrepresented as a consequence, but our chapters include references to many reviews that
can provide supplemental information on most of these topics.

Our aim has been to review the central neuronal components involved in autonomic
control, and it is in this context that the book should be judged. We asked our contributors
to provide both historical and contemporary accounts of their fields of interest while making
their chapters accessible in style and level of detail to graduate students, medical students,
interested clinicians, and neuroscientists in general. We hope that the material is of sufficient
value to benefit autonomic aficionados as well since this is probably the first text to focus on
the CNS aspects of the subject.

The first six chapters provide a comprehensive review of the basic anatomy, physiology,
and pharmacology of the autonomic nervous system. The organization and control of the
autonomic preganglionic neurons (Chapters 4 and 5) are emphasized, and an overview of the
complex central autonomic pathways (Chapter 6) is given. These topics are amplified at several stages throughout the book. The early chapters are intended to familiarize readers with
the essential background for an analysis of the more detailed material provided in subsequent
chapters. In particular, the role of the autonomic nervous system in cardiovascular homeostasis is discussed in some depth in Chapters 8, 9, 10, and 11, as well as in Chapters 13, 18, 19,
and 20, where it is placed in the context of behavioral activities. The relationship between the
autonomic regulation of the fluid and ionic composition of the extracellular environment of
the body and cardiovascular control is explored in Chapters 13 and 14. The sensory information arising from the viscera is outlined in Chapter 7, and the role of the cerebral cortex in
autonomic function is considered in Chapter 12. The latter two chapters give an indication of
the perceptual qualities of autonomic sensation and their potential in modifying behavior. The
importance of the autonomic nervous system in the expression of affective behavior is reviewed in Chapter 19. The changes that occur in autonomic function during sleep provide
considerable insight into the neural organization of this state (see Chapter 20). Together with
the understanding of affective behavior, these changes indicate the widespread role of the autonomic nervous system in natural activity. The more direct effects of the system in regulating
visceral and endocrine function are addressed in Chapters 15, 16, and 17, although in each
case there is an attempt to draw behavioral significance from the fundamental observations of
functional control.

We have been fortunate in persuading a number of distinguished scientists to contribute
to this endeavor. They have sustained their interest in the project through the protracted editorial process that allowed us to use a great number of independent reviewers. Each chapter

has undergone a number of revisions, and the final form in many cases reflects the expert and constructive comments of the reviewers. Their role cannot be overemphasized and our thanks to them are sincere and deeply felt. Many of these experts could easily have contributed valuable chapters themselves, but space constraints prevented us from expanding the text further.

For the two editors, the challenge posed by this venture has been stimulating, at times difficult, but also entertaining. The editorial process often operates at an interface between scientific fact and opinion, and this is always fraught with difficulties. We have insisted on balanced and accurate summaries of each field covered in this book by making stringent demands on our contributors and ourselves, and we believe that we have provided a critical review of each of the fields while preserving our friendships with our collaborators and with each other.

It is a pleasure to acknowledge our debts to colleagues, past and present, who have contributed, often unknowingly, to the development of our ideas and have supported our activities in many ways. A special note of thanks must go to Jeffrey House of Oxford University Press, who encouraged us to undertake the task and provided many constructive comments at all stages of this project. It has been an interesting experience and one that will ultimately be judged by its success, or otherwise, in fostering more interest in this field of neuroscience.

We wish to thank the many publishers who have permitted us to reproduce illustrations. A particular note of appreciation is due to George Paxinos and Charles Watson, and Jeremy Fisher the Managing Editor of Academic Press, for allowing us to use, often in modified form, several drawings from their atlas *The Rat Brain in Stereotaxic Coordinates,* 2nd ed. (Academic Press, Sydney, 1986).

Specific thanks go to Sue Eads in St. Louis, who retyped a large portion of the text, and to Shona Beer and Doreen Campbell in London, who have provided secretarial assistance. We also gratefully acknowledge the help we received from Ann Dillon, Director of the Computer Graphics Center at Washington University in St. Louis, and the staff members (Barbara Boughen, Sandra Cole, Bebe Davidson, Becky Hasen, Diane Ressler, and Patty Wilson) who provided expert artistic skill in constructing the graphics used in this volume.

St. Louis   A. D. Loewy
London   K. M. Spyer

CONTENTS

CONTRIBUTORS

J. B. CABOT, PH.D.
Department of Neurobiology and Behavior
State University of New York at Stony Brook
Stony Brook, New York 11794-5230

D. F. CECHETTO, PH.D.
Robarts Research Institute
University of Western Ontario
London, Ontario, Canada NGA 5K8

F. CERVERO, M.B., CH.B., PH.D.
Department of Physiology
University of Bristol
The Medical School
Bristol BS8 1TD, England

W. C. DE GROAT, PH.D.
Department of Pharmacology
University of Pittsburgh
Medical School
Pittsburgh, Pennsylvania 15261

A. V. EDWARDS, SC.D.
Physiological Laboratory
Cambridge University
Cambridge CB2 3EG, England

R. D. FOREMAN, PH.D.
Department of Physiology & Biophysics
University of Oklahoma College of Medicine
Oklahoma City, Oklahoma 73190

G. L. GEBBER, PH.D.
Department of Pharmacology and Toxicology
Michigan State University
East Lansing, Michigan 48824

P. G. GUYENET, PH.D.
Department of Pharmacology
University of Virginia School of Medicine
Charlottesville, Virginia 22908

M. C. HARRIS, PH.D.
Department of Physiology
The Medical School
University of Birmingham
Birmingham B15 2TJ, England

W. JÄNIG, M.D.
Physiologisches Institut
Christian-Albrechts-Universität zu Kiel
D-2300 Kiel, Federal Republic of Germany

A. K. JOHNSON, PH.D.
Department of Psychology
University of Iowa
Iowa City, Iowa 52242

D. JORDAN, PH.D.
Department of Physiology
Royal Free Hospital School of Medicine
London NW3 2PF, England

A. D. LOEWY, PH.D.
Department of Anatomy and Neurobiology
Washington University School of Medicine
St. Louis, Missouri 63110

A. R. MORRISON, DVM, PH.D.
Department of Animal Biology
University of Pennsylvania
School of Veterinary Medicine
Philadelphia, Pennsylvania 19104-6045

D. PARKINSON, PH.D.
Department of Cell Biology and Physiology
Washington University School of Medicine
St. Louis, Missouri 63110

P. L. PARMEGGIANI, M.D.
Istituto di Fisiologia Umana
Dell Università di Bologna
40127 Bologna, Italy

D. W. RICHTER, M.D.
Physiologisches Institut
Georg-August-Universität Göttingen
D-3400 Göttingen, Federal Republic of Germany

C. B. SAPER, M.D., PH.D.
Department of Pharmacology & Physiology
University of Chicago School of Medicine
Chicago, Illinois 60637

K. M. SPYER, D.SC.
Department of Physiology
Royal Free Hospital School of Medicine
London NW3 2PF, England

W. D. STEERS, M.D.
Department of Urology
University of Virginia
School of Medicine
Charlottesville, Virginia 22908

Central Regulation of Autonomic Functions

1

Anatomy of the Autonomic Nervous System: An Overview

A. D. LOEWY

The autonomic nervous system is traditionally described as a motor system that provides control over visceral functions critical for homeostasis. This system is responsible for the extrinsic regulation of cardiac muscle, smooth muscle, and all glandular secretions. Various metabolic processes are secondarily affected by this system due to its control over the release of hormones such as adrenaline and related chemical substances secreted by the adrenal gland, as well as insulin and glucagon liberated from the pancreas. However, the autonomic nervous system is not strictly an efferent motor system. Almost all visceral nerves have sensory fibers intermixed with the motor fibers. These sensory fibers arise from visceral sensory neurons lying either in dorsal root ganglia or in certain cranial nerve ganglia and they carry information from receptors located in the end organs to the central nervous system (CNS). These function as a feedback system. This information, in turn, is integrated and relayed by multineuronal pathways in the brain and/or spinal cord and eventually modulates the autonomic motor outflow that controls the end organ. Similarly, a sensory feedback system arising from specialized visceral receptors also influences the release of certain hormones such as vasopressin, which act on specific target tissues in a manner parallel with autonomic-induced changes. More detailed discussions of the sensory pathways affecting autonomic motor and hormonal output are presented in Chapters 6, 7, and 13.

GENERAL ORGANIZATION

The autonomic nervous system is composed of two major divisions: sympathetic and parasympathetic. A third division, the enteric nervous system, made up of a complex set of neurons in the wall of the gut, regulates gastrointestinal secretion and motility. It is now recognized as a separate division of the autonomic nervous system.

The motor portion of the sympathetic and parasympathetic systems is made up of two sets of serially connected neurons. Preganglionic neurons, whose cell bodies lie within the CNS, send their axons to specific ganglia located in the peripheral nervous system and synapse on second-order neurons called *ganglion cells* or *postganglionic neurons,*[1] which, in turn, innervate various target tissues (see Figure 1-1). This constitutes a major difference between the autonomic and somatic motor systems: the former always is made up of a two-neuron chain while somatic motor neurons directly innervate their target tissue.

Differences in the parasympathetic and sympathetic systems are illustrated in Figure 1-1. Parasympathetic ganglia lie either near or within the wall of the organ they innervate, and thus the axons of these ganglion cells are shorter than those arising from sympathetic ganglion cells. Although both types of preganglionic neurons use acetylcholine as a neurotransmitter, the postganglionic neurons differ. Almost all of the sympathetic postganglionic neurons use noradrenaline (norepinephrine) and all of the parasympathetic postganglionic neurons use acetylcholine. However, as we will see, this is an oversimplification because many of these neurons use multiple chemical messages as either transmitters or modulators and/or comediators.

Many organs are innervated by both the sympathetic and parasympathetic divisions of the autonomic nervous system. These control antagonistic functions. For example, the smooth muscles of the iris that dilate the pupil are activated by sympathetic nerves whereas those that constrict the pupil are activated by parasympathetic nerves. A second example of this dual innervation is seen in the heart, where stimulation of the sympathetic fibers causes

---

[1] Strictly speaking, the term *postganglionic neuron* is a misnomer, but it is used here to contrast these cells with preganglionic neurons. The two terms are used interchangeably in this chapter.

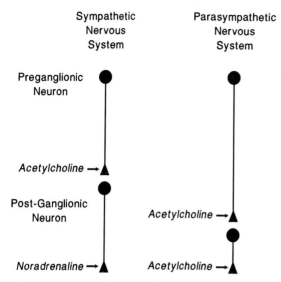

Figure 1-1 Schematic drawing illustrating the anatomical arrangement in the autonomic nervous system of preganglionic and postganglionic neurons and their transmitters.

tachycardia and excitation of the parasympathetic fibers produces bradycardia.

SYMPATHETIC NERVOUS SYSTEM

The motor outflow of the sympathetic nervous system arises predominantly from the intermediolateral cell column of the thoracic and upper lumbar spinal cord (Figure 1-2). This outflow originates from sympathetic preganglionic neurons that are segmentally organized in the spinal cord (Figure 1-3; also see Chapter 4). For this reason, this division of the autonomic nervous system is sometimes called the thoracolumbar outflow. The axons of the sympathetic preganglionic neurons leave the spinal cord at the same segment where their cell bodies lie and travel first in the ventral roots and then in the white communicating rami, either to gain access to the paravertebral sympathetic chain ganglia or other paravertebral ganglia (viz. superior cervical, middle cervical, and stellate sympathetic ganglia). However, some axons course through the sympathetic chain ganglia without synapsing to form the splanchnic nerves, which project to the preaortic (prevertebral) sympathetic ganglia (Figure 1-4).

Attempts have been made to provide quantitative data on the innervation ratio of sympathetic preganglionic neurons to sympathetic ganglion cells. Most of the studies have focused on the superior cervical ganglion in the rat, which is a functionally heterogeneous ganglion. The data obtained vary considerably from a 1:4 (Brooks-Fournier and Coggeshall, 1981) to a 1:20 sympathetic preganglionic neuron:ganglion cell ratio (see Gabella, 1985 for review and references). A more important statistic than total fiber counts would be a quantification of the relationship between sympathetic preganglionic neurons and ganglion cells in specific functional systems such as the iris and the heart. These might have lower ratios for finer control of the end organ than other tissues like sweat glands.

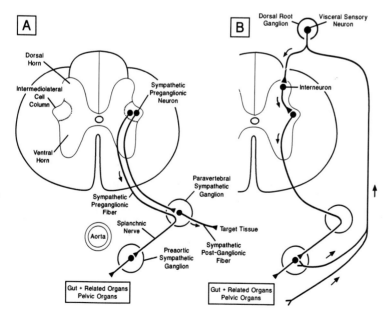

Figure 1-2 Drawing illustrating the organization of the sympathetic nervous system. (A) The sympathetic preganglionic neurons and sympathetic ganglion cells are shown. (B) Visceral sensory neurons originating in the dorsal root ganglia transmit sensory information from both the gastrointestinal viscera and the preaortic sympathetic ganglia to the dorsal horn.

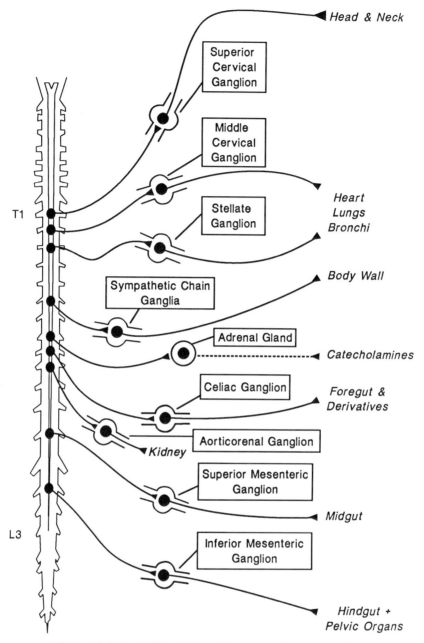

Figure 1-3 Schematic illustration of the sympathetic nervous system.

The sympathetic preganglionic neurons use acetylcholine as a neurotransmitter, although a small minority of these cells may use other neuroactive agents. Most of the sympathetic postganglionic neurons utilize noradrenaline as their neurotransmitter, with at least one notable exception—the neurons innervating the sweat glands use acetylcholine. In addition, in certain mammalian species, some of the postganglionic sympathetic nerves innervating the blood vessels of skeletal muscle may also use acetylcholine (Bolme et al., 1970).

Traditionally, it was thought that sympathetic postganglionic neurons used only one transmitter, but substantial anatomical and pharmacological evidence indicates that chemical transmission of these neurons employs multiple chemical agents (see reviews by Burnstock, 1986 and Lundberg and Hökfelt, 1986). Histochemical studies demonstrated that sympathetic postganglionic neurons contain immunoreactive neuropeptides colocalized in the same cells that produce noradrenaline (Hökfelt et al., 1977, see review by Schultzberg and Lindh, 1988).

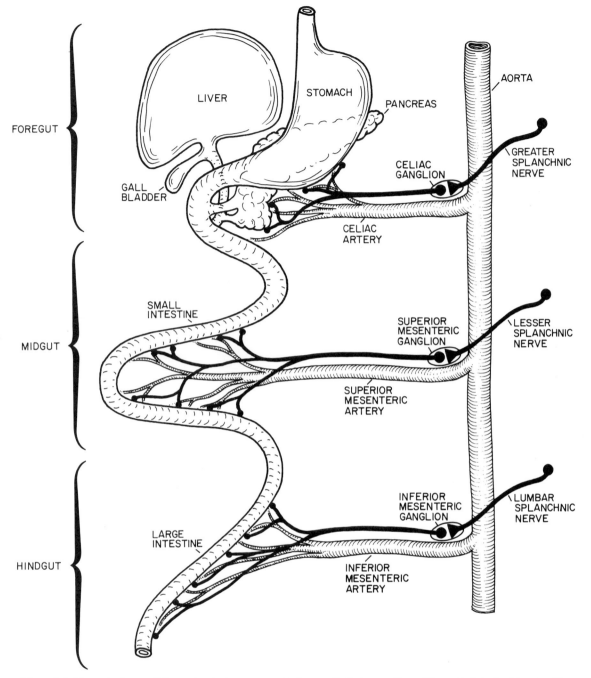

Figure 1-4 General scheme of the anatomical arrangement of sympathetic innervation of the gastrointestinal tract and its related organs, based on the embryonic pattern.

Some of these subpopulations of sympathetic post-ganglionic neurons innervate specific types of tissues. For example, noradrenergic–somatostatin immunoreactive sympathetic postganglionic neurons innervate the submucosal ganglia and gut mucosa (Costa and Furness, 1984) and noradrenergic–neuropeptide Y immunoreactive cells innervate the vasculature of the gut and hindlimb (Schmidt et al.,

1988a and b; Pernow and Lundberg, 1988). The cholinergic postganglionic neurons innervating the sweat glands contain immunoreactive calcitonin gene-related peptide and vasoactive intestinal polypeptide (Landis and Fredieu, 1986). Still other neuroactive chemicals have been shown to function as cotransmitters, modulators, or comediators along with noradrenaline. Adenosine-5′-triphosphate

(ATP), for example, has been implicated in the sympathetic control of blood vessels (Burnstock and Kennedy, 1986; Burnstock and Warland, 1987). The amount of release of many of these costored agents appears to be dependent on the firing frequency of the postganglionic neurons in both the parasympathetic and sympathetic systems (e.g., Lundberg, 1981; LaCroix et al., 1988a and b).

Sensory neurons associated with the sympathetic nervous system are located in dorsal root ganglia (Figure 1-2). These neurons are arranged segmentally and have projections to both sympathetic ganglia and peripheral targets. The density of the sensory innervation is variable. For example, it has been shown in the rat that the sympathetic ganglia innervating the gut and pelvic organs (viz. celiac, superior and inferior mesenteric ganglia) are also innervated by approximately 100–800 dorsal root ganglion cells, whereas the sympathetic ganglia controlling visceral structures in the head or thorax receive inputs from fewer than 100 dorsal root ganglion cells (Strack et al., 1988). This difference in the density of the dorsal root innervation of the preaortic ganglia may be related to the degree of control that these ganglia have on their end organs.

A chemical coding is suggested by the variety of neuropeptides that has been localized in some of the visceral dorsal root ganglion cells with immunohistochemical methods. The neuropeptides include angiotensin II, arginine-vasopressin, bombesin, calcitonin gene-related peptide (CGRP), cholecystokinin, galanin, substance P, enkephalin, oxytocin, somatostatin, and vasoactive intestinal polypeptide, (see Chapter 6 and reviews by Dockray and Sharkey, 1986 and Dalsgaard, 1988). Under certain circumstances, these peptides may function as a neurotransmitter or modulator at the end organ or within the sympathetic ganglion. For example, CGRP has been implicated in control of blood vessels in the skin (Brain and Williams, 1988) and in the gut (Kawasaka et al., 1988). Some of these neuropeptides have been shown to interact with other neuropeptides that may be coreleased from the sympathetic nervous system and some visceral responses are further modified by enzymes released from nearby mast cells (Brain and Williams, 1988).

PARASYMPATHETIC NERVOUS SYSTEM

Like the sympathetic nervous system, the motor portion of the parasympathetic division is organized as a two-neuron chain (Figures 1-1 and 1-5). The preganglionic neurons arise either from nuclei in the brain stem or from the intermediolateral cell column of the sacral spinal cord. They exit in either the oculomotor (IIIrd), facial (VIIth), glossopharyngeal (IXth), or vagal (Xth) cranial nerves or the 2nd, 3rd, and 4th sacral ventral roots, and because of this anatomical property, the parasympathetic nervous system is sometimes referred to as the *craniosacral outflow.*

The oculomotor (IIIrd cranial nerve) parasympathetic outflow originates from preganglionic neurons in the Edinger–Westphal nucleus (Figure 1-6) and other adjacent areas of the midbrain in nonprimate mammals (see Chapter 15). These neurons send their axons in the oculomotor nerve and project to the ciliary ganglion. Here, they synapse on the ganglion neurons that give rise to the parasympathetic fibers that control the pupilloconstrictor muscle of the iris and the ciliary muscle, which subserves accommodation. The sensory feedback for this system occurs via two separate multisynaptic central pathways originating from the retina. These pathways transmit information on luminosity and visual clarity to various visual centers. Then, after appropriate processing, they modulate the motor neurons controlling the iris and the ciliary muscle that affects the degree of tension exerted on the lens and hence controls accommodation. These pathways are discussed in Chapter 15.

The secretory glands of the head (lacrimal, mucous, and salivary glands) are controlled by the parasympathetic outflow of the facial (VIIth cranial) and glossopharyngeal (IXth cranial) nerves. These originate from parasympathetic preganglionic neurons localized in the medullary reticular formation (Figure 1-7). Two ill-defined areas that have been termed the *superior* and *inferior salivatory nuclei* are the main sources of these motor neurons. In addition, a few preganglionic neurons have also been reported to lie in the area near the nucleus tractus solitarius in the rat (Contreras et al., 1980). Although these cell groups are difficult to identify in routine histological material, since they are cholinergic, immunohistochemical preparations of the brain stem stained with antibodies to choline acetyltransferase have been used to reveal their location (Armstrong et al., 1983; Kimura et al., 1981). However, the most definitive evidence has been gathered by retrograde transport studies using horseradish peroxidase (Contreras et al., 1980; Hiura, 1977; Nicholson and Severin, 1981; Satoni et al., 1979).

The neurons of the superior salivatory nucleus send their axons out of the brain stem via the intermediate branch of the facial nerve. These axons synapse either on the pterygopalatine (formerly called sphenopalatine) or the submandibular ganglion cells. These ganglia give rise to postganglionic fibers that project to specific targets (Figure 1-7). The pterygopalatine ganglion cells innervate the lacrimal gland and the palatal, pharyngeal, and nasal mucous

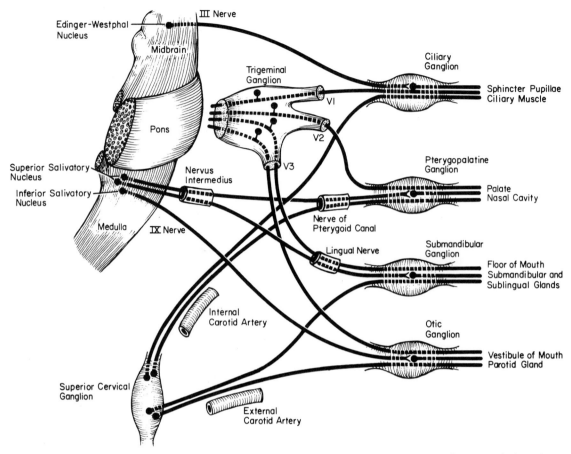

Figure 1-5 Drawing illustrating the parasympathetic innervation of the head and the accompanying sympathetic and sensory nerves. [Modified from Last, R. J. (1972). *Anatomy: Regional and Applied.* Churchill-Livingstone Medical Publishers, New York. With permission of the author and publisher.]

glands. In addition, some of these ganglion cells innervate the cerebral and ocular vasculature as well (e.g., Hara et al., 1985; Uddman et al., 1980). The submandibular ganglion cells innervate the submandibular and sublingual salivary glands as well as mucous glands in part of the oral cavity. Neurons of the inferior salivatory nucleus, lying just caudal to the superior salivatory nucleus, send their axons in the glossopharyngeal (IXth cranial) nerve to the otic ganglion (Figure 1-7). A few additional cells are also found in the vicinity of the nucleus tractus solitarius. The otic ganglion cells innervate the parotid salivary gland and mucous glands located in the vestibule of the mouth. In addition, they may also innervate the cerebral blood vessels of the posterior cranial fossa (Hara et al., 1985).

Sensory feedback from mucous membranes of the nasal and oral cavities is transmitted to the medulla oblongata by the trigeminal sensory fibers. Trigeminal fibers project to the nucleus tractus solitarius and the principal and spinal trigeminal nuclei (Beckstead and Norgren, 1979). While this afferent system is not strictly part of the autonomic nervous system, trigeminal sensory fibers innervating the cornea and the nasal and oral cavities reflexly trigger the appropriate lacrimal, nasal, and oral secretions via local brain stem pathways. The circuitry of these responses is not known, but it is likely to involve interneurons that originate either in the spinal trigeminal nucleus or the nucleus tractus solitarius and project to the respective parasympathetic preganglionic motor neurons.

The vagus nerve provides parasympathetic control of the heart, as well as of the smooth muscle and glands of the viscera of the neck, the thorax, and the gastrointestinal system, extending from the stomach to the left (splenic) colic flexure (Figure 1-8). It also innervates organs accessory to the gastrointestinal tract like the pancreas and the liver. Vagal preganglionic neurons originate from two nuclei in the medulla oblongata: the dorsal vagal nucleus and the nucleus ambiguus. The former is generally thought to control secretomotor functions and the latter visceromotor activities (see Chapter 5). The pregangli-

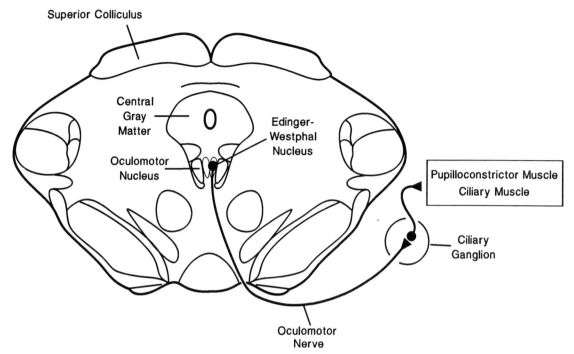

Figure 1-6 Transverse section of the midbrain illustrating the oculomotor parasympathetic system. [Drawing modified from Paxinos, G., and Watson, C. (1986). *The Rat Brain in Stereotaxic Coordinates,* 2nd ed. Academic Press, Sydney. With permission of the authors and publisher.]

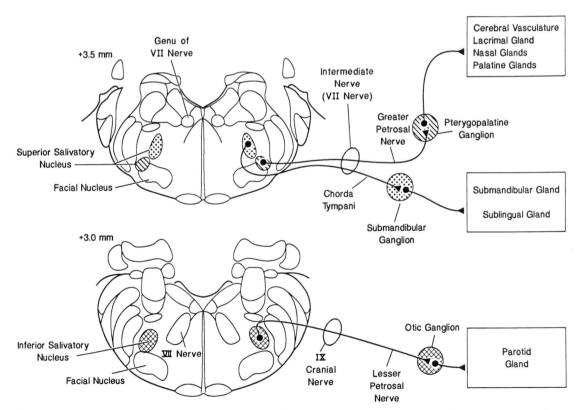

Figure 1-7 Transverse sections of the medulla oblongata illustrating the VIIth and IXth cranial nerve parasympathetic systems. Numbers in the left-hand corners indicate the distance from the calamus scriptorius. [Drawing modified from Paxinos, G., and Watson, C. (1986). *The Rat Brain in Stereotaxic Coordinates,* 2nd ed. Academic Press, Sydney. With permission of the authors and publisher.]

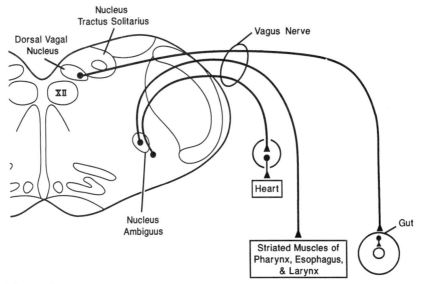

Figure 1-8 Transverse section of the medulla oblongata illustrating the vagal motor system.

onic fibers travel in the vagus nerve to their end organs and synapse in ganglia either embedded in the
wall of these structures or in close proximity to
them.

Vagal sensory ganglion cells that lie in the nodose
ganglion (inferior vagal ganglion) transmit sensory
information from the viscera of the neck, the thorax,
and most of the abdominal cavity to the nucleus
tractus solitarius. Further details are presented in
Chapters 6 and 10. A number of different neuropeptides, including calcitonin gene-related peptide, cholecystokinin, neurokinin A, somatostatin, substance
P, and vasoactive intestinal polypeptide have been

localized immunohistochemically in some of these
cells and probably code specific sensory messages
(Helke and Hill, 1988).

The sacral parasympathetic outflow controls the
pelvic organs (Figure 1-9) and is considered in Chapter 17. Cell bodies of the parasympathetic preganglionic neurons lie in the S2–S4 levels of the intermediolateral cell column and send their axons via the
ventral roots, and subsequently in the pelvic
splanchnic nerves, to the parasympathetic postganglionic neurons in the pelvic ganglia (Figure 1-8).
The postganglionic neurons innervate the descending colon, rectum, urinary bladder, and sexual or-

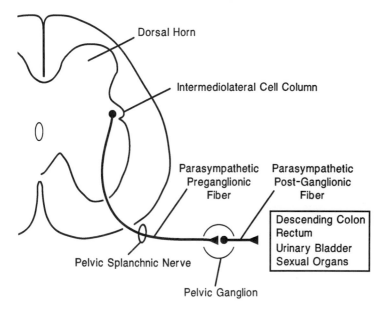

Figure 1-9 Transverse section of the sacral spinal cord illustrating the sacral
parasympathetic motor system.

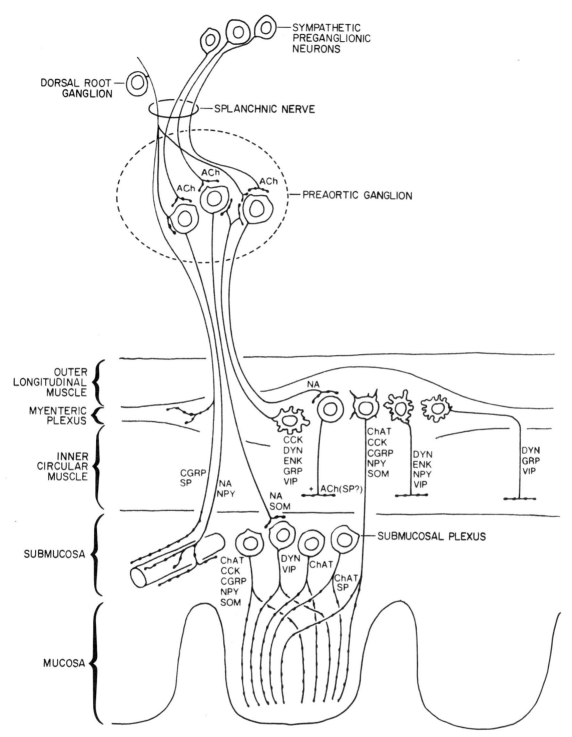

Figure 1-10 Schematic organization of the enteric nervous system. ACh, acetylcholine; CCK, cholecystokinin; CGRP, calcitonin gene-related peptide; ChAT, choline acetyltransferase; DYN, dynorphin; ENK, enkephalin; GRP, gastrin-related peptide; NA, noradrenaline; NPY, neuropeptide Y; SOM, somatostatin; SP, substance P; VIP, vasoactive intestinal poly-peptide. [Slightly modified from Costa, M., Furness, J. B., and Gibbons, I. L. (1986). *Progress in Brain Research* 68, 217–239, Elsevier Publications, Amsterdam. With permission of the authors and publisher.]

gans. Visceral sensory fibers arise in the S2–S4 dorsal root ganglia and are involved in control of colic, anorectal, and urogenital reflexes (see Chapter 17).

ENTERIC NERVOUS SYSTEM

Gastrointestinal functions are controlled by a system of intramural and extramural neurons. The intramural system, the major neural system that regulates gut motility and secretion, is made up of two sheets of neurons. The outer sheet, lying between the inner circular and outer longitudinal smooth muscle layers, is called the *myenteric plexus* and the inner sheet, lying in the submucosal layer of the gut, is called the *submucosal plexus* (Figure 1-10). The extramural system, formed by parasympathetic and sympathetic fibers, provides the motor commands that regulate gastrointestinal function and seems to subserve a secondary role, since almost all the basic functions of the gut may occur in the absence of an extrinsic innervation (see Furness and Costa, 1987, Furness et al., 1988, and Wood, 1987a,b for reviews). However, this does not negate the importance of the extrinsic innervation (see Gonella et al., 1987; Grundy, 1988; Jänig, 1988 for reviews).

A number of different functional types of neurons innervating the gut have been defined, and the scheme presented in Table 1-1 (Costa et al., 1986) is a useful summary. Figure 1-10 illustrates the diversity and complexity of these neurons and their putative neurotransmitters. Many of these neurons contain multiple neuropeptides and are thought to utilize these as neurotransmitters. Some general patterns can be summarized. The sympathetic postganglionic neurons comprise three anatomical subgroups: noradrenergic neurons that inhibit intestinal motility, noradrenergic–neuropeptide Y neurons that regulate blood flow, and the noradrenergic–somatostatin neurons that modulate intestinal secretions (see Costa et al., 1986, 1987 for reviews).

The neurons of the myenteric plexus regulate gastrointestinal motility. The neural circuitry controlling peristalsis involves at least five intrinsic enteric neurons (see Wood, 1987a for review). A command neuron that is sensitive to bowel distention regulates both inhibitory and excitatory interneurons. These interneurons control inhibitory and excitatory motor neurons (Figure 1-11). While the details of this circuit are unresolved, it is thought that the dynorphin–vasoactive intestinal polypeptide neurons function as inhibitory motor neurons and the cholinergic–substance P neurons may be the excitatory motor neurons. Whether separate types of excitatory motor neurons innervate the circular or longitudinal smooth muscles is unknown (for reviews, see Costa et al., 1986; Furness and Costa, 1987). In addition,

Table 1-1 Types of Neurons Innervating the Gut

Intrinsic motor neurons to gastrointestinal smooth muscle
    Excitatory cholinergic
    Excitatory noncholinergic (probably utilizing substance P)
    Inhibitory

Intrinsic secretomotor neurons
    Cholinergic
    Noncholinergic

Intrinsic vasomotor neurons
    Vasodilator neurons of unknown nature

Interneurons in myenteric ganglia
    Excitatory cholinergic
    Excitatory noncholinergic
    Inhibitory of unknown nature

Interneurons in submucosal ganglia
    Cholinergic excitatory
    Noncholinergic excitatory
    Inhibitory

Intrinsic sensory neurons

Extrinsic neurons
    Sympathetic noradrenergic neurons
        Inhibitory to myenteric ganglia
        Inhibitory to submucosal ganglia
        Excitatory to blood vessels
    Visceral afferent nerves from dorsal root ganglia

Intestinofugal neurons
    Excitatory enteric cholinergic neurons projecting to preaortic ganglia

Adapted from Costa et al. (1986).

there are neurons in the bowel that project to the sympathetic ganglia and are thought to function as part of the circuitry controlling sympathetic reflexes between different regions of the gastrointestinal tract (see Jänig, 1988 for review). These intestinofugal neurons contain at least five neuropeptides: cholecystokinin, dynorphin, enkephalin, gastrin releasing peptide, and vasoactive intestinal peptide (Costa et al., 1986). Very little information exists regarding these neurons and their role in modulating the activity of the preaortic sympathetic ganglion cells and how they affect sympathetically mediated gastrointestinal motor and/or vascular reflexes.

The intestinal epithelium plays a key role in body fluid homeostasis and specialized neurons in the submucosal plexus regulate this function. These neurons regulate ion and water transport across this epithelium, affect intestinal secretions of crypt cells, and provide a direct neural link to the myenteric plexus that affects gut motility (see Cooke, 1989 for review). When various toxins are present in the gut, specialized chemosensitive sensory neurons originating in the submucosal plexus trigger defensive reactions. Three events occur: absorption across the intestinal epithelium is inhibited, the crypt cells are

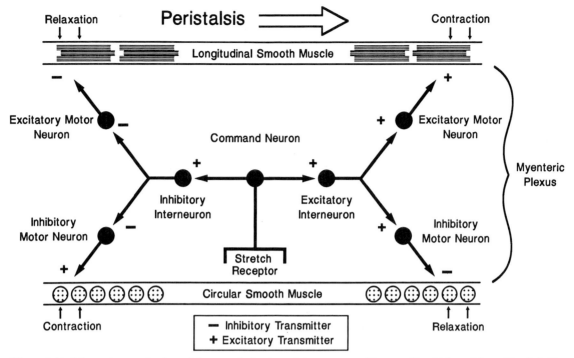

Figure 1-11 Schematic organization of the neural circuitry of the gut controlling motility. [Adapted from Wood, J. D. (1987). *Japanese Journal of Smooth Muscle Research* 23, 143–186. With permission of the author and publisher.]

stimulated to secrete water and ions, and gut motility is increased. Overall, the function of these changes is to eliminate the toxins by producing diarrhea. The neural basis of these three events is incompletely understood, but Ekblad et al. (1987; 1988) have produced detailed immunohistochemical maps of the rat small and large intestine. Their maps demonstrate that the neuropeptide-containing neurons of the submucosal plexus are organized in a highly specific chemically coded pattern. Although much of the detail of the plexus has not been studied, the individual actions of some of the neuropeptides on intestinal cell function have been examined (see Cooke, 1987, 1989 for reviews). It appears that many of these putative transmitters have complex functions involving the regulation of intestinal absorption and secretion as well as interactions with local lymphoid tissue affecting immune responses.

The external innervation of the gut comes from the sympathetic and parasympathetic divisions of the autonomic nervous system. For a long time, the prevailing view held that this extrinsic innervation served as a dual control system, but this view is an oversimplification of the complex neural mechanisms that regulate the gut. It appears more likely that the external nerves provide general commands over a heterogeneous set of intrinsic, highly specialized neurons (Figure 1-12; see Wood, 1987a and b for reviews). According to this hypothesis, the ex-

trinsic nerves can override the intrinsic system and produce profound changes in the gut. This is clearly illustrated under emergency conditions when the sympathetic innervation inhibits peristalsis and increases sphincter tone.

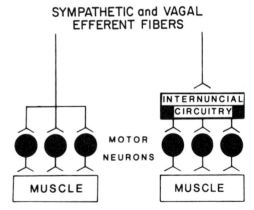

Figure 1-12 On the left, the older concept showing sympathetic and vagal efferent fibers synapsing directly on enteric motor neurons is illustrated. This view is no longer accepted and the current concept is illustrated on the right. According to this scheme, sympathetic and vagal efferent fibers transmit command signals to interneurons, which control the motor program circuitry of the enteric nervous system. [Adapted with modification from Wood, J. D. (1987). *Japanese Journal of Smooth Muscle Research* 23, 143–186. With permission of the author and publisher.]

SUMMARY

The autonomic nervous system is composed of both visceral motor and sensory nerve fibers that regulate homeostasis. This system can be subdivided into three major divisions: sympathetic, parasympathetic, and enteric. The first two provide dual, antagonistic control of many organs and directly innervate smooth muscle, cardiac muscle, and glands. The enteric nervous system is comprised of heterogeneous neurons within the gut itself that control gastrointestinal secretions and motility.

The sympathetic nervous system regulates most vital functions. When it is activated en masse, it functions to prepare the organism for the "fight or flight" response. Under these emergency conditions, heart rate and blood pressure increase, bronchioles dilate, gastrointestinal tract motility and secretions are inhibited, pupils dilate, and adrenaline is released from the adrenal gland to promote glycogenolysis. Under normal conditions, however, it provides the neural regulation of specific tissues.

The sympathetic preganglionic neurons lie in the intermediolateral cell column of the spinal cord and send their axons in the ventral roots to a series of topographically arranged sympathetic ganglia that contain the cell bodies of the sympathetic postganglionic neurons. These innervate specific target tissues. Associated with these motor nerves are sensory fibers whose cell bodies lie in the dorsal root ganglia. They provide some of the feedback for various autonomic reflexes.

The parasympathetic preganglionic neurons lie in several nuclei of the brain stem and in the intermediolateral cell column of the sacral spinal cord.

The head receives parasympathetic innervation from the oculomotor, facial, and glossopharyngeal nerves. The oculomotor preganglionic neurons lie in the Edinger–Westphal nucleus of the midbrain and send their axons in the oculomotor nerve to the orbit and synapse on the ciliary ganglion cells. This motor system controls the pupilloconstrictor muscle of the iris and the ciliary muscle that affects lens accommodation. The facial nerve preganglionic motor neurons lie in the superior salivatory nucleus and send their axons to the pterygopalatine or the submandibular ganglia. The former innervates the lacrimal gland and the mucous glands of the nasal cavity and the palate. In addition, it provides innervation of the ocular and cerebral vasculature. Submandibular ganglion cells innervate the sublingual and submandibular salivary glands and mucous glands of the mouth. The glossopharyngeal preganglionic neurons arise from the inferior salivatory nucleus and synapse on otic ganglion cells, which innervate the parotid salivary gland and the mucous glands of the mouth.

The vagus nerve provides parasympathetic control of smooth muscle and glands of viscera of the neck, thorax, and most of the gastrointestinal tract. Vagal preganglionic neurons originate from the dorsal vagal nucleus and the nucleus ambiguus in the medulla oblongata. The former is generally thought to control gastrointestinal secretomotor activity while the latter regulates visceromotor functions such as those related to bronchomotor tone and heart rate control. The preganglionic fibers travel to the end organ and synapse in ganglia that are either embedded in the wall of these structures or in close proximity to them. Vagal visceral sensory fibers originate from neurons in the nodose ganglion and travel with the motor fibers. They transmit visceral information to the nucleus tractus solitarius—the major visceral relay nucleus in the medulla oblongata.

The sacral parasympathetic system is involved in regulation of the descending colon, the rectum, the urinary bladder, and the sexual organs. It originates in the intermediolateral cell column of the S2–S4 spinal segments. The preganglionic fibers leave the spinal cord in the ventral roots and form the pelvic splanchnic nerves. They synapse in pelvic ganglia that lie close to or within the target organs of the pelvis. Associated with this motor system are sensory fibers that originate from the S2–S4 dorsal root ganglia.

The enteric nervous system is composed of two sheets of neurons that lie within the gut: the submucosal plexus and the myenteric plexus. Each is made up of specific types of sensory and motor neurons as well as interneurons. The enteric nervous system plays a major role in the control of water and ion movement across the intestinal epithelium and of gut motility. These two functions affect body fluid homeostasis and there are connections between the two sets of intrinsic neurons that serve this process. In addition, the extrinsic innervation plays an important role for reflex adjustments of large segments of the gastrointestinal tract that are needed for absorption of water and electrolytes and nutrients as well as dilution or elimination of gastrointestinal contents.

REFERENCES

Reviews

Burnstock, G. (1986). The changing face of autonomic neurotransmission. *Acta Physiologica Scandinavica* 126, 67–91.

Cooke, H. J. (1987). Neural and humoral regulation of small intestinal electrolyte transport. In: *Physiology of the Gastrointestinal Tract*, 2nd ed., L. R. Johnson (ed.), Raven Press, New York, Vol. 2, pp. 1307–1350.

Cooke, H. J. (1989). Role of the "little brain" in the gut in water and electrolyte homeostasis. *FASEB Journal* 3, 127–138.

Costa, M., Furness, J. B., and Gibbons, I. L. (1986). Chemical coding of enteric neurons. *Progress in Brain Research* 68, 217–239.

Costa, M., Furness, J. B., and Llewellyn-Smith, I (1987). Histochemistry of the enteric nervous system. In: *Physiology of the Gastrointestinal Tract*, 2nd ed., L. R. Johnson, Raven Press, New York, Vol. 1, pp. 1–40.

Dalsgaard, C. J. (1988). The sensory system. In: *Handbook of Chemical Neuroanatomy, Vol. 6: The Peripheral Nervous System.* A. Björklund et al. (eds.). Elsevier, Amsterdam, pp. 599–636.

Dockray, G. J., and Sharkey, K. A. (1986). The neurochemistry of visceral afferents. *Progress in Brain Research* 67, 133–148.

Furness, J. B., and Costa, M. (1987) *The Enteric Nervous System*, Churchill Livingstone, Edinburgh.

Furness, J. B., Llewellyn-Smith, I. J., Bornstein, J. C., and Costa, M. (1988). Chemical neuroanatomy and the analysis of neuronal circuitry in the enteric nervous system. In: *Handbook of Chemical Neuroanatomy, Vol. 6: The Peripheral Nervous System.* A. Björklund et al. (eds.). Elsevier, Amsterdam, pp. 161–218.

Gabella, G. (1985). Autonomic nervous system. In: *The Rat Nervous System,* Vol. 2, *Hindbrain and Spinal Cord,* G. Paxinos (ed.), Academic Press, Sydney, pp. 325–353.

Gonella, J., Bouvier, M., and Blanquet, F. (1987). Extrinsic nervous control of motility of small and large intestines and related sphincters. *Physiological Reviews* 67, 902–961.

Grundy, D. (1988). Vagal control of gastrointestinal function. *Baillière's Clinical Gastroenterology* 2, 23–43.

Jänig, W. (1988). Integration of gut function by sympathetic reflexes. *Baillière's Clinical Gastroenterology* 2, 45–62.

Lundberg, J. M., and Hökfelt, T. (1986), Multiple coexistence of peptides and classical transmitters in peripheral autonomic and sensory neuron-functional and pharmacological implications. *Progress in Brain Research* 68, 241–262.

Schultzberg, M., and Lindh, B. (1988). Transmitters and peptides in autonomic ganglia. In: *Handbook of Chemical Neuroanatomy, Vol. 6: The Peripheral Nervous System.* A. Björklund et al. (eds.). Elsevier, Amsterdam, pp. 297–326.

Wood, J. D. (1987a). Neurophysiological theory of intestinal motility. *Japanese Journal of Smooth Muscle Research* 23, 143–186.

Wood, J. D. (1987b). Physiology of the enteric nervous system. In: *Physiology of the Gastrointestinal Tract,* 2nd ed., L. R. Johnson, (ed.), Raven Press, New York, Vol. 1, pp. 67–109.

Research Articles

Armstrong, D. M., Saper, C. B., Levey, A. I., Wainer, B. H., and Terry, R. D. (1983). Distribution of cholinergic neurons in rat brain: Demonstrated by the immunocytochemical localization of choline acetyltransferase. *Journal of Comparative Neurology* 216, 53–68.

Beckstead, R. M., and Norgren, R. (1979). An autoradiographic examination of the central distribution of the trigeminal, facial, glossopharyngeal, and vagal nerves in the monkey. *Journal of Comparative Neurology* 184, 455–472.

Bolme, P., Novotny, J., Uvnas, B., and Wright, P. G. (1970). Species distribution of sympathetic cholinergic vasodilator nerves in skeletal muscle. *Acta Physiologica Scandinavica* 78, 60–64.

Brain, S. D., and Williams, T. J. (1988). Substance P regulates the vasodilator activity of calcitonin gene-related peptide. *Nature* 335, 73–75.

Brooks-Fournier, R., and Coggeshall, R. E. (1981). The ratio of preganglionic axons to postganglionic cells in the sympathetic nervous system of the rat. *Journal of Comparative Neurology* 197, 207–216.

Burnstock, G., and Kennedy, C. (1986). A dual function for adenosine-5′-triphosphate in the regulation of vascular tone. Excitatory co-transmitter with noradrenaline from perivascular nerves and locally released inhibitory intravascular agent. *Circulation Research* 58, 319–330.

Burnstock, G., and Warland, J. J. (1987). A pharmacological study of the rabbit saphenous artery *in vitro:* A vessel with a large purinergic contractile response to sympathetic nerve stimulation. *British Journal of Pharmacology* 90, 111–120.

Contreras, R. J., Gomez, M. M., and Norgren, R. (1980). Central origins of cranial nerve parasympathetic neurons in the rat. *Journal of Comparative Neurology* 190, 373–394.

Costa, M., and Furness, J. B. (1984). Somatostatin is present in a subpopulation of noradrenergic nerve fibers supplying the intestine. *Neuroscience* 13, 911–919.

Ekblad E., Ekman, R., Håkanson, R., and Sundler F. (1988). Projections of peptide-containing neurons in rat colon *Neuroscience* 27, 655–674.

Ekblad E., Winther C., Ekman R., Håkanson R. and Sundler F. (1987) Projections of peptide-containing neurons in rat small intestine. *Neuroscience* 20, 169–188.

Hara, H., Hamill, G. S., and Jacobowitz, D. M. (1985). Origin of cholinergic nerves to the rat cerebral arteries: Coexistence with vasoactive intestinal polypeptide. *Brain Research Bulletin* 14, 179–188.

Helke, C. J., and Hill, K. M. (1988). Immunohistochemical study of neuropeptides in vagal and glossopharyngeal afferent neurons of the rat. *Neuroscience* 26, 539–551.

Hiura, T. (1977). Salivatory neurons innervate the submandibular and sublingual glands in the rat: Horseradish peroxidase study. *Brain Research* 137, 145–149.

Hökfelt, T., Elfvin, L. G., Elde, R., Schultzberg, M., Goldstein, M., and Luft, R. (1977). Occurrence of somatostatin-like immunoreactivity in some peripheral sympathetic noradrenergic neurons. *Proceedings of the National Academy of Sciences USA* 74, 3587–3591.

Kawasaki, H., Takasaki, K., Saito, A., and Goto, K. (1988). Calcitonin gene-related peptide acts as a novel vasodilator neurotransmitter in mesenteric resistance vessels of the rat. *Nature* 335, 164–167.

Kimura, H., McGeer, P. L., Peng, J. H., and McGeer, E. G. (1981). The central cholinergic system studied by choline acetyltransferase immunohistochemistry in the cat. *Journal of Comparative Neurology* 200, 151–200.

LaCroix, J. S., Stjarne, P., Änggård, A., and Lundberg, J.

M. (1988a). Sympathetic vascular control of the pig nasal mucosa: (I) Increased resistance and capacitance vessel responses upon stimulation with irregular bursts compared to continuous impulses. *Acta Physiologica Scandinavica* 132, 83–90.

LaCroix, J. S., Stjarne, P., Änggård, A., and Lundberg, J. M. (1988b). Sympathetic vascular control of the pig nasal mucosa: (II) Reserpine-resistant, nonadrenergic nervous responses in relation to neuropeptide Y and ATP. *Acta Physiologica Scandinavica* 133, 183–197.

Landis, S. C., and Fredieu, J. R. (1986). Coexistence of calcitonin gene-related peptide and vasoactive intestinal polypeptide in cholinergic sympathetic innervation of rat sweat glands. *Brain Research* 377, 177–181.

Lundberg, J. M. (1981). Evidence for co-existence of vasoactive intestinal polypeptide (VIP) and acetylcholine in neurons of cat exocrine glands. Morphological, biochemical and functional studies. *Acta Physiologica Scandinavica* Suppl. 496, 1–57.

Nicholson, J. E., and Severin, C. M. (1981). The superior and inferior salivatory nuclei in the rat. *Neuroscience Letters* 21, 149–154.

Pernow, J., and Lundberg, J. M. (1988). Neuropeptide Y induces potent contraction of arterial vascular smooth muscle via an endothelium-independent mechanism. *Acta Physiologica Scandinavica* 134, 157–158.

Satoni, H., Takahashi, K., Ise, H., and Yamamoto, T. (1979). Identification of the superior salivatory nucleus in the cat as studied by the HRP method. *Neuroscience Letters* 14, 135–139.

Schmidt, R. E., McAtee, S. J., Plurad, D. A., Parvin, A., Cogswell, E., and Roth, K. A. (1988a). Differential susceptibility of prevertebral and paravertebral sympathetic ganglia to experimental injury. *Brain Research* 460, 214–226.

Schmidt, R. E., Plurad, D. A., and Roth, K. A. (1988b). Effects of chronic experimental streptozotocin-induced diabetes on the noradrenergic and peptidergic innervation of the rat alimentary tract. *Brain Research* 458, 353–360.

Strack, A. M., Sawyer, W. B., Marubio, L. M., and Loewy, A. D. (1988). Spinal origin of sympathetic preganglionic neurons in the rat. *Brain Research* 455, 187–191.

Uddman, R., Alvmets, J., Ehringer, B., Håkanson, R., Loren, I., and Sundler, F. (1980). Vasoactive intesitnal polypeptide nerves in ocular and orbital structures of the cat. *Investigative Ophthalmology and Visual Science* 19, 878–885.

2

Adrenergic Receptors in the Autonomic Nervous System

D. PARKINSON

The early history of adrenergic receptors, encompassing the first half of this century, is closely associated with the adrenal gland and the investigation of the effects of its major catecholamine, adrenaline. Although the high concentration of adrenaline facilitated its chemical identification, this focus on the chromaffin tissue of the adrenal gland diverted attention from the rest of the sympathetic nervous system. It was not until 1948 that it was shown that sympathetic nerves released noradrenaline rather than adrenaline. Since then, the study of how these catecholamines interact with the effector cells of the sympathetic nervous system has led the way for other neural and humoral chemical transmitters. The aim of this chapter is to describe briefly some of the early history of adrenergic receptors and review the current state of knowledge about the major receptor subtypes (i.e., α_1, α_2, β_1, β_2).

TWO SYMPATHETIC TRANSMITTERS OR TWO RECEPTOR TYPES ?

By the beginning of this century, the work of Langley, Elliot, and others had identified adrenaline as the agent in extracts of adrenal medulla that contracted some smooth muscles, relaxed others, and raised blood pressure. In 1911, Cannon and de la Paz observed the similarity between the physiological reactions to stress mediated by the sympathetic nervous system (cardioacceleration, inhibition of gut motility) and the effects of adrenaline. In an attempt to reconcile the inhibitory and excitatory actions produced by the sympathetic nervous system, Cannon and Rosenblueth (1933) proposed that two chemical transmitters were released during sympathetic stimulation: sympathin I produced the inhibitory effects and sympathin E produced the excitatory effects. However, it was subsequently deduced that these two different responses were the result of

different adrenergic receptors, not different chemical transmitters.

Probably the earliest indication for multiple adrenergic receptors was the demonstration by Dale (1906) that ergot extracts blocked, and in some cases reversed, the effects of adrenaline or sympathetic nerve stimulation. Two studies published at the end of the 1940s provided the foundation for our current understanding of sympathetic transmission.

In 1948, Ahlquist presented evidence for two adrenergic receptors. He used six different catecholamines and determined their relative potencies in over 20 intact and isolated animal preparations from four different species. When the six test compounds were arranged in order of potency, the data segregated into two groups. In the first, designated as α-receptor-mediated, adrenaline was the most potent, noradrenaline was the second most potent, and the synthetic agonist, isoproterenol, was the least potent (i.e., sixth in order). In the second group, designated as β-receptor-mediated, isoproterenol was most potent, adrenaline was second most potent, and noradrenaline was least potent.

This was probably the first time an agonist-based classification was used to demonstrate different receptor types. Ahlquist argued that adrenaline was the only sympathetic neurohormone and all the results of sympathetic stimulation could be explained in terms of adrenaline's action on either α- or β-receptors. However, at the same time von Euler (1948) and others demonstrated that noradrenaline, not adrenaline, was the predominant catecholamine released from stimulated sympathetic nerves. The α/β concept was further strengthened when Powell and Slater (1958) showed that dichloroisoproterenol was a selective antagonist/partial agonist of β-receptors. Ahlquist's work provided the model for future classifications of receptor subtypes from which derive current ideas about the four adrenergic receptors, their tissue distributions, and the responses they mediate (Table 2-1).

Table 2-1 Tissue Distribution and Responses Mediated by Adrenergic Receptors

Receptor	Tissue	Response
α_1	Smooth muscle: vascular, iris, radial ureter, pilomotor, uterus sphincters (gut, bladder)	Contraction
	Smooth muscle (gut)	Relaxation
	Heart	Positive inotropic ($\beta_1 \gg \alpha_1$)
	Salivary gland	Secretion
	Adipose tissue	Glycogenolysis
	Sweat glands	Secretion
	Kidney (proximal tubule)	Gluconeogenesis, Na^+ reabsorbed
α_2	Presynaptic autoreceptor on sympathetic nerve endings	Inhibition of NE release
	Platelets	Aggregation, granule release
	Adipose tissue	Inhibition of lipolysis
	Endocrine pancreas	Inhibition of insulin release
	Smooth muscle (vascular)	Contraction
	Kidney	Inhibition of renin release (?)
β_1	Heart	Positive inotropic effect; positive chronotropic effect
	Adipose tissue	Lipolysis
	Kidney	Renin release
β_2	Liver	Glycogenolysis, gluconeogenesis
	Skeletal muscle	Glycogenolysis, lactate release
	Smooth muscle: bronchi, uterus, gut vascular (skeletal muscle) detrusor, spleen capsule	Relaxation
	Endocrine pancreas	Insulin secretion (?)
	Salivary gland	Amylase secretion

α_1- AND α_2-RECEPTORS

Brown and Gillespie (1957) wanted to investigate the phenomenon of posttetanic facilitation (i.e., the increased response to a single stimulus that follows a high-frequency burst of stimuli) with a view to establishing its relationship to transmitter release. After treating a cat with dibenzyline or dibenamine (irreversible α-receptor antagonists), they found that the output of noradrenaline from the spleen at low stimulus frequencies increased about 5-fold. They explained these results by concluding that noradrenaline was metabolized on the adrenergic receptors, even though they also presented data that showed that these drugs had no effect on the metabolism of exogenous noradrenaline. With the availability of tritium-labeled noradrenaline, it has been possible to show that the release of noradrenaline is greater in the presence of α-blockade and the increased overflow of transmitter is not due to reduced inactivation of transmitter (Kirpekar et al., 1973). Alpha blockade also inhibits the response of the cat spleen to sympathetic stimulation, so the question remained whether this inhibition was related to the increased noradrenaline release. This problem was resolved when it was shown that α-blockade also increased stimulated noradrenaline release from cardiac tissue, where the sympathetic response is elicited primarily through β-receptors (Starke et al., 1971).

Langer (1974), considering that the concentrations of phenoxybenzamine needed to block the postsynaptic response differed from those required to enhance transmitter release, suggested that the postsynaptic receptors be referred to as α_1 and the presynaptic receptors be referred to as α_2.

ARE ALL α_2-RECEPTORS PRESYNAPTIC AUTORECEPTORS?

No! is the answer to this question. Exceptions to a subdivision of α-receptors on the basis of location were soon discovered. Alpha-mediated responses with similar pharmacology to the presynaptic α-receptor (i.e., α_2) have been found on adipocytes, platelets, vascular smooth muscle, and pancreatic islets. These receptors are functional. For example, Drew and Whiting (1979) demonstrated vasoconstriction due to postjunctional α_2-receptors.

Berthelsen and Pettinger (1977) suggested a classification on the basis of function: α_1 being excitatory and α_2 being inhibitory. However, classifying a receptor as inhibitory or excitatory is an arbitrary label dependent on the point of view. If binding of an agonist to an α_2-receptor in blood vessels first inhibits an enzymatic activity, but this subsequently leads to vasoconstriction, then α_2-receptors could be classified as either inhibitory or excitatory.

The current methods of subclassifying α-receptors employ a combination of biochemical and pharmacological approaches. Selective agonists and antagonists have been developed that can be used to classify α-adrenergic responses as either α_1- or α_2-receptor-mediated. A selection of these compounds is listed in Table 2-2. The biochemical approach to subclassification of α-receptors is discussed in the section on signal transduction and second messengers.

SIGNAL TRANSDUCTION AND SECOND MESSENGERS AS A MEANS TO CLASSIFY α-RECEPTORS

Even before the subclassification of α-receptors, Hokin and Sherwin (1957) had shown that adrenaline stimulated the turnover of phosphatidylinositol (PI) in salivary gland. This effect was blocked by dibenamine and ergotamine, indicating that an α-receptor was involved. Over the next 20 years, it was consistently found that increased phosphatidylinositol turnover stimulated by an adrenergic agonist was mediated by an α-receptor (see Michell, 1975 for review). Tolbert et al. (1980) showed that prazosin was much more potent than yohimbine as an inhibitor of the adrenaline-induced increase in phosphatidylinositol turnover in isolated hepatocytes. This pointed to α_1-receptor involvement in the response. Subsequent studies support the generalization that the primary response to activation

Table 2-2 The Pharmacology of α-Receptors

Receptor	Agonist	Antagonists
α_1	Methoxamine	Prazosin
	Phenylephrine	BE 2254
		Corynanthine
α_2	UK-14, 304	Yohimbine
	α-Methyl-NE	Idazoxan
	Tramazoline	Rauwolscine
	Xylazine	
	Clonidine[a]	

[a]Partial agonist.

of α_1-receptors is increased phosphatidylinositol turnover.

Michell (1975), in his review, noted that increased phosphatidylinositol turnover was often associated with calcium mobilization and deduced that the former preceded the latter. Our current understanding of how receptor-stimulated hydrolysis of phosphatidylinositol can lead to the generation of second messengers inside the cell is shown in Figure 2-1. It is unclear at the moment whether there is a G protein (i.e., a protein that binds guanine nucleotides; see Gilman, 1984 for review), analogous to those that link the other adrenergic receptors to adenylate cyclase, between the α_1-receptor and the phosphodiesterase that cleaves phosphatidylinositol-4,5-phosphate to diacylglycerol and inositol-1,4,5-phosphate. The end result is liberation of two compounds that are potential second messengers.

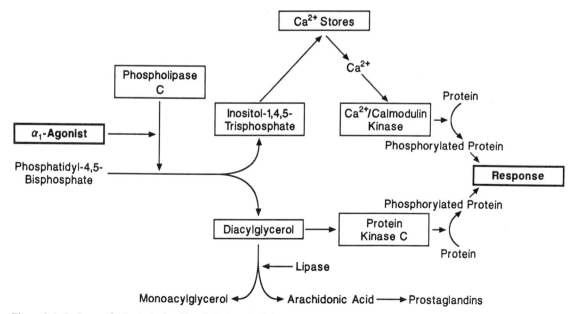

Figure 2-1 Pathways for hydrolysis of inositol phospholipids. (Adapted from Berridge, 1984, with permission of the author and publisher.)

The subsequent metabolism of inositol-1,4,5-phosphate becomes more complex as it is investigated, but the ultimate consequence is held to be release of calcium from internal stores such as the endoplasmic reticulum. Elevated intracellular calcium can then influence a range of cellular events, including vesicle-mediated secretion and contraction (in muscle cells), as well as increases in both synthesis and hydrolysis of cyclic nucleotides [cyclic adenosine monophosphate (cAMP) and cyclic guanosine monophosphate (cGMP)]. The effects on cyclic nucleotide metabolism can be attributed in part to binding of calcium to the ubiquitous calcium-binding protein calmodulin.

Diacylglycerol on the other hand remains in the membrane and acts as an anchored binding site for protein kinase C (for reviews, see Nishizuka, 1983; Blackshear et al., 1988). Protein kinase C activation also requires calcium and phosphatidylserine as cofactors. The tumor-promoting phorbol esters also stimulate protein kinase C. Activation of protein kinase C also seems to lead to its movement to a plasma membrane compartment and a parallel reduction in the concentration of soluble protein kinase C. Even while membrane bound, this kinase can still phosphorylate cytoplasmic proteins such as myosin light chains. As a further complication, diacylglycerol can be metabolized by one of two possible routes resulting in the liberation of arachidonic acid (which is usually esterified at the 2-position in diacylglycerol), from which prostaglandins can then be synthesized (see Berridge, 1984 for review).

The idea that α-adrenergic activation can lead to the inhibition of adenylate cyclase activity and reduced synthesis of cAMP also predates the α_1/α_2 subclassification (Robison et al., 1972). Adipocytes respond to adrenaline with an increase in cAMP synthesis (i.e., a β-receptor-mediated effect). The cAMP accumulated in response to a β-selective agonist (e.g., isoprenaline) or to adrenaline in the presence of an α_2-antagonist is up to 10-fold higher. Although α_2 activation will lower basal levels of cAMP

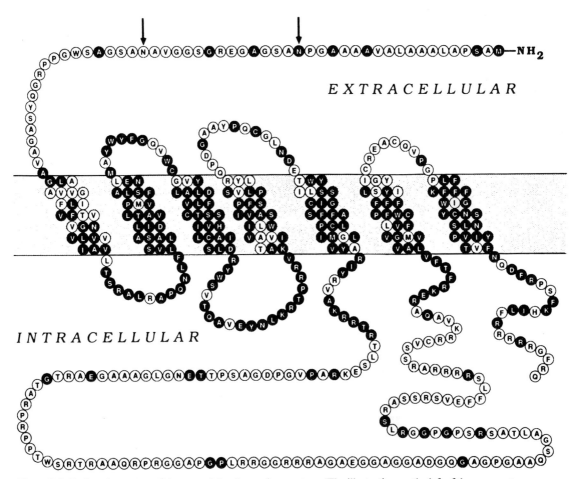

Figure 2-2 Deduced structure of the α_2- and β_2-adrenergic receptors. (The illustration on the left of the α_2-receptor sequence was taken from Regan et al., 1988, and the β_2-receptor sequence on the right was taken from Dohlman et al., 1987, with permission of the authors and publishers.)

synthesis, this is only by a factor of two. Thus, α_2-receptors are more effective at inhibiting stimulated than basal cAMP synthesis. In addition, this effect is not restricted to adrenergic mechanisms. Forskolin activates adenylate cyclase directly, apparently without a G protein intermediary, yet α_2 activation significantly inhibits its action (Burns et al., 1982).

α_2-Receptors appear to be similar to other receptors that are negatively coupled to adenylate cyclase in that they lower the maximum rate of cAMP synthesis but do not affect the affinity for substrate. The precise mechanism by which α_2-receptors inhibit cyclase has not been elucidated, though it appears that guanosine triphosphate (GTP) is necessary for function.

ARE THERE MORE THAN TWO α-RECEPTOR SUBTYPES?

The α_1/α_2 nomenclature continues to be a valuable classification scheme, but arguments have been made for further subdivisions of α-adrenergic receptors. These arguments have been based on agonist affinities, antagonist affinities, requirement for extracellular calcium rather than mobilization of intracellular calcium stores, and linkage to PI turnover (see Han et al., 1987 and Flavahan and Vanhoutte, 1986 for reviews). The subject is made confusing by the usage of subscript suffixes (e.g., α_{1H}, α_{1L}; α_{1a}, α_{1b}; α_{1A}, α_{1B}) that are neither consistent nor equivalent. Further investigations are needed to determine

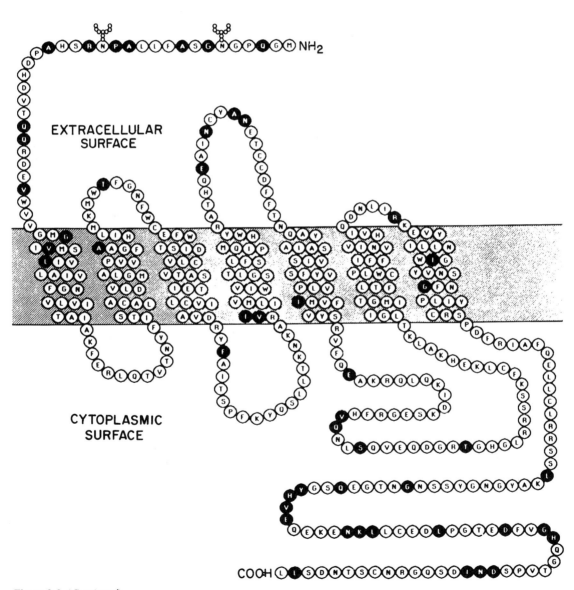

Figure 2-2 (*Continued*)

whether greater subclassification of α_1-receptors is needed, but the reader should keep this possibility in mind.

High- and low-affinity states of α_2-receptors have been described and are expected from the linkage of these receptors to G proteins (see below). There is, however, evidence for more than one kind of α_2-receptor. Subtypes of α_2-receptors have been suggested on the basis of differential affinity for the antagonist rauwolscine (Alabaster et al., 1986). Heterogeneity in α_2-receptors is supported by the discovery of two genes (one expressed in platelets, the other in the kidney) that are localized to different chromosomes (Regan et al., 1988). Inhibition of cAMP synthesis does not appear to reduce norepinephrine release (see Bylund and U'Prichard, 1983 for review). Thus, there is the possibility that there is a third gene encoding the presynaptic α_2-autoreceptor.

There is the potential for a number of α-receptor subtypes. Some of these problems may be resolved when the receptor proteins from the different tissues are cloned and their amino acid sequences are compared (Figure 2-2).

β-RECEPTORS STIMULATE ADENYLATE CYCLASE AND ELEVATE INTRACELLULAR cAMP

Sutherland and co-workers (reviewed in Sutherland et al., 1965) uncovered the link between adrenergic stimulation, cAMP synthesis, and hepatic glycogenolysis. The cAMP produced inside the cell activates protein kinase A, which in turn phosphorylates phosphorylase kinase. This step activates phosphor-

ylase kinase, which now converts inactive glycogen phosphorylase to the active form, resulting in the breakdown of glycogen into glucose-1-phosphate (Figure 2-3). The increase in cAMP also inhibits the synthesis of glycogen by stimulating the phosphorylation of an inhibitor that then binds to and inhibits a phosphatase. The role of the phosphatase is to dephosphorylate both phosphorylase kinase (to inactivate it) and glycogen synthase (to activate it).

From this work, Sutherland and co-workers suggested that activation of β-receptors increases cAMP synthesis by stimulating adenylate cyclase. The major components of this system have been isolated (see Gilman, 1984 for review) and are shown in Figure 2-4. As a result of the binding of agonist, the receptor undergoes a conformational change that allows it to bind to a G protein complex, in this case G_s because adenylate cyclase will ultimately be stimulated. The G protein is composed of three subunits: G_α, G_β, and G_γ. G_α also has bound GDP in the absence of agonist. After the agonist–receptor complex binds to the G protein complex, the GDP is replaced by GTP and G_α dissociates from the complex. This activated form of G_α now binds to and stimulates the catalytic subunit of adenylate cyclase to synthesize cAMP from ATP. When the GTP is hydrolyzed to GDP, G_α dissociates and now reforms the G protein complex with the other G subunits to await further binding to the agonist–receptor complex.

This process is not unique to β-receptors. In the liver, for example, glucagon stimulates cAMP synthesis through the same pool of G_s complex and adenylate cyclase, though it binds first to a different receptor protein. This is one reason why the response of a cell to adrenergic agonists can be affected by ex-

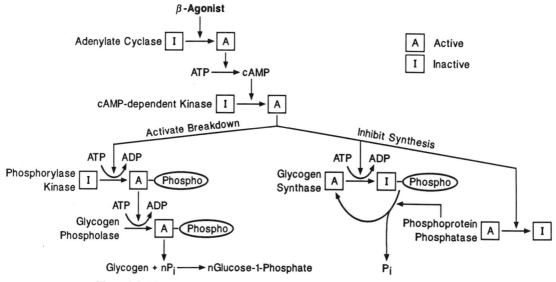

Figure 2-3 The regulation of glycogen metabolism by β-agonists through cAMP.

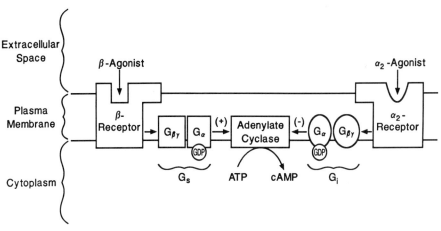

Figure 2-4 The components of the adenylate cyclase complex. (Adapted from Gilman, 1984.)

posure to other agents (see below). Before leaving the subject of adrenergic modulation of glycogenolysis, it is worth mentioning that the hyperglycemia produced by adrenergic agonists may not be simply due to activation of β-receptors in the liver. Adrenergic agonists can also increase the supplies of glucose by inhibiting the release of insulin, increasing the release of glucagon, and increasing the synthesis of glucose from lactate in skeletal muscles. There is also evidence that α-mediated glycogenolysis can be elicited from the liver, without changing cAMP levels. It has been claimed that this is the predominant mechanism in some species (Exton, 1985).

β_1- AND β_2-RECEPTORS

In a short report to *Nature (London)* in 1967, Lands et al. demonstrated that the actions of noradrenaline that had been assigned to β-receptors in Ahlquist's classification could be further subdivided. This work was also an agonist-based division, comparing the potencies of ten catecholamine derivatives in four tissue preparations. They showed that noradrenaline and adrenaline had similar affinities at β_1-receptors. The affinity of noradrenaline for β_2-receptors was similar to its affinity for β_1-receptors whereas the affinity of adrenaline was nearly 100-fold higher at β_2-receptors. This study laid the foundation for the development of a large array of selective agonists and antagonists for research and clinical use. A selection of these compounds is listed in Table 2-3.

The distribution of the β-receptor subtypes varies. Although one type may predominate in an organ or tissue, it is not unusual to find both types. The heart contains predominantly the β_1 types, which are responsible for both inotropic and chronotropic responses, but there are also β_2-receptors that may be linked to the inotropic response.

The β_1- and β_2-receptors are very similar; both stimulate cAMP synthesis and both are glycosylated proteins that have identical mobilities when analyzed by electrophoresis in polyacrylamide gels. Peptide maps of the two receptors are also are very similar (see Dohlman et al., 1987, for review). These observations raise the question of whether there are two different proteins, a common precursor that is modified in some way to yield one or other activity, or a single protein that is regulated in some way by its environment.

Molecular biological investigations have provided the answer to this question. Complementary DNA clones coding for β-receptors from several species have been isolated (Figure 2-2). These show that the β_1- and β_2-receptors are homologous, though different, proteins. The β-receptor cDNAs also show high homology with other G protein-coupled receptors, including rhodopsin (a receptor for "light"), the α_2-receptor, and some types of muscarinic cholinergic receptors (Dohlman et al., 1987). Common features of these proteins include seven α-helical membrane spanning regions connected by intra- and extracellular loops. There is a high degree of homology be-

Table 2-3 The Pharmacology of β-Receptors

Receptor	Agonist	Antagonists
β_1	Prenaterol	ICI 89,407
		CGP 26,505
		Betaxolol
		Atenolol
		Practolol
		Metoprolol
β_2	Terbutaline	ICI 118,551
	Salbutamol	IPS 339
	Rimiterol	
	Adrenaline	

tween these transmembrane regions in β_1- and β_2-receptors. Thus, these regions are probably involved in some common function such as binding to G proteins. Now that the β-receptor proteins have been cloned and expressed in cell lines that do not normally express them, we can expect that selective mutation experiments will reveal the agonist-binding sites and show why β_1- and β_2-receptors differ in their affinity for selective agonists and antagonists.

REGULATION OF ADRENERGIC RECEPTOR FUNCTION

Is there regulation of signaling in the sympathetic nervous system? In the face of fixed numbers of adrenergic receptors on effectors cells, the concentration of catecholamine, whether acting as a neurotransmitter at a synapse or as a hormone, will determine the magnitude of the respones. But there is good evidence that the adrenergic receptors are also dynamically regulated in response to the actions of adrenergic agonists and also to other agents. The regulation of signal transduction through β-adrenergic receptors has been most extensively studied, so they will be discussed first.

When a tissue containing β-receptors is first exposed to a β-agonist, the synthesis of cAMP increases due to activation of adenylate cyclase. After about 30 minutes the rate of cAMP synthesis declines and the tissue is said to be desensitized. If the response to only β-agonists is attenuated, then this is referred to as *agonist-specific* or *homologous desensitization* (see Sibley et al., 1987, for review). The activation of adenylate cyclase by agonists at other receptors or by nonreceptor activators such as fluoride ion or forskolin is not diminished. The mechanism of desensitization appears to involve both a reduction in the number of receptors on the cell surface and an uncoupling of the receptors from adenylate cyclase.

The mechanism underlying homologous desensitization appears to involve phosphorylation of the receptor. Phosphorylation begins within minutes of agonist occupation and leads to incorporation of about 2 mol of phosphate per mol of receptor. The phosphorylation does not appear to involve cAMP or require the coupling of receptor to G_s (Strasser et al., 1986). Rather, there is evidence for a cytosolic kinase (β-adrenergic receptor kinase) that appears to phosphorylate only the agonist-occupied receptor. Presumably the conformational change subsequent to agonist occupation reveals a phosphorylation site that would be otherwise hidden from the kinase. Phosphorylation of β-receptors uncouples them from the G_s protein (Sibley et al., 1986), impairing their ability to stimulate cAMP synthesis. Phosphor-

ylation also promotes internalization of β-receptors into intracellular compartments that are not yet fully characterized. In this compartment, a phosphatase appears to dephosphorylate the receptor so it can return to the cell surface (Sibley et al., 1986).

Desensitization of β-receptors can also occur in the absence of agonist. This is termed *heterologous desensitization* and also involves phosphorylation of the receptor but not internalization (see Sibley et al., 1987 for review). In part, the diminished response to agonists involves uncoupling of receptor from adenylate cyclase, and this can be correlated with cAMP-dependent receptor phosphorylation (Sibley et al., 1984b). Since the response to stimulation of other receptors and to agents that bypass receptors is also diminished, then there must be changes in the adenylate cyclase complex as well. Function impairment of G_s and increased activity of G_i have both been observed in association with heterologous desensitization of β-receptors (Kassis and Fishman, 1982; Garrity et al., 1983). Phosphorylation of β-receptors by cAMP-dependent kinases and protein kinase C appears to take place on the same serine residues (Bouvier et al., 1986). Muscarinic stimulation in the heart can lead to β-receptor desensitization (Limas and Limas, 1985). Some of the muscarinic receptors in heart are linked to elevated phosphatidylinositol breakdown, and this, in turn, leads to stimulation of protein kinase C. Therefore, this sequence of events illustrates how activity at one receptor (the muscarinic receptor) can modify the responsiveness of another receptor (the β receptor).

Although the discussion of receptor regulation has focused on β-receptors, there is also evidence that α-receptors are subject to regulation. It is known that α_2-receptors, and probably α_1-receptors also, are coupled to the next stage of signal transduction by G proteins, so the description of heterologous desensitization already given can be applied. It has been shown that α_1-agonists promote α_1-receptor desensitization that can be correlated with receptor phosphorylation and sequestration, i.e., homologous desensitization (Leeb-Lundberg et al., 1987). Although progress on the molecular biology of β-receptors has been ahead of that on the other adrenergic receptors, the gap is constantly being narrowed. We can soon expect to know as much about regulation of signaling through α-receptors as is known about that through β-receptors.

So far in this section, short-term regulation of adrenergic receptor function has been discussed. The regulation of adrenergic responsiveness over periods of days and weeks will now be considered. The relationship between circulating levels of thyroid hormone and the expression of β-receptors is a good example that has both physiological and clinical relevance.

Patients with pathological elevations of circulating thyroid hormones show manifestations typical of adrenergic activation: tachycardia, increased thermogenesis, and sweating (Bilezikian and Loeb, 1983). These symptoms can be successfully treated with β-receptor antagonists. Experimental studies point to increased numbers of β-receptors in some, though not all, tissues during thyrotoxicosis. Interestingly, α-receptor numbers appear to be reduced. Hypothyroid patients show some symptoms that could be attributed to impaired adrenergic function. In hypothyroidism, there appear to be fewer β-receptors.

Changes in the number of receptors on the cell surface cannot be extrapolated directly to an increased response of that cell to agonist because there may be "spare" receptors. The term *spare receptors* embodies the concept that the maximum biological response of a cell can be elicited when less than 100% of the receptors are occupied by agonist. Let us assume that there are 1,000 receptors per cell and the maximum increase in cAMP synthesis is elicited by only 10% occupancy: i.e., the maximum response is obtained when 100 receptors have bound agonist. What will be the consequence of increasing the number of receptors by 50%? The result is a shift in the dose–response curve to the left, i.e., the same effect as increasing the affinity for agonist. Direct assessment of agonist binding, for example, radioligand binding studies, would show increased numbers of binding sites but no change in affinity. The increased responsiveness at low concentrations can be demonstrated only by measuring the functional consequences of receptor occupancy. Conversely, if receptor concentration were reduced, the result would depend on the magnitude of the re-

duction. If the number of receptors did not fall below our hypothetical value of 100 receptors per cell needed to produce the maximum response, then we would see a right shift of the dose–response curve. Larger reduction would, however, lead to a reduction also in the maximum response that could be elicited. Thyroid hormone can regulate the level of expression of adrenergic receptors. This regulation is of physiological relevance during cold acclimation. Exposure of humans to a cold environment for several days results in increased serum levels of thyroid hormone. A part of the hypothalamus appears to be sensitive to core body temperature. If temperature falls, presumably the release of thyrotropin releasing hormone from the neurons in the hypothalamus and into the hypophyseal portal system is increased. This stimulates the release of thyrotropin from anterior pituitary cells, which in turn stimulates the synthesis and secretion of thyroid hormones from the thyroid gland. As already discussed, the response to adrenergic stimulation is then increased, in part by increasing the numbers of β-receptors. The effect of cold acclimation on the response to sympathetic stimulation is shown in Figure 2-5, taken from the work of Hseih and Carlson (1957). Administration of noradrenaline to a warm acclimated rat produces only a small increase in oxygen consumption and rectal temperature. After exposure to 5°C for 3–4 weeks, the same dose of noradrenaline produces much larger effects on oxygen consumption and rectal temperature.

Other hormones can also change the number of adrenergic receptors. In experimental studies α_1-adrenergic receptors on the myometrial cells of the rabbit uterus increased with elevation of plasma con-

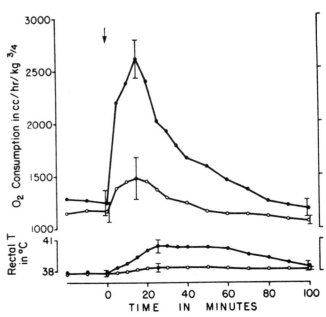

Figure 2-5 Effect of cold acclimation on noradrenaline-stimulated thermogenesis. (○, warm acclimated; ●, cold acclimated). Noradrenaline (0.2 mg/kg) was administered at the time indicated by the arrow. (From Hseih and Carlson, 1957, with permission of the authors and publisher.)

centrations of estrogens. This was accompanied by increased response to agonist. At the same time the number of α_2-receptors on platelets fell, providing a possible explanation for the increased incidence of thromboembolic disease in individuals receiving estrogens (e.g., women taking oral contraceptives).

In summary, the magnitude of the response of a tissue during sympathetic stimulation depends on several factors: previous exposure to adrenergic agonists (homologous desensitization), the biochemical state (heterologous desensitization), and the endocrine state of the individual.

SUMMARY

Considerable advances have been made in the last 100 years in our understanding of how the sympathetic nervous system elicits a response from its target tissues. Four concepts stand out that are important to understanding the physiological function of the sympathetic nervous system: (1) there are at least four receptor types, α_1, α_2, β_1 and β_2, (2) these receptors allow norepinephrine and adrenaline to elicit different responses by virtue of their linkage to different biochemical processes, (3) adrenaline is more potent than noradrenaline at all of these receptors, though it is most potent at β_2-receptors, and (4) most tissues contain more than one adrenergic receptor, so the response will depend on the agonist.

REFERENCES

Reviews

Berridge, M. J. (1984). Inositol trisphosphate and diacylglycerol as second messengers. *Biochemical Journal* 220, 345–360.

Bilezikian, J. P., and Loeb, J. N. (1983). The influence of hyperthyroidism and hypothyroidism on α- and β-adrenergic receptor systems and adrenergic responsiveness. *Endocrine Reviews* 4, 378–388.

Blackshear, P. J., Naim, A. C., and Kuo, J. F. (1988). Protein kinases 1988: A current perspective. *FASEB Journal* 2, 2957–2969.

Bylund, D. B., and U'Prichard, D. C. (1983). Characterization of α_1- and α_2-adrenergic receptors. *International Review of Neurobiology* 243, 343–431.

Dohlman, H. G., Caron, M. G., and Lefkowitz, R. J. (1987). A family of receptors coupled to guanine nucleotide regulatory proteins. *Biochemistry* 26, 2657–2664.

Gilman, A. E. (1984). G proteins and dual control of adenylate cyclase. *Cell* 36, 577–579.

Flavahan, N. A., and Vanhoutte, P. M. (1986). α_1-Adrenoceptor subclassification in vascular smooth muscle. *Trends in Pharmacological Sciences* 7, 347–349.

Langer, S. Z. (1974). Presynaptic regulation of catecholamine release. *Biochemical Pharmacology* 23, 1793–1800.

Michell, R. H. (1975). Inositol phospholipids and cell surface receptor function. *Biochimica et Biophysica Acta* 415, 81–147.

Nishizuka, Y. (1986). Studies and perspectives of protein kinase C. *Science* 233, 305–311.

Sibley, D. R., Benovic, J. L., Caron, M. G., and Lefkowitz, R. J. (1987). Regulation of transmembrane signaling by receptor phosphorylation. *Cell* 48, 913–922.

Sutherland, E. W., Oye, I., and Butcher, R. W. (1965). The action of epinephrine and the role of the adenyl cyclase system in hormone action. *Recent Progress in Hormone Research* 21, 623–646.

Research Papers

Ahlquist, R. P. (1948). A study of adrenotropic receptors. *American Journal of Physiology* 153, 586–600.

Alabaster, V. A., Keir, R. F., and Peters, C. J. (1986). Comparison of potency of α_2-adrenoceptor antagonists in vitro: Evidence for heterogeneity of α_2-adrenoceptors. *British Journal of Pharmacology* 88, 607–614.

Berthelsen, S., and Pettinger W. A. (1977). A functional basis for classification of α-adrenergic receptors. *Life Science* 21, 595–606.

Bouvier, M., Leeb-Lundberg, L. M. F., Benovic, J. L., Caron, M. G., and Lefkowitz, R. J. (1986). Regulation of adrenergic receptor function by phosphorylation. II. Effects of agonist occupancy on phosphorylation of α_1- and β_2-adrenergic receptors by protein kinase C and the cyclic AMP-dependent protein. *Journal of Biological Chemistry* 262, 3106–3113.

Brown, G. L., and Gillespie, J. S. (1957). The output of sympathetic transmitter from the spleen of the cat. *Journal of Physiology (London)* 138, 81–102.

Burns, T. W., Langley, P. E., Terry, B. E., Bylund, D. B., and Forte, L. R. (1982). Alpha-2 adrenergic activation inhibits forskolin-stimulated adenylate cyclase activity and lipolysis in human adipocytes. *Life Sciences* 31, 815–821.

Cannon, W. B., and de la Paz, D. (1911). Emotional stimulation of adrenal secretion. *American Journal of Physiology* 28, 64–70.

Cannon, W. B., and Rosenblueth, A. (1933). Studies on conditions of activity in endocrine organs. XXIX. Sympathin E and sympathin I. *American Journal of Physiology* 104, 557–574.

Dale, H. H. (1906). On some physiological actions of ergot. *Journal of Physiology (London)* 34, 163–206.

Drew, G. M., and Whiting, S. B. (1979). Evidence for two distinct types of postsynaptic α-adrenoceptor in vascular smooth muscle in vivo. *British Journal of Pharmacology* 67, 207–215.

Exton, J. H. (1985). Mechanism involved in α-adrenergic phenomena. *American Journal of Physiology* 248 (Endocrinology and Metabolism), E633–647.

Garrity, M. J., Andreasen, T. J., Storm, D. R., and Robertson, R. P. (1983). Prostaglandin E-induced heterologous desensitization of hepatic adenylate cyclase: Consequences on the guanyl nucleotide regulatory complex. *Journal of Biological Chemistry* 258, 8692–8697.

Han, C., Abel, P. W., and Minneman, K. P. (1987). α_1-Adrenoceptor subtypes linked to different mechanisms for increasing intracellular Ca^{2+} in smooth muscle. *Nature* 329, 333–335.

Hokin, M. R., and Hokin, L. E. (1953). Enzyme secretion and the incorporation of P32 into phospholipids of pancreas slices. *Journal of Biological Chemistry* 203, 967–977.

Hokin, L. E., and Sherwin, A. L. (1957). Protein secretion and phosphate turnover in the phospholipids in salivary glands in vitro. *Journal of Physiology (London)* 135, 18–29.

Hseih, A. C. L., and Carlson, L. D. (1957). Role of adrenaline and noradrenaline in chemical regulation of heat production. *American Journal of Physiology* 190, 243–246.

Kassis, S., and Fishman, P. H., (1982). Different mechanisms of desensitization of adenylate cyclase by isoproterenol by and prostaglandin E_1 in human fibroblasts: Role of regulatory components in desensitization *Journal of Biological Chemistry* 257, 5312–5318.

Kirpekar, S. M., Furchgott, R. F., Wakade, A. R., and Prat, J. C. (1973). Inhibition of sympathomimetic amines of the release of norepinephrine evoked by nerve stimulation in the cat spleen. *Journal of Pharmacology and Experimental Therapeutics* 187, 529–538.

Lands, A. M., Arnold, A., McAuliff, J. P., Luduena F. P., and Brown, T. G. (1967). Differentiation of receptor systems activated by sympathomimetic amines. *Nature* 214, 597–598.

Leeb-Lundberg, L. M. F., Cottechia, S., DeBlasi, A., Caron, M. G., and Lefkowitz, R. J. (1987). Regulation of adrenergic receptor function by phosphorylation. I. Agonist-promoted desensitization and phosphorylation of α_1-adrenergic receptors coupled to inositol phospholipid metabolism in DDT1 MF-2 smooth muscle cells. *Journal of Biological Chemistry* 262, 3098–3105.

Limas, C. J., and Limas, C. (1985). Carbachol induces desensitization of cardiac β-adrenergic receptors through muscarinic M_1 receptors. *Biochemical and Biophysical Research Communications* 128, 699–704.

Murad, F., Chi, Y.-M., Rall, T. W., and Sutherland, E. W. (1962). Adenyl cyclase. III. The effects of catecholamines and choline esters on the formation of adenosine 3′,5′-phosphate by preparations from cardiac muscle and liver. *Journal of Biological Chemistry* 237, 1233–1238.

Powell, C. E., and Slater, I. H. (1958). Blocking of inhibitory adrenergic receptors by a dichloro analog of isoproterenol. *Journal of Pharmacology and Experimental Therapeutics* 122, 480–488.

Regan, J. W., Kobilka, T. S., Yang-Feng, T. L., Caron, M. G., Lefkowitz, R. J., and Kobilka, B. K. (1988). Cloning and expression of a human kidney cDNA for an α_2-adrenergic receptor. *Proceedings of the National Academy of Sciences USA* 85, 6301–6305.

Robison, G. A., Langley, P. E., and Burns, T. W. (1972). Adrenergic receptors in human adipocytes—Divergent effects on adenosine 3′,5′-monophosphate and lipolysis. *Biochemical Pharmacology* 21, 589–592.

Sibley, D. R., Nambi, P., Peters, J. R., and Lefkowitz, R. J. (1984a). Phorbol esters promote β-adrenergic receptor phosphorylation and adenylate cyclase desensitization in duck erythrocytes. *Biochemical and Biophysical Research Communications* 121, 973–979.

Sibley, D. R., Peters, J. R., Nambi, P., Caron, M. G., and Lefkowitz, R. J. (1984b). Desensitization of turkey erythrocyte adenylate cyclase. *Journal of Biological Chemistry* 259, 9742–9749.

Sibley, D. R., Strasser, R. H., Benovic, J. L., Daniel, K., and Lefkowitz, R. J. (1986). Phosphorylation/dephosphorylation of the β-adrenergic receptor regulates its functional coupling to adenylate cyclase and subcellular distribution. *Proceedings of the National Academy of Sciences USA* 83, 9408–9412.

Starke, K., Montel, H., and Schumann, H. J. (1971). Influence of cocaine and phenoxybenzamine on noradrenaline uptake and release. *Naunyn-Schmiedebergs Archiv fur Pharmakologie* 270, 210–214.

Strasser, R. H., Sibley, D. R., and Lefkowitz, R. J. (1986). A novel catecholamine-activated adenosine cyclic 3′,5′-phosphate independent pathway for β-adrenergic receptor phosphorylation in wild-type and mutant S49 lymphoma cells: Mechanism of homologous desensitization of adenylate cyclase. *Biochemistry* 25, 1371–1377.

Tolbert, M. E. M., White A. C., Ospry, K., Cutts, J., and Fain, J. N. (1980). Stimulation by vasopressin and α-catecholamines of phosphatidylinositol formation in isolated rat liver parenchymal cells. *Journal of Biological Chemistry* 255, 1938–1944.

von Euler, U. S. (1948). Identification of the sympathomimetic ergone in adrenergic nerves of cattle (sympathin N) with laevo-noradrenaline. *Acta Physiologica Scandinavica* 16, 63–74.

3

Cholinergic Receptors

D. PARKINSON

Acetylcholine is used as a chemical transmitter at several parts of the peripheral and central nervous systems that are crucial for the functioning of the autonomic nervous system. The preganglionic neurons of both divisions of the autonomic nervous system release acetylcholine as their neurotransmitter; it is also used by all of the parasympathetic postganglionic neurons and the sympathetic neurons that innervate the sweat glands.

In the brain, cholinergic neurons appear to play a part in areas involved in central autonomic regulation, including the ventrolateral medulla, dorsal vagal nucleus, nucleus ambiguus, and nucleus tractus solitarius. Apart from these sites, acetylcholine is also a transmitter in nonautonomic CNS pathways such as those that project from the basal forebrain to cerebral cortex.

This chapter will focus on the receptor mechanisms that mediate the actions of acetylcholine in autonomic functions.

BACKGROUND

The discovery of acetylcholine as a neurotransmitter and the elucidation of two main cholinergic receptor types represent major advances in our understanding of the nervous system. Three early studies related to acetylcholine now appear as part of this intellectual cornerstone and provide the first clear insights into chemical transmission in the nervous system. In one of these classic experiments, Langley and Dickinson (1889) showed that application of nicotine to the superior cervical ganglion blocked synaptic transmission. After this treatment, electrical stimulation of the sympathetic fibers distal to the ganglion (i.e., postganglionic fibers) resulted in pupillary dilation and vasoconstriction in the ear, whereas stimulation proximal to the ganglion (i.e., the preganglionic fibers) did not produce this effect. The second major development came from studies by Dale (1914), who demonstrated that acetylcholine exhibited actions similar to those seen with stimulation of the parasympathetic nervous system. This observation confirmed and expanded the earlier findings by Dixon (1907), who first noted that the alkaloid, muscarine (Figure 3-1), which was derived from *Amanita* mushrooms, had actions similar to stimulation of the vagus nerve. In addition, Dale reexamined the action of nicotine (Figure 3-1) at autonomic ganglia and also studied its action on skeletal muscle (see Gilman, 1959, for a review of historical developments). These studies served as the basis for modern classification of cholinergic receptors and were performed some years before it was established by Loewi (1921) that a substance he termed *Vagusstoff* (i.e., acetylcholine) was released after stimulation of the vagus nerve.

From these observations, the actions of acetylcholine were divided into either nicotinic or muscarinic effects because, it was postulated, they were due to activation of nicotinic and muscarinic receptors, respectively. This classification has proved useful, but the recent advances in the study of cholinergic receptors have shown that a more complex scheme will be required. Much of this work is still in progress, and many of the ideas regarding cholinergic receptors are in flux. This means that a simplified overview cannot be given at this point. An attempt will be made to highlight the current status of this developing field.

MUSCARINIC RECEPTORS

Muscarinic receptors mediate all of the postganglionic actions of the parasympathetic division of the autonomic nervous system. These receptors are present on a wide variety of cell types, including cardiac muscle, endocrine and exocrine glands, smooth muscle of the gastrointestinal tract and bronchopulmonary tree, as well as sympathetic ganglion cells.

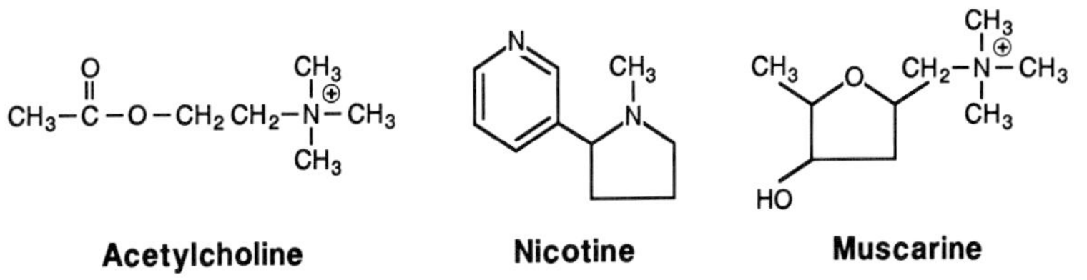

Figure 3-1 The chemical structures of acetylcholine, nicotine, and muscarine.

Acetylcholine   **Nicotine**   **Muscarine**

They also mediate the sympathetic innervation of the sweat glands. Muscarinic receptors are also abundant in the brain, much more so than nicotinic receptors.

Evidence for Multiple Muscarinic Receptors

If all of the physiological effects produced by both acetylcholine and muscarine were due to their interaction with a single muscarinic receptor, then this discussion would be brief. However, this is not the case. Evidence for multiple muscarinic receptors has come from three sources: radioligand-binding studies, receptor–response coupling, and molecular biology studies. At present, information is still flowing from research studies in all three areas.

Radioligand Binding Studies: Pirenzepine and the M_1/M_2 Classification

One of the first pieces of evidence for multiple muscarinic receptor sites came from displacement of radiolabeled antagonists (e.g., atropine or N-methylscopolamine) by cholinergic agonists. Initial experiments with the antagonists suggested that all of the muscarinic receptors were similar; e.g., atropine is equipotent at all muscarinic receptors. However, when agonists were used, complex inhibition curves were obtained. From this work, three sites that differed in their affinity for agonist were postulated: low, high, and superhigh (Birdsall et al., 1978). The properties of these sites could be modulated by guanine nucleotides and some divalent ions (Hulme et al., 1983).

The clearest evidence for multiple muscarinic receptors can be traced to the development of pirenzepine (Figure 3-2), an antimuscarinic drug that is considerably more effective at preventing the acetylcholine-induced secretion of gastric acid than it is at blocking acetylcholine-induced slowing of the heart. This result quickly led to the subclassification of muscarinic receptors into two groups on the basis of their affinity for pirenzepine: M_1 and M_2 (or M-1 and M-2). M_1 receptors show high affinity for pirenzepine, with dissociation constants in the 2–30 nM range (the affinity of anatagonists for muscarinic receptors determined by radioligand binding assays varies with ionic strength) (Hammer et al., 1980). M_2 receptors were defined by their low affinity for pirenzepine (0.7–10 μM). On this basis the muscarinic receptors in the stomach were classified as M_1, and those of the heart, lacrimal glands, and smooth muscle were classified as M_2. Both M_1 and M_2 receptor sites are also present in the brain (Gil and Wolfe, 1985).

It has been claimed that several muscarinic agonists distinguish between M_1 and M_2 receptors in both radioligand binding and functional studies (reviewed by Mitchelson, 1988). Of these compounds, pilocarpine and McN-A-343 were claimed to be M_1 selective and oxotremorine was suggested to exhibit M_2 selectivity. Interpretation of results with these compounds has been complicated by varying levels of partial agonist activity. There are no compounds yet available that show the degree of differentiation possible with some of the muscarinic antagonists.

Evidence for Multiple Types of M_2 Receptors: Cardiac Type and Glandular Type

The M_1/M_2 classification made possible by pirenzepine prompted the characterization of a wide variety of agonists and antagonists for their ability to discriminate between these subtypes. Pirenzepine consistently identified a single population of high-affinity (i.e., M_1) receptors. This was not the case with compounds that were not M_1 selective. Of these, a pirenzepine analog called AF-DX 116 (Figure 3-2) was one of the first compounds to provide good evidence for heterogeneity in the M_2 receptors. AF-DX 116 is more potent than pirenzepine as an antagonist at muscarinic sites in the heart. However, AF-DX 116 is less potent than pirenzepine at glandular

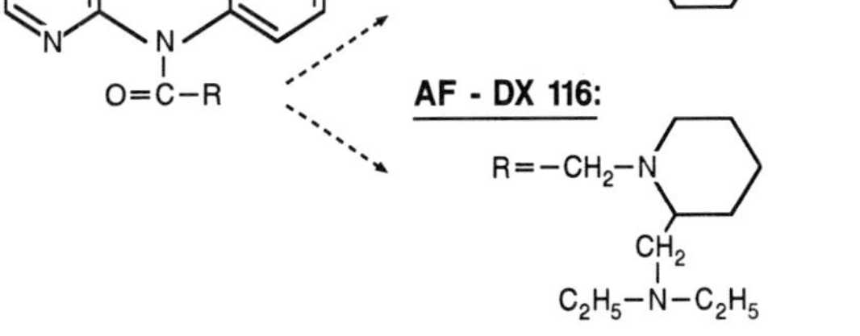

Figure 3-2 The chemical structures of pirenzepine and AF-DX 116. The common tricyclic ring structure is shown (left) with the structures of the two side-chains (R) that differ between pirenzepine and AF-DX 116.

muscarinic sites (e.g., lacrimal gland, submaxillary gland), which are also classified as M_2 sites because of their low affinity for pirenzepine. Methoctramine is a newer compound that is about 100-fold more selective for cardiac sites than for glandular sites. It is also more potent than AF-DX 116. The binding kinetics of AF-DX 116 in some tissues (e.g., smooth muscle from the gastrointestinal tract) argue that they contain both cardiac and glandular M_2 sites (see Ladinsky et al., 1988 for review).

This subclassification of M_2 sites is supported by studies with antagonists such as hexahydrosiladifenidol and 4-diphenylacetoxy-N-methyl piperidine. These compounds are complementary to AF-DX 116 in that they have higher affinity for the glandular M_2 subtype (see Ladinsky et al., 1988, for review).

Thus, the radioligand binding studies argue for at least three muscarinic receptor sites. Several schemes have been proposed for these sites. There is general agreement that M_1 should be used to identify those sites with high affinity for pirenzepine. The M_2 sites with high affinity for AF-DX 116 have been classified as either cardiac M_2 receptors (M_2c) or simply as M_2 receptors, whereas those with low affinity have been labeled as glandular M_2 receptors (M_2g) or M_3 receptors. Whether any of these systems continues in use will depend on future biochemical and molecular biology studies, as well as on ligand binding studies.

At Least Four Muscarinic Receptors from Molecular Cloning

The pharmacological heterogeneity of muscarinic receptors could be the result of a single receptor protein interacting with multiple effector systems, such as adenylate cyclase in one tissue and phosphatidylinositol turnover in another. Alternatively, multiple muscarinic receptor proteins might be produced in a tissue-specific manner. To address these questions, attempts have been made to distinguish between muscarinic receptor proteins from different tissues, either after purification or by selective labeling methods. The early result from these studies, using mostly porcine tissues, was that muscarinic receptors were glycosylated proteins of about 80 kDa. However, purification procedures that retained radioligand binding activity yielded proteins with a low affinity for pirenzepine, even if the receptor had high affinity in the native state. One conclusion from these results might be that muscarinic heterogeneity results from the interaction of a single receptor protein with different effector systems. Although other explanations, such as selective purification of one receptor protein from a mixed population, could explain some of these results, the importance of this work is that it made available purified receptor protein. Partial amino acid sequences were obtained that allowed molecular biologists to screen cDNA libraries to obtain clones encoding muscarinic receptor proteins.

The porcine M_1 receptor was the first muscarinic receptor protein to be cloned (Kubo et al., 1986a). The nucleotide sequence was obtained from a library of cDNA clones derived from porcine cerebrum. The deduced amino acid sequence is typical of the rhodopsin/adrenergic receptor family, with seven putative membrane-spanning regions (see Chapter 2). Expression of this sequence by injecting mRNA derived from this clone into *Xenopus laevis* oocytes demonstrated that it encoded for a protein that bound muscarinic antagonists with high affinity and could link with the endogenous mechanisms in the oocyte to modulate ion channels when specifically stimulated by muscarinic agonists.

The sequence for a porcine M_2 receptor has been determined from cDNA clones from the heart (Kubo et al., 1986b; Peralta et al., 1987a). The deduced amino acid sequence shows only 38% identity with the cerebral M_1 receptor. Hydropathicity analysis predicted six membrane spanning domains; a seventh membrane-spanning domain with less pronounced hydropathicity was suggested by sequence homology with the β-adrenergic receptor (Peralta et al., 1987a). The clone was identified as an M_2 receptor, not only because it originated from heart, which has a high M_2 expression, but because of the results from transfection experiments with Chinese hamster ovary cells. After transfection with the putative M_2 DNA, the hamster ovary cells expressed a protein that bound the nonselective muscarinic antagonist, quinuclidine benzilate, with high affinity while binding of pirenzepine was of relatively low affinity ($K_i = 0.35 \ \mu M$). Hybridization of this clone with restriction digests of porcine and human genomic DNAs indicated that this M_2 receptor was the product of a single gene.

Bonner et al. (1987) found four different genes encoding muscarinic receptors in rat brain: m1, m2, m3, and m4. The sequences of the m1 and m2 genes correspond, respectively, to the M_1 and M_2 receptors that were cloned from porcine tissues (see above). Expression of the m1, m3, and m4 types by transfection of cultured cells produced proteins with high affinity for pirenzepine with the rank order of m1 = m4 > m3. It was suggested that these three receptors would all be classified in the M_1 type if pirenzepine were used as the means of classification. The expression of these four muscarinic receptors in rat tissues outside of the brain needs to be determined so that their relationship to other classification schemes can be established.

There is evidence for four human muscarinic receptors, also on the basis of screening genomic libraries (Peralta et al., 1987b). These were labeled HM_1, HM_2, HM_3, and HM_4. As for the rat receptors, HM_1 and HM_2 correspond to porcine M_1 and M_2, respectively. HM_3 and HM_4 are probably also all M_1 types (but see the later section on second messengers). The labeling scheme may, however, lead to confusion in the future; rat m3 and m4 appear to be equivalent to HM_4 and HM_3, respectively. All four human genes are expressed in the brain, HM_2 is expressed in the heart, and HM_4 appeared to be the only gene expressed in the pancreas (Peralta et al., 1987b).

These molecular biology studies can be considered only a beginning. Although they strengthen the arguments for the existence of at least two kinds of muscarinic receptors, much remains to be done. The tissue distribution of both mRNA and functional proteins must still be determined. There appear to be multiple M_1 genes, but we do not yet know their levels of expression. If, for example, the m1 encodes the bulk of M_1 receptors then how important are the m3 and m4 types? Or are the m1, m3, and m4 types linked to different second messenger systems (see later). Finally, are there more than four muscarinic receptor genes or mRNAs (see Bonner et al., 1987)?

Muscarinic Receptor Subtypes and Effector Mechanisms

Many biochemical changes have been linked to activation of muscarinic receptors: phosphatidylinositol metabolism, cAMP metabolism, cGMP metabolism, and modulation of ion channels. None of these changes can be said to predominate in mediating the physiological actions of acetylcholine at muscarinic receptors. The data do not, at present, allow the unequivocal association of one type of muscarinic receptor with a specific biochemical change in the way such association has been possible for adrenergic receptors. This stems from our poor understanding of the molecular basis for muscarininc receptor diversity. From the sequence data available, it appears that all of the muscarinic receptors fit the general model for signaling systems that act through G protein intermediaries (see Chapter 2).

Stimulation of Phosphatidylinositol Turnover

The ability of muscarinic receptor activation to increase phosphatidylinositol metabolism was first shown by Hokin and Hokin (1954) in pancreas. The advent of the M_1/M_2 classification in the early 1980s led to the proposal that M_1 receptors could be identified by their high affinity for pirenzepine as well as their positive coupling to phosphatidylinositol turnover (Hammer and Giachetti, 1982; Gil and Wolfe,

1985). Further investigations have shown, however, that this concept is not universally applicable.

Muscarinic receptors in cardiac tissue are associated with both increased phosphatidylinositol metabolism and inhibition of adenylate cyclase. In chick cardiac cells, pirenzepine is more potent as an antagonist of the adenylate cyclase inhibition than of the phosphatidylinositol stimulation (Brown et al., 1985). These results are opposite those expected from the M_1/M_2 classification described in the previous paragraph. It now appears that part of the explanation can be attributed to different pharmacological properties of chick cardiac muscarinic receptors (Choo et al., 1988). Nevertheless, muscarinic receptors in mammalian cardiac cells stimulate phosphatidylinositol metabolism (Woodcock et al., 1987). Binding studies detect only M_2 sites in mammalian cardiac muscle; they have failed so far to detect M_1 sites (Hammer et al., 1980; Mattera et al., 1985). Analysis of muscarinic receptor mRNAs gives the same result; only M_2 proteins were detected in cardiac tissue. The implication is that cardiac M_2 receptors in heart are associated with increased phosphatidylinositol metabolism. Transfection experiments show that HM_2 receptors (e.g., the human cardiac muscarinic receptor, see above) are more efficiently coupled to inhibition of adenylate cyclase, at least in human embryonic kidney cells (Peralta et al., 1988). In this study, a small increase in phosphatidylinositol turnover was seen after expression of HM_2. Therefore it may be that cardiac M_2 receptors can couple to phosphatidylinositol turnover under some circumstances, and this may be the case for cardiac cells.

Coupling of M_2 receptors to phosphatidylinositol metabolism has been demonstrated in several other tissues, including pancreatic acinar cells (Korc et al., 1987), parotid gland (Ek and Nahorski, 1988), and smooth muscle preparations from trachea (Grandody et al., 1986), ileum (Ek and Nahorski, 1988), and colon and bladder (Noronha-Blob et al., 1987). Smooth muscle in the gut contains both glandular M_2 (20–30%) and cardiac M_2 (80–70%) receptor types but no detectable M_1 receptors (Giraldo et al., 1988). The muscarinic contraction of this smooth muscle has been attributed to the glandular M_2 receptors (see Ladinsky et al., 1988 for review). In tracheal smooth muscle, increased phosphatidylinositol metabolism has been correlated with contraction (Grandody et al., 1986; Meurs et al., 1988). Putting these two results together, it is tempting to suggest that glandular M_2 receptors are associated with phosphatidylinositol turnover. This idea is supported by data from a human astrocytoma cell line (Evans et al., 1984; Brown et al., 1985; Kunysz et al., 1989) and functional expression of the cloned human HM_4 muscarinic receptor (Peralta et al., 1988). HM_4

could be the putative glandular muscarinic receptor because it is the only mRNA expressed in pancreas. Further investigations are expected to show whether glandular M_2 receptors are always coupled to phosphatidylinositol turnover.

It is clear from these results that coupling of a muscarinic receptor to phosphatidylinositol turnover is not yet a reliable basis for classification.

Inhibition of Adenylate Cyclase

Soon after the discovery of cAMP and adenylate cyclase, Murad et al. (1962) found that muscarinic receptors could be negatively coupled to adenylate cyclase (i.e., occupation of the muscarinic receptor by acetylcholine leads to inhibition of adenylate cyclase activity with the resultant prevention of cAMP synthesis). Negative coupling of muscarinic receptors to adenylate cyclase has been demonstrated in the heart (Jakobs et al., 1979; Hazeki and Ui, 1981; Ehlert, 1985), GH$_3$ pituitary tumor cells (Wojcikiewicz et al., 1984), striatum (Olianas et al., 1983), cerebral cortex (Gil and Wolfe, 1985), and neuroblastoma-derived cell lines (Evans et al., 1984; McKinney et al., 1985).

A distinction should be made between "direct" muscarinic inhibition of adenylate cyclase through an inhibitory G protein (see Chapter 2) and apparent reductions in cAMP that can be attributed to "indirect" muscarinic actions. The "direct" inhibition of adenylate cyclase reduced cAMP synthesis in NG108-15 neuroblastoma $\times$ glioma cells (Kurose et al., 1983). In 1321 N1 astrocytoma cells, however, reductions in intracellular cAMP are due to calcium-dependent activation of phosphodiesterases that degrade cAMP (Meeker and Harden, 1983), presumably the result of increased phosphatidylinositol turnover (Hughes et al., 1984).

Muscarinic receptors can apparently inhibit both basal and stimulated synthesis of cAMP. Wojcikiewicz et al. (1984) found that muscarinic agonists inhibited growth hormone secretion from GH$_3$ pituitary tumor cells under two sets of conditions. One involved the "direct" inhibition of the stimulation of adenylate cyclase by vasoactive intestinal polypeptide. As a result, secretion was inhibited. GH$_3$ cells can also be stimulated to secrete by phosphodiesterase inhibitors that increase intracellular cAMP by preventing its catabolism. Muscarinic agonists also inhibit secretion caused by phosphodiesterase inhibitors. This result suggests that muscarinic receptors can also inhibit basal adenylate cyclase activity.

Can inhibition of adenylate cyclase be associated with any specific muscarinic receptor subtype? Binding and molecular studies have found evidence for expression of only M_2 receptors in cardiac cells (Mattera et al., 1985; Peralta et al., 1987b), which can be further classified as cardiac M_2 receptors that

are distinct from glandular M_2 receptors. Therefore muscarinic inhibition of adenylate cyclase in heart is probably mediated by cardiac M_2 receptors. There are not yet enough data to determine whether the other M_2 receptors negatively coupled to adenylate cyclase are always of the cardiac subtype.

Expression of the human muscarinic receptors in cell lines has shown that the HM$_2$ clone encodes a protein that can inhibit adenylate cyclase in the presence of a muscarinic agonist (Peralta et al., 1988). These same experiments show that the HM$_3$ product has the same capability. Therefore, inhibition of adenylate cyclase is unlikely to be restricted, within muscarinic receptors, to the cardiac M_2 receptor. Furthermore, cardiac muscarinic receptors have also been linked to stimulation of phosphatidylinositol metabolism (see above) and appear to be closely associated with potassium channels (see below), so not all cardiac M_2 receptors are negatively coupled to adenylate cyclase.

Modulation of Ion Channels

Muscarinic receptor modulation has been observed for several different ion channels, resulting in increases in potassium conductance, decreases in potassium conductance, decreases in calcium conductance, and increases in nonselective cation conductances (see Nathanson, 1987; Christie and North, 1988). For some of these channels, the conductance changes are probably secondary to muscarinic modulation of the intracellular concentrations of second messengers. The muscarinic inhibition of the heartbeat involves, in part, the closing of calcium channels. This has been attributed to reduced cAMP synthesis, which, in turn, reduced the cAMP-dependent phosphorylation of the calcium channel proteins (see Loffeholz and Pappano, 1985). Similarly, the increase in a nonselective cation conductance in pancreatic acinar cells appears to be linked to intracellular calcium concentration (Iwatsuki and Petersen, 1977; McCandless et al., 1980), which is presumably secondary to increased phosphatidylinositol turnover.

G Protein Coupling to Ion Channels. There is growing evidence that some neurotransmitter receptors are able to modulate ion fluxes by a G protein-linked interaction with ion channels rather than indirectly through second messenger systems. Some of the muscarinic actions of acetylcholine may be the result of direct effects on ion channels. The clearest evidence so far for muscarinic receptors comes from investigations in cardiac muscle.

The muscarinic receptor-induced slowing of the heart is the result of activation of a channel that has high permeability for potassium ions flowing into the cell. The resultant hyperpolarization slows pacemaker activity. The latency of this response is relatively long, ranging from 10 to several hundred milliseconds. This is much longer than the latency of channels that are thought to be activated by the binding of agonist to a site on the channel protein complex (e.g., nicotinic receptor, latency of 100–200 μsec). No evidence has been obtained to implicate any diffusible second messenger systems in this effect. Neither cGMP nor cAMP is involved in this response. Patch clamp studies with cell-attached patches revealed that acetylcholine was not effective in activating the potassium currents in the patch if applied in the bathing medium, i.e., outside the pipette (Sakmann et al., 1983). The interpretation of this result is that no diffusible second messengers in the cytoplasm are involved in muscarinic modulation of the channels within the isolated patch. Acetylcholine applied inside the pipette was effective. This result argues further that a diffusible second messenger is not involved in this muscarinic action.

Patch clamp studies with atrial cells showed that coupling of the muscarinic receptor to the potassium channel requires intracellular GTP (Pfaffinger et al., 1985). In the same study, pretreatment of the cells with pertussis toxin prevented the response to acetylcholine. Pertussis toxin is an enzyme that inactivates two G proteins (G_i and G_o) by specific ADP-ribosylation. Breitweiser and Szabo (1986) applied a nonhydrolyzable GTP analog alone to the inside of isolated bullfrog atrial cells and found no effect on channel activity. Subsequent addition of acetylcholine produced persistent activation of the potassium current. These are additional pieces of evidence that a G protein links the muscarinic receptor and the potassium channel. Since a diffusible second messenger does not seem to be involved in this action of acetylcholine, the most parsimonious model predicts that the G protein alone is sufficient for communication between receptor and channel.

Inhibition of the M Current. Stimulation of preganglionic fibers elicits two excitatory postsynaptic potentials in neurons in autonomic ganglia. Acetylcholine is presumed to be the neurotransmitter responsible for both potentials. The first potential is fast and is mediated by nicotinic receptors. The second is slower, is mediated by muscarinic receptors, and is due to inhibition of the M current. The M current is a time- and voltage-dependent potassium current that is active between −70 and 0 mV (Figure 3-3; Adams and Brown, 1982; Adams et al., 1982a). The slow excitatory potential appears to be due to suppression of the M current as a result of the closure of the potassium channels after the binding of muscarinic agonists. The M current is also inhibited by several neuropeptides, suggesting that there is a common intracellular pathway leading to closure of the potassium channels. Intracellular injections of a variety of possible second messengers, including cAMP, cGMP, and calcium (Adams et al., 1982b), do not affect the M current. However, compounds that inhibit the M current also stimulate phosphatidylinositol turnover (Pfaffinger et al., 1988). Phorbol esters do not appear to affect the M current in hippocampal neurons (Malenka et al., 1986), but they are able to partially suppress it in frog sympathetic neurons (Brown and Adams, 1987; Pfaffinger et al., 1988). Muscarinic stimulation of

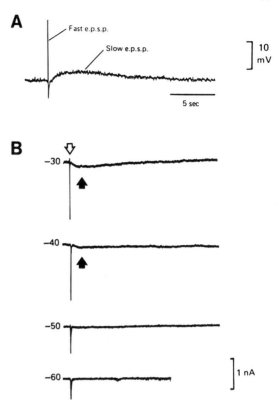

Figure 3-3 (A) An example of the excitatory postsynaptic potentials (e.p.s.p.) recorded from a bullfrog sympathetic ganglion neuron when a single electrical stimulus was applied to the preganglionic fibers. The time bar represents 5 seconds. (B) Electrophysiological demonstration of the voltage dependence of the M current in a bullfrog sympathetic ganglion neuron. The neuron was recorded under conditions of voltage clamp at several different holding potentials while the preganglionic neurons are stimulated electrically. The trace recorded at −30mV shows the current due to the fast excitatory current (open arrow), which is the result of acetylcholine binding to nicotinic receptors, and the slow excitatory current (i.e., M current, closed arrow), which is the result of acetylcholine binding to muscarinic receptors. As the membrane voltage is clamped at voltages less than −40 V, the M current is inhibited. The time bar represents 10 seconds. (From Adams and Brown, 1982.)

phosphatidylinositol turnover may be involved in modulating the inhibition of the M current, whereas alternative mechanisms such as G protein coupling of receptor to channel may be the primary muscarinic effector mechanism. Further work is needed before the mechanism underlying the muscarinic inhibition of the M current is understood.

Muscarinic regulation of M current is not unique to autonomic ganglia; it has also been demonstrated in neurons of spinal cord (Nowak and McDonald, 1983), hippocampus (Cole and Nicoll, 1984), and cerebral cortex (McCormick and Prince, 1985), as well as in smooth muscle cells (Sims et al., 1985). The consequence of inhibiting the M current is expected to be facilitation of the neuron's responsiveness to other inputs (Adams et al., 1982b).

Stimulation of cGMP Synthesis

Muscarinic effects on cGMP metabolism have been reported in a variety of cells and tissues (see Nathanson, 1987). Although acetylcholine will induce contraction of most smooth muscle, it causes relaxation of vascular smooth muscle apparently through cGMP. Investigation of this phenomenon in isolated tissue preparations demonstrated the importance of the endothelial cells (Furchgott and Zawadski, 1980). In the absence of functional endothelial cells, acetylcholine stimulated contraction. This suggested that the endothelial cells were stimulated by acetylcholine to produce a substance that was called endothelium-derived relaxing factor or EDRF. There is now good evidence that this factor is nitric oxide (see Moncada et al., 1988 for review) and that it is synthesized by the endothelial cells from arginine (Palmer et al., 1988). Nitric oxide is probably acting as a humoral mediator for acetylcholine (Figure 3-4). Diffusion of nitric oxide to the vascular smooth muscle appears to induce relaxation by stimulating guanylate cyclase (Murad et al., 1978). The increased cGMP levels result in the activation of a

cGMP-dependent protein kinase (Rapoport et al., 1983).

Use of nitric oxide as an intermediate is not unique to acetylcholine. Substance P, bradykinin, histamine, calcium ionophores, and many other vasodilators will also produce endothelium-dependent relaxation of vascular smooth muscle (Martin et al., 1985; Rees et al., 1989). The synthesis of nitric oxide is not restricted to the vasculature. There is evidence that some of the effects of glutamate in the cerebellum are due to nitric oxide-mediated increases in cGMP levels (Garthwaite et al., 1988). This result also raises the point that the effects of nitric oxide are not restricted to vasodilation; it also appears to have a role in controlling platelet function (Moncada et al., 1988).

The pharmacological properties of the muscarinic receptor on the endothelial cells that mediate the release of EDRF appear to be of the glandular M_2 type (McCormack et al., 1988). The observation that calcium ionophores mimic the effects of acetylcholine predicts that the mobilization of calcium will be involved. This, in turn, suggests that a muscarinic receptor linked to phosphatidylinositol turnover is most likely involved. This would further support the idea that glandular M_2 receptors are usually coupled to increased phosphatidylinositol turnover.

This unraveling of the EDRF story begs the question of whether the other reported increases in cGMP attributed to muscarinic receptors are due to nitric oxide. It would be interesting to see if any of the four muscarinic receptors transfected into cell lines (Peralta et al., 1988) are able to stimulate guanylate cyclase without generating nitric oxide as an intermediate.

Regulation of Muscarinic Receptors

Muscarinic receptors may be regulated by a variety of factors. Developmental changes, innervation, agonist exposure, and phosphorylation have all been associated with regulation of muscarinic receptors (see Nathanson, 1987 for review). These have mostly been phenomenological studies; very little has yet been discovered about the biochemical basis for these changes.

Administration of muscarinic agonists *in vivo* leads to a decrease in receptor number (Halvorsen and Nathanson, 1981; Marks et al., 1981). This reduction is accompanied by decreased response to muscarinic agonists. Similar results are obtained if the endogenous acetylcholine is allowed to persist by chronic inhibition of acetylcholinesterase (Gazit et al., 1979; Dawson and Jarrott, 1981).

Similarly, exposure of cells in culture to agonist leads to a loss of muscarinic receptors from the cell surface. This takes place in two phases. Initially

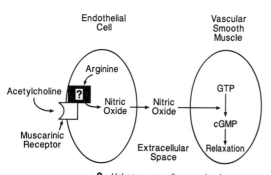

? - Unknown coupling mechanism

Figure 3-4 Acetylcholine stimulates the synthesis of a diffusible agent, nitric oxide, that causes relaxation of vascular smooth muscle.

there is a rapid removal of receptors from the cell surface, which appears to involve their sequestration in an intracellular compartment (Maloteaux et al., 1983; Feigenbaum and El-Fakahany, 1985). Removal of agonist permits the rapid return of receptors to the cell surface. In the continued presence of agonist, however, the receptors are degraded.

The molecular mechanism for this removal of muscarinic receptor is not known at present. Phosphorylation of the receptor protein is a possibility. Treatment of neuroblastoma cells with phorbol esters to activate protein kinase C causes a rapid initial internalization and subsequent degradation of muscarinic receptors in the absence of agonist (Liles et al., 1986). However, in some other cell lines phorbol esters inhibit the muscarinic response without changing the total number of receptors or the proportion on the cell surface (Misbahuddin et al., 1985; Orellana et al., 1985).

NICOTINIC RECEPTORS

Langley (1907) showed that nicotine stimulated the contraction of skeletal muscle. This result led him to put forward the idea of "receptive substances" for nicotine in skeletal muscle before acetylcholine was identified as the transmitter at the neuromuscular junction. Acetylcholine has been identified as the transmitter of the preganglionic fibers in the ganglia of both the sympathetic and parasympathetic divisions of the autonomic nervous system. The cholinergic receptors responsible for neurotransmission in these ganglia were shown to be nicotinic in nature; the effects of stimulation of the preganglionic fibers were mimicked by short-term exposure to nicotine (extended exposure to nicotine leads to receptor desensitization). Pharmacological studies with nicotine and compounds that were antagonists of nicotinic effects demonstrated that the ganglionic nicotinic receptors were clearly different from the nicotinic receptors at the neuromuscular junction.

Considerable effort has been expended in the last 20 years on the study of the nicotinic receptor at the neuromuscular junction (see McCarthy et al., 1986 for review). These efforts have yielded considerable insight into this receptor. It is known to be a channel for cations that is made up of five proteins, two α-subunits and one each of β-, γ-, δ-subunits (i.e., $\alpha_2\beta\gamma\delta$). The binding site for acetylcholine appears to be on the α-subunit. This work has also provided the starting point for studies of the other nicotinic receptors. Nicotinic receptors not at the neuromuscular junction are referred to as *neuronal* nicotinic receptors. This term includes nicotinic receptors in the brain, which are thought to have some properties in common with the receptors of the autonomic gan-

glia. The emphasis on the muscle receptor has led to a relative neglect of the neuronal receptors until recent years. Consequently, much of the work must still be considered "in progress."

How Many Nicotinic Receptors Are There?

Pharmacological Evidence

The snake toxin, α-bungarotoxin, has been the most important tool in the investigations of the muscle nicotinic receptor (Chiappanelli, 1986). Its high affinity binding has allowed receptor content, synthesis rate, and cellular location to be studied. α-Bungarotoxin is a potent inhibitor of neurotransmission at the neuromuscular junction. A high-affinity binding site is also found in the brains of several species, but this is not thought to be a nicotinic receptor for several reasons. With the possible exception of some lower vertebrates, α-bungarotoxin does not inhibit nicotinic effects in the brain (see Chiappanelli, 1986, for review). Furthermore, the distribution of binding sites is different from high-affinity sites for either acetylcholine or nicotine (Clarke et al., 1985). Thus, α-bungarotoxin is considered to be selective for the muscle receptor as opposed to the neuronal receptors.

Some preparations of α-bungarotoxin were found to inhibit the response of chick ciliary ganglion neurons to acetylcholine. This activity was found to be due to a peptide contaminant that has now been purified. It has been called bungarotoxin 3.1 (Ravdin and Berg, 1979), κ-bungarotoxin (Chiappanelli, 1983), and toxin F (Loring et al., 1984); all three terms apparently refer to the same substance. This toxin will inhibit neurotransmission at chick ciliary ganglia and rat superior cervical ganglia, though it is less potent in the latter preparation (see Chiappanelli, 1986 for review). α-Bungarotoxin is not effective in either of these preparations.

A large number of drugs have been synthesized that act as nicotinic antagonists. In a series of bisquaternary methonium compounds, the 6-carbon member of this series (hexamethonium) inhibits nicotinic actions at autonomic ganglia, whereas the 10-carbon member (decamethonium) is more potent as an antagonist at the muscle receptor. These observations have led to the distinction between C6 (ganglionic) and C10 (muscle) nicotinic receptors. Many of the ganglionic antagonists also inhibit the effects of nicotine in the brain, leading to the suggestion that the brain also contains C6 nicotinic receptors. Several observations suggest that this classification scheme is too simple. First, some compounds that would be classified as C10 antagonists, most notably *d*-tubocurare and dihydro-β-erythroidine, are also effective inhibitors at autonomic ganglia and in the brain (see Martin, 1986 for review). Second, the dissociation constant of ganglionic receptors for nicotine or acetylcholine is probably in the micromolar range (Kemp and Morely, 1986), yet binding studies show that there are binding sites in the brain that have low nanomolar affinities for acetylcholine and nicotine (Romano and Goldstein, 1980; Schwartz et al., 1982). Furthermore, some of the antagonists that inhibit nicotinic effects in the brain (e.g., hexamethonium, mecamylamine) are weak inhibitors of the high-affinity binding of nicotine or acetylcholine. These observations may point to the existence of subtypes of nicotinic receptors in the brain that would be distinguishable from one another by their affinity for agonists and/or antagonists.

Use of Antibodies to Determine Nicotinic Receptor Structure

The PC12 cell line has served as a model for postganglionic sympathetic neurons because it is derived from a tumor of the adrenal medulla (Greene and Tischler, 1976). These cells express nicotinic receptors that, when activated, stimulate the release of noradrenaline. Patrick and Stallcup (1977) were able to inhibit the function of these receptors with antiserum raised against nicotinic receptors from *Electrophorus electricus* electric organ (a tissue derived from modified muscle cells). This result indicates that the muscle and neuronal receptors may have some structural similarities.

Lindstrom and co-workers have used monoclonal antibodies to provide further insights into muscle and neuronal receptors. A monoclonal antibody called mAb 35 was obtained that bound to a site on the extracellular surface of the α-subunit of muscle receptors. The α-subunit is thought to carry the agonist binding site, though mAb 35 does not inhibit receptor function (Blatt et al., 1986). Immunohistochemical studies suggest that mAb 35 might also recognize neuronal nicotinic receptors in the chick. Specific staining was seen in the brain (Swanson et al., 1983) and at synapses in the ciliary ganglia (Jacob et al., 1984). mAb 35 was used in the immunoaffinity purification of nicotine-binding protein from chicken brain (Whiting and Lindstrom, 1986a,b). This protein was used to raise another monoclonal antibody, mAb 270, which was then used to purify a complex from rat brain that binds nicotine with high affinity (dissociation constant, 2 nM) and has some pharmacological properties expected of a nicotinic receptor (Whiting and Lindstrom, 1986b). The distribution of the epitope labeled by mAb 270 in rat brain is very similar to the distribution of [^{3}H]nicotine-binding sites revealed by autoradiography (Swanson et al., 1987). The complex purified with mAb 270 contained two proteins: a 51-kDa glycoprotein that contained the antibody-

binding epitope, and a 79-kDa glycoprotein that did not bind mAb 270 (Whiting and Lindstrom, 1987a). The 51-kDa protein was called the α-subunit because it was identified by antibodies initially directed to the α-subunit of the muscle receptor.

mAb 270 has provided evidence for two nicotinic receptors in chicken brain. These appeared to be composed of a common antibody-binding subunit called the α-subunit, and two proteins of different apparent molecular weight called β and β' (Whiting et al., 1987a). Unfortunately for this labeling scheme, affinity alkylating agents that are thought to label the agonist binding site react with the β and β' subunits, not the α-subunit (Whiting and Lindstrom, 1987b). Thus, this scheme is at odds with the naming scheme for muscle receptors where the agonist binding site is on the α-subunit.

It has been suggested that the neuronal receptors are assembled from two subunits into multimers of the form $\alpha_n \beta_n$ (where $n = 2$ or 3, Whiting et al., 1987a). Studies with cloned subunits support the idea that neuronal nicotinic receptors can be assembled from α- and β-subunits (see below). It is not known whether these two proteins represent the complete functional nicotinic receptor *in vivo*. Since the muscle receptor is composed of four subunits in a pentameric structure (i.e., $\alpha2\beta\gamma\delta$) there may be more components of the neuronal receptor that await discovery.

Molecular Cloning Studies

Molecular cloning studies have provided genetic evidence for diversity in neuronal nicotinic receptors. A cDNA clone was isolated from a PC12 library with a probe fragment derived from the α-subunit of the muscle receptor (Boulter et al., 1986). This clone hybridized to brain regions that also contain nicotine-binding sites. The protein predicted by this clone has considerable sequence and structural homology with the muscle α-subunit. Further work with this and other clones has identified several other potential α-subunits for neuronal nicotinic receptors. The naming scheme is now being formalized to include both muscle and neuronal receptors.

So far, evidence has been obtained for the expression of five α-subunits from four genes. The muscle receptor α-subunit was the first to be cloned and therefore is called $\alpha1$. Three other genes have been identified that encode proteins homologous to the $\alpha1$-subunits but are not expressed in muscle. Nef et al. (1988) obtained evidence for three α subunits in chicken brain: $\alpha2$, $\alpha3$, and $\alpha4$. Transcripts encoding $\alpha4$ are much more abundant than those for $\alpha2$ and $\alpha3$. Homologous genes have also been identified from rat tissues. The $\alpha3$ gene is expressed in some brain regions (Goldman et al., 1986), in PC12 cells (Boulter et al., 1986), and chick ciliary ganglia (Boyd et al., 1988). The $\alpha 4$-subunit is expressed in the brain and appears to give rise to two mRNAs (Goldman et al., 1987). The distribution of $\alpha 3$ in the brain differs from that of $\alpha 4$, though they overlap in some regions. Whiting et al. (1987b) have identified the $\alpha 4$ clone as coding for the β-subunit they isolated with mAb 270 (see above).

Several common properties can be identified by comparing the known or predicted α-subunit proteins. Two pairs of nearby cysteine residues are found in the amino-terminal half of the proteins; in the $\alpha 1$-subunit these are residues 128/142 and 192/193. The latter pair is thought to be very close to the agonist binding site. This region is also thought to be where α-bungarotoxin binds to the $\alpha 1$-subunit during blockade of muscle receptors. It is notable that there are many amino acid substitutions in this region when the $\alpha 1$-subunit is compared with the $\alpha 3$- or $\alpha 4$-subunits. This may explain why α-bungarotoxin does not bind to neuronal receptors. Other common properties are four putative membrane spanning regions with a high degree of homology in all subunits and the presence of an asparagine residue at position 141 for N-linked glycosylation.

The muscle receptor is composed of four different subunits. Probes derived from $\alpha 3$-subunit cDNAs have been used to search for the other non-α subunits of the neuronal receptors. Deneris et al. (1988) identified a sequence that is about 50% homologous to the $\alpha 3$ and $\alpha 4$ sequences. It is expressed in brain, spinal cord, and PC12 cells. The sequence predicts a protein of about 57 kDa that has two cysteine residues at positions equivalent to residues 128 and 142 of the muscle α-subunit. There are no paired cysteine residues around position 192/193, arguing that this is not another agonist-binding subunit. The sequence also predicts four membrane spanning regions with homology to the membrane spanning regions of the α-subunits. These properties are more like the β, γ, and δ subunits of the muscle receptor. Functional studies (described below) led Deneris et al. (1988) to call this new sequence the $\beta 2$-subunit, with the muscle receptor β-subunit called $\beta 1$. The $\beta 2$-subunit is probably the "non-α"-subunit identified by Nef et al. (1988) in chicken brain.

Molecular studies have clearly made significant progress in identifying potential components of the neuronal nicotinic receptors. To test whether any of these cloned sequences encode functional receptors, Xenopus oocytes were injected with combinations of mRNAs prepared from the different cloned cDNAs for the α- and β-subunits (Boulter et al., 1987; Wada et al., 1988; Deneris et al., 1988). The results of these studies are summarized in Table 3-1. Two major conclusions can be drawn from these results: (1) all five subunits of the muscle receptor form a functional channel, though the $\beta 2$-subunit can substitute

Table 3-1 Combinations of Nicotinic Subunits That Form Acetylcholine-Gated Channels When Injected into *Xenopus* Oocytes

Subunit mRNAs Injected	Functional Channels
$\alpha 1 + \beta 1 + \gamma + \delta$	Yes
$\alpha 1 + \gamma + \delta$	No
$\alpha 1 + \beta 2 + \gamma + \delta$	Yes
$\alpha 1 + \beta 2$	No
$\alpha 1$	No
$\beta 2$	No
$\alpha 1 + \beta 1 + \beta 2$	No
$\alpha 2 + \beta 2$	Yes
$\alpha 3 + \beta 2$	Yes
$\alpha 4 + \beta 2$	Yes

for the $\beta 1$-subunit; and (2) functional neuronal receptor channels can be assembled by pairing any of the $\alpha 2$-, $\alpha 3$-, or $\alpha 4$-subunits with the $\beta 2$-subunit. These results do not provide proof that the neuronal receptors are composed only of α- and β-subunits *in vivo*. Proteins endogenous to the *Xenopus* oocyte may be providing the functions for the neuronal subunits that are equivalent to the functions of the γ and δ muscle subunits. Nevertheless these results provide important evidence that the proteins identified by molecular cloning techniques are probably components of neuronal nicotinic receptors.

Results from injection of mRNAs into oocytes have provided further evidence that there are subtypes of neuronal nicotinic receptors. The channels formed by coinjection of either $\alpha 3$ or $\alpha 4$ with $\beta 2$ are sensitive to inhibition by κ-bungarotoxin but not by α-bungarotoxin. The combination of $\alpha 2$ and $\beta 2$, however, produces channels that are insensitive to both κ- and α-bungarotoxin (Deneris et al., 1988). This predicts that nicotinic responses in the parts of the brain that express $\alpha 2$-subunits may have a pharmacology that is different from other brain areas that express $\alpha 3$- and $\alpha 4$- subunits.

Can all of these results be combined to answer the question, how many nicotinic receptors are there? The answer must be conditional because use of the term *receptor* requires that a biological response be measured after binding of agonist. The safest answer would be to say that there are at least three nicotinic receptors: one muscle receptor and two neuronal receptors (one type in autonomic ganglia and the second in the brain). The molecular cloning studies argue for at least three neuronal receptors composed of different agonist-binding α-subunits and a common β-subunit. There is still a considerable amount of work to do before this idea can be integrated with the physiological and pharmacological observations to provide the complete picture of neuronal nicotinic receptors. The tools are in hand, so it is only a matter of time before this is achieved.

Regulation of Neuronal Nicotinic Receptors

A considerable amount is known about the regulation of nicotinic receptor biosynthesis and distribution in skeletal muscle (see Scheutze and Role, 1987 for review). Some of the important contributors to this regulation are development, innervation, and neurotransmission. Are neuronal nicotinic receptors also sensitive to these factors?

Nicotinic receptors on sympathetic ganglion neurons appear to be concentrated in regions of synapse formation (Harris et al., 1971). Localization with mAb 35 (Jacob et al., 1984) or κ-bungarotoxin (Loring et al., 1984) indicates that this is also true for cells of chick ciliary ganglion. Functional innervation of chick ciliary ganglia begins around embryonic day 5 (Landmesser and Pilar, 1972). mRNAs for $\alpha 3$-subunit were detected by day 6 (Boyd et al., 1988), and binding sites for mAb 35 increase progressively from day 8 to hatching (Smith et al., 1985). These data are insufficient to determine whether innervation induces the synthesis and clustering of nicotinic receptors on sympathetic neurons because the temporal relationship between receptor synthesis and the onset of neurotransmission has not been examined in sufficient detail. In tissue culture, however, innervation of embryonic chick sympathetic neurons is accompanied by a 10-fold increase in sensitivity to acetylcholine (Role, 1988).

The effect of denervation on neuronal nicotinic receptors has not been studied extensively. Denervation of frog parasympathetic ganglia was followed by increased sensitivity to acetylcholine and more uniform distribution of responsiveness over the neuron (Kuffler et al., 1971). On the other hand, denervation of frog sympathetic ganglia had no effect on the size or distribution of responses to acetylcholine (Dunn and Marshall, 1985). Denervation of chick ciliary ganglia produced a decline of greater than 50% in both the number of mAb 35 binding sites (Jacob and Berg, 1987) and in mRNA encoding the $\alpha 3$-subunit (Boyd et al., 1988). Denervation did not induce the expression of either $\alpha 2$ or $\alpha 4$ mRNAs in these ganglia (Boyd et al., 1988). One consequence of these changes would be a reduced sensitivity to acetycholine unless there are compensatory changes such as altered agonist affinity or some other factor such as inactivating mechanisms (Koelle and Ruch, 1983). These results may indicate that sympathetic and parasympathetic neurons respond differently to denervation. Further investigations are needed to establish the effects of denervation on neuronal nicotinic receptors in autonomic ganglia.

Second messenger systems can modulate neuronal nicotinic receptors. The effects of substance P provide one example. Substance P selectively inhibits nicotinic responses of Renshaw cells in the spinal cord (Ryall, 1982) and in parasympathetic and sympathetic neurons (Akasu et al., 1983; Role, 1984; Margiotta and Berg, 1986). Substance P receptors are linked to increased phosphatidylinositol turnover and, by implication, activation of protein kinase C. Phorbol esters, which activate protein kinase C, produce effects similar to that of substance P (Downing and Role, 1987). These results point to the involvement of a protein kinase C pathway and phosphorylation in the effects on nicotinic responses.

Effects attributable to cAMP have also been observed for neuronal nicotinic receptors. Exposure of chick ciliary ganglion neuron to membrane-permeant analogs of cAMP produces a 2- to 3-fold increase in the response to acetylcholine (Margiotta et al., 1987a,b). The effect of cAMP appears to be to increase the number of functional nicotinic receptors on the cell surface. This increase is not due to the synthesis of new receptor proteins or to the insertion of sequestered receptors. Rather, the effects of cAMP appear to be the activation of preexisting silent nicotinic receptors (Margiotta et al., 1987a,b; Halvorsen and Berg, 1987). Similar effects of cAMP have been reported for bovine adrenal chromaffin cells. For these cells, the age of the nicotinic receptors may be important (Higgins and Berg, 1988a,b)

In summary, there is evidence that neuronal nicotinic receptors are subject to regulation at several levels. The understanding of the mechanisms is still at an early stage, but rapid progress is expected now that there is a clearer picture of the structure and diversity of neuronal nicotinic recpetors.

SUMMARY

Over the last 5 years there has been a dramatic increase in the amount of knowledge that has accumulated on cholinergic receptors. The biggest advances have come from the application of molecular cloning techniques. There have also been significant advances in developing pharmacological tools to study cholinergic receptors, most notably for muscarinic receptors.

It seems clear at the moment that there are a least three functional muscarinic receptors. All three mediate the actions of acetylcholine in one autonomic function or another: M_1 in control of gastric acid secretion, M_2 (cardiac) in vagal-induced slowing of the heart, and M_2 (glandular) in contraction of smooth muscle of the gut. Muscarinic receptors appear to produce their physiological responses by modulation of a variety of transducing mechanisms, though a G protein intermediate always seems to be involved in linking the receptor to these mechanisms.

There are probably three functional nicotinic receptors also: the receptor at the neuromuscular junction, neuronal nicotinic receptors in autonomic ganglia, and nicotinic receptors in the brain. Of these, the ganglionic receptors are at crucial locations in the pathways for activation of both the sympathetic and parasympathetic divisions of the autonomic nervous system. There are many similarities among the three nicotinic receptors; they all appear to be composed of several different proteins that form both the acetylcholine binding site and an ion channel. There are more similarities between the ganglionic receptor and the receptor in the brain, but there are also clearly some differences.

Many questions regarding cholinergic receptors remain to be answered. Which tissues express which type of subtype of receptor? How is each receptor associated with the physiological response that it can elicit? How are the receptor proteins assembled and targeted to the appropriate part of the cell surface? What determines the time a receptor spends on the cell surface? The application of the reagents that have become available in the last few years is expected to provide answers to these and many other questions.

REFERENCES

Reviews

Chiappanelli, V. A. (1983). Kappa-bungarotoxin: A probe for the neuronal nicotinic receptor in the avian ciliary ganglion. *Brain Research* 277, 9–21.

Christie, M. J. and North, R. A. (1988). Control of ion conductances by muscarinic receptors. *Trends in Pharmacological Science* 9 (Suppl.), 30–34.

Gilman, A. (1959). The contribution of pharmacodynamics and pharmacology to basic physiological thought. In: *The Historical Development of Physiological Thought.* Hafner Publishing, New York, pp. 335–349.

Ladinsky, H., and Gralso, E., Monferini, E., Schiavi, G. B., Vigano, M. A., De Conti, L., Micheletti, R., Hammer, R. (1988). Muscarinic receptor heterogeneity in smooth muscle: Binding and functional studies with AF-DX 116. *Trends in Pharmacological Science* 9 (Suppl.), 44–48.

Loffeholz, K., and Pappano, A. J. (1985). The parasympathetic neuroeffector junction of the heart. *Pharmacological Reviews* 37, 1–24.

Martin, B. R. (1986). Nicotine receptors in the central nervous system. In: *The Receptors,* Vol. III, P. M. Conn (ed.), Academic Press, Orlando, Florida.

McCarthy, J. P., Earnest, J. P., Young E. F., Choe, S., and Stroud R. M. (1986). The molecular neurobiology of the acetylcholine receptor. *Annual Review of Neuroscience* 9, 383–413.

Mitchelson, F. (1988). Muscarinic receptor differentiation. *Pharmacology and Therapeutics* 37, 357–423.

Moncada, S., Radomski, M. W., and Palmer, R. M. J. (1988). Endothelium-derived relaxing factor: Identification as nitric oxide and role in the control of vascular tone and platelet function. *Biochemical Pharmacology* 37, 2495–2501.

Murad, F., Mittal, C. K., Arnold, W. P., Katsuki, S., and Kimura, H. (1978). Guanylate cyclase: Activation by azide, nitro compounds, nitric oxide, and hydroxyl radical and inhibition by hemoglobin and myoglobin. *Advances in Cyclic Nucleotide Research,* 9, 145–158.

Nathanson, N. M. (1987). Molecular properties of the muscarinic acetylcholine receptor. *Annual Reviews of Neuroscience* 10, 195-236.

Ryall, R. W. (1982) Modulation of cholinergic transmission by substance P. In: *Substance P in the Nervous System, CIBA Foundation Symposium* 9, 267–280.

Scheutze, S. M., Role, L. W. (1987). Developmental regulation of nicotinic acetylcholine receptors. *Annual Review of Neuroscience* 10, 403–457.

Research Papers

Adams, P. R., and Brown, D. A. (1982). Synaptic inhibition of the M-current: Slow excitatory post-synaptic potential mechanism in bullfrog sympathetic neurons. *Journal of Physiology (London)* 332, 263–272.

Adams, P. R., Brown, D. A., and Constanti, A. (1982a). M-currents and other potassium currents in bullfrog sympathetic neurones. *Journal of Physiology (London)* 330, 537–572.

Adams, P. R., Brown, D. A., and Constanti, A. (1982b). Pharmacological inhibition of the M-current. *Journal of Physiology (London)* 332, 223–262.

Akasu, T., Kojima, M., and Koketsu, K. (1983). Substance P modulates the sensitivity of the nicotinic receptor in amphibian cholinergic transmission. *British Journal of Pharmacology* 80, 123–131.

Birdsall, N. J. M., Burgen, A. S. V., and Hulme, E. C. (1978). The binding of agonists to brain muscarinic receptors. *Molecular Pharmacology* 14, 723–736.

Blatt, Y. M., Montal, M., Lindstron, J., and Montal, M. (1986). Monoclonal antibodies directed against epitopes in the β and γ subunits of the *Torpedo* cholinergic receptor block channel function. *Journal of Neuroscience* 6, 481–486.

Bonner, T. I., Buckley, N. J., Young, A. C., and Brann, M. R. (1987). Identification of a family of muscarinic acetylcholine receptor genes. *Science* 237, 527–532.

Boulter, J., Evans, K., Goldman, D., Martin, G., Treco, D., Heineman, S., and Patrick, J. (1986). Isolation of a cDNA clone coding for a possible neural nicotinic acetylcholine receptor alpha-subunit. *Nature* 319, 368–374.

Boulter, J., Connolly, J., Deneris, E., Goldman, D., Heineman, S., and Patrick, J. (1987). Functional expression of two neuronal nicotinic acetylcholine receptors from cDNA clones identifies a gene family. *Proceedings of the National Academy of Sciences USA* 84, 7763–7767.

Boyd, R. T., Jacob, M. H., Couturier, S., Ballivet, M., and Berg, D. K. (1988). Expression and regulation of neuronal acetylcholine receptor mRNA in chick ciliary ganglia. *Neuron* 1, 495–502.

Breitweiser, G. E., and Szabo, G. (1986). Uncoupling of cardiac muscarinic and β-adrenergic receptors from ion channels by a guanine nucleotide analogue. *Nature* 317, 538–540.

Brown, D. A., and Adams, P. R. (1987). Effects of phorbol dibutyrate on M currents and M current inhibition in bullfrog sympathetic neurons. *Cell and Molecular Neurobiology* 7, 255–269.

Brown, J. H., Goldstein, D., and Masters, S. B. (1985). The putative M_1 muscarine receptor does not regulate phosphoinositide hydrolysis. *Molecular Pharmacology* 27, 525–531.

Chiappanelli, V. A. (1986). Actions of snake venom toxins on neuronal nicotinic receptors and other neuronal receptors. *Pharmacology and Therapeutics* 31, 1–32.

Choo, L. K., Mitchelson, F., and Napier, P. (1988). Differences in antagonist affinities at muscarinic receptors in chick and guinea-pig. *Journal of Autonomic Pharmacology* 8, 259–266.

Clarke, P. B. S., Schwartz, R. D., Paul, S. M., Pert, C. B., and Pert, A. (1985). Nicotinic binding in rat brain: Autoradiographic comparison of [^{3}H]acetylcholine, [^{3}H]nicotine and [^{125}I]bungarotoxin. *Journal of Neuroscience* 5, 1307–1315.

Cole, A. E., and Nicoll, R. A. (1984). Characterization of a slow cholinergic post-synaptic potential recorded in vitro from rat hippocampal pyramidal cells. *Journal of Physiology (London)* 352, 173–188.

Dale, H. H. (1914). The action of certain esters and esters of choline, and their relation to muscarine. *Journal of Pharmacology and Experimental Therapeutics* 6, 147–190.

Dawson, R. M., and Jarrott, B. (1981). Response of muscarinic cholinoceptors of guinea pig brain and ileum to chronic administration of carbamate or organophosphate cholinesterase inhibitors. *Biochemical Pharmacology* 30, 2365–2368.

Deneris, E. S., Connolly, J., Boulter, J., Wada, E., Wada, K., Swanson, L. W., Patrick, J., and Heineman, S. (1988). Primary structure and expression of $\beta 2$: A novel subunit of neuronal nicotinic acetylcholine receptors. *Neuron* 1, 45–54.

Dixon, W. E. (1907). On the mode of action of drugs. *Medical Magazine (London)* 16, 454–457.

Downing, J. E. G., and Role, L. W. (1987). Activators of protein kinase C enhance acetylcholine receptor desensitization in sympathetic ganglion neurons. *Proceedings of the National Academy of Sciences USA* 84, 7739–7743.

Dunn, P. M., and Marshall, L. M. (1985) Lack of nicotinic supersensitivity in frog sympathetic neurones following denervation. *Journal of Physiology (London)* 363, 211–225.

Ehlert, F. J. (1985). The relationship between muscarinic receptor occupancy and adenylate cyclase inhibition in rabbit myocardium. *Molecular Pharmacology* 28, 410–428.

Ek, B., and Nahorski, S. (1988). Muscarinic receptor coupling to inositol phospholipid metabolism in guinea-pig cerebral cortex, parotid gland and ileal smooth muscle. *Biochemical Pharmacology* 17, 4461–4467.

Evans, T., Smith, M. M., Tanner, L., and Harden, T. K. (1984). Muscarinic cholinergic receptors of two cell lines that regulate cyclic AMP metabolism by different molecular mechanisms. *Molecular Pharmacology* 26, 395–404.

Feigenbaum, P., and El-Fakahany, E. E. (1985). Regulation of muscarinic cholinergic receptor density in neuroblastoma cells by brief exposure to agonist: Possible involvement in desensitization of receptor function. *Journal of Pharmacology and Experimental Therapeutics* 233, 134–140.

Furchgott, R. F., and Zawadski, J. V. (1980). The obligatory role of endothelial cells in the relaxation of arterial smooth muscle by acetylcholine. *Nature* 288, 373–376.

Garthwaite, J., Charles, S. L., and Chess-Williams, R. (1988). Endothelium-derived relaxing factor release on activation of NMDA receptors suggests role as intercellular messenger in brain. *Nature* 336, 385–388.

Gazit, H., Silman, I., and Dudai, Y. (1979). Administration of an organophosphate causes a decrease in muscarinic receptor levels in rat brain. *Brain Research* 174, 351–356.

Gil, D. W., and Wolfe, B. B. (1985). Pirenzepine distinguishes between muscarinic receptor-mediated phosphoinositide breakdown and inhibition of adenylate cyclase. *Journal of Pharmacology and Experimental Therapeutics* 23, 608–616.

Giraldo, E. Vigano, M. A., Hammer, R., and Ladinsky, H. (1988). Characterization of muscarinic receptors in guinea pig ileum longitudinal smooth muscle. *Molecular Pharmacology* 33, 617–625.

Goldman, D., Simmon, D., Swanson, L., Patrick, J., and Heineman, S. (1986). Mapping brain areas expressing RNA homologous to two different acetylcholine receptor alpha subunit cDNAs. *Proceedings of the National Academy of Sciences USA* 83, 4076–4080.

Goldman, D., Deneris, E., Luyten, W., Kochhar, A., Patrick, J., and Heineman, S. (1987). Members of a nicotinic acetylcholine receptor gene family are expressed in different regions of the mammalian central nervous system. *Cell* 48, 965–973.

Grandody, B. M., Cuss, F. M., Sampson, A. S., Palmer, J. B., and Barnes, P. J. (1986). Phosphatidylinositol response to cholinergic agonists in airway smooth muscle: Relationship to contraction and muscarinic receptor occupancy. *Journal of Pharmacology and Experimental Therapeutics.* 238, 273–279.

Greene, L. A., and Tischler, A. S. (1976). Establishment of a noradrenergic clonal line of rat adrenal pheochromocytoma cells which respond to nerve growth factor. *Proceedings of the National Academy of Sciences USA* 73, 2424–2428.

Halvorsen, S. W., and Berg, D. K. (1987). Affinity labeling of neuronal acetylcholine receptor subunits with an α-neurotoxin that blocks receptor function. *Journal of Neuroscience* 7, 2547–2555.

Halvorsen, S. W., and Nathanson, N. M. (1981). In vivo regulation of muscarinic acetylcholine receptor number and function in embryonic chick heart. *Journal of Biological Chemistry* 256, 7941–7948.

Hammer, R., and Giachetti, A. (1982). Muscarinic receptor subtypes: M_1 and M_2 biochemical and functional characterization. *Life Sciences* 31, 2991–2998.

Hammer, R., Berrie, C. P., Birdsall, N. J. M., Burgen, A. S. V., and Hulme, E. C. (1980). Pirenzepine distinguishes betweeen different subclasses of muscarinic receptors. *Nature* 283, 90–92.

Harris, A. J., Kuffler, S. W., and Dennis, M. J. (1971). Differential chemosensitivity of synaptic and extrasynaptic areas on the neuronal surface membrane in parasympathetic neurons of the frog, tested by microapplication of acetylcholine. *Proceedings of the Royal Society of London Series B* 177, 541–553.

Hazeki, O., and Ui, M. (1981). Modification by islet-activating protein of receptor-mediated regulation of cyclic AMP accumulation in isolated rat heart cells. *Journal of Biological Chemistry* 256, 2856–2862.

Higgins, L. S., and Berg, D. K. (1988a). Metabolic stability and antigenic modulation of nicotinic acetylcholine receptors on bovine adrenal chromaffin cells. *Journal of Cell Biology* 107, 1147–1156.

Higgins, L. S., and Berg, D. K. (1988b). Cyclic AMP-dependent mechanism regulates acetylcholine receptor function on bovine adrenal chromaffin cells discriminates between new and old receptors. *Journal of Cell Biology* 107, 1157–1165.

Hokin, M. R., and Hokin, L. E. (1954). Effects of acetylcholine on phospholipids in the pancreas. *Journal of Biological Chemistry* 209, 549–558.

Hughes, A. R., Martin, M. W., and Harden, T. K. (1984). Pertussis toxin differentiates between two mechanisms of attenuation of cyclic AMP accumulation by muscarinic receptors. *Proceedings of the National Academy of Sciences (USA)* 81, 5680–5684.

Hulme, E. C., Berrie, C. P., Birdsall, N. J. M., Jameson, M., and Stockton, J. J., (1983). Regulation of muscarinic agonist binding sites by cations and guanine nucleotides. *European Journal of Pharmacology* 94, 59–72.

Iwatsuki, N., and Petersen, O. H. (1977). Pancreatic acinar cells: Localization of acetylcholine receptors and the importance of chloride and calcium for acetylcholine-evoked depolarization. *Journal of Physiology (London)* 269, 723–733.

Jacob, M. H., and Berg, D. K. (1987). Effects of preganglionic denervation and postganglionic axotomy on acetylcholine receptors in the chick ciliary ganglion. *Journal of Cell Biology* 105, 1847–1854.

Jacob, M. H., Berg, D. K., and Lindstrom, J. M. (1984). A shared antigenic determinant between the *Electrophorus* acetylcholine receptor and a synaptic component on chick ciliary ganglion neurons. *Proceedings of the National Academy of Sciences USA* 81, 3223–3227.

Jakobs, K. H., Aktories, K., and Schultz, G. (1979). GTP-dependent inhibition of cardiac adenylate cyclase by muscarinic cholinergic agonists. *Naunyn-Schmiedeberg's Archives of Pharmacology* 310, 113–119.

Kemp, G., and Morely, B. J. (1986). Ganglionic nAChRs and high affinity nicotinic binding sites are not equivalent. *FEBS Letters* 205, 265–268.

Koelle, G. B., and Ruch, G. A. (1983). Demonstration of a neurotrophic factor for the maintenance of acetylcholinesterase and butylcholinesterase in the preganglionically denervated superior cervical ganglion of the cat. *Proceedings of the National Academy of Sciences USA* 80, 3106–3110.

Korc, M., Ackerman, M. S., and Roeske, W. R. (1987). A cholinergic antagonist identifies a subclass of muscarinic receptors in isolated rat pancreatic acini. *Journal of Pharmacology and Experimental Therapeutics* 240, 118–122.

Kubo, T., Fukuda, F., Mikami, A., Maeda, A., Takahashi, H., Michina, M., Haga, T., Haga, K., Ichiyama, A., Kangawa, K., Kojima, M., Matsuo, H., and Numa, S. (1986a). Cloning sequencing and expression of complementary DNA encoding the muscarinic acetylcholine receptor. *Nature* 323, 411–416.

Kubo, T., Maeda, A., Sugimoto, K., Akiba, I., Mikami, A., Takahashi, H., Haga, T., Haga K., Ichyama, A., Kangwa, K., Matsuo, H., Hirose, T., and Numa, S. (1986b). Primary structure of porcine cardiac muscarinic acetylcholine receptor deduced from the cDNA sequence. *FEBS Letters* 209, 367–372.

Kurose, H. T., Katada, T., Amano, T., and Ui, M. (1983). Specific uncoupling by islet-activating protein, pertussis toxin, of negative signal transduction via α-adrenergic, cholinergic and opiate receptors in neuroblastoma × glioma hybrid cells. *Journal of Biological Chemistry* 258, 4870–4875.

Kuffler, S. W., Dennis, M. J., and Harris, A. J. (1971). The development of chemosensitivity in extrasynaptic areas of the neuronal surface after denervation of parasympathetic ganglion cells in the heart of the frog. *Proceedings of the Royal Society of London Series B* 177, 555–563.

Kunysz, E. A., Michel, A. D., Whiting, R. L., and Woods, K. (1989). The human astrocytoma cell line 1321 N1 contains M_2-glandular type muscarinic receptors linked to phosphoinositide turnover. *British Journal of Pharmacology* 96, 271–278.

Landmesser, L., and Pilar, G. (1972). The onset and development of transmission in the chick ciliary ganglion. *Journal of Physiology (London)* 222, 691–713.

Langley, J. N. (1907). On the contraction of muscle, chiefly in relation to the presence of "receptive substances." *Journal of Physiology (London)* 36, 347–384.

Langley, J. N., and Dickinson, W. L. (1889). On the local paralysis of peripheral ganglia, and on the connexion of different classes of nerve fibers with them. *Proceedings of the Royal Society of London* 46, 423–431.

Liles, W. C., Hunter, D. D., Meier, K. E., and Nathanson, N. M. (1986). Activation of protein kinase C induces rapid internalization and subsequent degradation of muscarinic receptors in neuroblastoma cells. *Journal of Biological Chemistry* 261, 5307–5313.

Loewi, O. (1921). Uber humorale Ubertragbarkeit der Herznervenwirkung. *Pfluger's Archiv fur die gesamte Physiologie des Menschen und der Tiere* 189, 239–242.

Loring, R. H., Andrews, A., Lane, W., and Zigmond, R. E. (1984). Amino acid sequence of toxin F, a snake venom toxin that blocks neuronal nicotinic receptors. *Brain Research* 385, 30–37.

Malenka, R. C., Madison, D. V., Andrade, R., and Nicoll, R. A. (1986). Phorbol esters mimic some cholinergic actions in hippocampal pyramidal neurons. *Journal of Neuroscience* 6, 475–480.

Maloteaux, J. M., Gossuin, A., Pauwels, P. J., and Laduron, P. M. (1983). Short-term disappearance of muscarinic cell surface receptors in carbachol-induced desensitization. *FEBS Letters* 156, 103–107.

Margiotta, J. F., and Berg, D. K. (1986). Enkephalin and

substance P modulate synaptic properties of chick ciliary ganglion neurons in cell culture. *Neuroscience* 18, 175–182.

Margiotta, J. F., Berg, D. K., and Dionne, V. E. (1987a). Cyclic AMP regulates the proportion of functional acetylcholine receptors on chick ciliary ganglion neurons. *Proceedings of the National Academy of Sciences USA* 84, 8155–8159.

Margiotta, J. F., Berg, D. K., and Dionne, V. E. (1987b). The properties and regulation of functional acetylcholine receptors on chick ciliary ganglion neurons. *Journal of Neuroscience* 7, 3612–3622.

Marks, M. J., Artman, L. D., Patinkin, D. M., and Collins, A. C. (1981). Cholinergic adaptations to chronic oxotremorine infusion. *Journal of Pharmacology and Experimental Therapeutics* 218, 337–348.

Martin, W. Villani, G. M., Jothianandan, D., and Furchgott, R. F. (1985). Selective blockade of endothelium-dependent and glyceryl trinitrate-induced relaxation by hemoglobin and by methylene blue in the rabbit aorta. *Journal of Pharmacology and Experimental Therapeutics* 232, 708–716.

Mattera, R., Pitts, B. J. R., Entman, M. L., and Birnbauner, L. (1985). Guanine nucleotide regulation of a mammalian myocardial muscarinic receptor system. *Journal of Biological Chemistry* 260, 7410–7421.

McCandless, M., Nishiyama, A., Petersen, O. H., and Philpott, H. G. (1980). Mouse pancreatic acinar cells: Voltage clamp study of acetylcholine-evoked membrane current. *Journal of Physiology (London)* 318, 57–71.

McCormick, D. A., and Prince, D. A. (1985). Two types of muscarinic response to acetylcholine in mammalian cortical neurons. *Proceedings of the National Academy of Sciences USA* 82, 6344–6348.

McCormack, D. A., Mak, J. C., Minette, P., and Barnes, P. J. (1988). Muscarinic receptor subtypes mediating vasodilation in the pulmonary artery. *European Journal of Pharmacology* 158, 293–297.

McKinney, M., Stenstrom, S., and Richelson, E. (1985). Muscarinic responses and binding in a murine neuroblastoma clone (N1E-115). *Molecular Pharmacology* 27, 223–235.

Meurs, H., Roffel, A. F., Postema, J. B., Timmeremans, A., Elzinga, C. R. S., Kauffman, H. F., and Zaagsma, J. (1988). Evidence for a direct relationship between phosphoinositide metabolism and airway smooth muscle contraction induced by muscarinic agonists. *European Journal of Pharmacology* 156, 271–274.

Misbahuddin, M., Isosaki, M., Houchi, H., and Oka, M. (1985). Muscarinic receptor-mediated increase in cytoplasmic free Ca^{2+} in isolated bovine adrenal medullary cells. *FEBS Letters* 190, 25–28.

Murad, F., Chi, Y.-M., Ral, T. W., and Sutherland, E. W. (1962). Adenyl cyclase. II. The effect of catecholamines and choline esters on the formation of adenosine $3',5'$-phosphate by preparations from cardiac muscle and liver. *Journal of Biological Chemistry* 237, 1233–1238.

Nef, P., Oneyser, C., Alliod, C., Couturier, S., and Ballivet, M. (1988). Genes expressed in the brain define three distinct neuronal nicotinic acetylcholine receptors. *EMBO Journal* 7, 595–601.

Noronha-Blob, L., Lowe, V. C., Hansson, R. C., and U'Prichard, D. C. (1987). Heterogeneity of muscarinic receptors coupled to phosphoinositide breakdown in guinea pig brain and peripheral tissues. *Life Sciences* 41, 967–975.

Nowak, L. M., and McDonald, R. L. (1983). Muscarine-sensitive voltage-dependent potassium current in cultured murine spinal cord neurons. *Neuroscience Letters* 35, 85–91.

Olianas, M. C., Onali, P., Neff, N. H., and Costa, E. (1983). Adenylate cyclase activity of synaptic membranes from rat striatum. *Molecular Pharmacology* 23, 393–398.

Orellana, S. A., Solski, P. A., and Brown, J. H. (1985). Phorbol ester inhibits phosphoinositide hydrolysis and calcium mobilization in cultured astrocytoma cells. *Journal of Biological Chemistry* 260, 5236–5239.

Palmer, R. M. J., Ashton, D. S., and Moncada, S. (1988). Vascular endothelial cells synthesize nitric oxide from l-arginine. *Nature* 333, 664–666.

Patrick, J., and Stallcup, W. B. (1977). Immunological distinction between acetylcholine receptor and the alpha-bungarotoxin-binding component on sympathetic neurons. *Proceedings of the National Academy of Sciences USA* 74, 4689–4692.

Peralta, E. G., Winslow, J. W., Peterson, G. L., Smith, D. H., Ashkenazi, A., Ramachandran, J., Schimerlik, M. I., and Capon, D. J. (1987a). Primary structure and biochemical properties of an M_2 muscarinic receptor. *Science* 236, 600–605.

Peralta, E. G., Ashkenazi, A., Winslow, J. W., Smith, D. H., Ramachandran, J., and Capon D. J. (1987b). Distinct primary structures, ligand-binding properties and tissue specific expression of four human muscarinic acetylcholine receptors. *EMBO Journal* 6, 3923–3929.

Peralta, E. G., Ashkenazi, A. Winslow, J. W., Ramachandran, J., and Capon, D. J. (1988). Differential regulation of PI hydrolysis and adenylyl cyclase by muscarinic receptor subtypes. *Nature* 334, 434–437.

Pfaffinger, P. J., Martin, J. M., Hunter, D., Nathanson, N. M., and Hille, B. (1985). GTP-binding proteins couple cardiac muscarinic receptors to a K channel. *Nature* 317, 536–538.

Pfaffinger, P. J., Leibowitz, M. D., Subers, E. M., Nathanson, N. M., Almers, W., and Hille, B. (1988). Agonists that suppress M-current elicit phosphoinositide turnover and Ca^{2+} transients, but these events do not explain M-current suppression. *Neuron* 1, 447–484.

Rapoport, R. M., Draznin, M. B., and Murad, F. (1983). Endothelium-dependent relaxation in rat aorta may be mediated through cyclic GMP-mediated protein phosphorylation. *Nature* 306, 174–176.

Ravdin, P. M., and Berg, D. K. (1979). Inhibition of neuronal acetylcholine sensitivity by alpha-toxins from *Bungarus multicinctus* venom. *Proceedings of the National Academy of Sciences USA* 76, 2072–2076.

Rees, D. D., Palmer, R. M. J., Hodson, H. F., and Moncada, S. (1989). A specific inhibitor of nitric oxide formation from l-arginine attenuates endothelium-dependent relaxation. *British Journal of Pharmacology* 96, 418–424.

Role, L. W. (1984). Substance P modulation of acetylcholine-induced currents in embryonic chicken sympathetic and ciliary ganglion neurons. *Proceedings of the National Academy of Sciences USA* 81, 2924–2928.

Role, L. W. (1988). Neural regulation of acetylcholine sensitivity in embryonic sympathetic neurons. *Proceedings of the National Academy of Sciences USA* 85, 2825–2829.

Romano, C., and Goldstein, A. (1980). Stereospecific nicotine receptors on rat brain membranes. *Science* 210, 647–650.

Rotter, A., Birdsall, N. J. H., Burgen, A. S. V., Field, P. M., Hulme, E. C., and Raisman, G. (1979). Muscarinic receptors in the central nervous system of the rat. I. Technique for autoradiographic localization of the binding of [³H]-propylbenzilylcholine mustard and its distribution in the forebrain. *Brain Research Reviews* 1, 141–165.

Sakmann, B., Noma, A., and Trautwein, W. (1983). Acetylcholine activation of single muscarinic K^+ channels in isolated pacemaker cells of the mammalian heart. *Nature* 303, 250–253.

Schwartz, R. D., McGee, R., and Keller, K. J. (1982). Nicotinic cholinergic receptors labelled by [³H]-acetylcholine in rat brain. *Molecular Pharmacology* 22, 55–62.

Sims, S. M., Singer, J. J., and Walsh, J. V. (1985). Cholinergic agonists suppress a potassium current in freshly dissociated smooth muscle cells of the toad. *Journal of Physiology (London)* 367, 503–529.

Smith, M. A. J., Stollberg, J., Berg, D. K., and Lindstrom, J. (1985). Characterization of a component in chick ciliary ganglia that cross-reacts with monoclonal anitbodies to muscle and electric organ acetylcholine receptor. *Journal of Neuroscience* 5, 2726–2731.

Swanson, L. W., Lindstrom, J., Tzartos, S., Schmeud, L. C., O'Leary, D. D. M., and Cowan, W. M. (1983). Immunohistochemical localization of monoclonal antibodies to the nicotinic acetylcholine receptor in chick midbrain. *Proceedings of the National Academy of Sciences USA* 80, 4532–4536.

Swanson, L. W., Simmons, D., Whiting, P. J., and Lindstrom, J. (1987). Immunohistochemical localization of neuronal nicotinic receptors in the rodent central nervous system. *Journal of Neuroscience* 7, 3334–3342.

Wada, K. Ballivet, M., Boulter, J., Connolly, J., Wada, E.,

Deneris, E. S., Swanson, L. W., Heineman, S., and Patrick, J. (1988). Functional expression of a new pharmacological subtype of brain nicotinic acetylcholine receptor. *Science* 240, 330–334.

Whiting, P. J., and Lindstrom, J. M. (1986a). Purification and characterization of a nicotinic acetylcholine receptor from chick brain. *Biochemistry* 25, 2082–2093.

Whiting, P., and Lindstrom, J. (1986b). Pharmacological properties of immuno-isolated neuronal nicotinic receptors. *Journal of Neuroscience* 6, 3061–3069.

Whiting, P., and Lindstrom, J. (1987a). Purification and characterization of a nicotinic acetylcholine receptor from rat brain. *Proceedings of the National Academy of Sciences USA* 84, 595–599.

Whiting, P., and Lindstrom, J. (1987b). Affinity labelling of neuronal acetylcholine receptors localizes acetylcholine-binding sites to their β-subunits. *FEBS Letters* 213, 55–60.

Whiting P. J., and Liu R., Morley, B. J., and Lindstrom, J. M. (1987a). Structurally different neuronal nicotinic acetylcholine receptor subtypes purified and characterized using monoclonal anitbodies. *Journal of Neuroscience* 7, 4005–4016.

Whiting, P., Esch, F., Shimasaki, S., and Lindstrom, J. (1987b). Neuronal nicotinic acetylcholine receptor β-subunit is coded for by the cDNA clone α_4. *FEBS Letters* 219, 459–463.

Wojcikiewicz, R. J. H., Dobson, RPM., and Brown, B. L. (1984). Mucarinic acetylcholine receptor activation causes inhibition of cyclic AMP accumulation, prolactin and growth hormone secretion in GH3 rat anterior pituitary tumor cells. *Biochimica et Biophysica Acta* 805, 25–29.

Woodcock, E. A., Leung, E., and McLeod, J. K. (1987). A comparison of muscarinic acetylcholine receptor coupled to phosphatidylinositol turnover and to adenylate cyclase in guinea-pig atria and ventricles. *European Journal of Pharmacology* 133, 283–289.

4

Sympathetic Preganglionic Neurons:
Cytoarchitecture, Ultrastructure, and Biophysical Properties

J. B. CABOT

Sympathetic preganglionic neurons are found exclusively within spinal cord. They are the central nervous system's final common pathway responsible for the peripheral regulation of sympathetic function. Specifically, they are the last neuronal link contained within the central nervous system for the peripheral activation of sympathetic postganglionic neurons and adrenal chromaffin cells.

This idea of a final common pathway for autonomic function is an analogy with the α-motoneurons that innervate skeletal muscle. Other than this broad generalization, however, there are few similarities between these two populations of spinal cord motoneurons (for discussion on α-motoneurons see Burke et al., 1982; Cameron et al., 1983, 1985; Cullheim et al., 1987a,b; Ulfhake and Kellereth, 1981, 1983). In general, sympathetic preganglionic neurons are a far more heterogeneous population of cells than are α-motoneurons. Sympathetic preganglionic cells are found in four separate regions within the spinal gray matter. They exhibit significant variations in somal shape and size, have diverse dendritic arbors, and give rise to unmyelinated and myelinated axons. Moreover, the postsynaptic target for sympathetic preganglionic motoneurons, unlike α-motoneurons, is not singularly selective. Sympathetic preganglionic axons terminate on other neuronal elements (i.e., sympathetic postganglionic neurons), or on the secretory chromaffin cells of the adrenal medulla.

Currently it is impossible to assign functional significance to the nuclear and morphological differentiation displayed by sympathetic preganglionic neurons. Nevertheless, the existence of anatomical diversity suggests that there are substrates available to these neurons for the selective assembly of excitatory and inhibitory afferent inputs arriving from different levels of the neuraxis. The matching of specific afferent inputs with specific classes of sympathetic preganglionic neurons could endow spinal sympathetic networks with the ability to execute complex, differentiated, and patterned peripheral autonomic responses.

Functionally unrelated populations of sympathetic preganglionic neurons must be able to selectively alter their output from spinal cord. This statement is based on the fact that patterned peripheral autonomic responses accompany many simple animal behaviors. For example, animals and humans respond to life-threatening sensory stimuli with the following generalized, but differentiated peripheral autonomic responses (see Cannon, 1939, for review): (1) increased heart rate and cardiac contractility, (2) pupillary dilation, (3) increased adrenal medullary secretion of catecholamines, (4) vasoconstriction of the cutaneous and splanchnic vascular beds, (5) vasodilation within the skeletal muscle vascular beds, (6) bronchiolar dilation, (7) increased glucose metabolism, and (8) piloerection.

Qualitatively, quite different sympathomotor responses accompany orthostasis. Whether it be a giraffe raising its head from ground level to the tree tops or a man going from a supine to an erect stance, such postural changes precipitate a baroreceptor reflex due to a transient decrease in arterial blood pressure. Activation of this reflex elicits peripheral autonomic changes that purposefully ensure constancy of brain blood flow (see Heymans and Neil, 1958; Kircheim, 1976 for reviews). To accomplish this goal a patterned response occurs; the vascular beds in muscle constrict, heart rate increases, and there is a small increase in cutaneous vasoconstrictor tone. Importantly, the pattern is notably more selective than what occurs during fright: glucose metabolism does not increase, the pupils and bronchioles do not dilate, and piloerection does not occur.

Autonomic response patterns in spinal animals when compared to those in animals with an intact neuraxis illustrate further the complex integration of afferent information being performed by sympathetic preganglionic nuerons. With an intact neuraxis, the action potential discharge of sympathetic preganglionic neurons is largely unchanged, or marginally decreased, in response to innocuous muscle or skin indentation, or to light tapping and gentle brushing of the body surface (as long as the stimuli are not consciously perceived as being novel or threatening). In effect, these sensory stimuli are largely ignored. In contrast, each of these stimuli elicits mass sympathoexcitation when applied to cervically spinalized animals, including humans. The sympathoexcitatory responses include (1) profuse sweating, (2) intense, widespread cutaneous and muscle vascular bed constriction, (3) significant elevation of arterial blood pressure, and (4) tachycardia (for reviews, see Mathias and Frankel, 1988; Schramm, 1986). This pattern is so significantly abnormal as to be potentially life threatening. It would appear that sympathetic preganglionic neurons in spinal animals no longer receive, from supraspinal levels of the neuraxis, critical afferent feedback that is required for normal homeostatic adjustments.

As the above examples demonstrate, the execution of differentiated peripheral autonomic responses necessitates the selective patterning of action potential generation by populations of sympathetic preganglionic neurons. One of the principal goals of this chapter is to review some of the anatomical substrates and physiological mechanisms by which this may be accomplished, although these are far from well understood. Significant progress is being made and the approaches leading to this are discussed. Recent data on the cytoarchitectural organization, neuronal morphology, efferent connections, and biophysical properties of sympathetic preganglionic neurons will be reviewed. The observations begin to lay a solid foundation that will eventually lead to the elucidation of the primary principles that govern central neuronal regulation of sympathetic preganglionic neuronal function.

Throughout this chapter an attempt has been made to consolidate the salient features of sympathetic preganglionic neuronal structure and function. In so doing, specific contributions have not always been appropriately emphasized, or may not have been mentioned at all. Several comprehensive reviews can be consulted for more exhaustive discussions (Coote, 1988; Jänig, 1985, 1988; Laskey and Polosa, 1988; McCall, 1988; Polosa et al., 1988; Schramm, 1986).

LOCATIONS AND SPATIAL ARRANGEMENTS OF SYMPATHETIC PREGANGLIONIC NEURONS

It is rare when a single scientific publication lays down a fundamental framework that, after more than a decade of further investigation employing more refined and increasingly accurate methods, becomes only slightly modified. Just such a set of classic observations is epitomized in a paper by Petras and Cummings (1972). The essential elements of spinal autonomic cytoarchitecture were identified by these investigators and have since been repeatedly replicated in many other mammals and presumably can be generalized to humans (e.g., rat: Bacon and Smith, 1988; Barber et al., 1984; Rando et al., 1981; Schramm et al., 1975; Strack et al., 1988; guinea pig: McLachlan, 1985; McLachlan et al., 1985; Rubin and Purves, 1980; cat: Baron et al., 1985a,b,c; Chung et al., 1975, 1979; Jänig and McLachlan, 1986b; Morgan et al., 1986; Oldfield and McLachlan, 1981; dog: Petras and Cummings, 1978; Petras and Faden, 1978; additional references in review by Coote, 1988).

Sympathetic preganglionic neurons, in contrast to α- motoneurons, are not present along the entire longitudinal extent of the spinal cord, but rather are restricted to the caudal portions of the last cervical spinal segment (e.g., C8), the full length of thoracic spinal cord, and the upper lumbar spinal segments; thus, the origin of the term, *thoracolumbar sympathetic preganglionic neurons.* The caudal extension within lumbar spinal cord (L3–5) may be loosely related to the total number of lumbar spinal segments characteristic of a particular mammal (e.g., guinea pig vs. cat) (Jänig and McLachlan, 1986b; McLachlan, 1985).

Sympathetic preganglionic neurons are located in four topographically definable nuclei (Figure 4-1) within the intermediate spinal gray matter (i.e., zona intermedia). The most prominent division resides in the area defined classically as the *intermediolateral cell column* and occupies the lateral horn in the spinal gray matter. An alternative nomenclature for this region is nucleus intermediolateralis thoracolumbalis pars principalis. Quantitatively, the majority of sympathetic preganglionic cells are located in the intermediolateral cell column. Extending laterally and dorsally from this region and into the white matter of the lateral funiculus, a second segregation of sympathetic preganglionic neurons is found. This nucleus, the nucleus intermediolateralis thoracolumbalis pars funicularis is more simply termed the *lateral funicular area.* Neurons in the lateral funicular area are most numerous in upper thoracic and lumbar spinal segments. Lying medial to the intermediolateral cell column and coursing toward the central canal is a third nucleus, the *intercalated cell group.* The neurons in this nucleus are easily distinguished since the majority have their principal cell body axis, and some components of the dendritic arbor, aligned mediolaterally in the transverse plane. The fourth nuclear group of sympathetic pregangli-

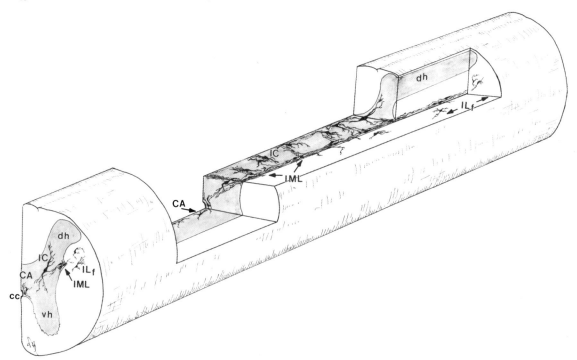

Figure 4-1 Schematic illustration showing the topography of the four principal sympathetic preganglionic nuclei (IL$_f$, IML, IC, CA) in the mammalian thoracic spinal cord. Proceeding from left to right the planes of section for the hemi-spinal cord are transverse, followed by two horizontal planes of sections and a sagittal view. Characteristically, the sympathetic preganglionic cell bodies and their dendritic arbors form a "ladder" arrangement (see text for further specifics). IL$_f$, lateral funicular nucleus; IML, intermediolateral nucleus; IC, intercalated nucleus; CA, central autonomic nucleus; dh, dorsal horn; vh, ventral horn; cc, central canal.

onic neurons is located dorsolateral to the central canal; this nucleus has been identified as the nucleus intercalatus pars paraependymalis by Petras and Cummings (1972) (also see Petras and Faden, 1978). More commonly, however, this region is referred to as the *central autonomic nucleus* (e.g., Barber et al., 1984; Chung et al., 1975; Cummings, 1969; Oldfield and McLachlan, 1981; Schramm, 1975; Rubin and Purves, 1980). This latter terminology, although prevalent, is ambiguous. This is especially true in the upper lumbar spinal cord of guinea pigs and rats (Baron et al., 1985a,b,c; Hancock and Peveto, 1979; Jänig and McLachlan, 1986b; McLachlan, 1985; Morgan et al., 1986; Nadelhaft and McKenna, 1987).

The longitudinal patterned arrangement of the lateral funicular, intermediolateral, intercalated, and central autonomic preganglionic neurons resembles a "ladder" (Figure 4-1; cf. Petras and Cummings, 1972). In a view of the spinal cord in the horizontal or longitudinal plane, the "side supports" are the bilateral columns of sympathetic preganglionic neurons in the intermediolateral cell columns. Within these columns sympathetic preganglionic cells tend to cluster periodically in groups of 20–100 neurons to form what have been frequently termed *nests*

(e.g., Oldfield and McLachlan, 1981). Depending on the mammalian species, the inter-nest distance varies from 200 to 500 μm throughout the thoracic spinal cord and characteristically shortens in the lumbar spinal cord, where it approaches 100–300 μm (Barber et al., 1984; Morgan et al., 1986; Oldfield and McLachlan, 1981; Rando et al., 1981). In transverse section, the "rope-like ladder rungs" connecting the "side supports" are formed, in part, by the intercalated neurons. The intercalated nucleus is continuous laterally with the intermediolateral cell column, and courses medially, merging often indistinguishably with central autonomic cells at the level of the central canal. "Inter-rung" distances vary across mammalian species. They differ in frequency within and between spinal segments, do not share a 1–1 correspondence with intermediolateral cell column nests, and often correlate with distinctive patterns of afferentation (e.g., Bernstein-Goral and Bohn, 1988; Davis et al., 1984; Glazer and Ross, 1980; Krukoff et al., 1985; McLachlan and Oldfield, 1981; Newton and Hamill, 1989; Newton et al., 1989; Oldfield and McLachlan, 1981; Romagnano et al., 1987; Rubin and Purves, 1980). Continuation of the "ladder rung" across the midline occurs via the paired (right and left sides) central autonomic neurons. The absolute number of central autonomic neurons is variable, with more being present in guinea pig than in rat, cat, and dog.

TOPOGRAPHICAL DIFFERENTIATION OF SYMPATHETIC PREGANGLIONIC NEURONS

A central issue regarding the spinal organization of sympathetic preganglionic neurons is whether their spatial distribution is of functional significance (McLachlan et al., 1985). This problem remains largely unresolved. Anatomical studies have been unsuccessful, for the most part, because of limitations inherent in the methods that have been used. Specifically, the retrograde cell body labeling methods (e.g., with horseradish peroxidase, fast blue, or fluorogold) do not distinguish between labeling due to uptake by damaged axons of passage or that resulting from exclusive uptake by intact synaptic terminals. Further, none of the methods provides for the selective labeling of sympathetic preganglionic neurons that innervate specific end-organs (with one potential exception, the adrenal gland). Correlations of sympathetic preganglionic structure, location, and function will be established only when neuroanatomical methods are developed that provide for the retrograde transsynaptic specification of neuronal connectivity. Such a methodological breakthrough may cccur soon, as several groups are actively experimenting with proteins and viruses capable of retrograde transneuronal labeling of specific sets of neurons.

Despite the existing methodological shortcomings, it is important not to lose sight of the fact that significant progress has been achieved in the last 20 years. Relatively complete descriptions of the nuclear and topographic distribution of sympathetic preganglionic cells whose axons pass through or terminate within paravertebral ganglia (superior cervical, stellate, T3–8 segmental, lumbar sympathetic trunk), prevertebral ganglia (superior and inferior mesenteric ganglia), terminal ganglia (indirectly via labeling from the hypogastric nerve), and the adrenal medullae have been reported in the rat (Appel and Elde, 1988; Bacon and Smith, 1988; Hancock and Peveto, 1979; Holets and Elde, 1982; Nadelhaft and McKenna, 1987; Rando et al., 1981; Schramm et al., 1975; Strack et al., 1988), guinea pig (Dalsgaard and Elfvin, 1979, 1981; McLachlan, 1985; McLachlan et al., 1985; Rubin and Purves, 1980), and cat (Baron et al., 1985a–c; Chung et al., 1979; Holets and Elde, 1983; Jänig and McLachlan, 1986b; Morgan et al., 1986; Oldfield and Mc-

Lachlan, 1981; Pardini and Wurster, 1984). The results may be generalized as follows.

First, lateral funicular, intermediolateral, intercalated and central autonomic cells are distributed bilaterally and in a symmetrical manner. Neurons originating from the right side of the spinal cord affect autonomic functions on the right side of the body and those on the left affect the left side. There are, however, important exceptions; namely, sympathetic preganglionic neurons innervating the prevertebral and terminal ganglia that control the intestine and pelvic viscera are not unilaterally distributed.

The symmetry within spinal cord is matched by the bilateral placement of paravertebral ganglia and adrenal medullae (see Pick, 1970 for review). For several widely dispersed, bilaterally located peripheral autonomic targets, such as the resistance vessels in skin and muscle, the symmetrical location of sympathetic preganglionic neurons within spinal cord provides the necessary anatomical substrate to accomplish complete, coordinated control of these targets. It is important to recognize, however, that anatomical symmetry is, first and foremost, an organizational principle. This principle is not a strong predictor of functional organization. For example, activation of sympathetic preganglionic neurons in the right half of the upper thoracic spinal cord effects large increases in cardiac chronotropy and has little or no effect on cardiac contractility; in contrast, activation of sympathetic preganglionic neurons located on the left side of upper thoracic spinal cord effects large increases in cardiac contractility and only minor increases in chronotropy (see Armour and Hopkins, 1984; Randall, 1984; Schwartz, 1984 for reviews).

Second, like α-motoneuron pools in spinal cord (see Burke, 1981 for review), sympathetic preganglionic cells exhibit a topographically organized, rostrocaudal pattern of efferent connections. For example, sympathetic preganglionic neurons innervating postganglionic neurons in superior cervical ganglia, the output of which affects autonomic function to the head and neck region, are located in spinal segments C8–T5; sympathetic preganglionic neurons innervating the more caudally located adrenal medullary chromaffin cells arise from spinal segments T4–T12. This is a unique example in many respects, but it exemplifies the general finding that sympathetic ganglia receive sympathetic preganglionic inputs from several spinal segments; as the location of peripheral autonomic targets moves progressively more caudal, the contributing spinal segments are systematically located more caudally (Figure 4-2). Further, the dominant sympathetic preganglionic input to any particular peripheral autonomic ganglion originates within a single (or at

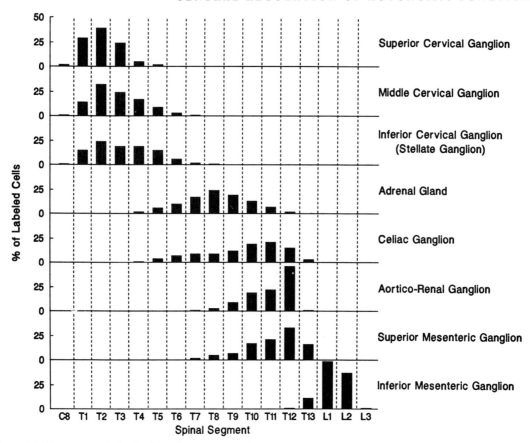

Figure 4-2 The segmental distribution of retrogradely labeled sympathetic preganglionic neurons after Fluoro-gold injections into the major peripheral sympathetic ganglia and adrenal glands of rats. Examination of the histograms reveals two principal observations: (1) most peripheral sympathetic ganglia receive dominant input from a single thoracic or lumbar spinal cord segment; and (2) more caudally located peripheral sympathetic ganglia receive sympathetic preganglionic input from neurons located more caudally in the spinal cord. (Reproduced with permission from Strack et al., 1988.)

most two) spinal segment (Figure 4-2; Jänig and McLachlan, 1986a,b; Purves et al., 1986; Strack et al., 1988). The general pattern ignores nuclear divisions. This conservative anatomical framework is deceptive, however, since it obscures a much more elaborate and finely tuned physiological organization. In physiological terms, differences in spinal sympathetic segmental outflow to a single peripheral ganglion often correlate with differences in the magnitude or relative exclusivity of particular end-organ responses (Lichtman et al., 1979; Nja and Purves, 1977; for reviews, see Pick, 1970; Purves and Lichtman, 1985).

Third, while sympathetic preganglionic neurons from several spinal segments contribute to the innervation of a single sympathetic ganglion (see Figure 4-2), the neurons themselves are segmentally organized (Figure 4-3; Oldfield and McLachlan, 1981; Rubin and Purves, 1980). That is, each preganglionic neuron gives rise to an axon that courses along the lateral margin of, or through, the ventral horn and exits the spinal cord via the ventral rootlets as-

sociated with the same spinal segment in which the neuron resides (Bogan and Cabot, 1985; Cabot and Bogan, 1987; Dembowsky et al., 1985a; Forehand, 1985; Oldfield and McLachlan, 1981; Rubin and Purves, 1980).

On exiting the ventral root, sympathetic preganglionic axons enter rami communicantes. In most vertebrates these are white in coloration in fresh tissue, indicating the presence of myelin. These axons then follow one of several divergent courses (Figure 4-3; see section on Properties of Sympathetic Preganglionic Axons for further detail). (1) They branch, synapsing on one or more sympathetic postganglionic neurons in the segmental paravertebral ganglia and then continue rostrally or caudally along the sympathetic chain, ultimately terminating on postganglionic neurons in one or more other paravertebral ganglia. (2) They pass through the segmental paravertebral ganglion and course rostrally or caudally to contact several postganglionic neurons in one or more other paravertebral ganglia. (3) They bypass the segmental paravertebral ganglia alto-

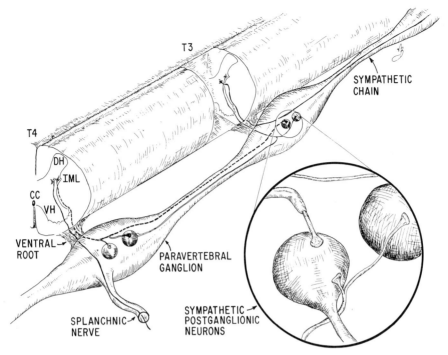

Figure 4-3 Schematic illustration showing that: (1) Sympathetic preganglionic neurons are segmentally organized; preganglionic axons exit the ventral root of the spinal segment where the preganglionic cell body is located. (2) The axons of sympathetic preganglionic neurons are either myelinated (————) or unmyelinated (- - -). (3) Sympathetic preganglionic axons can assume several trajectories on exiting the spinal cord via the ventral rootlets; the axons course through the ventral rootlets and into white rami (not shown) before entering the peripheral autonomic ganglia (see text for specific details). (4) In the periphery sympathetic preganglionic axons terminate on many separate sympathetic postganglionic neurons (divergence). (5) Sympathetic postganglionic neurons receive input from several sympathetic preganglionic neurons (convergence, see Table 4-3 and discussion of neural unit size for more details). T3-4, thoracic spinal cord segments; DH, dorsal horn; IML, intermediolateral nucleus; CC, central canal; VH, ventral horn.

gether and enter one of the major splanchnic nerves, eventually synapsing on postganglionic neurons in prevertebral or terminal ganglia. Other combinations of trajectory exist, but the above three predominate. An important new observation is that individual sympathetic preganglionic neurons within a single spinal segment give rise to axons that, upon exiting spinal cord, assume either a rostral or a caudal trajectory, but only infrequently (<2%) does an axon split to go in both directions (Forehand and Rubin, 1986).

There are two fundamental functional consequences that can be deduced from the anatomical organization discussed above. The first is that sympathetic preganglionic cells within a single spinal segment can control peripheral autonomic targets both rostral and caudal to the spinal segment in which the sympathetic preganglionic neurons reside. Since the axons of individual sympathetic preganglionic neurons only rarely project rostrally and caudally along the sympathetic chain, this control of the periphery is achieved almost entirely by altering the neuronal discharge of separate populations of sympathetic preganglionic neurons within a single spinal

segment. Furthermore, as sympathetic preganglionic neurons do not have pacemaker properties, the coordination of such changes in neuronal discharge must be a direct result of the integration of afferent information by separate populations of sympathetic preganglionic cells within a single spinal segment. The second functional implication follows directly from the first. Specifically, peripheral divergence of sympathetic preganglionic axon terminations is a necessary, but not a sufficient, anatomical substrate to ensure the proper coordination of generalized peripheral sympathetic responses (see section on Properties of Sympathetic Preganglionic Axons for further details on convergence and divergence).

Fourth, the spinal sympathetic outflow to the mammalian hindlimb and the pelvic organs is topographically organized (see Figure 18-2 in Jänig, this volume). Sympathetic preganglionic axons coursing in the hypogastric nerve, which is the source of sympathetic fibers to the pelvic organs, have spinal cells of origin located medial to those providing sympathetic preganglionic input to the sympathetic postganglionic innervation of hindlimb muscles and skin (Baron et al., 1985a,b; Hancock and Peveto, 1979;

Jänig and McLachlan, 1986b; McLachlan, 1985; McLachlan et al., 1985; Morgan et al., 1986; Nadelhaft and McKenna, 1987; Neuhuber, 1982). Interestingly, there are species-specific differences in the spinal locations of sympathetic preganglionic neurons that give rise to this general topography. In rats, for example, the sympathetic preganglionic neurons whose axons course in the hypogastric nerve are located in the region dorsal to the central canal. Despite the central location of these sympathetic preganglionic neurons in the rat, it is unlikely that they represent a caudal continuation of sympathetic preganglionic neurons of the central autonomic nucleus; indeed, these neurons were originally named dorsal commissural neurons (Hancock and Peveto, 1979; also see McLachlan, 1985). The other extreme is represented in cat. In this vertebrate, the homologous sympathetic preganglionic neurons projecting out of the hypogastric nerve are found in the region of the intermediolateral cell column (Jänig and McLachlan, 1986b; also see Figure 18-2 in Jänig, this volume). The observations in the cat and rat suggest that in the lumbar spinal cord of some mammals there may be a fifth nuclear division of sympathetic preganglionic neurons. This issue will not be settled unequivocally, however, until physiologi-

cal data on the properties of these neurons have been obtained in the two vertebrates.

SOMATIC AND DENDRITIC DIFFERENTIATION OF SYMPATHETIC PREGANGLIONIC NEURONS

It is now well documented that sympathetic preganglionic neurons are located in four spinal cord nuclei (see previous sections). However, the functional organization of sympathetic preganglionic neurons and the relationship this may have with the spinal cord anatomy have not been established. For example, it is unknown whether cardiac-related sympathetic preganglionic neurons reside in more than one nucleus. It also remains to be determined if functionally related sympathetic preganglionic cells constitute a single morphologically homogenous class of neurons or whether functionally unrelated sympathetic preganglionic neurons are morphologically distinct. It has been shown, however, that sympathetic preganglionic neurons exhibit considerable structural diversity within and across spinal cord nuclei.

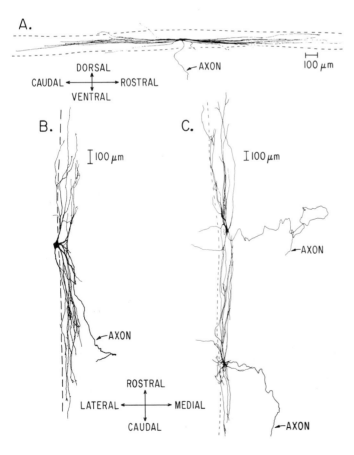

Figure 4-4 Camera lucida drawings of four intracellularly labeled sympathetic preganglionic neurons located in the intermediolateral cell column of the cat. (A) A parasagittal view; (B and C) horizontal views. These examples illustrate the facts that perikaryal shape varies and that the dendrites of many sympathetic preganglionic neurons in the intermediolateral cell column are aligned planarly in the rostrocaudal axis of the spinal cord. The dashed lines demarcate the border between the intermediolateral cell column and the adjacent lateral white matter. (Reproduced with permission from Figures 3 and 4 of Dembowsky et al., 1985a.)

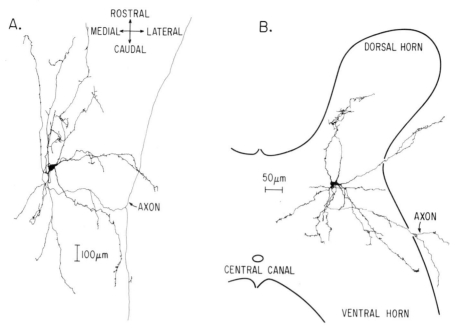

Figure 4-5 Camera lucida drawings of an intracellularly labeled sympathetic preganglionic neuron located within the intercalated nucleus of the pigeon. (A) A horizontal view; (B) a transverse view. The dendritic arbors of intercalated neurons are more radially complex than the dendritic trees of most sympathetic preganglionic neurons located within the intermediolateral cell column. (See Cabot and Bogan, 1987 for more details.)

Sympathetic preganglionic perikarya display at least four distinctly different shapes (Figures 4-4 and 4-5) (Barber et al., 1984; Cabot and Bogan, 1987; Chung et al., 1975; Dembowsky et al., 1985a; Forehand, 1985; Morgan et al., 1986; Nadelhaft and Mc-Kenna, 1987; Oldfield and McLachlan, 1981; Petras and Cummings, 1972). On average, sympathetic preganglionic perikarya are larger than those of most dorsal horn neurons, but significantly smaller (40–50%) than α-motoneuron cell bodies. Somal dimensions vary considerably, with the majority of sympathetic preganglionic neurons being classifed as small to medium sized. Large multipolar cells are less frequently observed, but are present within lateral funicular, intermediolateral, and intercalated nuclei. Major axes diameters vary over a 4-fold range, measuring approximately 15–60 μm; minor axes dimensions are less expansive, varying 3-fold with a range of 10–40 μm. Perikaryal shape, per se, does not specify nuclear location. Somal differentiation appears to be most conspicuous within the intermediolateral cell column.

The surface area of a mature sympathetic preganglionic perikaryon can be conservatively estimated to be less than 15% of the total membrane surface area of the neuron. A direct consequence of this is that any significant differences in the biophysical parameters (e.g., membrane resistance, rheobase) of sympathetic preganglionic neurons are likely to be correlated with differences in total dendritic membrane surface area rather than somal surface area. The importance of defining dendritic orientation, structure, and expanse is reinforced when one considers the fact that sympathetic preganglionic perikarya are postsynaptic to few afferent inputs (see section on Fine Structure of the Sympathetic Preganglionic Neuropil). Consequently, the majority of spatial and temporal summation of incoming information to sympathetic preganglionic neurons is occurring within the dendritic trees. This suggests that any future models of sympathetic preganglionic function will have to incorporate data on dendritic topology as it relates to patterns of afferentation. Within this functional context, the accumulation of morphometric data on sympathetic preganglionic dendritic arborizations becomes important; more so, perhaps, than data on cell body shape and size.

Many sympathetic preganglionic neurons in the intermediolateral cell column have dendritic trees that are oriented principally in the rostrocaudal axis of the spinal cord (Figure 4-4). The longitudinal distances traversed by these dendrites are sizable. The rostrocaudal dendritic trajectory in the adult cat ranges from 1.5 to 2.5 mm (Dembowsky et al., 1985a), in the young rat (9–13 days of age) the spread is approximately 0.6 mm (Forehand, 1985), and in the pigeon, the distances extend 0.5–1.0 mm (Cabot and Bogan, 1986). The longitudinal dendritic extent is greater than, by a factor of 2 or more, the inter-nest cell cluster distances within the intermediolateral cell column. These dendritic arbors are often monoplanar to the extent that their dorsoventral excursions are restricted (<150 μm) (Figure 4-4). This dendritic pattern has long been appreciated and contributes to the "ladder" image as the "side support" (Petras and Cummings, 1972; Rethelyi, 1972). This arrangement has been hypothesized to be a potential structural substrate for dendrodendritic interactions (Dembowsky et al., 1985a).

Some dendrites of sympathetic preganglionic neurons in the intermediolateral cell column project in the mediolateral plane of the spinal cord. Medial projections are most often observed in cells located within the medial aspects of the intermediolateral nucleus. These dendritic branches extend medially into the zona intermedia and overlap laterally directed dendrites that emanate from intercalated cells (Bacon and Smith, 1988; Barber et al., 1984; Baron et al., 1985a,b; Krukoff et al., 1985; Oldfield and McLachlan, 1981). Less frequently, intermediolateral neurons have dendrites that extend into the lateral white matter, or dorsolaterally along the lateral margin of the dorsal horn, or ventrally into the ventral portion of the lateral part of lamina VII (Bacon and Smith, 1988). Within the lumbar spinal cord, a notable shift occurs in preferred dendritic orientation; intermediolateral cells exhibit dominant dendritic extensions in the mediolateral and dorsoventral directions (Baron et al., 1985a; Morgan et al., 1986; Torigoe et al., 1985).

The dendritic patterns of neurons within the intercalated nucleus are significantly different, and more radially complex, than those observed within the intermediolateral cell column (Figure 4-5). The most frequently described dendritic extensions are those that course medially toward the central canal and laterally toward the intermediolateral cell column. This pattern is easily observed in either horizontal or transverse planes of section and contributes to the formation of the "ladder-rung" (e.g., Bacon and Smith, 1988; Barber et al., 1984; Morgan et al., 1986; Nadelhaft and McKenna, 1987; Petras and Faden, 1978). The laterally directed dendrites commingle with medially projecting dendrites that arise from intermediolateral cell column neurons. Medially traveling dendrites sometimes penetrate the central autonomic region; occasionally the dendrites of intercalated neurons extend across the mid-sagittal plane of the spinal cord. Intercalated neurons also have extensive dorsoventral dendritic extensions. These dendrites course obliquely through the transverse plane (Cabot and Bogan, 1987; Forehand, 1985). The dorsally directed dendritic branches end in the base of the dorsal horn, and the ventrally projecting branches terminate in the ventromedial and ventrolateral portions of lamina VII (Cabot and Bogan, 1987; Forehand, 1985).

The dorsal extensions do not, as far as is known, significantly overlap dendritic elements originating from sympathetic preganglionic neurons within other sympathetic preganglionic nuclei. There have been no reported functional correlations; indeed, nothing is known about the physiology of intercalated neurons.

There are no data on the distal dendritic arbors of lateral funicular, central autonomic, and dorsal commissural preganglionic neurons. There are several reports on proximal dendritic orientation. Lateral funicular neurons have dendritic trees that extend in several directions; the most frequently noted projections are those that are oriented rostrocaudally; less frequently, dendrites have been observed to extend medially toward and through the intermediolateral cell column; a few reports indicate that some lateral funicular cells give rise to transversely aligned dendritic processes that project for considerable distances into the dorsolateral white matter (Bacon and Smith, 1988; Barber et al., 1984; Chung et al., 1975; Oldfield and McLachlan, 1981; Petras and Cummings, 1972; Rando et al., 1981). Very little is known about the dendritic structure of central autonomic cells. These neurons are most commonly described as having dendritic arborizations with no particular directional preference (Barber et al., 1984; Dalsguaard and Elfvin, 1981; Oldfield and McLachlan, 1981; Petras and Cummings, 1972; Petras and Faden, 1978). Dorsal commissural cells tend to display prominent mediolateral somatic and dendritic orientations (Hancock and Peveto, 1979; Nadelhaft and McKenna, 1987). As is true for the intercalated neurons, there are no reported structure–function correlations since there are no physiological data on neurons in the lateral funicular, central autonomic, and dorsal commissural nuclei.

CHEMICAL PHENOTYPIC DIFFERENTIATION OF SYMPATHETIC PREGANGLIONIC NEURONS

Sympathetic preganglionic neurons exhibit a cholinergic phenotype. That is, they synthesize acetylcholine and release this neurotransmitter from synaptic terminals in peripheral sympathetic ganglia (e.g., Barber et al., 1984; Cabot and Bogan, 1987; Felberg and Gaddum, 1934). The postsynaptic effects of acetylcholine are complex and involve the activation of both nicotinic and muscarinic receptors in the membrane of postganglionic neurons (see Karczmar et al., 1986 for reviews).

Recent evidence indicates that sympathetic preganglionic neurons also express other neurotransmitter phenotypes. Specifically, vertebrate sympathetic preganglionic cells contain enkephalins, substance P, lutenizing hormone-releasing hormone, neurotensin, and somatostatin (Dalsgaard et al., 1982; Jan and Jan, 1982; Kondo et al., 1985; Krukoff et al., 1985; Warden and Young, 1988). Putative mechanisms of transmitter action on postganglionic cells and/or the presynaptic release from preganglionic axon terminals have been postulated for all but one of these substances; the lone exception is somatostatin (Bachoo et al., 1987; Konishi et al., 1981; see Jones and Adams, 1988; Karczmar et al., 1986 for reviews). Codistribution of more than one of these peptides with acetylcholine has not been established.

It is unknown whether colocalization of putative neurotransmitters within sympathetic preganglionic cells is a general or specific characteristic. The latter is a distinct possibility, however, since in mammals substance P, neurotensin, and enkephalins are found only in a very small percentage of sympathetic preganglionic neurons. This implies indirectly the existence of specialized classes of sympathetic preganglionic neurons. These specialized classes may have unique functional roles. In lower vertebrates this has already been shown to be true. In bullfrog sympathetic ganglia differences in sympathetic preganglionic terminal neurotransmitter contents correlate with connectional specificity (see Jones and Adams, 1988 for review).

This area of research is rapidly expanding, and undoubtedly the list of putative neurotransmitters coexisting with acetylcholine in sympathetic preganglionic neurons will continue to grow. Revisions in the chemical phenotypic classifications of sympathetic preganglionic neurons are likely to be ongoing for some time to come.

FINE STRUCTURE OF THE SYMPATHETIC PREGANGLIONIC NEUROPIL

Relatively little is known about the ultrastructural architecture of sympathetic preganglionic neurons. Solid data on the classes and types of terminal configurations synapsing on their somas and dendritic processes and on the chemical identification of presynaptic terminal contents are just beginning to be consolidated. It is not yet possible, using terminal ultrastructural criteria alone, to predict (1) intraterminal neurotransmitter–neuromodulator contents, (2) relationships with specific membrane-bound receptor-ion channel proteins, or (3) the locations of the cell bodies of origin giving rise to a particular class of bouton.

General Observations

Two basic experimental approaches have been used. The least definitive protocol involves electron microscopic examination of tissue sampled from the lateral horn region of the thoracic spinal cord. Observations have been made in this way in the monkey (Wong and Tan, 1980), cat (Rethelyi, 1972), guinea pig (Chiba and Masuko, 1987), and rat (Chiba and Masuko, 1986; Chiba and Murata, 1981; Hwang and Williams, 1982; Milner et al., 1988; Tan and Wong, 1975). An implicit assumption underlying these investigations is that the lateral horn contains only sympathetic preganglionic cells, their dendrites, and afferent terminations onto these neuronal elements. Recent data suggest that this assumption is not completely justified. For example, studies of the GABAergic innervation of sympathetic preganglionic neurons in the rat reveal that GABAergic perikarya and dendrites are found within the lateral horn (Bogan et al., 1989; see Mugnani and Oertal, 1985 for review).

The second approach has been to study the ultrastructural features of afferent terminations on retrogradely labeled sympathetic preganglionic neurons (cat: Chung et al., 1980; guinea pig: Chiba and Masuko, 1987; rat: Bacon and Smith, 1988; Chiba and Murata, 1981; Hwang and Williams, 1982; Milner et al., 1988; Bogan et al., 1989; and pigeon: Bogan et al., 1989). The principal limitation of this method has been the failure to obtain labeling of distal dendritic branches. Recent experiments using choleratoxin–horseradish peroxidase conjugates or intracellular horseradish peroxidase injections indicate that this obstacle can eventually be surmounted (Bacon and Smith, 1988; Cabot and Bogan, 1987; Dembowsky et al., 1985a; Forehand, 1985; McIlhinney et al., 1988).

Despite the limitations associated with both experimental methods, certain observations have been repeatedly verified. First, sympathetic preganglionic perikarya contain the usual array of intracellular organelles (free ribosomes, Golgi apparatus, mitochondria, lysosomes, etc.), prominent accumulations of rough endoplasmic reticulum are prevalent, and occasionally the nuclear membrane is invaginated. Primary cilia have also been observed within the cell bodies of some sympathetic preganglionic neurons.

Second, the perikaryal surface of sympathetic preganglionic neurons receives few synapses. Regions free of synaptic input are often ensheathed by fibrous astrocytic processes. To date, four classes of axosomatic terminations have been described (Table 4-1).

Third, synaptic input onto proximal sympathetic preganglionic dendrites is dense and, in some cases, may be compartmentalized. Five classes of bouton

Table 4-1 Ultrastructural Characteristics of Synapses on Sympathetic Preganglionic Neurons[a]

Terminal Vesicle Contents	Synaptic Specialization	Terminal Location
Small, round, clear (agranular)	Symmetric	Somal; dendrites
Small, round, clear; one to several dense cores	Symmetric (Gray's type 2)	Somal; large and small dendrites
	Asymmetric (Gray's type 1)	Somal; dendrites
	Asymmetric with Taxi bodies	Dendrites
Flattened or pleomorphic, clear	Symmetric	Somal; dendrites

[a]This tabulation lists the cytological characteristics of terminals synapsing on identified sympathetic preganglionic processes. The table is not a comprehensive catalog of all terminal classes found within the sympathetic preganglionic neuropil. The terminal classes listed have been observed in the monkey, cat, guinea pig, rat, and pigeon. For more specific details see the following papers: Bogan et al. (1989), Chiba and Masuko (1987), Chiba and Murata (1981), Chung et al. (1980), Milner et al. (1988), Rethelyi (1972), and Wong and Tan (1980).

have been found to synapse on sympathetic preganglionic dendrites (Table 4-1). With a single exception, all are similar to axosomatic profiles.

In the monkey and rat intermediolateral neuropil, it has been suggested that synaptic glomeruli are present; that is, the evidence indicates that there are clusters of terminals completely surrounded by astrocytic processes (Milner et al., 1988; Tan and Wong, 1975; Wong and Tan, 1980). The generality of this organizational feature remains to be more fully documented as glomeruli are observed only rarely in the guinea pig intermediolateral cell column (Chiba and Masuko, 1987). Quantitative estimates of the frequency of occurrence of glomerular aggregates or correlations with cellular source(s) of origin are not available.

Identification of Transmitter-Specific Synapses on Sympathetic Preganglionic Neurons

Light microscopic observations reveal that the sympathetic preganglionic neuropil contains more than 20 putative transmitter substances (Table 4-2). An important next step is to establish, using electron microscopic analyses, the relationships between terminal morphology, terminal location, and chemical neurotransmitter. Until relatively recently, most electron microscopic efforts were directed toward determining the synaptic relationships between bulbospinal catecholaminergic inputs and sympathetic preganglionic processes. Several different protocols have been used.

The least specific ultrastructural information on catecholaminergic afferents has been generated

using a method that "loads" synaptic terminals with an osmiophilic marker. This type of terminal labeling has been achieved by pretreating animals with 5-hydroxydopamine (guinea pig: Chiba and Masuko, 1987; rat: Chiba and Masuko, 1986; Chiba and Murata, 1981; Hwang and Williams, 1982). The data gathered in such experiments are difficult to interpret, however, since the labeling that occurs within a bouton does not provide evidence for the presence of a particular catecholamine. A labeled bouton may contain dopamine and/or noradrenaline and/or adrenaline. This is so because 5-hydroxydopamine uptake by synaptic terminals is selective for amine-containing terminals, but not specific for a single amine. The strongest conclusions that can be made are that sympathetic preganglionic perikarya and dendrites receive monosynaptic catecholamine-containing inputs. Both asymmetric and symmetric prepostsynaptic terminal specializations are formed. More direct data on noradrenaline-containing terminals (i.e., exhibiting noradrenaline-like immunoreactivity) within the intermediolateral cell column have been reported, but the postsynaptic elements were not unequivocally identified (guinea pig: Chiba and Masuko, 1987).

The most conclusive work on catecholamine afferentation is that of Milner et al. (1988) (Figure 4-6). Their results indicate that phenylethanolamine N-methyltransferase (PNMT)-containing terminals (therefore, presumably adrenaline-containing) rarely synapse on somas in the adult rat intermediolateral cell column; when an axosomatic contact has been observed, only symmetric specializations are formed. The boutons contain numerous clear, spherical vesicles, and one to several large dense core vesicles. PNMT-containing axodendritic synapses are more prevalent and have vesicular contents iden-

Table 4-2 Neurotransmitter Candidates within the Sympathetic Preganglionic Neuropil[a]

Glutamate	Vasopressin
	Calcitonin gene-related
GABA	peptide
	Corticotropin-releasing
Glycine	factor
Noradrenaline	Somatostatin
Adrenaline	Neurotensin
Dopamine	Galanin
Serotonin	Cholecystokinin
Substance P	Avian pancreatic polypeptide
	Vasoactive intestinal
Enkephalin	polypeptide
Oxytocin	Angiotensin II
Thyrotropin-releasing	Neurophysin
hormone	
Neuropeptide Y	Bombesin

[a]See reviews by Coote (1988), McCall (1988), Loewy and McKellar (1980), Nishi et al. (1987), and Schramm (1986).

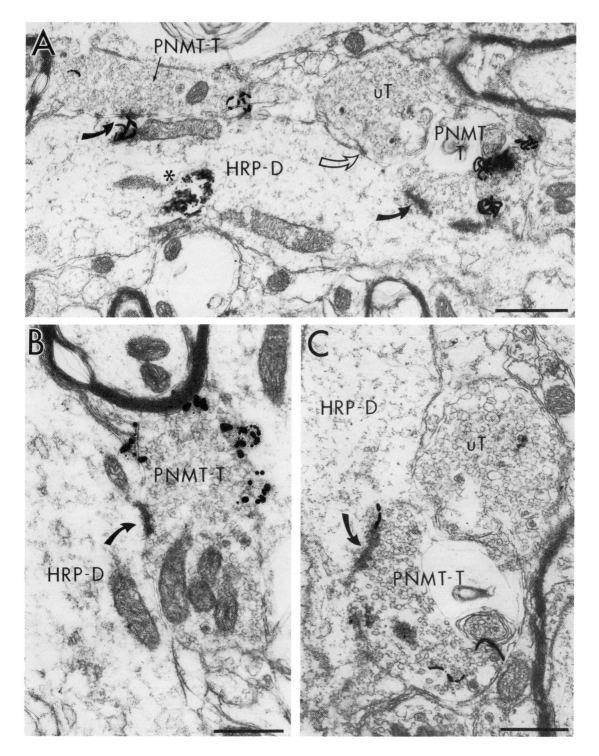

Figure 4-6 Three electron micrographs showing phenylethanolamine *N*-methyltransferase-containing terminals (PNMT-T) synapsing on a horseradish peroxidase labeled (*) sympathetic preganglionic dendrite (HRP-D) in the intermediolateral cell column of the rat. (B and C) Serial sections through the two PNMT-T terminals identified in A. Asymmetric contacts are formed by both terminals. uT, unlabeled terminals. Calibration bar = 0.5 μm. (Reproduced with permission from Figures 7 and 8 of Milner et al., 1988.)

tical to those present on perikarya. A most interesting observation is that the type of axodendritic synaptic specialization differs as a function of the caliber of dendrite contacted. Large proximal sympathetic preganglionic dendrites were contacted by PNMT-containing boutons that formed symmetric specializations, while smaller diameter dendritic elements received inputs that formed an asymmetric synaptic specialization. These data suggest strongly that, within the sympathetic preganglionic neuropil, terminal morphology, per se, may be of marginal value if one desires to use such information to predict neurotransmitter contents.

Ultrastructural observations on other chemically

definable inputs to sympathetic preganglionic neurons have also been reported. Specifically, there are electron microscopic data on GABAergic, serotonergic, substance P, and enkephalinergic inputs to the sympathetic preganglionic neuropil. The GABAergic innervation of sympathetic preganglionic neurons has been studied in the rat and pigeon (Figure 4-7; Bacon and Smith, 1988; Bogan et al., 1989). In both of these vertebrates it was observed that terminals containing GABA-like immunoreactivity (1) synapsed on sympathetic preganglionic perikarya and proximal dendrites in all the spinal cord nuclei, (2) exhibited uniform intraterminal vesicular content (numerous clear, spherical vesicles,

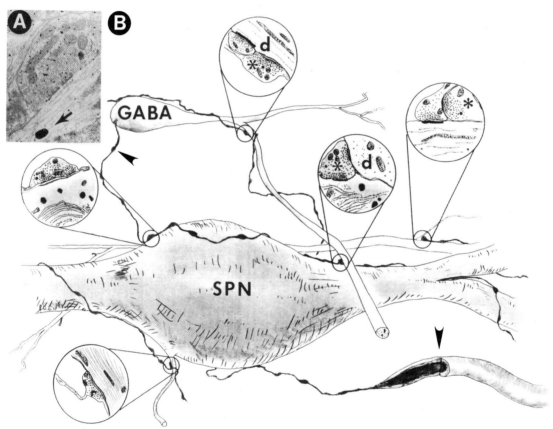

Figure 4-7 The organization of GABAergic processes within the vertebrate sympathetic preganglionic neuropil. (A) Electron micrograph of an immunogold-labeled GABA-like immunoreactive (GABA-LIR) bouton synapsing on a horseradish peroxidase-labeled (HRP, arrow points to an HRP granule) dendrite within the rat nucleus intercalatus. (B) Schematic illustration showing the various morphological arrangements of GABAergic (i.e., GABA-LIR) cells, dendrites, axons, and terminals within the sympathetic preganglionic neuropil of the rat and pigeon. The magnified views depict (beginning in the lower left hand corner and proceeding in a clockwise direction) the following principal observations: (1) GABAergic axon terminals synapse on the initial segment region of some sympathetic preganglionic axons; (2) GABAergic boutons terminate on sympathetic preganglionic somas (SPN); (3) GABAergic dendrites (d) are present within the SPN neuropil and are postsynaptic to GABAergic (*) and non-GABAergic synaptic input; (4) GABAergic boutons (*) synpase on GABA-containing dendrites (d) as well as proximal sympathetic preganglionic dendrites; (5) GABAergic (*) terminals synapse on other non-GABA terminals that in turn are presynaptic to sympathetic preganglionic dendrites; (6) myelinated and unmyelinated GABA-containing axons (arrowheads) enter the sympathetic preganglionic neuropil. GABA terminals contain round, electron-lucent as well as one to several dense core vesicles. GABAergic synaptic contacts are symmetric in configuration. (From Bogan et al., 1989.)

and one to several dense core vesicles), and (3) formed symmetric prepostsynaptic specializations, exclusively. In the rat, there also appears to be another population of GABAergic terminals that contain pleomorphic or flattened vesicles (Bacon and Smith, 1988). Ultrastructural data on serotonergic afferent input to intermediolateral cell column neurons in the rat suggest that this amine is localized within terminals that contact somas as well as dendrites (Bacon and Smith, 1988). Moreover, there are two types of boutons that contain serotonin-like immunoreactivity; one has small vesicles while the other contains a mixture of dense core vesicles and larger clear vesicles (Bacon and Smith, 1988). Substance P-like immunoreactive inputs onto identified and presumed sympathetic preganglionic processes have been observed in the guinea pig (Chiba and Masuko, 1987), rat (Bacon and Smith, 1988), and pigeon (Davis et al., 1988). For this afferent population there may be vertebrate class-specific variation in the types of synaptic specialization. In these vertebrates, however, substance P-like immunoreactive boutons appeared similar and contained small, clear spherical vesicles and a sparse distribution of large dense core vesicles. Enkephalin-like immunoreactive afferent terminals synapse on guinea pig intermediolateral cell somas and dendrites and have intraterminal contents similar to those described for substance P. Enkephalin-like immunoreactive terminals form asymmetric as well as symmetric synaptic specializations (Chiba and Masuko, 1987).

BIOPHYSICAL PROPERTIES OF SYMPATHETIC PREGANGLIONIC NEURONS

Anatomical comparisons of sympathetic preganglionic neurons suggest the presence of significant individual variations. As discussed in the sections that follow, data on the intrinsic biophysical properties of these neurons indicate that, across several dimensions (e.g., axon conduction velocity, input resistance), substantial differences exist within this domain as well. There appears to be enough variability, across morphological and biophysical attributes, that one cannot help but wonder whether the patterning of spinal sympathetic autonomic output might be influenced by a modified form of the "size principle" (see Stuart and Enoka, 1983, for review).

Properties of Sympathetic Preganglionic Axons

There are three well-established properties of sympathetic preganglionic axons that generalize across vertebrate phylogeny.

First, the axons arise from several loci: cell bodies, primary dendrites, and, less frequently, second-order dendrites (cat: Dembowsky et al., 1985a; Rethelyi, 1972; pigeon: Cabot and Bogan, 1987). The biophysical and physiological implications of this arrangement have not been investigated. The finding that some axons originate from dendritic processes raises an interesting query: Are some sympathetic preganglionic neurons biophysically polarized despite the fact that they may otherwise appear to be architecturally symmetrical? (Bras et al., 1987).

Second, some sympathetic preganglionic axons are myelinated and others are unmyelinated (Cabot and Bogan, 1987; Coote and Westbury, 1979b; Dembowsky et al., 1985b, 1986; Fernandez de Molina et al., 1965; Gilbey et al., 1982, 1986; Lebedev, 1972; McLachlan and Hirst, 1980; Nishi et al., 1965; Polosa, 1967; Taylor and Gebber, 1973). Although the absolute or relative percentages of unmyelinated and myelinated axons across vertebrate classes have not been systematically tabulated, available data in cat suggest that in this species approximately 60% of preganglionic axons are myelinated in the white rami (Coggeshall and Galbraith, 1978). However, electron microscopic examination of the splanchnic nerve in cat indicates that this percentage can vary substantially within the same species; the ratio of myelinated to unmyelinated preganglionic fibers is <1 in this peripheral nerve (Kuo et al., 1982). Electrophysiological and anatomical data show that in the rat the majority of preganglionic axons are unmyelinated (Brooks-Fournier and Coggeshall, 1981; Gilbey et al., 1982, 1986). It follows directly that the absence or presence of myelination accounts for the broad range of reported conduction velocities across vertebrate classes: 0.3–15 m/second (see Table 4-4).

The biological significance of the broad spectrum of conduction velocities is something of a mystery: there is a 20- to 30-fold range across vertebrate species, and a 50-fold range across vertebrate classes. Furthermore, preganglionic conduction velocity is not an accurate predictor of peripheral connectivity and, therefore, does not appear to correlate with the activation of specific peripheral autonomic functions (Bahr et al., 1986a–c; Dodd and Horn, 1983; Horn and Stoffer, 1988; Lichtman et al., 1979; Nishi et al., 1965; Nja and Purves, 1977; Robertson, 1987; see Jänig, 1988 for review).

Third, the terminations of sympathetic preganglionic axons are widely divergent (Table 4-3). That is, individual axons branch in the periphery and synapse on many different sympathetic postganglionic neurons. The anatomical evidence for divergence is supported by the facts that (1) there are many more sympathetic postganglionic neurons than sympathetic preganglionic neurons; and (2) all sympathetic postganglionic neurons are innervated (Brooks-

Table 4-3 Divergence and Convergence of Sympathetic Preganglionic Axons

Species	Number of Postganglionic Cells/ Number of Preganglionic Cells (Divergence)	Mean Number of Preganglionic Neurons Innervating One Postganglionic Cell (Convergence)	Neural Unit Size[a]
Mouse[b]	14.2	4.5	64
Hamster	25	7.2	180
Rat	27.2	8.7	237
Guinea pig	26.8	12.3	330
Rabbit	27.2	15.5	422
Monkey[c]			
Squirrel	28 ($n = 1$)[d]		
Macaca	50 ($n = 2$; 41–59[e])		
Stumptail	55 ($n = 2$; 52–57)		
Baboon	62 ($n = 2$; 47–77)		
Chimpanzee	102 ($n = 2$; 87–123)		
Man	122 ($n = 3$; 63–196)		

[a]Neural unit size = divergence × convergence (see Purves et al., 1986).

[b]Data for mouse, hamster, rat, guinea pig, and rabbit reproduced from Tables 1–3 in Purves et al. (1986).

[c]Data for monkey and man are averages of values from Table 1 in Ebbesson (1968).

[d]n = number of animals.

[e]Range of values.

Fournier and Coggeshall, 1981; Ebbesson, 1968; Purves et al., 1986). This simple anatomical relationship tends to obscure the far more relevant physiological issue concerning the precision of the connectivity. The concept of "neural unit size" addresses this problem more directly (Table 4-3; Purves and Wigston, 1983; Purves and Lichtman, 1985; Purves et al., 1986). Neural unit size, by analogy to α-motoneuron–skeletal muscle fiber innervation ratios (motor-unit size; see Burke, 1981 for review), is a calculated prediction of how many sympathetic postganglionic cells are innervated by a single sympathetic preganglionic neuron; to provide the most accurate estimate one must know not only the ratio of postganglionic neurons to preganglionic cells but also the extent of sympathetic preganglionic convergence (Purves and Lichtman, 1985).

Neural unit size calculations have lead to the development of several organizational rules. (1) In all mammals examined to date, including nonhuman primates and man (Ebbesson, 1968), neural unit size has a value greater than 1. (2) In scaling the phylogenetic hierarchy from mouse to rabbit, neural unit size increases approximately 7-fold, from 64 to 422, but not as a linear function of body mass. (3) Increases in neural unit size are not solely a consequence of absolute increases in the ratios of the numbers of postganglionic neurons to the numbers of preganglionic neurons. (4) That is, increases in neural unit size across phylogeny also reflect the fact that sympathetic postganglionic neurons receive more sympathetic preganglionic axonal input: there is a significant increase in convergence (Purves and Lichtman, 1985). It is important to understand that these rules do not address whether the peripheral

convergence and divergence of sympathetic preganglionic output are physiologically defined processes. For example, we do not know if postganglionic vasoconstrictor neurons are innervated exclusively by sympathetic preganglionic axons whose collateral branches terminate exclusively on other vasoconstrictor postganglionic neurons.

There are two additional characteristics of sympathetic preganglionic axons that merit mention. First, some sympathetic preganglionic axons increase significantly the velocity at which they conduct action potentials. This occurs as the axons exit the central nervous system and proceed toward their sympathetic postganglionic cell targets. In fact, the conduction velocity of sympathetic preganglionic axons, when measured in the periphery (e.g., in the white rami), can exceed intraspinal conduction velocity by as much as 80% (Lebedev, 1972; Yoshimura et al., 1986a). The precise physiological importance of this remains unclear. The anatomical substrate, however, may be increased myelination within the spinal cord. This has recently been shown to occur in an electron microscopic study of preganglionic axons in the pigeon spinal cord (Bogan and Cabot, 1985). Second, some sympathetic preganglionic axons branch within the spinal cord (Figure 4-5; Bogan and Cabot, 1985; Cabot and Bogan, 1987; Forehand, 1985). The presence or absence of intraspinal axon collaterals has been the subject of a long-standing debate (Dembowsky et al., 1985a; Rethelyi, 1972). Past failures to anatomically demonstrate intraspinal axon branching are likely due to technical limitations in combination with the fact that collateralization probably occurs only within a restricted subset of sympathetic preganglionic neurons. Physiological observations have long predicted the presence of collaterals and, indeed, they are proposed to be integrally involved in recurrent inhibitory phenomena (deGroat, 1976; Lebedev, 1980; McKenna and Schramm, 1985; see Barman, 1984; Coote, 1988; Polosa et al., 1982; Schramm, 1986 for reviews). Although this hypothesis may ultimately prove to be true, there is at least one type of spinal circuit that is not involved. Intracellular recordings have repeatedly failed to show the presence of inhibitory postsynaptic potentials impinging on sympathetic preganglionic neurons after orthodromic or antidromic activation (Coote and Westbury, 1979a; Dembowsky et al., 1985b; Ma and Dun, 1986; McLachlan and Hirst, 1980; Yoshimura et al., 1986a). Thus, sympathetic preganglionic axon collaterals are probably not involved in the activation of a recurrent inhibitory pathway analogous to the inhibitory feedback circuit activated by α-motoneuron axon collaterals (for a discussion of Renshaw cell inhibition of α-motoneurons see Burke and Rudomin, 1977). Recurrent disfacilitatory mechanisms (e.g., presynaptic inhibition of excitatory inputs) have not been excluded as alternative explanations of existing data. The confounding irony is that the morphological findings fail to resolve the physiological issues, except insofar as it appears certain that recurrent collaterals, when present, do not contact any somatic or dendritic processes belonging to the sympathetic preganglionic cell of origin.

Properties of Sympathetic Preganglionic Neuron Action Potential Generation

Levels of Activity

In all vertebrates studied, a remarkably consistent observation has been that sympathetic preganglionic neurons exhibit, *in vivo,* low levels of maintained activity. The reported mean discharge rates range typically from less than 1 Hz to no greater than 4 Hz (Backman and Henry, 1984; Bahr et al., 1986c; Bartel et al., 1986; Coote and Westbury, 1979b; Jänig and Szulczyk, 1980; Gilbey et al., 1982; Guyenet and Cabot, 1981; for reviews, see Jänig, 1988; Polosa et al., 1979, 1982). Moreover, most sympathetic preganglionic neurons recorded extracellularly or intracellularly in anesthetized or unanesthetized decerebrate preparations, are silent; that is, no action potential activity is observed. Why this is so and its potential physiological relevance are matters for speculation (for reviews, see Polosa et al., 1982; Jänig, 1988). On the basis of intracellular data, however, it now seems very clear that such behavior is not indicative of total quiescence; silent neurons are continuously being bombarded by subthreshold excitatory and, to a lesser extent, inhibitory synaptic input (Dembowsky et al., 1985b; McLachlan and Hirst, 1980).

A second, well-conserved physiological property of sympathetic preganglionic neuronal discharge activity is that these neurons do not show sustained, high-frequency patterns of action potential generation when appropriately activated by electrical or physiological stimuli (somatic, visceral, baroreceptor, and/or brainstem systems) that are known to elicit excitatory changes in sympathetic outflow. In fact, instantaneous frequency within such evoked bursts of activity rarely exceeds 20 Hz. The physiological mechanisms responsible for this behavior are incompletely understood, but it appears that intrinsic membrane properties contribute to (see below), but do not entirely account for, the observed rate-limiting discharge behavior (Dembowsky et al., 1985b; Yoshimura et al., 1986a,b, 1987). Indeed, intracellularly applied depolarizing current pulses cause sympathetic preganglionic neurons to fire action potentials at initial instantaneous rates approaching 100 Hz; sympathetic preganglionic neurons soon accommodate to this artificial stimulus, but rates of 70–80 Hz can be sustained. When one considers the weight of all of the evidence, the low levels of preganglionic neuron discharge activity, *in vivo,* appear to be a direct result of the integration of excitatory and inhibitory postsynaptic events, and not a consequence of intrinsic membrane property constraints.

Membrane Properties

The rising phase of the action potential, whether recorded extracellularly or intracellularly, frequently displays a notable inflexion that reflects depolarization of the axon initial segment (IS) (Figure 4-8). Somadendritic (SD) depolarization accounts for the remaining upstroke in potential, which typically has an overshoot of 10–20 mV (i.e., mV above 0 relative to a resting potential of approximately −60). Depolarization events are due to an increase in membrane permeability to Na^+ (increase in membrane conductance, g_{Na+}).

Repolarization (downstroke or falling phase) of the action potential is a more complex series of events involving (1) increases in membrane permeability to both K^+ (classic delayed rectifier; see Rudy, 1988 for review) and Ca^{2+} ions; and (2) a decrease in permeability to Na^+. The most noteworthy, visually discernible, feature is the presence of a distinctive hump on the falling phase that reflects the slowing of the rate of repolarization (see dV/dt in Figure 1 of Dembowsky et al., 1986). This is a result of the membrane depolarizing effects caused by inward movement of extracellular Ca^{2+} ions to the sympathetic preganglionic neuronal intracellular space (Yoshimura et al., 1986a). Were it not for this

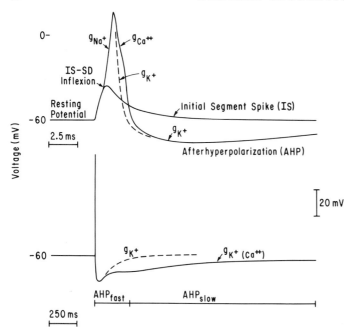

Figure 4-8 Schematic illustration showing a typical action potential of a sympathetic preganglionic neuron located within the intermediolateral cell column. The established changes in ion permeabilities associated with the various phases of the action potential are also indicated. See text for further details.

increase in Ca^{2+} permeability, the action potential would repolarize more rapidly and lack the hump (Figure 4-8, dotted line). The resultant splaying leads to an action potential duration (excluding the afterhyperpolarization phase) which is relatively long, with reported mean values ranging from 3.0 to 4.9 msec in cat (Table 4-4).

The action potential after-hyperpolarization phase (i.e., period of repolarization when the membrane potential is more negative than the resting potential) is of long duration (Yoshimura et al., 1986b; see Polosa et al., 1988 for review). The best estimates of afterhyperpolarization duration in adult sympathetic preganglionic neurons have been obtained in a cat *in vitro* preparation (Yoshimura et al., 1986a,b; Table 4-4); total mean duration is $2,800 \pm 300$ msec. This is substantially longer, on average, than values reported *in vivo* (e.g., 678 ± 8.4 msec, range 50–4,260 msec; Table 4-4). The shorter duration, *in vivo*, may partially reflect current shunting effects due to ever-present changes in membrane permeability resulting from incoming excitatory synaptic input; or perhaps be partially artifactual because of current shunting due to microelectrode impalement-induced damage (Dembowsky et al., 1985b; see Polosa et al., 1988 for review).

There are two other significant characteristics of the afterhyperpolarization phase that are likely to be integrally involved in the regulation of sympathetic preganglionic neuron firing rate, spike frequency adaptation, and burst termination (see Table 1 in Rudy, 1988, for a description of K^+ channels and their functions). First, successive periods of afterhyperpolarization summate temporally (Yoshimura et

al., 1986a; see Polosa et al., 1988 for review). It follows directly that as summation proceeds, neuronal refractory period (absolute and/or relative times of inexcitability) becomes increasingly long and, concomitantly, instantaneous firing frequency decreases; this may ultimately contribute to a silent or postexcitatory depression period of discharge (McKenna and Schramm, 1985; Polosa, 1967; see Polosa et al., 1982 for review). Second, there is not just one phase of afterhyperpolarization, but at least two. In both phases, changes in K^+ permeability are ongoing, but different mechanisms are invoked.

There is an initial fast afterhyperpolarization phase (AHP$_{fast}$; Figure 4-8) that lasts approximately 300 msec (range 150–600 msec). During this time, voltage-dependent, delayed rectifier K^+ channels remain open. K^+ continues to flow out of the sympathetic preganglionic neuron, driving the membrane to levels more negative than the resting potential and toward the K^+ equilibrium potential (approximately -90 mV). The relatively slow repolarization rate of AHP$_{fast}$ back toward the resting potential is the result of the slow inactivation of these delayed rectifier channels. However, the duration of AHP$_{fast}$ is frequently more prolonged than can be accounted for by the inactivation of delayed rectifier channels; consequently there may be a separate increase in K^+ permeability that is due to the activation of a fast, voltage-dependent, rapidly inactivating K^+ current, the so-called "A" current (see Rudy, 1988 for review). The presence of this "A" current requires further confirmation and still is considered speculative (Dembowsky et al., 1986; Yoshimura et al., 1986b, 1987; see Polosa et al., 1988 for review). The second

Table 4-4 Electrophysiological and Biophysical Properties of Sympathetic Preganglionic Neurons

Property	Mean ± SD or SEM (Range)
Axonal conduction velocity (m/sec)	
Cat[a]	(0.6–15)
Rat[b]	0.2–3.3)
Bird[c]	(0.3–5.6)
Frog[d]	(0.4–2.4)
Resting potential (mV)	
Cat, in vitro [e]	−61.3 ± 1.6 (−50 to −68)
Cat, in vivo [f]	−59.7 ± 6.9[g] (−40 to −86)
Rat, in vitro[h]	−58.0 ± 7 (−40 to −75)
Input resistance (MΩ)	
Cat, in vitro	67.5 ± 3.7 (31–117)
Cat, in vivo	23.7 ± 5.0[g] (12–50)
Rat, in vitro	110 ± 34 (45–280)
Membrane time constant (msec)	
Cat, in vitro	11.5 ± 1.2 (7–20)
Cat, in vivo	(4–26)
Rat, in vitro	8.9 ± 2.7
Action potential amplitude (mV)	
Cat, in vitro	77.4 ± 2.3
Cat, in vivo	85.9 ± 6.4[g] (70–107)
Rat, in vitro	59 ± 11 (40–85)
Action potential duration (msec)	
Cat, in vitro	3.03 ± 0.16
Cat, in vivo	4.85 ± 0.05[i] (3–15)
Rat, in vitro	2.20 ± 0.8 (1.2–5)
Afterhyperpolarization amplitude (mV)	
Cat, in vitro	16.6 ± 0.7
Cat, in vivo	9.03 ± 0.94[g] (3–17)
Rat, in vitro	5.8 ± 2.4
Afterhyperpolarization duration (msec)	
Cat, in vitro	2800 ± 300 (AHP$_{fast}$, 330, range 150–600)
Cat, in vivo	678 ± 298[g] (50–4260)
Rat, in vitro	59 ± 16.8

[a]Backman and Henry (1984), Bahr et al. (1986c), Coote and Westbury (1979b), Dembowsky et al. (1986), Fernandez de Molina et al. (1965), Hongo and Rall (1966), Jänig (1988), McLachlan and Hirst (1980), Polosa (1967), Taylor and Gebber (1973), and Yoshimura et al. (1986a).
[b]Gilbey et al. (1982), Gilbey et al. (1986), and McKenna and Schramm (1983, 1985).
[c]Cabot and Bogan (1987).
[d]Dodd and Horn (1983) and Nishi et al. (1965).
[e]Yoshimura et al. (1986a).
[f]Coote and Westbury (1979a), Dembowsky et al. (1986), and McLachlan and Hirst (1980).
[g]Average of Type A, B, and C neurons in Dembowsky et al. (1986).
[h]Dun and Mo (1988) and Ma and Dun (1985, 1986).
[i]Average of Type A and C neurons in Dembowsky et al. (1986).

well-defined phase, AHP$_{slow}$, is very long in duration (>2 seconds) and is the result of an increase in K$^+$ permeability that is dependent on Ca^{2+} entry from the extracellular environment (Ca^{2+}-activated, K$^+$ channel opening).

At this time it is a matter of pure conjecture whether all, or most, or just some sympathetic preganglionic neurons share membrane and action potential properties identical to those described above. Indeed, the in vivo work of Dembowsky et al. (1986) suggests that variations are discernible if one considers an ensemble of properties: resting membrane potential, input resistance, resting discharge activity, and shapes of upstroke and repolarization phases of

the action potential. Considerably more information will have to be accumulated, however, to warrant acceptance that actual differences in biophysical properties across the population of sympathetic preganglionic neurons are physiologically relevant.

Nevertheless, this possibility should probably not be summarily dismissed. Repeated measurements, both in vivo and in vitro, of the input resistance of sympathetic preganglionic neurons have consistently demonstrated wide-ranging variability: cat, 12–117 MΩ; rat, 45–280 MΩ (Table 4-4). Interestingly, this variable is well established as being a relatively sensitive (albeit indirect) barometer of cell size (cell membrane surface area; see Rall, 1977 for review). The within-species range of values is not easily explained as being exclusively due to experimentally induced artifact; moreover, the spreads are sizable (6- to 10-fold) and, accordingly, may be indicative of significant differences. By comparison, a 4-fold difference in input resistance is sufficient to help differentiate between α-motoneurons innervating fast contracting, highly fatigable muscle fibers from those innervating slow contracting, slowly fatigable muscle fibers (see Stuart and Enoka, 1983 for review). The reported across-species differences in preganglionic input resistance (cat vs. rat) indirectly lends further credence to the "size" argument; it is conceivable that the significantly higher observed values in rat reflect the fact that immature preganglionic neurons (*in vitro* data gathered in 8- to 15-day-old animals) have not completely expressed their adult dendritic arbor and thus are smaller (less total membrane surface area) (Bernstein-Goral and Bohn, 1988; Schramm et al., 1976). Smaller cells characteristically have higher input resistances.

SUMMARY

The peripheral expression of patterned, autonomic responses remains an undefined, complex function of preceding alterations in the neuronal discharge of functionally related, spatially dispersed populations of sympathetic preganglionic neurons. The physiological specificity that is reflected in the final common pathway output must be correlated, at least in part, with the morphological, neurochemical, and biophysical properties of sympathetic preganglionic cells and their inputs.

Sympathetic preganglionic neurons are located in four nuclei throughout the thoracic and upper lumbar spinal cord. The nuclear divisions separate sympathetic preganglionic neurons into lateral funicular, intermediolateral, intercalated, and central autonomic cell populations. The functional sequelae of the spinal nuclear subdivision of sympathetic preganglionic neurons have not been determined. Independent of the spinal nuclear organization, sympathetic preganglionic neurons are segmentally organized. This arrangement provides the anatomical substrate for a more general rostrocaudal functional topography. For example, sympathetic preganglionic neurons affecting the sympathetic outflow to the head and neck are located in the upper thoracic spinal cord segments, whereas those affecting changes in the hindlimb are located within lumbar spinal cord segments.

Sympathetic preganglionic neurons have several different somal shapes and give rise to simple as well as complex dendritic trees. Differences in perikaryal shape are most conspicuous in the intermediolateral

cell column. Somal shape does not predict nuclear locus. Simple dendritic arbors are characteristic of many neurons within the intermediolateral cell column. The dendritic extensions of intermediolateral cell column neurons are frequently restricted to a narrow plane of section within the horizontal axis of the spinal cord. More complex, dorsoventrally directed, dendritic arbors single out neurons within the intercalated nucleus. It remains to be determined whether differential dendritic patterns provide an adequate anatomical substrate for exclusive patterns of afferentation.

Sympathetic preganglionic neurons are cholinergic cells. That is, they synthesize and release the neurotransmitter acetylcholine. Some sympathetic preganglionic neurons express at least one additional chemical phenotype. In particular, subpopulations of sympathetic preganglionic neurons contain the putative neurotransmitters substance P, neurotensin, somatostatin, enkephalin, or luteinizing hormone-releasing hormone. Colocalization of more than one of these neurotransmitters with acetylcholine has not yet been established. It is likely that chemical differentiation of sympathetic preganglionic neurons has significant functional consequences.

Ultrastructural data on the location, cytological features, and chemical identity of afferent inputs to sympathetic preganglionic neurons are elementary. Synapses on sympathetic preganglionic neurons that contain adrenaline, GABA, serotonin, enkephalin, and substance P have been identified. In general, it appears that ultrastructural criteria, in the absence of other types of data, have little or no discriminative value.

Anatomical diversification of sympathetic preganglionic neuronal organization is paralleled by interneuronal differences in the neurophysiological and biophysical properties of these neurons. For example: (1) The axonal conduction velocity of sympathetic preganglionic neurons varies over a 50-fold range; this property correlates with the fact that some sympathetic preganglionic axons are myelinated and others are not. (2) Few sympathetic preganglionic neurons exhibit low levels of maintained activity; the majority are silent. (3) Some sympathetic preganglionic neurons have low input resistances and others have very high input resistances. (4) Single sympathetic preganglionic neurons only rarely generate a burst of action potentials that has an instantaneous frequency greater than 20 Hz. This rate-limiting behavior is not a direct consequence of intrinsic membrane property constraints. Rather, the temporal regulation of evoked discharge activity is significantly modulated by the duration of the early and late after-hyperpolarization phases of the action potential. The temporal regulation of after-hyperpolarization duration is determined by the efficacy of the activation of multiple K^+ channels.

It is certain that sympathetic preganglionic neurons are not a homogeneous population of spinal neurons. One clear challenge for the future is to try to understand the significance of this fact by establishing correlative relationships between anatomical, physiological, and biophysical parameters.

ACKNOWLEDGMENTS

The author thanks N. Bogan for his photographic and creative contributions. J. B. C. is an Established Investigator of the American Heart Association and is supported in part by grant HL24103 from the National Heart, Lung and Blood Institute.

REFERENCES

Reviews

Armour, J. A., and Hopkins, D. A. (1984). Anatomy of the extrinsic efferent autonomic nerves and ganglia innervating the mammalian heart. In: *Nervous Control of Cardiovascular Function,* W. C. Randall (ed.), Oxford University Press, New York, pp. 21–45.

Barman, S. M. (1984). Spinal cord control of the cardiovascular system. In: *Nervous Control of Cardiovascular Function,* W. C. Randall (ed.), Oxford University Press, New York, pp. 321–345.

Burke, R. E. (1981). Motor units: Anatomy, physiology, and functional organization. In: *Handbook of Physiology, Section 1: The Nervous System,* V. Brooks (ed.), American Physiological Society, Bethesda, MD, pp. 325–343.

Burke, R. E., and Rudomin, P. (1977). Spinal neurons and synapses. In: *Handbook of Physiology, Section 1: The Nervous System,* J. M. Brookhart and V. B. Mountcastle (eds.) American Physiological Society, Bethesda, MD., pp. 877–944.

Cannon, W. B. (1939). *The Wisdom of the Body,* 2nd ed. Norton, New York.

Coote, J. H. (1988). The organisation of cardiovascular neurons in the spinal cord. *Reviews of Physiology, Biochemistry and Pharmacology* 110, 148–285.

Heymans, C., and Neil, E. (1958). *Reflexogenic Areas of the Cardiovascular System.* Churchill, London.

Jänig, W. (1985). Organization of the lumbar sympathetic outflow to skeletal muscle and skin of the hindlimb and tail. *Reviews of Physiology, Biochemistry and Pharmacology* 102, 119–213.

Jänig, W. (1988). Pre- and postganglionic vasoconstrictor neurons: Differentiation, types and discharge properties. *Annual Review of Physiology* 50, 525–539.

Jones, S. W., and Adams, P. R. (1988). Peptides and slow synaptic potentials. In: *Molecular Neurobiology: Endocrine Approaches,* J. F. Strauss and D. W. Pfaff (eds.), Academic Press, New York.

Karczmar, A. G., Koketsu, K., and Nishi, S. (1986). *Autonomic and Enteric Ganglia. Transmission and Its Pharmacology.* Plenum, New York.

Kircheim, H. R. (1976). Systemic arterial baroreceptor reflexes. *Physiological Reviews* 56, 100–176.

Laskey, W., and Polosa, C. (1988). Characteristics of the sympathetic preganglionic neuron and its synaptic input. *Progress in Neurobiology* 31, 47–84.

Loewy, A. D., and McKellar, S. (1980). The neuroanatomical basis of central cardiovascular control. *Federation Proceedings* 39, 2495–2503.

Mathias, C. J., and Frankel, H. L. (1988). Cardiovascular control in spinal man. *Annual Review of Physiology* 50, 577–592.

McCall, R. B. (1988). Effects of putative neurotransmitters on sympathetic preganglionic neurons. *Annual Review of Physiology* 50, 553–564.

Mugnani, E., and Oertel, W. H. (1985). An atlas of the distribution of GABAergic neurons and terminals in the rat CNS as revealed by GAD immunohistochemistry. In: *Handbook of Chemical Neuroanatomy, Volume 4, GABA and Neuropeptides in the CNS, Part I,* A. Björklund and T. Hökfelt (eds.), Elsevier, New York, pp. 436–608.

Nishi, S., Yoshimura, M., and Polosa, C. (1987). Synaptic potentials and putative transmitter actions in sympathetic preganglionic neurons. In: *Organization of the Autonomic Nervous System: Central and Peripheral Mechanisms,* J. Ciriello, F. R. Calaresu, L. P. Renaud, and C. Polosa (eds.), Liss, New York, pp. 15–26.

Pick, J. (1970). *The Autonomic Nervous System.* Lippincott, Philadelphia.

Polosa, C., Mannard, A., and Laskey, W. (1979). Tonic activity of the autonomic nervous system: Functions, properties, origins. In: *Integrative Functions of the Autonomic Nervous System,* C. McC. Brooks, K. Koizumi, and A. Sato (eds.), University of Tokyo Press, Elsevier, New York, pp. 342–354.

Polosa, C., Schondorf, R., and Laskey, W. (1982). Stabilization of the discharge rate of sympathetic preganglionic neurons. *Journal of the Autonomic Nervous System* 5, 45–54.

Polosa, C., Yoshimura, M., and Nishi, S. (1988). Electrophysiological properties of sympathetic preganglionic neurons. *Annual Review of Physiology* 50, 541–551.

Purves, D., and Lichtman, J. W. (1985). *Principles of Neural Development.* Sinauer Associates, Sunderland, MA.

Rall, W. (1977). Core conductor theory and cable properties of neurons. In: *Handbook of Physiology, Section 1: The Nervous System,* J. M. Brookhart and V. B. Mountcastle (eds.), American Physiological Society, Bethesda, MD, pp. 39–97.

Randall, W. C. (1984). Selective autonomic innervation of the heart. In: *Nervous Control of Cardiovascular Function.* W. C. Randall (ed.), Oxford University Press, New York, pp. 46–67.

Rudy, B. (1988). Diversity and ubiquity of K channels. *Neuroscience* 25, 729–749.

Schramm, L. P. (1986). Spinal factors in sympathetic regulation. In: *Central and Peripheral Mechanisms of Cardiovascular Regulation,* A. Mafro, W. Osswald, D. Reis, and P. Vanhoutte (eds.), Plenum, New York, pp. 303–352.

Schwartz, P. J. (1984). Sympathetic imbalance and cardiac arrhythmias. In: *Nervous Control of Cardiovascular Function,* W. C. Randall, (ed.), Oxford University Press, New York, pp. 225–252.

Stuart, D. G., and Enoka, R. M. (1983). Motoneurons, motor units, and the size principle. In: *The Clinical Neurosciences, Neurobiology, Volume 5,* W. D. Willis (ed.), Churchill Livingstone, New York, pp. 471–517.

Research Articles

Appel, N. M., and Elde, R. P. (1988). The intermediolateral cell column of the thoracic spinal cord is comprised of target-specific subnuclei: Evidence from retrograde transport studies and immunohistochemistry. *Journal of Neuroscience* 8, 1767–1775.

Bachoo, M., Ciriello, J., and Polosa, C. (1987). Effect of preganglionic stimulation on neuropeptide-like immunoreactivity in the stellate ganglion of the cat. *Brain Research* 400, 377–382.

Backman, S. B., and Henry, J. L. (1984). Physiological properties of sympathetic preganglionic neurones in the thoracic intermediolateral nucleus of the cat. *Canadian Journal of Physiology and Pharmacology* 62, 1183–1193.

Bacon, S. J., and Smith, A. D. (1988). Preganglionic sympathetic neurones innervating the rat adrenal medulla: immunocytochemical evidence of synaptic input from nerve terminals containing substance P, GABA, or 5-hydroxytryptamine, *Journal of the Autonomic Nervous System* 24, 97–122.

Bahr, R., Bartel, B., Blumberg, H., and Jänig, W. (1986a). Functional characterization of preganglionic neurons projecting in the lumbar splanchnic nerves: neurons regulating motility. *Journal of the Autonomic Nervous System* 15, 109–130.

Bahr, R., Bartel, B., Blumberg, H., and Jänig, W. (1986b). Functional characterization of preganglionic neurons projecting in the lumbar splanchnic nerves: vasoconstrictor neurons. *Journal of the Autonomic Nervous System* 15, 131–140.

Bahr, R., Bartel, B., Blumberg, H., and Jänig, W. (1986c). Secondary functional properties of lumbar visceral preganglionic neurons. *Journal of the Autonomic Nervous System* 15, 141–152.

Barber, R. P., Phelps, P. E., Houser, C. R., Crawford, G. D., Salvaterra, P. M., and Vaughn, J. E. (1984). The morphology and distribution of neurons containing choline acetyltransferase in the adult rat spinal cord: An immunocytochemical study. *Journal of Comparative Neurology* 229, 329–346.

Baron, R., Jänig, W., and McLachlan, E. M. (1985a). The afferent and sympathetic components of the lumbar spinal outflow to the colon and pelvic organs in the cat. I. The hypogastric nerve. *Journal of Comparative Neurology* 238, 135–146.

Baron, R., Jänig, W., and McLachlan, E. M. (1985b). The afferent and sympathetic components of the lumbar spinal outflow to the colon and pelvic organs in the cat. II. The lumbar splanchnic nerves. *Journal of Comparative Neurology* 238, 147–157.

Baron, R., Jänig, W., and McLachlan, E. M. (1985c). The afferent and sympathetic components of the lumbar spinal outflow to the colon and pelvic organs in the cat. III. The colonic nerves, incorporating an analysis of all components of the lumbar prevertebral outflow. *Journal of Comparative Neurology* 238, 158–168.

Bartel, B., Blumberg, H., and Jänig, W. (1986). Discharge patterns of motility-regulating neurons projecting in the lumbar splanchnic nerves to visceral stimuli in spinal cats. *Journal of the Autonomic Nervous System* 15, 153–163.

Bernstein-Goral, H., and Bohn, M. C. (1988). Ontogeny of adrenergic fibers in rat spinal cord in relationship to adrenal preganglionic neurons. *Journal of Neuroscience Research* 21, 333–351.

Bogan, N., and Cabot, J. B. (1985). Light and electron microscopic observations on axon collaterals of sympathetic preganglionic neurons. *Neuroscience Abstracts* 11, 35.

Bogan, N., Mennone, A., and Cabot, J. B. (1989). Light microscopic and ultrastructural localization of GABA-like immunoreactive input to retrogradely labeled sympathetic preganglionic neurons. *Brain Research* 505, 257–270.

Bras, H., Gogan, P., and Tyc-Dumont, S. (1987). The dendrites of single brain-stem motoneurons intracellularly labelled with horseradish peroxidase in the cat. Morphological and electrical differences. *Neuroscience* 22, 947–970.

Brooks-Fournier, R., and Coggeshall, R. E. (1981). The ratio of preganglionic axons to postganglionic cells in the sympathetic nervous system of the rat. *Journal of Comparative Neurology* 197, 207–216.

Burke, R. E., Dun, R. P., Fleshman, J. W., Glenn, L. L., Lev-Tov, A., O'Donovan, M. J., and Pinter, M. J. (1982). An HRP study of the relation between cell size and motor unit type in cat ankle extensor motoneurons. *Journal of Comparative Neurology* 209, 17–28.

Cabot, J. B., and Bogan, N. (1987). Light microscopic observations on the morphology of sympathetic preganglionic neurons in the pigeon, *Columba livia. Neuroscience* 20, 467–486.

Cameron, W. D., Averill, D. B., and Berger, A. J. (1983). Morphology of cat phrenic motoneurons as revealed by intracellular injection of horseradish peroxidase. *Journal of Comparative Neurology* 219, 70–80.

Cameron, W. D., Averill, D. B., and Berger, A. J. (1985). Quantitative analysis of the dendrites of cat phrenic motoneurons stained intracellularly with horseradish peroxidase. *Journal of Comparative Neurology* 230, 91–101.

Chiba, T., and Masuko, S. (1986). Direct contacts of catecholamine axons on the preganglionic sympathetic neurons in the rat thoracic spinal cord. *Brain Research* 380, 405–408.

Chiba, T., and Masuko, S. (1987). Synaptic structure of the monoamine and peptide nerve terminals in the intermediolateral nucleus of the guinea pig thoracic spinal cord. *Journal of Comparative Neurology,* 262, 242–255.

Chiba, T., and Murata, Y. (1981). Architecture and synaptic relationships in the intermediolateral nucleus of the thoracic spinal cord of the rat: HRP labelling, catecholamine histochemistry and electron microscopic studies. *Journal of Neurocytology* 10, 315–329.

Chung, J. M., Chung, K., and Wurster, R. D. (1975). Sympathetic preganglionic neurons of the cat spinal cord: Horseradish peroxidase study. *Brain Research* 91, 126–131.

Chung, K., Chung, J. M., LaVelle, F. W., and Wurster, R. D. (1979). Sympathetic neurons in the cat spinal cord projecting to the stellate ganglion. *Journal of Comparative Neurology* 185, 23–29.

Chung, K., LaVelle, F. W., and Wurster, R. D. (1980). Ultrastructure of HRP-identified sympathetic preganglionic neurons in cats. *Journal of Comparative Neurology* 190, 147–155.

Coggeshall, R. E., and Galbraith, S. L. (1978). Categories of axons in mammalian rami communicantes, Part II. *Journal of Comparative Neurology* 181, 349–359.

Coote, J. H., and Westbury, D. R. (1979a). Intracellular recordings from sympathetic preganglionic neurones. *Neuroscience Letters* 15, 171–175.

Coote, J. H., and Westbury, D. R. (1979b). Functional grouping of sympathetic preganglionic neurons. *Brain Research* 179, 367–372.

Cummings, J. F. (1969). Thoracolumbar preganglionic neurons and adrenal innervation in the dog. *Acta Anatomica* 73, 27–37.

Cullheim, S., Fleshman, J. W., Glenn, L. L., and Burke, R. E. (1987a). Membrane area and dendritic structure in type-identified triceps surae alpha motoneurons. *Journal of Comparative Neurology* 255, 68–81.

Cullheim, S., Fleshman, J. W., Glenn, L. L., and Burke, R. E. (1987b). Three-dimensional architecture of dendritic tree in type identified α-motoneurons. *Journal of Comparative Neurology* 255, 82–96.

Dalsgaard, C.-J., and Elfvin, L.-G. (1979). Spinal origin of preganglionic fibers projecting onto the superior cervical ganglion and inferior mesenteric ganglion of the guinea pig, as demonstrated by the horseradish peroxidase technique. *Brain Research* 172, 139–143.

Dalsgaard, C.-J., and Elfvin, L.-G. (1981). The distribution of the sympathetic preganglionic neurons projecting onto the stellate ganglion of the guinea pig. A horseradish peroxidase study. *Journal of the Autonomic Nervous System* 4, 327–337.

Dalsgaard, C.-J., Hokfelt, T., Elfvin, L.-G., and Terenius, L. (1982). Enkephalin-containing sympathetic preganglionic neurons projecting to the inferior mesenteric ganglion: Evidence from combined retrograde tracing and immunohistochemistry. *Neuroscience* 7, 2039–2050.

Davis, B. M., Krause, J. E., McKelvy, J. F., and Cabot, J. B. (1984). Effects of spinal lesions on substance P levels in the rat sympathetic preganglionic cell column: Evidence for local spinal regulation. *Neuroscience* 13, 1311–1326.

Davis, B. M., Krause, J. E., Bogan, N., and Cabot, J. B. (1988). Intraspinal substance P containing projections to the sympathetic preganglionic neuropil in pigeon, *Columba livia:* HPLC, radioimmunoassay and electron microscopic evidence. *Neuroscience* 26, 655–668.

DeGroat, W. C. (1976). Mechanisms underlying recurrent inhibition in the sacral parasympathetic outflow to the urinary bladder. *Journal of Physiology (London)* 257, 503–513.

Dembowsky, K., Czachurski, J., and Seller, H. (1985a). Morphology of sympathetic preganglionic neurons in the thoracic spinal cord of the cat: An intracellular horseradish peroxidase study. *Journal of Comparative Neurology* 238, 453–465.

Dembowsky, K., Czachurski, J., and Seller, H. (1985b). An intracellular study of the synaptic input to sympathetic preganglionic neurones of the third thoracic segment of the cat. *Journal of the Autonomic Nervous System* 13, 201–244.

Dembowsky, K., Czachurski, J., and Seller, H. (1986). Three types of sympathetic preganglionic neurones with different electrophysiological properties are identified by intracellular recordings in the cat. *Pflugers Archives* 406, 112–120.

Dodd, J., and Horn, J. P. (1983). A reclassification of B and C neurones in the ninth and tenth paravertebral sympathetic ganglia of the bullfrog. *Journal of Physiology (London)* 334, 255–269.

Dun, N. J., and Mo, N. (1988). *In vitro* effects of substance P on neonatal rat sympathetic preganglionic neurones. *Journal of Physiology (London)* 399, 321–333.

Ebbesson, S. O. E. (1968). Quantitative studies of superior sympathetic ganglia in a variety of primates including man. I. The ratio of preganglionic fibers to ganglionic neurons. *Journal of Morphology* 124, 117–124.

Feldberg, W., and Gaddum, J. H. (1934). The chemical transmitter at synapses in a sympathetic ganglion. *Journal of Physiology (London)* 81, 305–319.

Fernandez de Molina, A., Kuno, M., and Perl, E. R. (1965). Antidromically evoked responses from sympathetic preganglionic neurones. *Journal of Physiology (London)* 180, 321–335.

Forehand, C. J. (1985). Morphology of sympathetic preganglionic neurons in the rat spinal cord revealed by intracellular staining with horseradish peroxidase. *Neuroscience Abstracts* 11, 34.

Forehand, C. J., and Rubin, E. (1986). Specificity of sympathetic preganglionic projections: Rat preganglionic neurons project to either rostral or caudal ganglia along the sympathetic chain. *Neuroscience Abstracts* 12, 1056.

Gilbey, M. P., Peterson, D. F., and Coote, J. H. (1982). Some characteristics of sympathetic preganglionic neurones in the rat. *Brain Research* 241, 43–48.

Gilbey, M. P., Numao, Y., and Spyer, K. M. (1986). Discharge patterns of cervical sympathetic preganglionic neurones related to central respiratory drive in the rat. *Journal of Physiology (London)* 378, 253–265.

Glazer, E. J., and Ross, L. L. (1980). Localization of noradrenergic terminals in sympathetic nuclei of the rat: Demonstration by immunocytochemical localization of dopamine-β-hydroxylase. *Brain Research* 185, 39–49.

Guyenet, P. G., and Cabot, J. B. (1981). Inhibition of sympathetic preganglionic neurons by catecholamines and clonidine: Mediation by an alpha-adrenergic receptor. *Journal of Neuroscience* 1, 908–917.

Hancock, M. B., and Peveto, C. A. (1979). A preganglionic autonomic nucleus in the dorsal gray commissure of the lumbar spinal cord of the rat. *Journal of Comparative Neurology* 183, 65–72.

Holets, V., and Elde, R. (1982). The differential distribution and relationship of serotonergic and peptidergic fibers to sympathoadrenal neurons in the intermediolateral cell column of the rat: A combined retrograde axonal transport and immunofluorescence study. *Neuroscience* 7, 1155–1174.

Holets, V., and Elde, R. (1983). Sympathoadrenal preganglionic neurons: their distribution and relationship to chemically–coded fibers in the kitten intermediolateral cell column. *Journal of the Autonomic Nervous System* 7, 149–163.

Hongo, T., and Ryall, R. W. (1966). Electrophysiological and micro-electrophoretic studies on sympathetic preganglionic neurons in the spinal cord. *Acta Physiologica Scandinavica* 68, 96–104.

Horn, J. P., and Stofer, W. D. (1988). Spinal origins of preganglionic B and C neurons that innervate paravertebral sympathetic ganglia nine and ten of the bullfrog. *Journal of Comparative Neurology* 268, 71–83.

Hwang, B. H., and Williams, T. H. (1982). Fluorescence microscopy used in conjunction with horseradish peroxidase localization and electron microscopy for studying sympathetic nuclei of the rat spinal cord. *Brain Research Bulletin* 9, 171–177.

Jan, L. Y., and Jan, Y. N. (1982). Peptidergic transmission in sympathetic ganglia of the frog. *Journal of Physiology (London)* 327, 219–246.

Jänig, W., and McLachlan, E. M. (1986a). The sympathetic and sensory components of the caudal lumbar sympathetic trunk in the cat. *Journal of Comparative Neurology* 245, 62–73.

Jänig, W., and McLachlan, E. M. (1986b). Identification of distinct topographical distributions of lumbar sympathetic and sensory neurons projecting to end organs with different functions in the cat. *Journal of Comparative Neurology* 246, 104–112.

Jänig, W., and Szulczyk, P. (1980). Functional properties of lumbar preganglionic neurons. *Brain Research* 186, 115–131.

Kondo, H., Kuramoto, H., Wainer, B. H., and Yanaihara, N. (1985). Evidence for the coexistence of acetylcholine and enkephalin in sympathetic preganglionic neurons of rats. *Brain Research* 335, 309–314.

Konishi, S., Tsunoo, A., and Otsuka, M. (1981). Enkephalin as a transmitter for presynaptic inhibition in sympathetic ganglia. *Nature* 294, 81–83.

Krukoff, T. I., Ciriello, J., and Calaresu, F. R. (1985). Segmental distribution of peptide-like immunoreactivity in cell bodies of the thoracolumbar sympathetic nuclei of the cat. *Journal of Comparative Neurology* 240, 90–102.

Kuo, D. C., Yang, G. C. H., Yamasaki, D. S., and Krauthamer, G. M. (1982). A wide field electron microscopic analysis of the fiber constituents of the major splanchnic nerve in cat. *Journal of Comparative Neurology* 210, 49–58.

Lebedev, V. P. (1972). Properties of axons of sympathetic preganglionic neurones of the lower thoracic spinal cord. *Neuroscience Behavior Physiology* 5, 377–384.

Lebedev, V. P. (1980). Do sympathetic preganglionic neurones have a recurrent inhibitory mechanism? *Pflugers Archives* 383, 91–97.

Lichtman, J. W., Purves, D., and Yip, J. (1979). On the purpose of selective innervation of guinea-pig superior cervical ganglion cells. *Journal of Physiology (London)* 292, 69–84.

Ma, R. C., and Dun, N. J. (1985). Vasopressin depolarizes lateral horn cells of the neonatal rat spinal cord in vitro. *Brain Research* 348, 36–43.

Ma, R. C., and Dun, N. J. (1986). Excitation of the lateral horn cells of the neonatal rat spinal cord by 5-hydroxytryptamine. *Developmental Brain Research* 24, 89–98.

McIlhinney, R. A. J., Bacon, S. J., and Smith, A. D. (1988). A simple and rapid method for the production of cholera B-chain coupled to horseradish peroxidase for neuronal tracing. *Journal of Neuroscience Methods* 22, 189–194.

McKenna, K. E., and Schramm, L. P. (1983). Sympathetic preganglionic neurons in the isolated spinal cord of the neonatal rat. *Brain Research* 269, 201–210.

McKenna, K. E., and Schramm, L. P. (1985). Mechanisms mediating the sympathetic silent period. Studies in the isolated spinal cord of the neonatal rat. *Brain Research* 329, 233–240.

McLachlan, E. M. (1985). The components of the hypogastric nerve in male and female guinea pigs. *Journal of the Autonomic Nervous System* 13, 327–342.

McLachlan, E. M., and Hirst, G. D. S. (1980). Some properties of preganglionic neurons in upper thoracic spinal cord of the cat. *Journal of Neurophysiology* 43, 1251–1265.

McLachlan, E. M., and Oldfield, B. J. (1981). Some observations on the catecholaminergic innervation of the intermediate zone of the thoracolumbar spinal cord of the cat. *Journal of Comparative Neurology* 200, 529–544.

McLachlan, E. M., Oldfield, B. J., and Sittiracha, T. (1985). Localization of hindlimb vasomotor neurones in the lumbar spinal cord of the guinea pig. *Neuroscience Letters* 54, 269–275.

Milner, T. A., Morrison, S. F., Abate, C., and Reis, D. J. (1988). Phenylethanolamine N-methyltransferase containing terminals synapse directly on sympathetic preganglionic neurons in the rat. *Brain Research* 448, 205–222.

Mo, N., and Dun, N. J. (1987). Is glycine an inhibitory transmitter in rat lateral horn cells? *Brain Research* 400, 139–144.

Morgan, C., deGroat, W. C., and Nadelhaft, I. (1986). The spinal distribution of sympathetic preganglionic and visceral primary afferent neurons that send axons into the hypogastric nerves of the cat. *Journal of Comparative Neurology* 243, 23–40.

Nadelhaft, I., and McKenna, K. E. (1987). Sexual dimorphism in sympathetic preganglionic neurons of the rat hypogastric nerve. *Journal of Comparative Neurology* 256, 308–315.

Newton, B. W., and Hamill, R. W. (1989). Immunohistochemical distribution of serotonin in spinal autonomic nuclei: I. Fiber patterns in the adult rat. *Journal of Comparative Neurology* 279, 68–81.

Newton, B. W., Burkhart, A. B., and Hamill, R. W. (1989). Immunohistochemical distribution of serotonin in spinal autonomic nuclei: II. Early and late postnatal ontogeny in the rat. *Journal of Comparative Neurology* 279, 82–103.

Neuhuber, W. (1982). The central projection of visceral primary afferent neurones of the inferior mesenteric plexus and hypogastric nerves and the location of the related sensory and preganglionic cell bodies in the rat. *Anatomy and Embryology* 164, 413–425.

Nja, A., and Purves, D. (1977). Specific innervation of guinea-pig superior cervical ganglion cells by preganglionic fibres arising from different levels of the spinal cord. *Journal of Physiology (London)* 264, 565–583.

Nishi, S., Soeda, H., and Koketsu, K. (1965). Studies on sympathetic B and C neurons and patterns of preganglionic innervation. *Journal of Cell and Comparative Physiology* 66, 19–32.

Oldfield, B. J., and McLachlan, E. M. (1981). An analysis of the sympathetic preganglionic neurons projecting from the upper thoracic spinal roots of the cat. *Journal of Comparative Neurology* 196, 329–345.

Pardini, B. J., and Wurster, R. D. (1984). Identification of the sympathetic preganglionic pathway to the cat stellate ganglion. *Journal of the Autonomic Nervous System* 11, 13–25.

Petras, J. M., and Cummings, J. F. (1972). Autonomic neurons in the spinal cord of the rhesus monkey. A correlation of the findings of cytoarchitectonics and sympathectomy with fiber degeneration following dorsal rhizotomy. *Journal of Comparative Neurology* 146, 189–218.

Petras, J. M., and Cummings, J. F. (1978). Sympathetic and parasympathetic innervation of the urinary bladder and urethra. *Brain Research* 153, 363–369.

Petras, J. M., and Faden, A. I. (1978). The origin of sympathetic preganglionic neurons in the dog. *Brain Research* 144, 353–357.

Polosa, C. (1967). The silent period of sympathetic preganglionic neurons. *Canadian Journal of Physiology and Pharmacology* 45, 1033–1045.

Purves, D., and Lichtman, J. W. (1985). Geometrical differences among homologous neurons in mammals. *Science* 228, 298–302.

Purves, D., and Wigston, D. J. (1983). Neural units in the superior cervical ganglion of the guinea-pig. *Journal of Physiology (London)* 334, 169–178.

Purves, D., Rubin, E., Snider, W. D., and Lichtman, J. (1986). Relation of animal size to convergence, divergence and neuronal number in peripheral sympathetic pathways. *Journal of Neuroscience* 6, 158–163.

Rando, T. A., Bowers, C. W., and Zigmond, R. E. (1981). Localization of neurons in the rat spinal cord which project to the superior cervical ganglion. *Journal of Comparative Neurology* 196, 73–83.

Rethelyi, M. (1972). Cell and neuropil architecture of the intermediolateral (sympathetic) nucleus of the cat spinal cord. *Brain Research* 46, 203–213.

Robertson, D. R. (1987). Sympathetic preganglionic neurons in frog spinal cord. *Journal of the Autonomic Nervous System* 18, 1–11.

Romagnano, M. A., Braiman, J., Loomis, M., and Hamill, R. W. (1987). Enkephalin fibers in autonomic nuclear

regions: Intraspinal vs. supraspinal origin. *Journal of Comparative Neurology* 266, 332–359.

Rubin, E., and Purves, D. (1980). Segmental organization of sympathetic preganglionic neurons in the mammalian spinal cord. *Journal of Comparative Neurology* 192, 163–174.

Schramm, L. P., Adair, J. R., Stribling, J. M., and Gray, L. P. (1975). Preganglionic innervation of the adrenal gland of the rat: A study using horseradish peroxidase. *Experimental Neurology* 49, 540–553.

Schramm, L. P., Stribling, J. M., and Adair, J. R. (1976). Developmental reorientation of sympathetic preganglionic neurons in the rat. *Brain Research* 106, 166–171.

Strack, A. M., Sawyer, W. B., Marubio, L. M., and Loewy, A. D. (1988). Spinal origin of sympathetic preganglionic neurons in the rat. *Brain Research* 455, 187–191.

Taylor, D. G., and Gebber, G. L. (1973). Sympathetic unit responses to stimulation of cat medulla. *American Journal of Physiology* 225, 1138–1146.

Tan, C. K., and Wong, W. C. (1975). An ultrastructural study of the synaptic glomeruli in the intermediolateral nucleus of the rat. *Experientia* 31, 201–203.

Torigoe, Y., Cernucan, R. D., Nishimoto, J. A. S., and Blanks, R. H. I. (1985). Sympathetic preganglionic efferent and afferent neurones mediated by the greater splanchnic nerve in rabbit. *Experimental Neurology* 87, 334–348.

Ulfhake, B., and Kellerth, J.-O. (1981). A quantitative light microscopic study of the dendrites of cat spinal α-motoneurons after intracellular staining with horseradish peroxidase. *Journal of Comparative Neurology* 202, 571–584.

Ulfhake, B., and Kellereth, J.-O. (1983). A quantitative morphological study of HRP-labeled cat α-motoneurons supplying different muscles. *Brain Research* 264, 1–20.

Warden, M. K., and Young, W. S. III (1988). Distribution of cells containing mRNAs encoding substance P and neurokinin B in the rat central nervous system. *Journal of Comparative Neurology* 272, 90–113.

Wong, W. C., and Tan, C. K. (1980). The fine structure of the intermediolateral nucleus of the spinal cord of the monkey *(Macaca fascicularis). Journal of Anatomy* 130, 263–277.

Yoshimura, M., Polosa, C., and Nishi, S. (1986a). Electrophysiological properties of sympathetic preganglionic neurons in the cat spinal cord in vitro. *Pflugers Archives* 406, 91–98.

Yoshimura, M., Polosa, C., and Nishi, S. (1986b). Afterhyperpolarization mechanisms in cat sympathetic preganglionic neuron in vitro. *Journal of Neurophysiology* 55, 1234–1246.

Yoshimura, M., Polosa C., and Nishi, S. (1987). A transient outward rectification in the cat sympathetic preganglionic neuron. *Pflugers Archives* 408, 207–208.

5

Vagal Preganglionic Neurons

A. D. LOEWY AND K. M. SPYER

Vagal parasympathetic preganglionic fibers arise from two main nuclei in the medulla oblongata: (1) the dorsal vagal nucleus and (2) the nucleus ambiguus. These fibers innervate parasympathetic ganglia that lie near, on the surface, or within the muscular walls of cervical, thoracic, and abdominal visceral organs. The vagus nerve supplies motor fibers that control the mucous glands and muscles of the pharynx, esophagus, stomach, and the rest of the gastrointestinal tract, up to the point where the descending colon begins. The remaining lower gastrointestinal tract is innervated by the sacral parasympathetic fibers. The dorsal vagal nucleus is probably the sole source of the preganglionic fibers in the abdominal portion of the vagus nerve, and it functions in control of gastrointestinal motility and secretion. In addition, it regulates the exocrine and endocrine pancreatic secretions. The nucleus ambiguus gives rise to motor fibers that innervate the striated muscle of the soft palate, pharynx, esophagus, and larynx; this nucleus functions as the final common pathway in swallowing and provides the motor control used in vocalization. Parasympathetic preganglionic fibers innervating the cardiac ganglia arise from the ventrolateral nucleus ambiguus. These fibers are the main source of inhibitory fibers affecting heart rate.

In this chapter, the cytoarchitecture, the efferent and afferent connections, and the function of these two nuclei will be summarized. The discussion will focus mainly on results dealing with the rat, because this species has been the mammalian prototype for neuroanatomical investigations.

DORSAL VAGAL NUCLEUS

The dorsal vagal nucleus lies in the dorsomedial portion of the caudal medulla oblongata close to the floor of the fourth ventricle (Figure 5-1). It extends caudally to the first cervical spinal segment lying dorsolateral to the central canal. In histological preparations of the brain stem stained for cell bodies, this nucleus is distinctive because it is composed of a densely packed, homogeneous collection of darkly stained neurons. This is a characteristic feature of this cell group in all mammals.

Efferent Projections

The majority of the neurons in the dorsal vagal nucleus (80%) give rise to the parasympathetic preganglionic fibers of the vagus nerve (see Hopkins, 1987 for review). Almost all of these neurons are cholinergic (Houser et al., 1983). The remaining 20% of the neurons in this nucleus may be centrally projecting neurons or interneurons. In the cat, some neurons found in the dorsal vagal nucleus project to the parabrachial nucleus (King, 1980), and others project to the cerebellar cortex and the deep cerebellar nuclei (Zheng et al., 1982). The projection to the cerebellar cortex is arranged in a topographical manner: the rostral part of the nucleus projects to the posterior cerebellar lobe and the caudal part projects to the anterior lobe (Zheng et al., 1982). Whether these are vagal motor neurons or a dispersed group of cells with properties equivalent to those of the nucleus tractus solitarius is unclear. In addition, it is not known yet if the dorsal vagal nucleus of other mammals also contains centrally projecting cells.

Catecholamine-Containing Neurons

One controversy regarding the dorsal vagal nucleus in the rat is whether the catecholamine-containing neurons found in this nucleus contribute to the vagal outflow. Catecholaminergic vagal motor neurons have been retrogradely labeled after either immersing the cut proximal end of the vagus nerve in horseradish peroxidase or injecting horseradish peroxidase (HRP) into the stomach wall (Gwyn et al., 1985; Kalia et al., 1984). However, Blessing et al. (1985) failed to confirm these results using similar

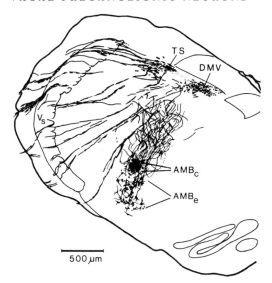

Figure 5-1 Transverse section of rat medulla oblongata showing retrograde cell body labeling of vagal motor neurons after injection of horseradish peroxidase into the cervical vagus nerve. Vagal motor neurons lie in the dorsal vagal nucleus (DMV) as well as within two portions of the nucleus ambiguus (the compact part—AMB_c and the ventrolateral or external division—AMB_e). TS, tractus solitarius; V_s, spinal trigeminal tract. (Reproduced from Bieger and Hopkins, *Journal of Comparative Neurology* 262, 546–562, 1987, with permission of the authors and publisher.)

techniques. To explain this difference, it was suggested that the earlier observations represent a false positive artifact due to the use of a double chromagen histochemical procedure. In these earlier studies, the HRP reaction product produced by the diaminobenzidine reaction was intensified by cobalt to produce a black granular reaction product. Then, in a sequential histochemical step, the catecholamine-synthesizing enzyme tyrosine hydroxylase was stained by the standard diaminobenzidine reaction to produce a brown reaction product in the nerve cell bodies. Blessing and co-workers contended that distinguishing black granular product against a brown background provided equivocal results because of discrimination difficulties, whereas the double fluorescence procedure used by them enhanced their ability to observe double cell body labeling.

In further support of their contention, Blessing et al. (1985) pointed out that the catecholamine histofluorescence that is normally seen in the vagus nerve disappears after superior cervical ganglionectomy (see Blessing et al., 1985, for references). This suggests that the source for these catecholamine fibers is the sympathetic nervous system and not the central nervous system.

However, this controversy remains as Sawchenko et al. (1987) report that after immersing the proximal end of the transected cervical vagus nerve in the

fluorescent tracer True Blue, the retrogradely labeled cells in the rostral portion of the dorsal vagal nucleus stain with antibodies against dopamine-β-hydroxylase (DBH: the enzyme marker for noradrenergic neurons). Assuming that the antibodies used in these studies are specific, these may be atypical catecholamine neurons because the same cells fail to stain with antibodies to tyrosine hydroxylase (TH: the enzyme marker for all catecholamine cells). In the middle region of the nucleus, a group of TH-positive (but DBH-negative) cells was labeled, suggesting that these may be dopamine-containing neurons. In the caudal third of the nucleus, some of the retrogradely labeled cells stained positively for either TH or DBH, indicating that part of the vagal outflow from this level may be from dopaminergic and/or noradrenergic neurons.

Some of the dorsal vagal neurons appear to contain multiple putative transmitters. For example, the caudal cholinergic vagal neurons also exhibit tyrosine hydroxylase immunoreactivity (Manier et al., 1987). Galanin-containing vagal neurons that lie in the lateral part of the nucleus are thought to be cholinergic as well, but direct proof of this point is lacking (see Sawchencko et al., 1987, for review).

Viscerotopic Organization in the Dorsal Vagal Nucleus

The dorsal vagal nucleus is the principal (if not the sole) source of vagal fibers that innervate the subdiaphragmatic visceral organs (stomach, small intestine, liver, gallbladder, pancreas, ascending and transverse colon). It also innervates cervical organs (viz. pharynx, larynx) and thoracic viscera (viz. trachea, bronchi, lungs, heart, esophagus) (see Kalia, 1981, for review). This motor outflow is organized in a visceral topographical manner. The cells that innervate abdominal organs lie in the medial two-thirds of the nucleus. The cells that innervate the heart and the lungs lie in the lateral third of the nucleus, mainly at the caudal levels (see Hopkins, 1987, for review).

A distinct viscerotopic pattern has been demonstrated for the motor innervation of the stomach (Figure 5-2). The neurons innervating the fundus lie laterally and those controlling the pylorus and antrum are situated medially (Pagani et al., 1988). Fox and Powley (1985) found a similar specific viscerotopic pattern of innervation that follows the embryonic body plan. During development, the gastrointestinal tract begins as a simple tube. The upper end of the foregut differentiates into the stomach by enlarging and rotating 90° in the rostrocaudal axis, so the original embryonic right side of the stomach becomes the posterior (or dorsal) surface in the adult. The gastric branches of the posterior trunk arise

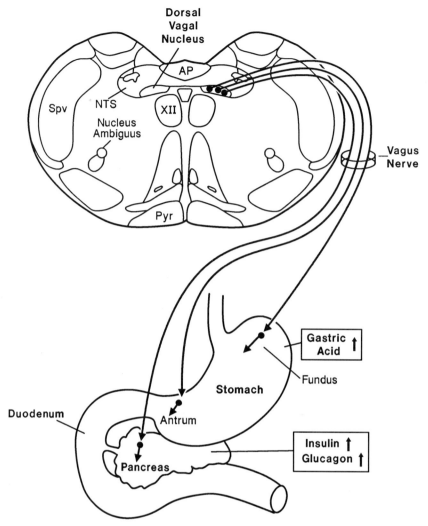

Figure 5-2 Schematic drawing illustrating the topographic organization of the projection from the dorsal vagal nucleus to the stomach and pancreas in the rat. AP, area postrema NTS, nucleus tractus solitarius; Pyr, pyramidal tract; Spv, superior paraventricular nucleus.

from the medial-most portion of the right dorsal vagal nucleus, and the gastric branch of the anterior trunk originates from the medial portion of the left dorsal vagal nucleus. At the more rostral levels, neurons contributing to the anterior and posterior gastric branches of the vagus nerve occupy the full mediolateral extent of the nucleus. The motor column that gives rise to the celiac branch of the vagus nerve lies lateral to the gastric motor column; it is composed of fewer cell bodies and displays the same geometrical pattern of being columnar at caudal levels and tending to be wider in mediolateral extent at rostral levels. The hepatic branch arises only from cell bodies in the left dorsal vagal nucleus, and it is coextensive with the cells that give rise to the anterior gastric branch.

Comparable data for the viscera of the head, neck,

and thorax are not available. However, experiments by Hopkins (1987) suggest that some of these organs are innervated by neurons in the lateral one-third of the caudal dorsal vagal nucleus.

Afferents of the Dorsal Vagal Nucleus

Axonal transport techniques have been used to determine the afferent inputs to the dorsal vagal nucleus. These arise from both peripheral and central neurons.

Vagal sensory afferents arising from the nodose ganglion project directly to the dorsal vagal nucleus of the rat (Shapiro and Miselis, 1985). The projection is sparse and restricted to the dorsal and lateral edges of the nucleus. These afferents potentially affect both cell bodies and dendrites of vagal preganglionic neurons, although electron microscopic evidence that these fibers terminate on these neurons is lacking. However, some vagal preganglionic neurons have dendrites that extend dorsally, beyond the border of the dorsal vagal nucleus into the nucleus tractus solitarius. This region receives a dense input from the vagus nerve. It is quite likely that this projection may provide the anatomical substrate for vago-vagal reflexes that are involved in cardiac and gastrointestinal control.

Central afferents arise from at least 12 sites in the brain (Figure 5-3). These include (1) the insular region of the cerebral cortex (mouse: Shipley, 1982), (2) the central nucleus of the amygdala (cat: Hopkins and Holstege, 1978; monkey: Price and Amaral, 1981; rabbit: Schwaber et al., 1982), (3) the paraventricular hypothalamic nucleus (rat: Luiten et al., 1985), (4) the lateral hypothalamic area (rat: Berk and Finkelstein, 1982), (5) the dorsomedial hypothalamic nucleus (rat: Luiten et al., 1987), (6) the posterior hypothalamus (rat: Luiten et al., 1987), (7) the mesencephalic central gray matter (rat: Rogers et al., 1980; Luiten et al., 1987), (8) the parabrachial nucleus (rat: Luiten et al., 1987), (9) the A5 catecholamine cell group (rat: Loewy et al., 1979), (10) the nucleus tractus solitarius (rat: Luiten et al., 1987), (11) the medullary reticular formation (rat: Rogers et al., 1980; Luiten et al., 1987), and (12) the raphe obscurus nucleus (rat: Rogers et al., 1980; Luiten et al., 1987).

Neurochemical Classification of Afferents to the Dorsal Vagal Nucleus

A variety of neurotransmitters are present in the dorsal vagal nucleus (see Table 5-1). The source(s) of these neurochemicals is incompletely known, and the discussion in this section will focus on three main classes of putative transmitters: monoamines, opioid peptides, and nonopioid neuropeptides.

Monoamines

The dorsal vagal nucleus receives inputs from various aminergic containing fiber systems, but the cells of origin for most of these projections are unknown.

The A5 noradrenergic cell group of the rostral ventrolateral medulla projects to the dorsal vagal nucleus in the rat (Loewy et al., 1979). It has not been determined whether this is the only source of noradrenergic fibers present in this nucleus. Other nearby noradrenergic neurons found in the area postrema or the A2 region within the nucleus tractus solitarius may contribute to this innervation, but anatomical evidence is lacking in support of this point. There is no evidence that the A1 cell group, the locus coeruleus, or subcoeruleus nuclei project to this nucleus.

The issue of whether the dorsal vagal nucleus receives a dopaminergic innervation has not been clearly addressed. In regional surveys of the rat brain for dopamine (Versteeg et al., 1976), relatively high amounts of dopamine were demonstrated in the dorsomedial region of the medulla oblongata. Since both the dorsal vagal nucleus and nucleus tractus solitarius were assayed together it is uncertain if the dorsal vagal nucleus contains this catecholamine. When horseradish peroxidase is injected into the dorsal vagal nucleus, three areas in the hypothalamus that are known to contain dopaminergic neurons are labeled: posterior, dorsomedial, and paraventricular hypothalamic nuclei (Luiten et al., 1987). Dopamine-containing neurons in the paraventricular hypothalamic nucleus are labeled after fluorochrome dye injections into the dorsomedial portion of the medulla oblongata (Sawchenko and Swanson, 1982), but it is not known if this is due to a projection to the nucleus tractus solitarius and/or dorsal vagal nucleus.

Similar uncertainties exist regarding the projections of the other monoamine-containing neurons that send fibers to the dorsal vagal nucleus. Serotonin immunoreactive fibers are present in the dorsal vagal nucleus in moderate concentration (Steinbusch, 1981). These fibers probably originate from neurons of the nucleus raphe obscurus. These neurons may also contain other putative neurotransmitters such as thyrotropin-releasing hormone and/or substance P. Fibers containing immunoreactive phenylethanolamine N-methyltransferase, the enzyme marker for adrenaline, and immunoreactive histidine decarboxylase, the histamine-synthesizing enzyme, have been identified in the dorsal vagal nucleus (Hökfelt et al., 1974; Watanabe et al., 1984), but the cells of origin of these fibers are unknown. The histidine decarboxylase immunoreactive fibers arise probably from neurons in the posterior or dorsomedial hypothalamic regions because these areas are known to contain histidine decarboxylase immunoreactive cell bodies and also project to the dorsal vagal nucleus. Direct evidence for this inference is lacking.

Opioid Peptides

The dorsal vagal nucleus is innervated by a variety of opioid peptide-containing fiber systems. Both met-enkephalin and leu-enkephalin immunoreactive-containing fibers have been found in this nucleus in the rat (Sar et al., 1978; Yamazoe et al., 1984). Fibers stained for dynorphin A (dynorphin 1–8), a peptide derived from the pro-dynorphin precursor, and met-enkephalin-Arg-Gly-Leu, a peptide derived from the pro-enkephalin precursor, have been found in the nucleus (Fallon and Leslie, 1986; see Yaksh, 1987 for review of opioid nomenclature),

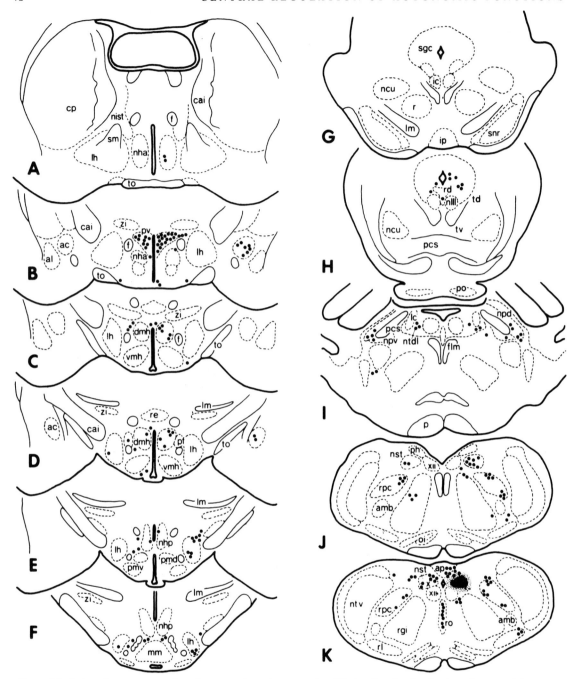

Figure 5-3 Series of transverse sections from anterior (A) to posterior (K) showing the distribution of retrogradely labeled cells indicated by solid black dots following an HRP injection in the dorsal motor vagus nucleus. ac, central amygdaloid nucleus; al, lateral amygdaloid nucleus; amb, nucleus ambiguus; ap, area postrema; cai, internal capsule; cp; caudate putamen; dmh, dorsomedial hypothalamic nucleus; f, fornix; flm, medial longitudinal fasciculus; ip, interpeduncular nucleus; lc, locus coeruleus; lh, lateral hypothalamic area; lm, lateral lemniscus; mm, mammillary nuclei, ncu, cuneiform nucleus; nha, anterior hypothalamic nucleus; nhp, posterior hypothalamic nucleus; nist, interstitial nucleus of stria terminalis; npd, dorsal parabrachial nucleus; npv, ventral parabrachial nucleus; nst, solitary tract nucleus; ntdl, dorsal tegmental nucleus, pars lateralis; oi, inferior olivary nucleus; p, pyramidal tract; pf, perifornical nucleus; pmd, dorsal premammillary nucleus; pmv, ventral premammillary nucleus; po, pons; psc, superior cerebellar peduncle; pv, paraventricular nucleus; r, red nucleus; rd, dorsal raphe nucleus; re, reuniens thalamic nucleus; rgi, nucleus reticularis gigantocellularis; rl, lateral reticular nucleus; ro, nucleus raphe obscuris; rpc, nucleus reticularis parvocellularis; sgc, substantia grisea centralis; snr, substantia nigra, pars reticulata; vmh, ventromedial hypothalamic nucleus; zi, zona incerta; X, dorsal motor vagus nucleus. (Reproduced from ter Horst et al., *Journal of the Autonomic Nervous System* 11, 59–75, 1984, with permission of the authors and publisher.)

Table 5-1 Neuroactive Substances in Dorsal Vagal Nucleus of the Rat

Amino acids
 Aspartate
 GABA
 Glutamate
 Glycine

Biogenic amines or related synthetic enzymes
 Adrenaline
 Noradrenaline
 Histamine
 Serotonin

Neuropeptides
 TRH
 CRF
 Somatostatin
 Vasopressin
 Oxytocin
 ACTH
 α-MSH
 β-Endorphin
 Met-enkephalin
 Met-enkephalin-Arg, Phe
 Leu-enkephalin
 FMRF amide
 Dynorphin A
 α-Neo-endorphin
 Neuropeptide Y
 Vasoactive intestinal polypeptide
 Substance P
 Bombesin
 Neurotensin

Adapted from Palkovits (1985).

but the source of these opioid peptidergic fibers is unknown. Other types of immunoreactive opioid fibers such as β-endorphin (Finley et al., 1981a), ACTH (Romagnano and Joseph, 1983), α-melanocyte-stimulating hormone (O'Donohue et al., 1979), and β- and γ-lipotropin (Schwartzberg and Nakane, 1983) have not been detected in the dorsal vagal nucleus.

Nonopioid Peptides

Nonopioid neuropeptide-containing fibers have been localized in the dorsal vagal nucleus of the rat by immunohistochemistry, including cholecystokinin-8 (Yamazoe et al., 1984), corticotropin-releasing factor (Swanson et al., 1983), neuropeptide Y (De Quidt and Emson, 1986), neurotensin (Higgins et al., 1984), oxytocin (Sawchenko and Swanson, 1982), somatostatin (Higgins and Schwaber, 1983), substance P (Yamazoe et al., 1984), thyrotropin-releasing hormone (Kubek et al., 1983), and vasopressin (Sawchenko and Swanson, 1982).

The paraventricular hypothalamic nucleus provides both a vasopressinergic and an oxytocinergic input to the dorsomedial portion of the rat medulla oblongata (Sawchenko and Swanson, 1982). The dorsal vagal nucleus receives a part of this projec-

tion; the nucleus tractus solitarius receives the rest. The oxytocin input is denser than vasopressin projection. Although it is clear that the paraventricular hypothalamic nucleus is the sole source of the oxytocinergic input, it has not been established that the paraventricular hypothalamic nucleus is the only source of the vasopressin fibers found in the nucleus tractus solitarius or the dorsal vagal nucleus. It is possible, although as yet not demonstrated, that a portion of the input could originate from the vasopressin neurons of the dorsomedial hypothalamic nucleus and the bed nucleus of the stria terminalis (Caffe and van Leeuwen, 1983).

The thyrotropin-releasing hormone-containing fibers present in the dorsal vagal nucleus (Kubek et al., 1983) probably originate from neurons in the nucleus raphe obscurus. Three observations support this view: (1) the raphe obscurus nucleus projects to the dorsal vagal nucleus (Luiten et al., 1987); (2) some of the raphe obscurus neurons contain thyrotrophin-releasing hormone as well as serotonin (Johannsson et al., 1981); and (3) knife cuts ventral to the dorsal vagal nucleus, but not rostral to it, reduce the thyrotropin-releasing hormone content and the number of immunoreactive fibers in this nucleus (Palkovits et al., 1986). These observations provide circumstantial evidence for this projection. Stronger evidence is needed to establish this neuronal connection, such as combined retrograde transport, immunohistochemistry, and biochemical assays following lesions of the cell bodies in this area.

The dorsal vagal nucleus contains sparse numbers of somatostatin immunoreactive fibers (Finley et al., 1981b). Fluorescent dye injections into the dorsomedial medulla oblongata of rabbits label somatostatin-containing neurons of the central nucleus of the amygdala (Higgins and Schwaber, 1983). However, the somatostatinergic projection from the central nucleus of the amygdala may be directed to the nucleus tractus solitarius rather than to the dorsal vagal nucleus. Additional experiments will be required to determine the source of this somatostatinergic input.

In summary, although the dorsal vagal nucleus contains a variety of different neuropeptide-containing fibers, the cell groups of the brain that give rise to these projections are unknown except for the oxytocin input, which originates from the paraventricular hypothalamic nucleus, and is likely to be an excitatory transmitter (Charpak et al., 1984; Raggenbass et al., 1987).

Receptor Binding

In vitro autoradiography has revealed the presence of binding sites for numerous ligands within the dorsal vagal nucleus. Muscarinic cholinergic receptors have been identified extending throughout the nucleus (Wamsley et al., 1981; Cox et al., 1986). Both opiate and α_2-adrenergic receptors are also localized to the nucleus (Dashwood et al., 1985; Unnerstall et al., 1984).

With regard to the opiate receptors, Dashwood et al. (1988b) have shown that the predominant receptor subtype localized within the nucleus in the cat is of the μ category, with little or no evidence of the presence of any δ or κ opioid receptor subtypes. The density of μ receptors was unaffected by section of the ipsilateral vagus nerve, although the number of these receptors in the nucleus tractus solitarius was reduced significantly (Dashwood et al., 1988b).

The binding of noradrenaline to the dorsal vagal nucleus appears to be via α_2-adrenergic receptors in both the cat and rat (Dashwood et al., 1985; Unnerstall et al., 1984).

There is also evidence for an abundance of serotonin receptors in the dorsal vagal nucleus of the rat (Pazos and Palacios, 1985), and from the results of preliminary studies in the cat, these appear to be of the 5-HT$_{1A}$ class (Dashwood et al., 1988a). The functional role of these receptors remains to be resolved.

Physiological Studies of the Dorsal Vagal Nucleus

The dorsal vagal nucleus functions mainly in the control of gastrointestinal and pancreatic secretions. Its role in the control of other visceral functions such as smooth muscle motility and cardioinhibition is uncertain and is discussed below.

Gastrointestinal Function

Gastric acid secretion can be induced by chemical or electrical stimulation of the dorsal vagal nucleus (see Taché, 1988, for review). The first experiments to suggest this idea were performed by Kerr and Preshaw (1969). They demonstrated in the cat that insulin-induced gastric acid secretion was dependent on the integrity of the dorsal vagal nucleus. Destruction of this nucleus prevented increases in gastric secretion following intravenous injections of insulin.

More contemporary studies have used the microinjection technique to study the function of the dorsal vagal nucleus. Microinjections of either thyrotropin-releasing hormone or oxytocin into this nucleus cause gastric acid secretions, but comparable injections of vasopressin are without effect (Rogers and Hermann, 1985). Oxytocin-induced gastric acid release can be blocked by central injections of an oxytocin antagonist or by peripheral administration of atropine. These findings imply that the descending oxytocin pathway originating from the paraventricular hypothalamic nucleus functions in regulating gastric acid secretion. The source for the thyrotropin-releasing hormone fibers is unknown.

The dorsal vagal nucleus may also be involved in the control of gastrointestinal smooth muscle. Electrical stimulation of the rostral part of the dorsal vagal nucleus in the cat increases gastric motility (Pagani et al., 1985). In contrast, microinjections of L-glutamate in the dorsal vagal nucleus of the rat cause decreased gastric smooth muscle tone (Spencer and Talman, 1986). It is difficult to explain the differences in results of these two studies. However, a major concern with both sets of experiments is the fact that in neither case were the investigators able to document that they were not concomitantly activating the nucleus tractus solitarius. Until this can be done, the interpretation of experiments of this nature remains unclear.

In summary, the above discussion has assumed that gastrointestinal motility and secretion are separate, neurally controlled phenomena. This may be an overly simplistic view. Motility may provide the sensory stimulus for reflexly activated secretion (see Greenwood and Davison, 1987, for review). This link between motility and secretion involves an integration between the vagal and intrinsic neural systems. However, the circuitry for this potential physiological coupling is still obscure.

Pancreatic Function

Claude Bernard (1855) reported that puncture wounds of the medulla oblongata caused diabetes mellitus. This famous experiment of *piqûre diabétique* provided the first evidence that the medulla oblongata was involved in the control of carbohydrate metabolism (see Chapter 16). Even to this date, the critical site destroyed in these experiments and the mechanism causing diabetes in these animals remain still uncertain.

Interest in this problem had remained dormant for over a century, until Laughton and Powley (1987) demonstrated that electrical stimulation of the dorsal vagal nucleus in the rat causes an increase in insulin and glucagon secretion. The response appeared to be quite specific, because stimulation of the more lateral aspect of the nucleus caused insulin and glucagon secretion, whereas stimulation of the more medial aspects of the nucleus caused gastric acid release. No information exists regarding the CNS cell groups that regulate these target-specific vagal preganglionic neurons.

The neural mechanisms involved in the regulation of exocrine pancreatic secretions are complex and poorly understood (see Solomon, 1987, for review).

Cardiovascular Function

The role of the dorsal vagal nucleus in cardiac control remains a controversial issue. There is, however, no doubt that some dorsal vagal neurons project to the heart, although the great majority arise from the region of the nucleus ambiguus. This conclusion has been drawn on the basis of two main lines of evidence (Figure 5-4). First, retrogradely labeled neurons can be identified in this nucleus after HRP is injected into the cardiac branch(es) of the vagus (rat: Nosaka et al., 1979; cat: Bennett et al., 1981). Second, dorsal vagal neurons are antidromically activated by electrical stimulation of the cardiovagal nerve (McAllen and Spyer, 1976; Jordan et al., 1986;

Nosaka et al., 1982). A third line of evidence exists, but it is regarded as inconclusive; namely, electrical stimulation of the dorsal vagal nucleus evokes a bradycardia (rat: Nosaka et al., 1979; Rogers and Herman, 1985). Similar conclusions have been made from equivalent studies in the cat (Calaresu and Pearce, 1965, among others), and a claim has also been made that such stimulation elicits a decrease in myocardial contractility (Geis and Wurster, 1980).

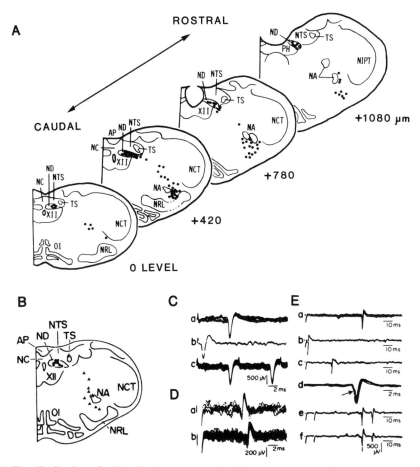

Figure 5-4 (A) The distribution of cell bodies in the medulla oblongata of the rat that were retrogradely labeled after application of horseradish peroxidase into the cardiac branch of the vagus nerve. The sections show the rostrocaudal distribution of labeled neurons. The 0 level is at the calamus scriptorius and the subsequent sections are 420, 780, and 1080 µm rostral to this level as indicated. AP, area postrema; NA, nucleus ambiguus; NC, commissural nucleus; NCT, spinal trigeminal nucleus, caudal part; ND, dorsal vagal nucleus; NIPT, spinal trigeminal nucleus, interpolaris part; NRL, lateral reticular nucleus; NTS, nucleus tractus solitarius; OI, inferior olivary nucleus; PH, prepositus hypoglossal nucleus; TS, solitary tract; XII, hypoglossal nucleus. (Reproduced from Nosaka et al., *Journal of Comparative Neurology,* 186, 79–92, 1979, with permission and slight modification from the original figures.) (B) Distribution of vagal cardiac preganglionic neurons in the rat medulla oblongata localized by antidromic activation. Solid circles represent cells that showed antidromic responses of long latencies (greater than 44 msec) to stimulation of the cardiac branch of the vagus nerve. Solid triangles represent cells that showed antidromic responses of short latencies (less than 10 msec). (B–E are reproduced from Nosaka et al., *American Journal of Physiology* 243, R92–R98, 1982, with permission.) (C) Antidromic response of a cell in the nucleus ambiguus following stimulation of the cardiac branch of the vagus nerve. a, Superimposed records; b, cancellation of the antidromic response by a spontaneous spike; c, capability of following high-frequency stimulations (100/second). (D) Antidromic response of a cell in the intermediate zone. a, Superimposed recordings at stimulus repetition rate of 1 m/second; b, those at 50/second. (E) Antidromic response of a cell in the dorsal vagal nucleus. a, Superimposed recordings; b and c, cancellation of the antidromic spike by spontaneous spikes; d, temporal expansion of the antidromic spike. Note a notch in positively going phase of spike (arrow). e and f, Effect of paired stimulations. Note a complete somadendritic block in the second spike in f. Negativity is shown as downward deflection.

Unfortunately, little can justifiably be concluded from these latter observations since they could have resulted from current spread to the adjacent nucleus tractus solitarius. Further, negative inotropic effects can be confirmed only if the heart rate is controlled, and this was not the case in this study.

Even the results obtained using the retrograde cell body labeling method are often viewed critically. Some workers claim that in the rat it is rare to label dorsal vagal neurons from the injection of HRP into the myocardium near the sinoatrial and atrioventricular nodes, or into the ventricular myocardium (Stuesse, 1982). In contrast, using the retrograde transport of cholera toxin-conjugated HRP, clear evidence of clusters of labeled cells in the caudal regions of the dorsal vagal nucleus was obtained when injections were made in the vicinity of the postganglionic vagal neurons on the atria of the rat (Bradd et al., 1989).

Interestingly, in both the rat (Nosaka et al., 1982) and the cat (McAllen and Spyer, 1976), it has been shown that C-fiber axons arising from the dorsal vagal nucleus project to the heart. In contrast, the cardiac-projecting neurons of the nucleus ambiguus have axons that conduct action potentials in the range of B-fibers (see below), which are traditionally believed to be the most important vagal efferent fibers for eliciting cardiac slowing (Middleton et al., 1950). In the rabbit, many dorsal vagal neurons with axons in the range of B-fibers have properties compatible with negative chronotropic function, and in relation to physiological properties they appear to be indistinguishable from their counterparts in the nucleus ambiguus (Jordan et al., 1986). These neurons have a low level of ongoing activity in anesthetized animals (2–20 spikes/second) and are excited at short latency on electrical stimulation of the aortic nerve (latency 6–25 msec). They also show a pulse rhythm in their discharge, presumably resulting from an excitatory input from the arterial baroreceptors, and tend to fire during expiration; when they are excited by the iontophoretic application of an excitatory amino acid D,L-homocysteatic acid, a measurable bradycardia can be demonstrated. Similar studies have not been performed in other species, and so it remains to be resolved whether cardioinhibitory neurons are present in the dorsal vagal nucleus in other than the rabbit.

In summary, part of the vagal input to the heart arises from neurons in the dorsal vagal nucleus. Whether this is a source of cardioinhibitory preganglionic fibers or of other cardiac vagal fibers with different functions, such as those involved in control of myocardial contractility or the coronary artery circulation (Van Charldorp et al., 1987), is unresolved.

Biophysical Properties of the Dorsal Vagal Nucleus

The biophysical properties of the dorsal vagal neurons have been studied (Yarom et al., 1985a,b; Champagnet et al., 1986; Fukuda et al., 1987; Plata-Salamán et al., 1988; Nabekura et al., 1989). Using an *in vitro* slice preparation of the guinea pig medulla oblongata, Yarom et al. (1985b) demonstrated that these neurons have many properties that are similar to those of spinal motoneurons with regard to a fast initial sodium spike. They have, however, a prominent after-depolarization on the falling phase of their action potential that may be the consequence of a calcium current generated at the dendritic level (see Figure 5-5). Equally, they have a prominent all-or-none calcium spike when sodium currents are blocked with tetrodotoxin. This and the normal action potential are followed by a prolonged after-hyperpolarization. A particularly powerful calcium-activated potassium current appears to generate this unusually long duration after-hyperpolarization that is often in excess of 1 sec (Figure 5-5D). This is sensitive to acetylcholine, which appears to block both voltage- and calcium-dependent potassium currents when injected into the cells (Yarom et al., 1985a). In addition to this current, which will have major consequences for the firing pattern of dorsal vagal neurons, there is also evidence for a voltage-dependent potassium current that is inactivated at potentials around the resting membrane potential, but becomes deinactivated at hyperpolarized

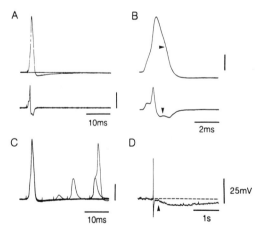

Figure 5-5 Antidromic activation of vagal motoneurons. (A, B) Intracellular recording of an antidromic action potential at two different sweep speeds. The time derivative is shown in the lower traces. Note the three different components of the action potential. Arrowheads indicate the after-depolarization. (C) Paired antidromic responses at different intervals, superimposed to show the three types of "all-or-none" response. (D) Antidromic response at a slow-sweep speed illustrating the early and late after-hyperpolarization, separated by the arrowhead. (Reproduced from Yarom et al., *Neuroscience* 16, 719–737, 1985, with permission of the authors and publisher.)

levels of the potential. This has the effect of delaying the onset of discharge when vagal neurons are rapidly depolarized from a hyperpolarized level. The activation of this current is both time and voltage dependent and appears to involve a specific potassium channel.

The membrane effects of noradrenaline have been investigated in a slice preparation of the rat brain stem (Fukuda et al., 1987). These studies indicate that an α_1-mediated depolarization of identified vagal neurons is observed in some 55% of neurons. The α_2-receptors appear to mediate a hyperpolarization of membrane potential in approximately 32% of vagal neurons. Of particular importance was the fact that the specific α_2-antagonist, yohimbine, blocked the normal inhibitory influence of focal electrical stimulation of the commissural area of the nucleus tractus solitarius on the activity of these vagal neurons. Since the A2 cell group lies within this area, this suggests that these noradrenergic neurons may be involved in the control of vagal activity (Fukuda et al., 1987).

Similar types of studies have examined the effects of various peptides on dorsal vagal neurons. For example, cholecystokinin octapeptide was shown to cause excitation of rat vagal neurons (Plata-Salamán et al., 1988) and somatostatin 14 to inhibit these cells (Nabekura et al., 1989). This inhibition is caused by a membrane hyperpolarization mediated by an increase in potassium conductance (Nabekura et al., 1989). However, the data derived from one species may not apply to other species. A good example of this is found in a study published by Raggenbass et al. (1987). They found that when oxytocin was applied to rat dorsal vagal neurons it caused excitation. In contrast, oxytocin had no effect on homologous neurons from the guinea pig. This finding underscores the potential problem related to making generalizations based on studies of a single species.

NUCLEUS AMBIGUUS

The nucleus ambiguus lies in the ventrolateral portion of the medullary reticular formation beginning posterior to the facial nucleus and extending caudally to the C1 level of the spinal cord. This nucleus was so named because it lacks distinct cytoarchitectonic borders. Three distinct parts of the nucleus have been recognized: nucleus retrofacialis, nucleus ambiguus, and nucleus retroambigualis, but this distinction is confusing because these terms have been applied arbitrarily by various investigators (see Bieger and Hopkins, 1987 for discussion). Because the three nuclei are continuous with one another, Bieger and Hopkins (1987) have recommended using the term *nucleus ambiguus* to describe the entire cell column. In this chapter, their nomenclature is followed. This column consists of two main parts: (1) a dorsal division that is made up of a longitudinal column of motor neurons innervating the soft palate, pharynx, esophagus, and larynx; and (2) a ventrolateral subdivision that contains parasympathetic preganglionic neurons that innervate the heart and possibly other viscera (Figure 5-1). Each of the subdivisions is organized topographically with regard to the end organs it innervates and the morphological characteristics of the neurons that make up the nucleus; these features are summarized below.

Efferent Projections

The neurons of the nucleus ambiguus or the adjacent reticular formation project to five different targets: (1) vagus nerve (see Hopkins, 1987, for review), (2) cervical and thoracic intermediate gray matter and ventral horn (cat: Feldman et al., 1985; rat: Saether et al., 1987; for review, see Long and Duffin, 1984), (3) parabrachial nucleus (cat: King, 1980), (4) facial nucleus (rabbit: Bystrzycka and Nail, 1983), and (5) nucleus tractus solitarius (cat: Kalia et al., 1979).

After immersion of the cervical vagus nerve of the cat or monkey in HRP, only about 50% of the neurons in the nucleus ambiguus are retrogradely labeled (Hopkins, 1987). Although this result implies that the rest of the neurons project to other levels in the central nervous system or are interneurons, it should be noted that this technique may not label all cells. In addition, these studies were hampered by the fact that the exact cytoarchitectonic borders of the nucleus are extremely difficult to define. Thus, the samples used in these studies may include variable portions of the adjacent reticular formation and so may falsely skew the data.

The dorsal division of the nucleus ambiguus is organized in a viscerotopic fashion with three subdivisions: (1) a rostral group of cells innervates the esophagus, forming a compact group of cells; (2) the intermediate group innervates the pharynx and larynx; and (3) the caudal group innervates the larynx (Figure 5-6).

Each of the regions is made up of motor neurons with their own distinctive dendritic architecture. The rostral part contains closely packed clusters of cells, and dendrites of these cells are organized in special bundles; this area has been termed the "compact" region. The function of these dendritic bundles is unclear, but the region functions in control of swallowing (Bieger, 1984). Activation of these cells may trigger a sequential pattern of activation of other nearby neurons controlling the swallowing reflex. This region also contains the motor neurons that innervate the soft palate (cat: Holstege et al., 1983; van Loveren et al., 1983). The middle portion

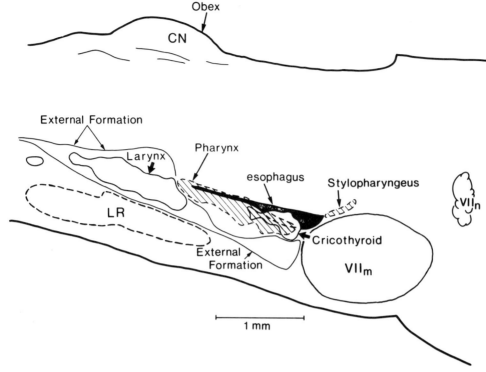

Figure 5-6 Schematic drawing of a parasagittal section of the rat medulla illustrating the topographic organization of vagal motor neurons in the nucleus ambiguus. (Reproduced from Bieger and Hopkins, *Journal of Comparative Neurology* 262, 546–562, 1987, with permission of the authors and publisher.)

of the nucleus is the source of the motor neurons that innervate the middle and inferior pharyngeal constrictor muscles and the cricothyroid muscle. This region has been termed the "semicompact" portion because of the arrangement of the motor neurons. The neurons of the caudal portion innervate the intrinsic laryngeal musculature (with the exception of the cricothyroid muscle). The neurons are spaced relatively far apart, and hence this region has been described as the "loose" portion.

Pulmonary-projecting vagal efferents, which will include those with either secretomotor and bronchomotor function, have been identified in the cat by studying the retrograde transport of HRP (Jordan et al., 1986). They are distributed widely through the full extent of the nucleus ambiguus, particularly within its dorsal extremes and in the "loose" formation more caudally. The greatest density is in the area from 1 mm caudal to 1 mm rostral to the obex, and a particularly dense aggregation is seen at the most rostral levels of the nucleus. Equivalent neurons are found also in less profusion in the dorsal vagal nucleus, but only at levels rostral to the obex. Electrophysiological studies (McAllen and Spyer, 1978a) had earlier described the presence of pulmonary projecting vagal motor neurons in the rostral regions of the nucleus and had distinguished them

also on the basis of their inspiratory discharge pattern. These were considered to have properties indicating a bronchomotor function.

The ventrolateral division of the nucleus ambiguus is the main site of origin of the cardioinhibitory neurons in most mammals (Hopkins, 1987). There is a distinct clustering of cardiac preganglionic cells in this area. Electrophysiological recordings in the cat revealed the same clustering of cardioinhibitory neurons (McAllen and Spyer, 1976).

Vagal Motor Neurons Use Acetylcholine as a Neurotransmitter

In 1921, Loewi reported that a chemical mediator, which he termed Vagusstoff, and was later shown to be acetylcholine, was released in the region of the heart during stimulation of the vagus nerve in frogs and toads. This was the first evidence of chemical transmission in the nervous system and is regarded as one of the most historically important experiments in neurobiology. In a subsequent study, acetylcholine was shown to have an inhibitory action on the heart (Loewi and Navratil, 1926).

Choline acetyltransferase immunoreactive cell bodies are present in the nucleus ambiguus (Houser et al., 1983). Other types of immunoreactive substances are found in the cell bodies of this nucleus and, in all likelihood, are colocalized in the cholinergic neurons. For example, calcitonin gene-related peptide and galanin immunoreactive neurons are found in the nucleus ambiguus and form part of the vagal outflow (Sawchenko et al., 1987). The former group of cells is concentrated within the compact part of the nucleus, and a lesser number were found at the caudal levels of the nucleus ambiguus. The galanin immunoreactive cells are more evenly distributed in the rostrocaudal axis of the nucleus. Whether these cells also synthesize acetylcholine is unknown. Somatostatin cell bodies have also been identified in the area (Finley et al., 1981b) but as yet have not been shown to be part of the vagal outflow.

Afferents to the Nucleus Ambiguus

The nucleus ambiguus, or the intermediate surrounding region of medullary reticular formation of the rat, receives afferents from at least 13 different regions in the brain (Figure 5-7). These include (1) the bed nucleus of the stria terminalis, (2) the substantia innominata, (3) the central nucleus of the amygdala, (4) the paraventricular hypothalamic nucleus, (5) the dorsomedial hypothalamic nucleus, (6) the lateral hypothalamic area, (7) the zona incerta, (8) the posterior hypothalamus, (9) the mesencephalic central gray matter, (10) the mesencephalic reticular formation, (11) the parabrachial nucleus including the Kölliker–Fuse nucleus, (12) the nucleus tractus solitarius, and (13) the medullary reticular formation (ter Horst et al., 1984; see Luiten et al., 1987 for review). Because the nuclear boundaries of this nucleus are ill defined, current tract tracing studies have not established whether the above connections are to the vagal motor neurons, the vagal parasympathetic preganglionic neurons, or the adjacent reticular formation.

Few studies have been directed at studying the inputs to functionally defined regions of the nucleus ambiguus. The cardioinhibitory region of the nucleus ambiguus in the rat has been identified electrophysiologically and injected with HRP (Stuesse and Fish, 1984). On the basis of retrograde cell body labeling, it appears that the major input to this region arises from the medial nucleus of the nucleus tractus solitarius. Smaller numbers of labeled cells were seen in the paraventricular hypothalamus nucleus, medial and lateral parabrachial nuclei, Kölliker–Fuse nucleus, ventrolateral nucleus of the solitary tract, caudal portion of the nucleus ambiguus, and contralateral rostral nucleus ambiguus. A cautionary note should be included: It is not clear from these experiments that all the labeled cells represent cardiovascular neurons because HRP can be taken up by fibers of passage as well as by axon terminals. In

addition, it has not yet been established that specific regions of the nucleus ambiguus are composed of functional unique parasympathetic preganglionic neurons. Some overlap, such as with cardiac and bronchiomotor preganglionic neurons, may exist, which would result in difficulties in interpretation of retrograde cell body labeling patterns.

Two areas in the brain stem project to the rostral part of the nucleus ambiguus containing the motor neurons involved in swallowing: the rostral part of the medial nucleus of the nucleus tractus solitarius and the pontine reticular formation. A small cluster of cells in the medial nucleus of the solitary tract termed the *central subnucleus* projects to the compact region of the nucleus ambiguus—the neurons that innervate the esophagus (Beiger, 1984). This central subnucleus appears to be part of the neural circuitry involved in control of swallowing. Holstege et al. (1983), using the autoradiographic anterograde tracing technique in the cat, described a projection from the pontine reticular formation to the compact portion of the contralateral dorsal nucleus ambiguus (the area containing motor neurons innervating the muscles of the soft palate and pharynx). This area also projects to the contralateral motor trigeminal nucleus in the area innervating the mylohyoid muscle and to the contralateral hypoglossal nucleus to the area innervating the geniohyoid muscle. On the basis of these connections, Holstege et al. (1983) have hypothesized that this area of the pontine reticular formation is a swallowing center.

Two additional neuroanatomical studies have provided evidence of topographic projections to the nucleus ambiguus, although their functions are unclear. Sawchenko et al. (1987) made injections of the plant lectin *Phaseolus vulgaris* leucoagglutinin (PHA-L) into the different rostrocaudal levels of the medial nucleus of the tractus solitarius in the rat and found a topographic pattern of innervation. The rostral part of the medial nucleus of nucleus tractus solitarius projects heavily to the compact formation of nucleus ambiguus (i.e., the region that contains esophageal motor neurons). An injection in the middle part of the medial nucleus at the level of the area postrema results in minimal axonal labeling in the nucleus ambiguus, but labels a dense projection to the nearby region containing the A1 and C1 catecholamine cell groups. Injections into the commissural nucleus result in light labeling in the region of the nucleus ambiguus.

The lateral hypothalamic area projects in a differential fashion to the nucleus ambiguus (ter Horst, 1986). The lateral hypothalamic area lying at the level of the ventromedial hypothalamus nucleus projects heavily to the caudal part of the nucleus ambiguus and A1 region, whereas the anterior part (i.e., anterior to the ventromedial nucleus) projects to the

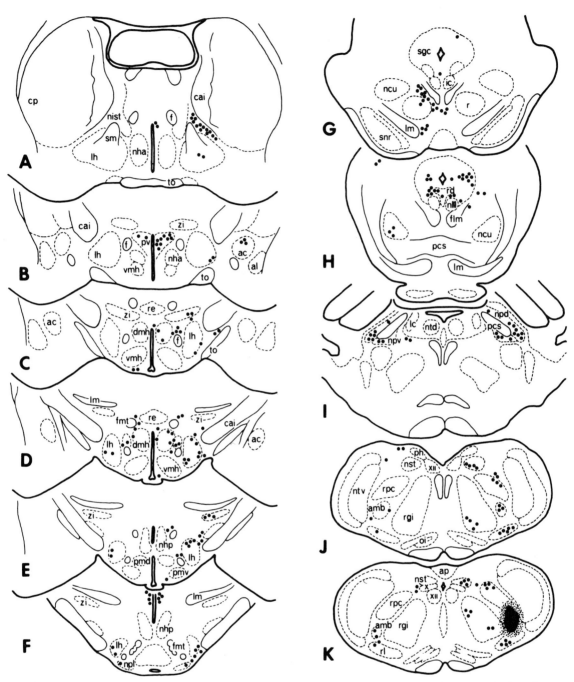

Figure 5-7 Diagrammatic charting of transverse sections from anterior (A) to posterior (K) giving the distribution of HRP-positive somata resulting from an HRP injection in the nucleus ambiguus in the rat. al, lateral amygdaloid nucleus; ac, central amygdaloid nucleus; amb, nucleus ambiguus; ap, area postrema; cai, internal capsule; cp, caudate putamen; dmh, dorsomedial hypothalamic nucleus; flm, medial longitudinal fasciculus; f, fornix; fmt, ; ic, internal capsule; lc, locus coeruleus; lh, lateral hypothalamic area; lm, lateral lemniscus; ncu, cuneiform nucleus; nha, anterior hypothalamic nucleus; nhp, posterior hypothalamic nucleus; nist, interstitial nucleus of stria terminalis; npd, dorsal parabrachial nucleus; npl, lateral mammillary nucleus, pars posterior; npv, ventral parabrachial nucleus; nst, solitary tract nucleus; ntd, dorsal tegmental nucleus; ntdl, dorsal tegmental nucleus, pars lateralis; oi, inferior olivary nucleus; pcs, superior cerebellar peduncle; pmd, dorsal premammillary nucleus; pmv, ventral premammillary nucleus; pv, paraventricular nucleus; rd, dorsal raphe nucleus; re, reunicus thalamic nucleus; rgi, nucleus reticularis gigantocellularis; rl, lateral reticular nucleus; rpc, nucleus reticularis parvocellularis; sgc, substantia grisea centralis; sl, lateral septal nucleus; snr, substantia nigra, pars reticulata; vmh, ventromedial hypothalamic nucleus; zi, zona incerta; X, dorsal motor vagus nucleus. (Reproduced from ter Horst et al., *Journal of the Autonomic Nervous System* 11, 59–75, 1984, with permission of the authors and publisher.)

rostral nucleus ambiguus and C1 cell group. The functional significance of this differential pattern of innervation is unknown.

Neurochemical Classification of Afferents

Although numerous immunohistochemical studies have reported the presence of various putative neurotransmitters in the lower brain stem, only a few have noted the distribution of immunoreactive fibers in the nucleus ambiguus.

Monoamines do not appear to play a prominent role in the innervation of the nucleus ambiguus. Sparse numbers of noradrenergic (Swanson and Hartman, 1975) and a moderate concentration of serotonergic (Steinbusch, 1981) fibers are found in this area of the brain in the rat. There is no evidence of adrenergic (Hökfelt et al., 1974) or histaminergic (Watanabe et al., 1984) fibers. Further, the nucleus ambiguus contains few substance P (Ljungdahl et al., 1978), somatostatin (Finley et al., 1981b), or thyrotropin-releasing hormone (Kubek et al., 1983) immunoreactive fibers.

Peptides from all three of the opioid peptide families (pro-enkephalin, pro-dynorphin, and pro-opiomelanocortin; see Yaksh, 1987 for review) are present in the nucleus ambiguus. Peptide fragments from all three prohormones have been localized immunohistochemically in the rat nucleus ambiguus. Met-enkephalin Arg-Gly-Leu (pro-enkephalin family) immunoreactive fibers and cell bodies are found in the nucleus ambiguus (Fallon and Leslie, 1986). Dynorphin A (1–8) and dynorphin B (pro-dynorphin family) immunoreactive fibers and cell bodies are also found in this area (Fallon and Leslie, 1986). α-neo-endorphin (pro-dynorphin family) immunoreactive fibers are also present in this nucleus (Zamir et al., 1984). Peptides of the pro-opiomelanocortin family are poorly represented. Scant numbers of immunoreactive adrenocorticotropic hormone (Romagnano and Joseph, 1983; Schwartzberg and Nakane, 1983) fibers have been described. Other peptides from the pro-opiomelanocortin group such as β-endorphin (Finley et al., 1981a), α-melanocyte-stimulating hormone (O'Donohue et al., 1979), and β-lipotrophin (Watson et al., 1978) cannot be detected here but are present in the nucleus tractus solitarius.

Physiological Studies of the Nucleus Ambiguus

This section will be restricted to a consideration of the cardiovascular and gastrointestinal role of the nucleus ambiguus. The respiratory and certain aspects of the cardiovascular role of the nucleus are detailed in Chapter 11. An important consideration is the close proximity of the ventrolaterally placed cell groups that are considered to exert such marked influences on autonomic control (see Chapters 9, 10, and 13). Accordingly, much of the literature concerning the effects of electrical stimulation within this area is of little use in attributing function to various components of the nucleus ambiguus.

Some of the earliest observations to indicate a visceromotor function for this nucleus were the result of a study in which Kerr (1969) demonstrated that certain functions could be preserved in situations where the dorsal vagal nucleus had been destroyed. In the cat, the dorsal nucleus was destroyed by electrolytic lesioning and, after allowing a sufficient period of time for degeneration of efferent fibers in the vagus originating here, Kerr was able to demonstrate that bronchomotor, esophageal, duodenal, and cardiac effects could still be elicited from the vagus on electrical stimulation. With regard to bronchomotor control, McAllen and Spyer (1978a) have provided evidence for the presence of neurons in the nucleus ambiguus in the cat that could be antidromically activated on electrical stimulation of pulmonary projecting intrathoracic vagal branches. Further, the widespread distribution of such neurons throughout the nucleus has since been confirmed using the retrograde transport of HRP (Bennett et al., 1981; Jordan et al., 1986). With regard to gastrointestinal function, the question must remain open since it is unlikely that the lesions of the dorsal nucleus would have included the caudal-most regions of the nucleus. Equally, the assessment of degenerative damage was crude when compared with the techniques that are now available. There is now little doubt that in all species the nucleus ambiguus has a major role in cardiomotor control.

Cardiovascular Functions

Cardioinhibitory neurons arise mainly from the ventrolateral subdivision of the nucleus ambiguus (for reviews, see Hopkins, 1987, and Spyer and Jordan, 1987). They appear to form a distinct group of neurons that has a relatively low level of ongoing activity, at least in the anesthetized cat (McAllen and Spyer, 1978a,b), rabbit (Jordan et al., 1982), and rat (Nosaka et al., 1982) and to have axons in the B fiber class. They are powerfully excited by activation of the arterial baroreceptors and when active show a pulse rhythm in their discharge that depends in large part on this input (Figure 5-8). Their ongoing discharge is also patterned by a respiratory-related input (see Chapter 11). A most interesting observation is that those neurons that are normally silent under the conditions of the experiment in the anesthetized animal, and those with ongoing activity, are excited by the iontophoresis of excitatory amino acids and a bradycardia ensues. The fact that a mea-

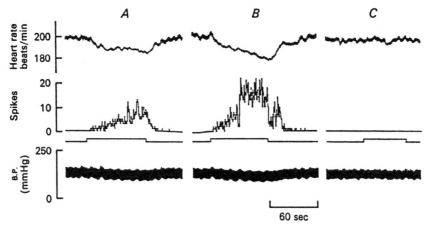

Figure 5-8 Iontophoretic application of an excitatory amino acid onto a cardiovagal neuron in the nucleus ambiguus elicits bradycardia. Traces from top downward: heart rate derived from the arterial pulse, neural activity of a single cardiovagal motor neuron is plotted as spikes in 200-msec bins, event marker showing application of D,L-homocysteic acid (DLH), and lastly femoral arterial blood pressure. (A) The response of cat cardiovagal motor neuron to application of DLH at 60 nA. (B) Response after DLH application at 80 nA. Note the accompanying fall in heart rate and the similarity in time course of the two effects. (C) The effects can be attributed to the influence of DLH, since passing 80 nA of direct current through a micropipette barrel containing a solution of pontamine blue, while recording through the DLH barrel caused no change in neural activity of the cardiovagal motor neuron or heart rate. (Reproduced from McAllen and Spyer, *Journal of Physiology (London)* 282, 353–362, 1978, with permission of the authors and publisher.)

surable decrease in heart rate accompanies the discharge of potentially a single vagal neuron (see McAllen and Spyer, 1978a; Jordan et al., 1982) indicates that these neurons must have a marked divergence among the pool of postganglionic vagal neurons, which also must receive a highly convergent input from several such nucleus ambiguus neurons. This arrangement is highlighted by the relative paucity of specific cardiomotor vagal neurons in the nucleus, and the large number of ganglionic cells (Calaresu and Pearce, 1965). Whether these neurons exert inotropic and dromotropic influences that are independent of their chronotropic influence remains to be resolved. Equally, it is known that different patterns of cardiac response accompany stimulation of the left and right vagi in the dog (Thompson et al., 1987) so that there may be an asymmetric arrangement between the nuclei on each side of the medulla. It is claimed, for instance, that electrical stimulation of the right nucleus ambiguus evokes a pronounced atrial bradycardia while the equivalent stimulus delivered to the left side provokes a ventricular bradycardia (Thompson et al., 1987).

Pharmacology of Cardioinhibitory Neurons

Attempts have been made to determine the pharmacology of the control of the vagal cardioinhibitory neurons of the nucleus ambiguus. These have concentrated on the potential role of γ-aminobutyric acid (GABA), acetylcholine, opioid peptides, and monoamines.

With regard to GABA, there is evidence from microinjection studies that cardioinhibitory neurons are under a tonic GABA-mediated inhibitory control. The injection of the GABA antagonist bicuculline into the nucleus evokes a dose-dependent fall in heart rate in artificially ventilated anesthetized cats (DiMicco et al., 1979), an effect that was reversed by the injection of the GABA agonist muscimol. Also, the microiontophoretic application of GABA onto antidromically identified cardioinhibitory neurons evokes an inhibition that is antagonized by the iontophoretic application of bicuculline (Gilbey et al., 1985). The location of the GABAergic neurons that exert this control has yet to be resolved, but the nucleus ambiguus contains two to three times the GABA content and density of [3H]GABA binding than the surrounding reticular formation (Gale et al., 1980). The potential role of GABA-mediated inhibition in the nucleus ambiguus has been reviewed elsewhere (see Spyer and Jordan, 1987 for review).

The inspiratory related inhibition of cardioinhibitory neurons is not antagonized by the iontophoretic application of either bicuculline or the glycine antagonist strychnine, although the appropriate agonists do indeed inhibit these neurons (Jordan and Spyer, 1987). Conversely, the iontophoretic application of acetylcholine does inhibit these neurons, and this effect is antagonized by the application of atropine, which also blocks the inspiratory-related inhibition (Gilbey et al., 1984, 1985). Whether this implies a direct action of acetylcholine on receptors on the vagal neuron or an action on a local inhibitory interneuron, it does not seem likely that either GABA or glycine can be mediating the influence.

The question of excitatory transmitters is less well

investigated. There is plentiful evidence that cardio-inhibitory neurons are excited by amino acids such as glutamate and D,L-homocysteic acid, but there is not yet any evidence that these have a physiological role. In addition, there is a good evidence that the microinjection of the opioids fentanyl and met-enkephalin amide into the nucleus ambiguus leads to cardiac slowing (see Laubie et al., 1979). These latter studies failed to control for the possibility that the response was a result of inhibition of the descending excitatory pathways that control the sympathetic outflow to the heart. Nevertheless, the nucleus ambiguus has a high density of receptors for [^{3}H]naloxone (Dashwood et al., 1985; Wamsley, 1983). Whether there are opioid-containing neurons innervating the cardio-inhibitory neurons remains unknown.

There is now evidence that the nucleus ambiguus in the cat has a high density of receptors for 5HT and that these have the characteristics of $5HT_{1A}$ subtype (Dashwood et al., 1988a). Further, there is immunocytochemical evidence at both the light and electron microscopic levels for 5HT in the terminal boutons on retrogradely labeled cardioinhibitory neurons (Izzo et al., 1988). The microinjection of 5HT, or specific agonists of the $5HT_{1A}$ receptor into the nucleus ambiguus at sites where excitant amino acids evoke cardiac slowing, shows that these are also effective. Clearly, 5HT alone, or coliberated with another transmitter, is a probable transmitter regulating cardioinhibitory activity.

Gastrointestinal Functions

Few studies have been directed at determining the role of the nucleus ambiguus in gastrointestinal function. Microinjections of glutamate or acetylcholine into the rostral division of the nucleus ambiguus in rats causes contractions of the pharynx and esophagus (Bieger, 1984). This effect could also be produced by microinjections in the nucleus tractus solitarius. The esophageal motor activity elicited in these experiments was blocked by systemic administration of the antimuscarinic drug scopolamine. This drug was probably causing a central cholinergic blockade, because the vagal motor outflow to the esophagus utilizes nicotinic cholinergic receptors.

Microinjections of the GABA receptor antagonist bicuculline in the nucleus ambiguus of the cat causes an increase in gastric smooth muscle activity, and the GABA agonist muscimol produces the opposite effect (Williford et al., 1981). This is a vagally mediated change.

The nucleus ambiguus has been reported to be involved in control of insulin secretion, although the evidence is weak. Increases in plasma insulin occur after microinjections of bicuculline, a GABA antagonist, are made in the ventral medulla of rats in an area that included the nucleus ambiguus (Bereiter et al., 1982). During these experiments, plasma glucose levels did not change, indicating that the responses were not due to a secondary effect of glucose release. Since the rats were given the α-adrenergic blocker phentolamine, the response was thought by these investigators not to be a sympathetically mediated effect. One interpretation of the data presented in this study is that GABA inhibitory interneurons in the nucleus ambiguus control insulin release. It is important, however, to stress that the parasympathetic innervation of the pancreas is derived solely from the dorsal vagal nucleus (Rinnamon and Miselis, 1987). Moreover, since neurons that lie around the nucleus ambiguus project to the dorsal vagal nucleus (see Figure 5-2), it is quite possible that it is these periambigual neurons that were affected by the bicuculline in these experiments.

SUMMARY

Vagal preganglionic parasympathetic neurons lie in the dorsal vagal nucleus and in the region ventrolateral to the nucleus ambiguus. These neurons are cholinergic, although some may contain other neurotransmitters.

The dorsal vagal nucleus lies in the dorsomedial portion of the medulla oblongata, and its neurons provide part of the vagal preganglionic outflow involved in regulating the gastrointestinal tract. Other dorsal vagal neurons innervate the viscera of the head, neck, and thorax. The lateral third of the nucleus innervates the heart, but it is not certain what function these cells serve. The dorsal vagal nucleus receives a wide range of afferent inputs. These come from the cerebral cortex, amygdala, hypothalamus, central gray matter, and lower brain stem. The nucleus plays an important role in regulating gastrointestinal and pancreatic secretions and provides motor commands affecting gastrointestinal motility.

The nucleus ambiguus consists of two major cell columns in the ventrolateral medulla that contribute axons to the vagus nerve. The main group of motor neurons innervates striated muscle in the soft palate, pharynx, larynx, and esophagus and is involved in the control of swallowing as well as vocalization. A second group of preganglionic parasympathetic neurons lies ventrolateral to the main cell column and is the main site of the origin of the cardioinhibitory neurons. This area of the medulla oblongata receives inputs from the forebrain areas, hypothalamus, central gray matter, and lower brain stem. The neurotransmitters involved in the control of the nucleus ambiguus are a matter of current investigation, but few firm conclusions can yet be drawn from the literature, although both GABA and serotonin appear to be strong candidates.

REFERENCES

Reviews

Greenwood, B., and Davison, J. S. (1987). The relationship between gastrointestinal motility and secretion. *American Journal of Physiology* 252, G1–G7.

Hopkins, D. A. (1987). The dorsal motor nucleus of the vagus nerve and the nucleus ambiguus: Structure and connections. In: *Cardiogenic Reflexes*, R. Hainsworth, P. N. McWilliam, and D. A. S. G. Mary (eds.), Oxford University Press, Oxford, pp. 185–203.

Kalia, M. (1981). Brain stem localization of vagal preganglionic neurons. *Journal of the Autonomic Nervous System* 3, 451–481.

Long, S. E., and Duffin, J. (1984). The medullary respiratory neurons: A review. *Canadian Journal of Physiology and Pharmacology* 62, 161–182.

Luiten, P. G. M., ter Horst, G. J., and Steffens, A. B. (1987). The hypothalamus, intrinsic connections and outflow pathways to the endocrine system in relation to the control of feeding and metabolism. *Progress in Neurobiology* 28, 1–54.

Palkovits, M. (1985). Distribution of neuroactive substances in the dorsal vagal complex of the medulla oblongata. *Neurochemistry International* 7, 213–219.

Sawchenko, P. E., Cunningham, E. T., Jr., and Levin, M. C. (1987). Anatomic and biochemical specificity in central autonomic pathways. In: *Organization of the Autonomic Nervous System: Central and Peripheral Mechanisms,* J. Ciriello, F. R. Calaresu, L. P. Renaud, and C. Polosa (eds.), Liss, New York, pp. 267–281.

Solomon, T. E. (1987). Control of exocrine pancreatic secretion. In: *Physiology of the Gastrointestinal Tract,* 2nd edition, L. R. Johnson (ed.), Raven Press, New York, pp. 1173–1207.

Spyer, K. M., and Jordan, D. (1987). Electrophysiology of the nucleus ambiguus. In: *Cardiogenic Reflexes,* R. Hainsworth, P. N. McWilliam, and D. A. S. G. Mary (eds.), Oxford University Press, Oxford, pp. 237–249.

Taché, Y. (1988). CNS peptides and regulation of gastric acid secretion. *Annual Review of Physiology* 50, 19–39.

Wamsley, J. K. (1983). Opioid receptors: Autoradiography. *Pharmacological Reviews* 35, 69–83.

Yaksh, T. (1987). Opioid receptor systems and the endorphins: A review of their spinal organization. *Journal of Neurosurgery* 67, 157–176.

Research Papers

Bennett, J. A., Kidd, C., Latif, A. B., and McWilliam, P. N. (1981). A horseradish peroxidase study of vagal motoneurones with axons in cardiac and pulmonary branches of the cat and dog. *Quarterly Journal of Experimental Physiology* 66, 145–154.

Bereiter, D. A., Berthoud, H. R., Becker, M. J. A., and Jeanrenaud, B. (1982). Brain stem infusion of the gamma aminobutyric acid antagonist bicuculline increases plasma insulin levels in the rat. *Endocrinology* 11, 324–328.

Berk, M. L., and Finkelstein, J. A. (1982). Efferent connections of the lateral hypothalamic area of the rat: An autoradiographic investigation. *Brain Research Bulletin* 8, 511–526.

Bernard, C. (1855–1856). *Leçons de Physiologie* 1 (1855), pp. 288–373.

Bieger, D. (1984). Muscarinic activation of rhombencephalic neurones controlling oesophageal peristalsis in the rat. *Neuropharmacology* 23, 1451–1464.

Bieger, D., and Hopkins, D. A. (1987). Viscerotopic representation of the upper alimentary tract in the medulla oblongata in the rat: The nucleus ambiguus. *Journal of Comparative Neurology* 262, 546–562.

Blessing, W. W., Willoughby, J. O., and Joh, T. H. (1985). Evidence that catecholamine-synthesizing perikarya in rat medulla oblongata do not contribute axons to the vagus nerve. *Brain Research* 348, 397–400.

Bradd, J., Dubin, J., Due, B., Miselis, R. R., Montor, S., Rogers, W. T., Spyer, K. M., and Schwaber, J. (1989). Mapping of carotid sinus inputs and vagal cardiac outputs in the rat. *Society of Neuroscience Abstracts* 15(1), 593..

Bystrzycka, E. K., and Nail, B. S. (1984). The source of the respiratory drive to nasolabialis motoneurones in the rabbit: A HRP study. *Brain Research* 266, 183–191.

Caffe, A. R., and van Leeuwen, F. W. (1983). Vasopressin-immunoreactive cells in the dorsomedial hypothalmic region, medial amygdaloid nucleus and locus coeruleus of the rat. *Cell and Tissue Research* 233, 23–33.

Calaresu, F. R., and Pearce, J. W. (1965). Effects on heart rate of electrical stimulation of medullary vagal structures in the cat. *Journal of Physiology (London)* 176, 241–251.

Champagnat, J., Denavit-Saubie, M., Grant, K., and Shen, K. F. (1986). Organization of synaptic transmission in the mammalian solitary complex studied *in vitro. Journal of Physiology (London)* 381, 551–573.

Charpak, S., Armstrong, W. E., Muhlethaler, M., and Dreifuss, J. J. (1984). Stimulatory action of oxytocin on neurones of the dorsal motor nucleus of the vagus nerve. *Brain Research* 300, 83–89.

Cox, G. E., Dashwood, M. R., Jordan, D., and Spyer, K. M. (1986). An autoradiographic and iontophoretic study of muscarinic receptors in the dorsomedial medulla of the rabbit. *Journal of Physiology (London)* 371, 119P.

Dashwood, M. R., Gilbey, M. P., and Spyer, K. M. (1985). The localization of adrenoceptors and opiate receptors in regions of the cat central nervous system involved in cardiovascular control. *Neuroscience* 15, 537–552.

Dashwood, M. R., Gilbey, M. P., Jordan, D., and Ramage, A. (1988a). Autoradiographic localization of $5HT_{1A}$ binding sites in the brainstem of the cat. *British Journal of Pharmacology* 94(s), P386.

Dashwood, M. R., Muddle, J. R., and Spyer, K. M. (1988b). Opiate receptor subtypes in the nucleus tractus solitarii of the cat: The effect of vagal section. *European Journal of Pharmacology* 155, 85–92.

De Quidt, M. E., and Emson, P. C. (1986). Distribution of neuropeptide Y-like immunoreactivity in the rat central nervous system. II. Immunohistochemical analysis. *Neuroscience* 18, 545–618.

DiMicco, J. A., Gale, K., Hamilton, B., and Gillis, R. A. (1979). GABA receptor control of parasympathetic outflow to the heart: Characterization and brainstem localization. Science 204, 1106–1109.

Fallon, J. H., and Leslie, F. M. (1986). Distribution of dynorphin and enkephalin peptides in the rat brain. *Journal of Comparative Neurology* 249, 293–336.

Feldman, J. L., Loewy, A. D., and Speck, D. F. (1985). Projections from the ventral respiratory group to phrenic and intercostal motoneurons in cat: An autoradiographic study. *Journal of Neuroscience* 5, 1993–2000.

Finley, J. W. C., Lindstrom, P., and Petrusz, P. (1981a). Immunocytochemical localization of beta-endorphin-containing neurons in the rat brain. *Neuroendocrinology* 33, 28–42.

Finley, J. W. C., Maderdrut, J. L., Roger, L. J., and Petrusz, P. (1981b). The immunocytochemical localization of somatostatin-containing neurons in the rat central nervous system. *Neuroscience* 6, 2173–2192.

Fox, E. A., and Powley, T. L. (1985). Longitudinal columnar organization within the dorsal motor nucleus represents separate branches of the abdominal vagus. *Brain Research* 341, 269–282.

Fukuda, A., Minami, T., Nabekura, J., and Oomura, Y. (1987). The effects of noradrenaline on neurons in the rat dorsal motor nucleus of the vagus *in vitro. Journal of Physiology (London)* 393, 213–231.

Gale, K., Hamilton, B. L., Brown, S. C., Norman, W. P., Souza, J. D., and Gillis, R. A. (1980). GABA and specific GABA binding sites in brain nuclei associated with vagal outflow. *Brain Research Bulletin* 5, Suppl. 2, 325–328.

Geis, G. S., and Wurster, R. D. (1980). Cardiac responses during stimulaton of the dorsal motor nucleus and nucleus ambiguus in the cat. *Circulation Research* 46, 606–611.

Gilbey, M. P., Jordan, D., Richter, D. W., and Spyer, K. M. (1984). Synaptic mechanisms involved in the inspiratory modulation of the vagal cardioinhibitory neurons in the cat. *Journal of Physiology (London)* 356, 65–78.

Gilbey, M. P., Jordan, D., Spyer, K. M., and Wood, L. M. (1985). The inhibitory action of GABA on cardiac vagal motoneurons in the cat. *Journal of Physiology (London)* 361, 49P.

Gwyn, D. G., Ritchie, T. C., and Coulter, J. D. (1985). The central distribution of vagal catecholaminergic neurons which project into the abdomen in the rat. *Brain Research* 328, 139–144.

Higgins, G. A., and Schwaber, J. S. (1983). Somatostatinergic projections from the central nucleus of the amygdala to the vagal nuclei. *Peptides* 4, 669–672.

Higgins, G. A., Hoffman, G. E., Wray, S., and Schwaber, J. S. (1984). Distribution of neurotensin-immunoreactivity within baroreceptor portions of the nucleus of the tractus solitarius and the dorsal vagal nucleus of the rat. *Journal of Comparative Neurology* 226, 155–164.

Hökfelt, T. Fuxe, K., Goldstein, M., and Johansson, O. (1974). Immunohistochemical evidence for the existence of adrenaline neurons in the rat brain. *Brain Research* 66, 235–251.

Holstege, G., Graveland, G., Bijker-Biemond, C., and Schuddeboom, I. (1983). Location of motoneurons innervating the soft palate, pharynx, and upper esophagus. Anatomical evidence for a possible swallowing center in the pontine reticular formation. An HRP and autoradio-

graphic tracing study. *Brain, Behavior, and Evolution* 23, 47–62.

Holstege, G., Meiners, L., and Tan, K. (1985). Projections of the bed nucleus of the stria terminalis to the mesencephalon, pons, and medulla oblongata in the cat. *Experimental Brain Research* 58, 379–391.

Hopkins, D. A., and Holstege G. (1978). Amygdaloid projections to the mesencephalon, pons, and medulla oblongata in the cat. *Experimental Brain Research* 32, 529–547.

Houser, C. R., Crawford, G. D., Barber, R. P., Salvaterra, P. M., and Vaughn, J. E. (1983). Organization and morphological characteristics of cholinergic neurons: An immunocytochemical study with a monoclonal antibody to choline acetyltransferase. *Brain Research* 266, 97–119.

Izzo, P. N., Jordan, D., and Ramage, A. (1988). Anatomical and pharmacological evidence supporting the involvement of serotonin in the central control of cardiac vagal motoneurons in the anesthesized cat. *Journal of Physiology (London)* 406, 19P.

Johansson, O., Hökfelt, T., Pernow, B., Jeffcoate, S. L., White, N., Steinbusch, H. W. M., Verhofstad, A. A. J., Emson, P. C., and Spindel, E. (1981). Immunohistochemical support for three putative transmitters in one neuron: Co-existence of 5-hydroxytryptamine, substance P and thyrotropin releasing hormone-like immunoreactivity in medullary neurons projecting to the spinal cord. *Neuroscience* 6, 1857–1881.

Jordan, D., Spyer, K. M., Withington-Wray, D., and Wood, L. M. (1986). Histochemical and electrophysiological identification of cardiac and pulmonary preganglionic neurons in the cat. *Journal of Physiology (London)* 372, 87P.

Kalia, M., Feldman, J. L., and Cohen, M. I. (1979). Afferent projections to the inspiratory neuronal regions of the ventrolateral nucleus of the tractus solitarius in the cat. *Brain Research* 171, 135–141.

Kalia, M., Fuxe, K., Goldstein, M., Harfstrand, A., Agnati, L. F., and Coyle, J. T. (1984). Evidence for the existence of putative dopamine-, adrenaline-, and noradrenaline-containing vagal motor neurons in the brainstem of the rat. *Neuroscience Letters* 50, 57–62.

Kerr, F. W. L. (1969). Preserved vagal visceromotor function following destruction of the dorsal motor nucleus. *Journal of Physiology (London)* 202, 755–769.

Kerr, F. W. L., and Preshaw, R. M. (1969). Secretomotor function of the dorsal motor nucleus of the vagus. *Journal of Physiology (London)* 205, 405–415.

King, G. W. (1980). Topology of ascending brainstem projections to nucleus parabrachialis in the cat. *Journal of Comparative Neurology* 191, 615–638.

Kubek, M. J., Rea, M. A., Hodes, Z. I., and Aprison, M. H. (1983). Quantitation and characterization of thyrotropin-releasing hormone in vagal nuclei and other regions of the medulla oblongata of the rat. *Journal of Neurochemistry* 40, 1307–1313.

Laubie, M., Schmitt, H., and Vincent, M. (1979). Vagal bradycardia produced by microinjections of morphine-like drugs into the nucleus ambiguus in anesthetized dogs. *European Journal of Pharmacology* 59, 287–291.

Laughton, W. B., and Powley, T. L. (1987). Localization of efferent function in the dorsal motor nucleus of the vagus. *American Journal of Physiology* 252, R13–R25.

Loewi, O. (1921). Uber humorale Ubertragbarkeit der Herznervenwirkung. *Pflugers Archives* 189, 239–242. (On the humoral propagation of cardiac nerve action, translated into English by I. Cooke and M. Lipkin, Jr., 1972. *Cellular Neurophysiology. A Source Book.* Holt, New York, pp. 464–466.)

Loewi, O., and Navratil, E. (1926). Uber humorale Ubertragbarkeit der Herznerven wirkung. X. Uber das Schicksal des Vagusstoffs. *Pflugers Archives* 214, 678–688. (On the humoral propagation of cardiac nerve action. X. The fate of the vagus substance, translated into English by I. Cooke and M. Lipkin, Jr., *Cellular Neurophysiology. A Source Book.* Holt, New York, pp. 478–485.)

Loewy, A. D., McKellar, S. and Saper, C. B. (1979). Direct projections from A5 catecholamine cell group to the intermediolateral cell column. *Brain Research* 174, 309–314.

Ljungdahl, A., Hökfelt, T., and Nilsson, G. (1978). Distribution of substance P-like immunoreactivity in the central nervous system of the rat. I. Cell bodies and nerve terminals. *Neuroscience* 3, 861–943.

Luiten, P. G. M., ter Horst, G. J., Karst, H., and Steffens, A. B. (1985). The course of paraventricular efferents to autonomic structures in medulla and spinal cord. *Brain Research* 329, 283–297.

Manier, M., Mouchet, P., and Feuerstein, C. (1987). Immunohistochemical evidence for the coexistence of cholinergic and catecholamine phenotypes in neurones of the vagal motor nucleus in the adult rat. *Neuroscience Letters* 80, 141–146.

McAllen, R. M., and Spyer, K. M. (1976). The location of cardiac vagal preganglionic motoneurons in the medulla of the cat. *Journal of Physiology (London)* 258, 187–204.

McAllen, R. M., and Spyer, K. M. (1978a). Two types of vagal preganglionic motoneurones projecting to the heart and lungs. *Journal of Physiology (London)* 282, 353–364.

McAllen, R. M., and Spyer, K. M. (1978b). The baroreceptor input to cardiac vagal motoneurones. *Journal of Physiology (London)* 282, 365–374.

Middleton, S., Middleton, H. H., and Grundfest, H. (1950). Spike potentials and cardiac effects of mammalian vagus nerve. *American Journal of Physiology* 162, 553–559.

Nabekura, J., Mizuno, Y., and Oomura, Y. (1989). Inhibitory effect of somatostatin on vagal motoneurons in the rat brain stem in vitro. *American Journal of Physiology* 256, C155–C159.

Nosaka, S., Yamamoto, T., and Yasunaga, K. (1979). Localization of vagal cardioinhibitory preganglionic neurons within rat brain stem. *Journal of Comparative Neurology* 186, 79–92.

Nosaka, S., Yamamoto, T., and Tamai, S. (1982). Vagal cardiac preganglionic neurons; distribution, cell types, and reflex discharge. *American Journal of Physiology* 243, R92–R98.

O'Donohue, T. L., Miller, R. L., and Jacobowitz, D. M. (1979). Identification, characterization and stereotaxic mapping of intraneuronal alpha-melanocyte stimulating hormone-like immunoreactive peptides in discrete regions of the rat brain. *Brain Research* 176, 101–123.

Pagani, F. D., Norman, W. P., Kasbekar, D. K., and Gillis, R. A. (1985). Localization of sites within dorsal motor nucleus of vagus that affect gastric motility. *American Journal of Physiology* 249, G73–G84.

Pagani, F. D., Norman, W. P., and Gillis, R. A. (1988). Medullary parasympathetic projections innervate specific sites in the feline stomach. *Gastroenterology* 95, 277–288.

Palkovits, M., Mezery, E., Eskay, R. L., and Brownstein, M. J. (1986). Innervation of the nucleus of the solitary tract and the dorsal vagal nucleus by thyrotropin releasing hormone containing raphe neurons. *Brain Research* 373, 246–251.

Pazos, A., and Palacios, J. M. (1985). Quantitative autoradiographic mapping of serotonin receptors in the rat brain. I. Serotonin-1 receptors. *Brain Research* 346, 205–230.

Plata-Salamán, C., Fukuda, A., Oomura, Y., and Minami, T. (1988). Effects of sulphated cholecystokinin octapeptide (CCK-8) on the dorsal motor nucleus of the vagus. *Brain Research Bulletin* 21, 839–842.

Price, J. L., and Amaral, D. G. (1981). An autoradiographic study of the projectiosn of the central nucleus of the monkey amygdala. *Journal of Neuroscience* 1, 1242–1259.

Raggenbass, M., Dubois-Dauhin, M., Charpak, S., and Dreifuss, J. J. (1987). Neurons in the dorsal motor nucleus of the vagus nerve are excited by oxytocin in the rat but not in the guinea pig. *Proceedings of the National Academy of Sciences USA* 84, 3926–3930.

Rinaman, L., and Miselis, R. R. (1987). The organization of vagal innervation of rat pancreas using cholera toxin-horseradish peroxidase conjugate. *Journal of the Autonomic Nervous System* 21, 109–125.

Rogers, R. C., Kita, H., Butcher, L. L., and Novin, D. (1980). Afferent projections to the dorsal motor nucleus of the vagus. *Brain Research Bulletin* 5, 365–373.

Rogers, R. C., and Hermann, G. E. (1985). Dorsal medullary oxytocin, vasopressin, oxytocin antagonist, and TRH effects on gastric acid secretion and heart rate. *Peptides* 6, 1143–1148.

Romagnano, M. A., and Joseph, S. A. (1983). Immunocytochemical localization of ACTH 1–39 in the brainstem of the rat. *Brain Research* 276, 1–16.

Saether, K., Hilaire, G., and Monteau, R. (1987). Dorsal and ventral respiratory groups of neurons in the medulla of the rat. *Brain Research* 419, 87–96.

Sar, M., Stumpf, W. E., Miller, R. J., Chang, K. J., and Cuatrecasas, P. (1978). Immunohistochemical localization of enkephalin in rat spinal cord. *Journal of Comparative Neurology* 182, 17–38.

Sawchenko, P. E., and Swanson, L. W. (1982). Immunohistochemical identification of neurons in the paraventricular nucleus of the hypothalamus that project to the medulla or to the spinal cord in the rat. *Journal of Comparative Neurology* 205, 260–272.

Schwaber, J. S., Kapp, B. S., Higgins, G. A., and Rapp, P. R. (1982). Amygdaloid and basal forebrain direct connections with the nucleus of the solitary tract and the dorsal motor nucleus. *Journal of Neuroscience* 2, 1424–1438.

Schwartzberg, D. G., and Nakane, P. K. (1983). ACTH-related peptide containing neurons with the medulla oblongata of the rate. *Brain Research* 276, 351–356.

Shapiro, R. E., and Miselis, R. R. (1985). The central organization of the vagus nerve innervating the stomach of the rat. *Journal of Comparative Neurology* 238, 473–488.

Shipley, M. T. (1982). Insular cortex projection to the nucleus of the solitary tract and brain stem visceromotor regions in the mouse. *Brain Research Bulletin* 8, 138–148.

Spencer, S. E., and Talman, W. T. (1986). Modulation of gastric and arterial pressure by nucleus tractus solitarius in rat. *American Journal of Physiology* 250, R996–R1002.

Steinbusch, H. W. M. (1981). Distribution of serotonin-immunoreactivity in the central nervous system of the rat. Cell bodies and terminals. *Neuroscience* 6, 557–618.

Stuesse, S. L. (1982). Origins of cardiac vagal preganglionic fibers: A retrograde transport study. *Brain Research* 236, 15–25.

Stuesse, S. L., and Fish, S. E. (1984). Projections to the cardioinhibitory region of the nucleus ambiguus of rat. *Journal of Comparative Neurology* 229, 271–278.

Swanson, L. W., and Hartman, B. K. (1975). The central adrenergic system. An immunofluorescence study of the location of cell bodies and their efferent connections in the rat utilizing dopamine-beta-hydroxylase as a marker. *Journal of Comparative Neurology* 163, 467–506.

Swanson, L. W., Sawchenko, P. E., Rivier, J., and Vale, W. W. (1983). Organization of bovine corticotropin-releasing factor immunoreactive cells and fibers in the rat brain: An immunohistochemical study. *Neuroendocrinology* 36, 165–186.

ter Horst, G. J. (1986). *The Hypothalamus, Intrinsic Connections and Outflow Pathways to the Pancreas*. University of Groningen, The Netherlands.

ter Horst, G. J., Luiten, P. G. M., and Kuipers, F. (1984). Descending pathways from hypothalamus to dorsal motor vagus and ambiguus nuclei in the rat. *Journal of the Autonomic Nervous System* 11, 59–75.

Thompson, M. E., Felstein, G., Yavorsky, J., and Natelson, B. H. (1987). Differential effect of stimulation of nucleus ambiguus on atrial and ventricular rates. *American Journal of Physiology* 253, R150–R157.

Unnerstall, J. R., Kopajtic, T. A., and Kuhar, M. J. (1984). Distribution of α_2-agonist binding sites in the rat and human central nervous system: analysis of some functional, anatomic correlates of the pharmacologic effects of clonidine and related adrenergic agents, *Brain Research Reviews* 7, 69–101.

Van Charldorp, K. J., De Jonge, A., Davidesko, D., Rinner, I., Doods, H. N., and Van Zwieten, P. A. (1987). Coronary constriction induced by vagal stimulation in the isolated rat heart. *European Journal of Pharmacology* 136, 135–136.

van Loveren, H., Saunders, M. C., and Keller, J. T. (1983). Localization of motoneurons innervating the levator veli palatini muscle in the cat. *Brain Research Bulletin* 11, 303–307.

Versteeg, D. H. G., Van der Gugten, J., DeJong, W., and Palkovits, M. (1976). Regional concentrations of noradrenaline and dopamine in rat brain. *Brain Research* 113, 563–574.

Wamsley, J. K., Lewis, M. S., Young, W. S., and Kuhar, M. J. (1981). Autoradiographic localization of muscarinic cholinergic receptors in the rat brainstem. *Journal of Neuroscience* 1, 176–191.

Watanabe, T., Taguchi, Y., Shiosaka, S., Tanaka, J., Kuboata, H., Terano, Y., Tohyama, M., and Wada, H. (1984). Distribution of the histaminergic neuron system in the central nervous system of rats; a fluorescent immunohistochemical analysis with histidine decarboxylase as a marker. *Brain Research* 295, 13–25.

Watson, S. J., Richard, C. W. III, and Barchas, J. D. (1978). Adrenocorticotropin in rat brain: Immunocytochemical localization in cells and axons. *Science* 200, 1180–1182.

Williford, D. J., Ormsbee, H. S., Norman, W., Harmon, J. W., Garvey, T. Q., DiMicco, J. A., and Gillis, R. A. (1981). Hindbrain GABA receptors influence parasympathetic outflow to the stomach. *Science* 214, 193–194.

Yamazoe, M., Shiosaka, S., Shibasaki, T., Ling, N., Tateishi, K., Hashimura, E., Hamaokaka, T., Kimmel, J. R., Matsuo, H., and Tohyama, M. (1984). Distribution of six neuropeptides in the nucleus tractus solitarii of the rat: An immunohistochemical analysis. *Neuroscience* 13, 1243–1266.

Yarom, Y., Brecha, O., and Werman, R. (1985a). Intracellular injection of acetylcholine blocks various potassium conductances in vagal motoneurons. *Neuroscience* 16, 739–752.

Yarom, Y., Sugimari, M., and Llinas, R. (1985b). Ionic currents and firing patterns of mammalian vagal motoneurons *in vitro*. *Neuroscience* 16, 719–737.

Zamir, N., Palkovits, M., and Brownstein, M. J. (1984). The distribution of immunoreactive alpha neo-endorphin in the central nervous system of the rat. *Journal of Neuroscience* 4, 1240–1247.

Zheng, Z. H., Dietrichs, E., and Walberg, F. (1982). Cerebellar afferent fibres from the dorsal vagal nucleus in the cat. *Neuroscience Letters* 32, 113–118.

6

Central Autonomic Pathways

A. D. LOEWY

Our understanding of the central pathways involved in the control of autonomic functions has been advanced by many technical developments in the neurosciences. In particular, neuroanatomy has undergone a renaissance following the development of highly sensitive techniques for tracing of neural pathways and immunohistochemical methods for the biochemical characterization of neurons. As a result of these advances, a large body of data has been collected regarding the neuroanatomical organization of central autonomic pathways.

The objective of this chapter is to provide an overview of central autonomic pathways with an emphasis on two general principles of organization. First, some central autonomic circuits are organized in the form of reflex arcs to produce highly ordered control of end organ function. Second, other pathways connect to a central CNS autonomic network that is capable of producing widespread autonomic, neuroendocrine, and behavioral responses.

The present discussion will focus almost exclusively on neuroanatomical studies that have been performed on rats. Although it is quite likely that all mammals exhibit similar patterns of neuronal organization, it is premature to make such a broad generalization, because only limited observations exist concerning other mammalian species. The lack of information in nonhuman primates is particularly noteworthy. While it is probable that there are broad parallels in the organization of these pathways across vertebrate lines, further studies will have to address this issue specifically before observations can be extrapolated to humans.

GENERAL ORGANIZATION

In Figure 6-1, the two levels of organization are illustrated schematically showing how some auto-nomic pathways are organized for reflex adjustments of the end organ and others for integrative functions involving more complex changes that affect multiple systems. Reflex pathways involve relatively simple neuronal circuits. For example, most cardiovascular reflexes may involve as few as five neurons. This appears to be the case for both the sympathetic and parasympathetic limbs of the baroreceptor reflex (see Figure 9-9 of Chapter 9). Afferent neurons with endings in specialized pressure-sensitive mechanoreceptors lying in the carotid sinus and aortic arch send information to the nucleus tractus solitarius (NTS). From here, information is sent via interneurons to brain stem neurons that project either directly to the vagal neurons or the sympathetic preganglionic neurons or indirectly via the local interneurons that regulate them. The vagal and sympathetic preganglionic neurons project subsequently to ganglion cells in their respective autonomic ganglia, which in turn innervate specific target tissues. These and other reflexes are considered in more detail in Chapters 9 and 10.

The second general way in which central autonomic pathways are organized is illustrated in Figure 6-1. An ascending NTS projection system carries visceral information that includes taste sensations (a consciously perceived modality) and a spectrum of general visceral sensations (modalities that are not consciously perceived, such as baroreceptor and chemoreceptor information) to a variety of brain stem and forebrain nuclei that integrate this information and, then, command specific autonomic motor and neuroendocrine responses. This central network may also affect certain complex behavioral activities such as those involving food, water, and sodium intake, as well as the pathways that influence other functions by virtue of its connections with the cerebral cortex and limbic system. In essence, this is the critical neural machinery needed to keep an organism functioning within a homeostatic range.

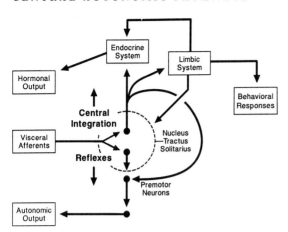

Figure 6-1 Drawing illustrating how visceral afferent information is processed either for reflex responses or as part of a central autonomic circuit that can affect autonomic, hormonal, and behavioral activities.

VISCEROTOPIC PATTERN OF ORGANIZATION IN THE NUCLEUS TRACTUS SOLITARIUS

The nucleus tractus solitarius (NTS) is the major visceral sensory relay cell group in the brain and, as such, it receives inputs from all the major organs of the body. Prior to discussing the organization of this nucleus, some background information is useful. Figure 6-2 presents a schematic drawing of a dorsal view of the medulla oblongata in the rat, illustrating the location of the three major regions of the NTS. Similar zones are recognized in other mammals. The three NTS regions are defined with reference to their position relative to the area postrema: rostral, intermediate, and caudal. These zones do not correspond

exactly with the underlying nuclei but are useful surface landmarks that have been used by investigators as a guide for the placement of electrodes in the NTS.

The NTS is an ovoid shaped nucleus that lies just ventral to the dorsal column nuclei and is composed of a number of different cytoarchitectonic subnuclei. These subnuclei can be classified on the basis of their position relative to the solitary tract into two main groups: medial and lateral. Other subnuclei are especially prominent at the intermediate level and are also defined relative to the solitary tract, which is a central fiber bundle formed by the incoming sensory axons of the VIIth, IXth, and Xth cranial nerves.

The incoming primary visceral afferent fibers that project to the NTS are organized in two ways. The first involves an organ-specific projection pattern to individual NTS subnuclei (Figure 6-3) and the second is subserved by a set of overlapping afferents that project to a common NTS region—the commissural NTS (Figure 6-4). The output of these NTS regions appears to be organized for two modes of responses. The "organ-specific" NTS subnuclei project probably only to specific lower brain stem nuclei that control reflex adjustments of the end organ, but experimental evidence for this is still incomplete. Most, if not all, visceral afferents make connections with other NTS subnuclei besides their main "organ-specific" receptive one. The details of these connections have been studied by Altschuler et al. (1989) and others as well (see review by Jordan and Spyer, 1986, and discussion below). One NTS area in particular is unique in that it receives inputs from all of the major visceral systems except those related to the pelvic organs; this region is the commissural nucleus, and its rostral continuation is the medial

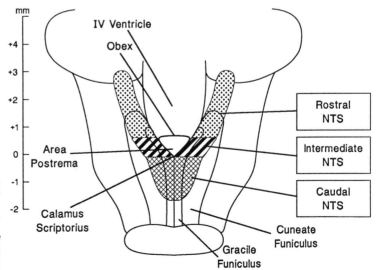

Figure 6-2 Schematic drawing of the dorsal medulla illustrating three zones of the nucleus tractus solitarius. [Modified from an illustration published by Zanberg, P., and deJong, W. (1980). In: *Arterial Baroreceptor and Hypertension*, P. Sleight, (ed.), Oxford University Press, Oxford, pp. 436–442.]

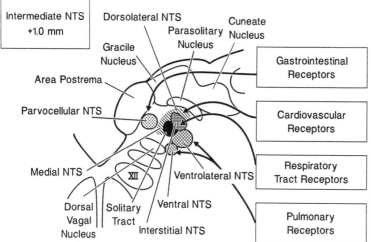

Figure 6-3 Drawing showing the viscerotopic pattern of innervation of the nucleus tractus solitarius. This drawing illustrates the nucleus tractus solitarius of the cat in the transverse plane and the number given indicates the distance from the obex. The nomenclature used follows that presented by Loewy and Burton (1978).

NTS subnucleus.[1] Thus, visceral afferents from the cardiovascular, respiratory, and gastrointestinal systems project in an overlapping, and possibly convergent fashion, to neurons in the commissural-medial NTS region.

Although there is no physiological evidence to support the idea that individual neurons in the commissural-medial NTS receive convergent inputs from the different organ systems, it is well documented that the neurons in this region contribute most of the axons that project to forebrain areas. This pathway forms the ascending link to the central autonomic network. Although unproven, it is highly probable that this ascending projection system is organized in a viscerotopic fashion. Some NTS neurons, especially those in the rostral part of the medial

[1]The commissural and medial NTS regions have often been considered as separate subnuclei, however, it is clear from cytoarchitectonic (Loewy and Burton, 1978) and connectional studies (Ricardo and Koh, 1978) that these two regions are essentially the same.

NTS, relay taste information along specific neural lines to forebrain nuclei. Other cells in the commissural nucleus relay cardiovascular information along similar neural pathways to some of the same forebrain areas, but to functionally different areas within some of the same cell groups.

A hypothesis that will be developed in the remainder of this section is that the incoming sensory fibers carrying visceral sensations are organized in a viscerotopic fashion with two modes of fiber sorting in the NTS: one is involved in reflex modification of the end organs, and the other contributes to an ascending pathway responsible for more complex integrative functions. The two following sections will further elaborate this idea.

Taste Pathways

The central gustatory pathways are organized at two levels of complexity. The first controls reflex func-

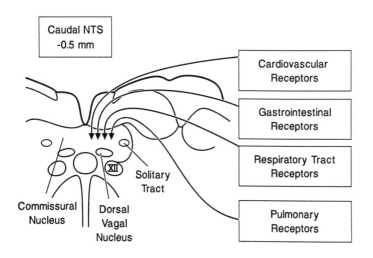

Figure 6-4 Drawing illustrating a common site of projection for various visceral afferents in the nucleus tractus solitarius in the cat. As explained in the text, it is not yet certain whether this common area of projection receives overlapping projections or whether the fibers carrying different visceral modalities converge on specific commissural-medial NTS neurons. The number indicates the position relative to the obex.

tions and the second subserves integrative activities. The reflex functions involve NTS projections to lower brain stem nuclei that provide the motor output for chewing, swallowing, and salivation. The rostral NTS receives gustatory inputs (see below) and projects to the perinuclear zones of the medullary motor nuclei controlling chewing and swallowing (Norgren, 1978; Travers, 1988; Travers and Norgren, 1983). In rats, this lower brain stem circuitry appears to be the minimal set of neural components needed for selection or rejection of food substances because these functions have been shown to be preserved in midbrain transected rats (Grill, 1980). However, the neural circuitry controlling swallowing involves forebrain sites as well and, in certain mammals, these areas may play a more critical role (see Jean, 1984, for review).

Gustatory Afferents

Taste afferents arise from four main gustatory receptor fields: (1) fungiform papillae on the anterior two-thirds of the tongue, (2) circumvallate and foliate papillae on the posterior one-third of the tongue, (3) soft palate region, and (4) laryngeal surface of the epiglottis. Each of these areas is innervated by a specific gustatory nerve that transmits sensory infor-

mation to a specific zone in the rostral portion of the NTS (Figure 6-5). The chorda tympani, a branch of the VIIth nerve, innervates taste buds on the anterior two-thirds of the tongue. The greater petrosal nerve, another branch of the VIIth nerve, innervates taste buds on the roof of the oral cavity. The cell bodies of both of these nerves lie in the geniculate ganglion. Taste receptors located on the posterior one-third of the tongue are innervated by the lingual branch of the IXth nerve. This nerve originated from cell bodies that lie in the petrosal ganglion. The superior laryngeal branch of the Xth cranial nerve innervates the taste receptors on the epiglottis. The cell bodies forming this nerve lie in the nodose ganglion (see Norgren, 1984, for review).

The central axonal processes of the gustatory nerves terminate in a viscerotopic pattern in the rostral NTS (Figure 6-5). VIIth nerve fibers synapse in the rostral-most pole of the NTS. The two branches of the VIIth nerve—the chorda tympani and greater petrosal nerve—have overlapping areas of termination. The IXth and Xth nerves project to the NTS area immediately caudal to this region. Somatosensory fibers from the oral cavity also project to the rostral NTS and terminate in the same area as the gustatory afferents (Hamilton and Norgren, 1984).

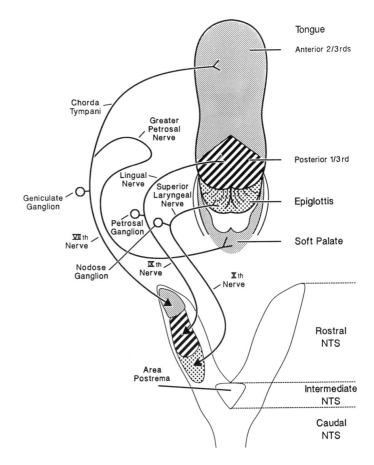

Figure 6-5 Schematic drawing illustrating the gustatory sensory nerves and their central sites of termination in the nucleus tractus solitarius.

Central Projections of Taste Region of the NTS

The ascending gustatory NTS pathway projects to pontine, diencephalic, and telencephalic centers. In particular, the NTS projects heavily to the medial parabrachial nucleus in a restricted area that has been called the pontine taste area; this region serves as a secondary relay center for taste afferent information. The ascending gustatory pathways arising from the rostral NTS and the medial parabrachial nucleus give rise to parallel pathways that project to the diencephalon and telencephalon. One part of this parallel pathway synapses in the ventroposterior thalamic nucleus. Both the NTS and the parabrachial neurons that comprise this projection arise from neurons that are immunoreactive for cholecystokinin, enkephalin, neurotensin, somatostatin, and substance P (Mantyh and Hunt, 1984). The ventroposterior thalamic area relays information to the taste region of the cerebral cortex (see Chapter 12). In addition, the ascending taste NTS pathway also projects to the lateral hypothalamic area, the paraventricular hypothalamic nucleus, the central nucleus of the amygdala, the bed nucleus of the stria terminalis, and the substantia innominata (Norgren, 1984). Similar projections arise from the medial parabrachial region (Saper and Loewy, 1980). These forebrain areas are involved in complex aspects of food intake, but the details regarding their functions are sketchy. However, pharmacological studies have implicated both the lateral and paraventricular hypothalamic areas as regulatory sites for the control of uptake of specific types of food, but the neuronal sources for chemically coded messages are unknown (see Leibowitz, 1986, for review).

General Visceral CNS Pathways

The NTS receives specific information from various visceral organs. Afferent fibers from cardiovascular, pulmonary, respiratory tract, and gastrointestinal receptors project to specific areas in the NTS (Figure 6-3; see Jordan and Spyer, 1986, for review). Afferents from air passages (pharynx, larynx, trachea, bronchi) project mainly to the interstitial NTS, cardiovascular afferents are sent predominantly to the dorsolateral NTS, pulmonary receptors terminate in the ventral and ventrolateral NTS, and gastric afferents synapse heavily in the parvocellular NTS (also termed subgelatinosa or subpostrema NTS), whereas the commissural-medial NTS region receives inputs from all of these ograns (Kalia and Mesulam, 1980; Altschuler et al., 1989). Whether the individual neurons lying in the commissural-medial NTS receive convergent or overlapping inputs has not yet been established (Figure 6-4). Nevertheless, these two modes of fiber sorting within individual NTS sub-

nuclei and a common recipient area lend support for the main thesis of this chapter: certain afferents may function as part of the neural circuitry for reflex responses whereas others serve to transmit visceral information to higher neural centers for more integrated responses.

Cardiovascular Afferents

Cardiovascular afferents arising from the heart and great vessels project to specific NTS areas. For example, the carotid sinus and aortic depressor nerves that transmit high-pressure baroreceptor and chemoreceptor afferent information project to three NTS areas: (1) the dorsolateral NTS, (2) the medial NTS, (3) the commissural nucleus (see Housley et al., 1987, for a recent research report). The baro- and chemoreceptor projections overlap in the medial and commissural NTS, although baroreceptor fibers terminate in a more highly restricted area of the medial NTS than the chemoreceptor afferents (Czachurski et al., 1988). Cardiac afferents terminate in the lateral NTS, with lighter projections to the medial and commissural NTS (Kalia and Mesulam, 1980). It is still not certain how this cardiovascular afferent information is processed within the NTS, and the role of the individual NTS nuclei that receive cardiovascular afferents also needs to be elucidated. However, the output from the commissural-medial NTS is directed, in part, to brain stem and hypothalamic nuclei that project directly to the sympathetic preganglionic neurons, as well as to other CNS regions of the autonomic network (see below).

Respiratory Tract Afferents

Vagal afferents originating from receptors in the trachea, larynx, and bronchi project to the interstitial, ventrolateral, medial, and commissural NTS, with the densest projection found in the interstitial NTS (see Figures 3D and E, 5D, and 7D of Kalia and Mesulam, 1980). These afferents may function to control the motor activity of the respiratory tree and regulate mucus secretion (see Widdicombe, 1982 for review). Although the details of this circuitry are unknown, it is reasonable to hypothesize that the interstitial NTS region projects directly or indirectly to the vagal nuclei controlling the mucous glands and the muscle tone in the airway passages.

Pulmonary Afferents

Lung afferents project to the ventrolateral, ventral, medial, and commissural NTS (Kalia and Mesulam, 1980). Two classes of mechanoreceptor afferents have been described: slowly and rapidly adapting lung stretch afferents (see Chapter 10 for discussion). On the basis of intracellular recordings made in the NTS of the cat, it has been suggested that the slowly adapting lung stretch receptor afferents make monosynaptic connections with a specific type of respiratory neurons in the ventrolateral NTS called *inspiratory β-NTS neurons*. These cells increase their neural activity during inspiration and project to the phrenic respiratory motor neurons (Backman et al., 1984; Berger and Dick, 1987). In contrast, rapidly adapting lung receptor afferents project mainly to the commissural and medial NTS and may subserve different pulmonary functions than the direct modulation of respiratory motor neurons (Davies and Kubin, 1986).

Gastrointestinal Afferents

Gastrointestinal afferents terminate in the parvocellular NTS, but some fibers also project to the medial and commissural NTS (Gwyn et al., 1985; Leslie et al., 1982; Shapiro and Miselis, 1985). A viscerotopographic organization for the upper alimentary tract has been demonstrated (Altschuler et al., 1989). Similarly, afferents carried in the subdiaphragmatic part of the vagus nerve project to discrete regions of the parvocellular NTS; hepatic afferents project dorsal and medial to the gastric afferents (Rogers and Hermann, 1980; Shapiro and Miselis, 1985).

The gastrointestinal receptors provide information necessary for sodium and water balance and for general metabolism. In addition, the liver itself may possess specialized sodium, glucose, and osmolality sensitive receptors (see Lautt, 1980 for review). Portal vein receptors monitor plasma sodium concentration and osmolarity (Contreras and Kosten, 1981). Glucose receptors in the small intestine transmit information via the vagus nerve to the NTS; this is thought to serve as an important link for the central mechanisms that control carbohydrate metabolism (see Niijima and Mei, 1987, for review; see also Chapter 16).

Convergence of General Visceral Afferents

Afferents from thoracic and abdominal viscera converge on neurons in the commissural-medial NTS, thus providing information regarding the physiological state of major visceral organs. This information is then transmitted via the ascending NTS pathways to a CNS autonomic network to produce a broad range of autonomic, endocrine, and behavioral effects.

CENTRAL AUTONOMIC NETWORK

The NTS receives a variety of sensory inputs. Some of these come from autonomic sensory nerves that project directly to the nucleus, others involve multisynaptic ascending spinal pathways as well as projections from various nuclei of the brain, and still other inputs come from the area postrema, which is a circumventricular organ and functions as a sensor of the chemical environment of the plasma and of the cerebrospinal fluid (Figure 6-6; see also Chapter 14). This information is processed and used to affect a number of autonomic, neuroendocrine, and behavioral functions. Thus, it is not surprising that the NTS projects to a number of key nuclei in the lower

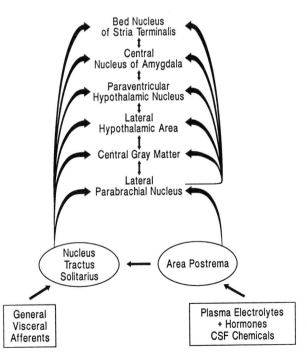

Figure 6-6 Drawing showing how afferent information from the internal environment of the body is transmitted in the central autonomic network of the brain.

brain stem that regulate the autonomic preganglionic neurons of the sympathetic and vagal systems as well as projecting to forebrain nuclei in the central autonomic network that are capable of regulating both autonomic and neuroendocrine functions. This network also provides connections to limbic and neocortical areas and quite probably affects behavioral and cognitive functions. In this section, the discussion will focus on anatomical and physiological data that support this concept.

Central Projections of the NTS

The ascending NTS pathways illustrated in Figures 6-7 and 6-8 are based on the anatomical studies of Beckstead et al. (1980), Loewy and Burton (1978), Norgren (1978), and Ricardo and Koh (1978). These ascending projections transmit a wide range of visceral information to the forebrain nuclei. For example, baroreceptor and chemoreceptor information reaches the central nucleus of the amygdala (Cecchetto and Calaresu, 1985) and paraventricular hypothalamic nucleus (Ciriello and Calaresu, 1980). Some of these NTS pathways also project to forebrain nuclei that regulate the release of vasopressin, especially the median preoptic nucleus (see Chapters 13 and 14). Other NTS pathways transmit osmoreceptor signals to the paraventricular hypothalamic nucleus, lateral hypothalamic area, and zona incerta (Kobashi and Adachi, 1988). Other fibers in this pathway most likely affect ingestive functions.

The commissural NTS is the main medullary site that receives general visceral sensations via the IXth and Xth cranial nerves and transmits this information to the pontine, mesencephalic, and forebrain cell groups that control the autonomic and neuroendocrine systems. This area also receives afferent inputs from the spinal cord, brain stem, forebrain, and cerebral cortex. Spinal inputs originate from neurons in the laminae I, V, and X and project mainly to the commissural nucleus (Menetrey and Basbaum, 1987). This ascending pathway may carry both somatic and visceral afferent information and represent an important sensory linkage whereby both visceral and somatic information from both the internal and external environments of the body may be transmitted to higher neural centers for autonomic and endocrine responses (see Chapter 7). Similarly, the spinal trigeminal nucleus, which receives somatic afferents from the head, the tongue, the soft palate, and the pharynx, also projects to the NTS (Menetrey and Basbaum, 1987).

The commissural NTS is reciprocally connected to a number of CNS cell groups that provide direct inputs to sympathetic and vagal preganglionic neurons. These reciprocal connections may function as a feedback mechanism. The reciprocally linked regions include the A5 cell group, caudal raphe nuclei, rostral ventrolateral medulla, central gray matter, and paraventricular and lateral hypothalamic areas (Loewy et al., 1979, 1986; Thor and Helke, 1987, 1988; Luiten et al., 1985; also see review by Luiten et al., 1987; see Fig. 6-10). Other forebrain centers that are reciprocally connected to the NTS

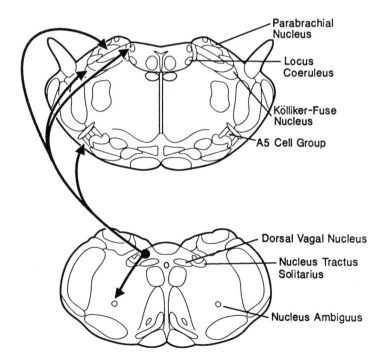

Parabrachial Nucleus

Locus Coeruleus

Kölliker-Fuse Nucleus

A5 Cell Group

Dorsal Vagal Nucleus

Nucleus Tractus Solitarius

Nucleus Ambiguus

Figure 6-7 Drawing illustrating the nucleus tractus solitarius projections to the lower brain stem.

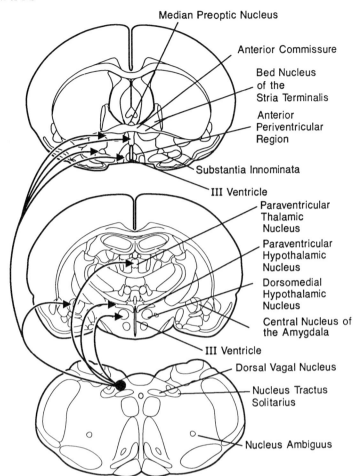

Figure 6-8 Drawing illustrating the nucleus tractus solitarius projections to the forebrain.

like the central amygdaloid nucleus, bed nucleus of the stria terminalis, and insular cortex seem to project mainly to the dorsal vagal nucleus, and thus influence the vagal outflow to the gastrointestinal system (Hopkins and Holstege, 1978; Holstege et al., 1985).

Parabrachial Nucleus:
A Source of Ascending Forebrain Pathways
That Parallels the NTS Pathways

The parabrachial nucleus is a second major brain stem relay center for visceral information. Its major afferents arise from specific regions in the NTS (Herbert et al., 1989). The gustatory region of the NTS projects to the medial parabrachial nucleus, the general visceroreceptive portion of the NTS projects to the lateral parabrachial area, and the respiratory part of the NTS projects to the ventral parabrachial nucleus (Kölliker–Fuse nucleus). As would be predicted, the medial and lateral parabrachial nuclei project in topographic fashion to higher areas of the brain. These connectional patterns are summarized

later. In contrast, the ventral parabrachial nucleus is part of a network in the lower brain stem that controls respiration (Caille et al., 1981). It must be recognized that this scheme is an oversimplification. Each of the parabrachial regions possesses many individual subnuclei with unique afferent and efferent connections. More detailed discussions of the ascending projections of the parabrachial nucleus can be found in Saper and Loewy (1980), Fulwiler and Saper (1984), Moga and Gray (1985), and Herbert et al. 1990).

Although the pathways arising from the lateral parabrachial nucleus are thought to function mainly in the control of autonomic and neuroendocrine responses, it is clear that more complex functions may be effected because this region provides direct and indirect connections with the cerebral cortex. One major linkage to the cerebral cortex occurs via pathways that project to the intralaminar thalamic nuclei, which include the parafascicular, the paracentral, and the central lateral thalamic nuclei. The parabrachial–thalamic pathway may influence cortical functions in a highly selective way because the parafascicular thalamic nucleus projects to the frontal cortex and the paracentral and central lateral thalamic nuclei project to the parietal areas of the cerebral cortex. The lateral parabrachial nucleus also has connections with the centromedial thalamic nucleus, which, in turn, projects to the cingulate and anterior limbic areas. It also projects to the paraventricular thalamic nucleus, which may produce widespread alterations in cortical function. Apart from these indirect pathways, the medial parabrachial nucleus provides direct projections to the frontal, infralimbic, and insular regions of the cerebral cortex (Saper and Loewy, 1980; see also Chapter 12).

One area in the lateral parabrachial nucleus, which is made up of cholecystokinin immunoreactive and/or calcitonin gene-related peptide immunoreactive neurons (Fulwiler and Saper, 1985; Shimada et al., 1985), projects predominantly to the ventromedial hypothalamic nucleus and may be part of the major ascending pathways affecting food intake since this hypothalamic nucleus has clearly been shown to regulate food intake (Shimizu et al., 1987).

The lateral parabrachial nucleus also projects to (1) the zona incerta, (2) the lateral hypothalamic area, (3) the paraventricular hypothalamic nucleus, (4) the substantia innominata, (5) the median preoptic nucleus, (6) the central nucleus of the amygdala, and (7) the bed nucleus of the stria terminalis (Fulwiler and Saper, 1984). These ascending projections parallel those that arise from the commissural-medial NTS. Undoubtedly, this region is involved in the processing of general visceral information.

The medial parabrachial nucleus, an area thought to be involved in gustatory functions, projects to a number of the forebrain sites such as the ventroposterior thalamic nucleus, zona incerta, central nucleus of the amygdala, bed nucleus of the stria terminalis, and infralimbic cortex. The higher centers involved in processing gustatory information are discussed in Chapter 12.

LOCUS COERULEUS

The locus coeruleus (A6 cell group) is a group of noradrenergic neurons located in the dorsolateral pons that projects in a highly divergent pattern throughout the entire CNS (Jones and Yang, 1985 as well as others). As a result, it has been implicated in almost every brain function that is known. In contrast to its extensive efferent projections, the afferents to the locus coeruleus originate from two sites in the medulla oblongata: the nucleus prepositus hypoglossi and the rostral ventrolateral medulla (Aston-Jones et al., 1986; Ennis and Aston-Jones,

1986, 1987), with the latter region being a site strongly implicated as a cardiovascular control center (see Chapter 9).

The function of the locus coeruleus is unknown, but a variety of views have been presented (see reviews by Aston-Jones, 1985; Aston-Jones et al., 1984; Foote et al., 1983). One idea that has emerged is that the locus coeruleus acts as a relay center that monitors afferent information from both the external and the internal environment and that the level of activity of its neurons covaries with different stages of the sleep–wakefulness cycle. Locus coeruleus neurons fire at a higher rate during the waking state and at a progressively slower rate during deeper stages of sleep (see Chapter 20). During paradoxical non-REM sleep, almost all neuronal activity in the locus coeruleus neurons ceases (Aston-Jones, 1985). However, the firing patterns of these cells are more complex than simple neuronal indicators of the state of consciousness. During different behavioral conditions such as grooming or drinking, locus coeruleus neurons decrease their ongoing neural activity (Aston-Jones, 1985). This activity is not simply related to arousal level; it tends to correlate more directly with the level of vigilance or surveillance of the external environment (Aston-Jones, 1985). However, the locus coeruleus neurons also receive afferent information via multisynaptic pathways from a wide variety of different internal receptors such as the splanchnic, pelvic, and vagal nerves (Elam et al., 1984, 1986; Svensson and Thoren, 1979).

Microinjections of L-glutamate into the locus coeruleus of rats cause a decrease in blood pressure and heart rate, which is eliminated by local 6-hydroxydopamine injections (Sved and Felsten, 1987). Although these experiments may be interpreted as evidence that the locus coeruleus neurons are part of the central autonomic network, this view still must be tempered because it is unclear which CNS nucleus is responsible for the response. Since the locus coeruleus does not project directly to the autonomic preganglionic nuclei like the intermediolateral cell column, the vagal preganglionic neurons (Jones and Yang, 1985), or the NTS (Thor and Helke, 1987), there is no straightforward way to explain the anatomical basis of this response unless it produces changes via indirect pathways. For example, its ascending projections to the lateral hypothalamic area and to the bed nucleus of stria terminalis (Jones and Yang, 1985)—two areas implicated in the central autonomic control—may be the critical links in this circuit. Although it is highly speculative, it is possible that activation of the locus coeruleus causes cardiovascular changes due to excitation or inhibition of these two central sites.

FOREBRAIN AUTONOMIC NUCLEI

Several forebrain nuclei, including the paraventricular hypothalamic nucleus (PVH), lateral hypothalamic area, central nucleus of the amygdala, and bed nucleus of the stria terminalis have been implicated as nuclei that are part of a central autonomic circuit. These nuclei are reciprocally connected to the NTS and the parabrachial nucleus. In addition, the two hypothalamic nuclei project both to the dorsal vagal preganglionic neurons and to sympathetic preganglionic neurons, whereas the latter two nuclei project to the dorsal vagal preganglionic neurons. In fact, these nuclei form an interconnected network. Unfortunately, our knowledge of the specific functions of most of these nuclei is primitive. Because so few studies have been done, it is difficult to provide more than cursory comments about each of them. Nevertheless, a brief catalog of our current knowledge is useful.

The PVH is composed of several functionally distinct subnuclei that affect both endocrine and autonomic responses (see Chapter 13 and Swanson, 1987, for review). Specific sets of PVH neurons contain peptides involved in anterior and pituitary regulation, and other neurons are involved in autonomic control. Some PVH neurons contain corticotropin-releasing hormone, which acts via the hypophysial portal system to regulate ACTH release from the anterior pituitary. Other PVH neurons release vasopressin into the vascular system. Still others give rise to descending autonomic pathways to the brain stem and spinal cord, which are illustrated in Figure 6-9.

The descending PVH pathway projects to the central gray matter, locus coeruleus, parabrachial nucleus, NTS, dorsal vagal nucleus, nucleus ambiguus and intermediolateral cell column (Luiten et al., 1985). Although all of these areas have been implicated in autonomic control, it is not clear what functions are regulated by the descending PVH pathways. Anatomical evidence suggests that the PVH is one of a few places in the brain that regulates the entire sympathetic outflow (Strack et al., 1989b). However, the control appears not to be uniform. For example, microinjections of L-glutamate in the PVH evoke an increase in adrenal nerve activity and a decrease in renal nerve activity and blood pressure (Katafuchi et al., 1988). In addition, the PVH has also been linked to control of food intake because lesions and injections of various peptides into this nucleus cause overeating and obesity in rats (Leibowitz et al., 1981; Leibowitz, 1986 for review). It is likely that there are multiple chemically coded neurons in the PVH that regulate a large variety of autonomic and visceral functions.

The amygdala has been implicated in a wide range of autonomic, neuroendocrine, and behavioral functions (see review by Price et al., 1987). This area of the brain is made up of heterogeneous collections of neurons with a variety of inputs and outputs. The bulk of the neuroanatomical evidence favors the view that the central nucleus of the amygdala is involved in processing autonomic information. This conclusion has been derived from anatomical studies that have revealed that the central nucleus of the amygdala receives dense inputs from the NTS (Ricardo and Koh, 1978; Norgren, 1978) and from the parabrachial nucleus (e.g., Saper and Loewy, 1980), as well as a number of other areas (Russchen, 1982). It also projects to a number of key nuclei known to be involved in autonomic processing such as the lateral hypothalamic area, central gray matter, and autonomic nuclei of the lower brain stem (Hopkins and Holstege, 1978; Krettek and Price, 1978; Price and Amaral, 1981; Wallace et al., 1989). The projections to the lower brain stem arise from separate cells within the central nucleus of the amygdala (Thompson and Cassell, 1989), and some project directly to the C1 adrenergic neurons that have been implicated in vasomotor control (Cassell and Gray, 1989; see Chapter 9). The descending central amygdaloid projections to the lower brain are illustrated in Figure 6-10; the projections are predominantly to autonomic centers such as the parabrachial nucleus, NTS, and vagal motor nuclei. In addition, the central nucleus of the amygdala also projects to the dopamine neurons of the substantia nigra and of the ventral tegmental area—areas in which it may subserve motor functions and possibly other functions as well (Wallace et al., 1989).

Since the central nucleus of the amygdala receives direct inputs from the orbital, frontal, and insular regions of the cerebral cortex, areas implicated in autonomic function (see Chapter 12), and indirect cortical connections via interamygdaloid projections arising from the lateral amygdaloid nucleus, which receives inputs from the sensory areas of the cerebral cortex, it is most likely that a wide range of convergent information modulates the activity of these neurons (see Price et al., 1987, for review). Although the inputs from the lower brain stem nuclei, such as those to the parabrachial nucleus and the NTS, most surely transmit autonomic information, the function of the other inputs may subserve motor functions.

The physiological data published to date have not provided insight into the functions of this nucleus (see Chapter 19). Although single units related to taste and to cardiovascular functions have been recorded in the central nucleus (Azuma et al., 1984; Cechetto and Calaresu, 1985), we are currently in

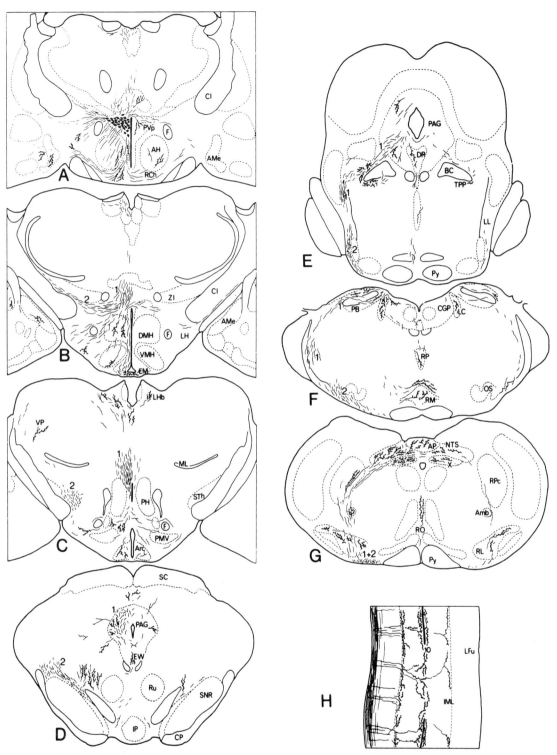

Figure 6-9 Series of drawings illustrating the descending projections arising from the paraventricular hypothalamic nucleus. AH, anterior hypothalamic nucleus; Amb, nucleus ambiguus; AP, area postrema; Arc, arcuate nucleus; DMH, dorsomedial hypothalamic nucleus; DR, dorsal raphé; LHb, lateral habenula; LL, lateral lemniscus; NTS, solitary tract nucleus; PAG, periaqueductal grey; PVp, parvocellular paraventricular nucleus; RL, lateral reticular nucleus; RM, raphé magnus; RO, raphé obscuris; RP, raphé pontis; RPc, parvocellular reticular nucleus; TPP, pedunculo-pontine tegmental nucleus; X, dorsal motor vagus nucleus; 10, layer 10 of Rexed. (Reproduced from Luiten et al., 1985, with permission of the authors and publisher.)

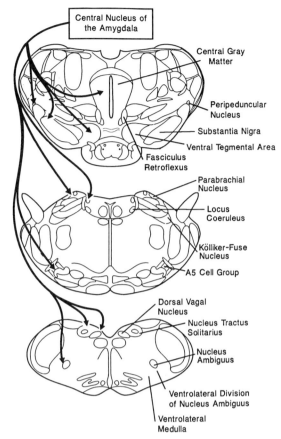

Figure 6-10 Series of drawings showing the descending projections from the central nucleus of the amygdala that innervate the brain stem.

the position of knowing almost nothing about the function(s) of this nucleus. Similar problems exist for the bed nucleus of the stria terminalis, another forebrain nucleus that has inputs and outputs similar to the central nucleus of the amygdala (Weller and Smith, 1982; Holstege et al., 1985). For the lateral hypothalamic area, more information exists, which has been reviewed by Swanson (1987); but, as he points out, many of the techniques employed to study this area fail to provide definitive evidence. Thus, particular functions attributed to the lateral hypothalamic area may not really be due to the neurons of the lateral hypothalamic area as opposed to neural pathways that project through this area. To avoid this problem, Spencer et al. (1989) made microinjections of L-glutamate in the lateral hypothalamic area of rats and showed that this caused a decrease in blood pressure, heart rate, and cardiac output. The two latter changes were mediated by both parasympathetic and β-adrenergic mechanisms.

RECIPROCAL CONNECTIONS

As mentioned earlier in the chapter, a general feature of the central autonomic network is the reciprocal nature of its connections. Almost every CNS site that receives an NTS input also sends a projection back to the NTS. An example of this is illustrated in Figure 6-11 which shows the reciprocal brain stem connections of the A5 cell group. Similarly, the other nuclei are reciprocally connected with the NTS. This form of connectional arrangement implies that some type of feedback system exists at almost all levels within the network.

DESCENDING PATHWAYS REGULATING THE SYMPATHETIC OUTFLOW

The central autonomic network may function like a microprocessor. After receiving information about the internal environment of the body, it affects the specific output systems whether they involve release of specific hormones or changes in the autonomic preganglionic neurons. In this section, the discussion will focus on the CNS cell groups that regulate the sympathetic outflow. Discussion of the control of

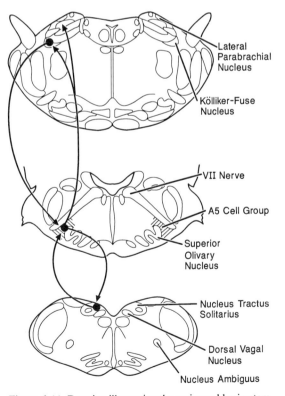

Figure 6-11 Drawing illustrating the reciprocal brain stem connections of the A5 cell group.

the parasympathetic outflow of the vagus nerve is found in Chapter 5, and the control of vasopressin release is found in Chapters 13 and 14.

The sympathetic preganglionic neurons represent the final CNS output of the autonomic network. These neurons produce the changes that maintain homeostasis as a result of multiple CNS inputs that have been modified by the central processing of visceral afferent information. As a result, considerable interest has been generated in determining the CNS sites that give rise to the neuronal pathways that innervate the sympathetic preganglionic neurons and in determining the chemical transmitters involved (see Coote, 1988, for review).

The sympathetic outflow is controlled directly by descending pathways that originate in various nuclei of the brain stem and hypothalamus (see review by Coote, 1988). In general, the tract tracing methods that have been used to analyze these pathways fail to provide information on the innervation of functionally defined sympathetic preganglionic neurons. To circumvent this problem, the retrograde transneuronal viral cell body labeling method has been used to study the central pathways that regulate specific sympathetic ganglia (Figure 6-12). Five key areas of the brain innervate all levels of the sympathetic preganglionic outflow (Strack et al., 1989b). These areas include the paraventricular hypothalamic nucleus, A5 noradrenergic cell group, caudal raphe region, rostral ventrolateral medulla, and ventromedial medulla (Figure 6-13). It is not certain if these results mean that there are neurons in each of these nuclei capable of regulating the entire sympathetic outflow or whether these projections are topographically organized as was demonstrated in the paraventricular hypothalamic nucleus (Strack et al., 1989b). However, these findings do not exclude the possibility that particular CNS regions control the entire sympathetic outflow in order to produce global sympathetic changes as seen in the defense reaction or in the sleep/wakefulness cycle.

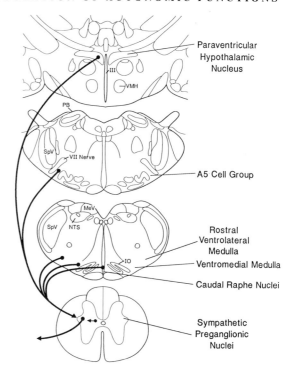

Figure 6-13 The general pattern of innervation of the sympathetic outflow as demonstrated by the retrograde transneuronal viral cell body labeling technique. III, third ventricle; NTS, nucleus tractus solitarius; MeV, medial vestibular nucleus; PB, parabrachial nucleus; SpV, spinal trigeminal nucleus; VMH, ventromedial hypothalamic nucleus. (Reproduced from Strack et al., 1989a.)

The neurons that give rise to these descending projections are chemically coded. For example, Strack et al. (1989a) found that a variety of different neuropeptide-containing neurons in the medulla and paraventricular hypothalamic nuclei innervate the sympathoadrenal preganglionic neurons (see Figure 16-7, Chapter 16). It is quite probable that specific chemically coded patterns of innervation exist for all of the descending sympathetic pathways.

One final point needs to be stressed: Local interneurons in the intermediate gray matter of the spinal cord (laminae VII and X) also innervate the sympathetic preganglionic neurons at all levels of the sympathetic outflow (Strack et al., 1989a). Interneurons are also probably present in the dorsal horn as well. The presence of local interneurons implies that there are additional descending and intrinsic spinal pathways that indirectly control the sympathetic outflow, but relatively little is known about these pathways (see Schramm, 1986, for review). To understand completely how the sympathetic outflow is regulated, studies will need to elucidate the function as well as the transmitter and receptor mechanisms

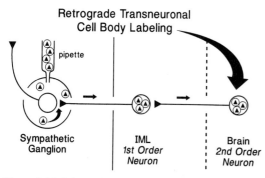

Figure 6-12 Schematic drawing illustrating the retrograde transneuronal viral cell body labeling technique.

of the interneurons in reference to functionally defined sets of neurons in a manner analogous to our level of knowledge regarding α and γ motoneurons.

SUMMARY

Central autonomic pathways are organized at two levels of complexity. Some pathways are organized for reflex adjustments of the end organ, and others are organized in a more complex fashion by connecting to higher neural centers that form a central autonomic circuit capable of producing widespread autonomic, endocrine, and behavioral responses.

Sensory fibers that innervate visceral organs project to the nucleus tractus solitarius (NTS) in a viscerotopic fashion. Nerves carrying gustatory information project to the rostral part of the NTS. They synapse on NTS neurons that project to lower brain stem centers controlling chewing, swallowing, and salivation, and to other neurons in the same NTS region which project to higher neural centers involved in food sensation. Similarly, general visceral afferents project to specific NTS regions. Some project to NTS subnuclei that control lower brain stem neurons for reflex adjustment of the end organ. Others project to a common site in the NTS called the commissural-medial NTS, which acts as a relay center and projects to higher CNS regions. This connects to a central autonomic network that is made up of a collection of interrelated CNS nuclei, including the parabrachial nucleus, the central gray matter, the lateral and paraventricular hypothalamic nuclei, the central nucleus of the amygdala, and the bed nucleus of the stria terminalis. This central network probably functions like a microprocessor to integrate a wide range of autonomic afferent information and then causes output changes in the autonomic nervous system, the neuroendocrine system, and possibly behavioral activities.

REFERENCES

Reviews

Aston-Jones, G. (1985). Behavioral functions of locus coeruleus derived from cellular attributes. *Physiological Psychology* 13, 118–126.

Aston-Jones, G., Foote, S. L., and Bloom, F. E. (1984). Anatomy and physiology of locus coeruleus neurons: Functional implications. In: *Frontiers in Clinical Neuroscience,* Vol. 2. *Norepinephrine,* M. Ziegler and C. Lake (eds.), Williams & Wilkins, Baltimore, pp. 92–116.

Coote, J. H. (1988). The organization of cardiovascular neurons in the spinal cord. *Reviews in Physiology, Biochemistry, and Pharmacology* 110, 148–285.

Foote, S. L., Bloom, F. E., and Aston-Jones, G. (1983). The nucleus locus coeruleus: New evidence of anatomical and physiological specificity. *Physiological Reviews* 63, 844–914.

Jean, A. (1984). Brainstem organization of the swallowing network. *Brain, Behaviour, and Evolution* 25, 109–116.

Jordan, D., and Spyer, K. M. (1986). Brainstem integration of cardiovascular and pulmonary afferent activity. *Progress in Brain Research* 67, 295–314.

Lautt, W. W. (1980). Hepatic nerves: A review of their functions and effects. *Canadian Physiology and Pharmacology* 58, 105–123.

Leibowitz, S. F. (1986). Brain monoamines and peptides: Role in the control of eating behavior. *Federation Proceedings* 45, 1396–1403.

Luiten, P. G. M., ter Horst, G. J., and Steffens, A. B. (1987). The hypothalamus, intrinsic connections and outflow pathways to the endocrine system in relation to the control of feeding and metabolism. *Progress in Neurobiology* 28, 1–54.

Niijima, A., and Mei, N. (1987). Glucose sensors in viscera and control of blood glucose level. *News in Physiological Sciences* 2, 164–167.

Norgren, R. (1984). Central neural mechanisms of taste. In: *Handbook of Physiology; The Nervous System, III. Sensory Processes,* I. Darien-Smith (ed.), American Physiological Society, Washington, DC, pp. 1087–1128.

Palkovits, M. (1985). Distribution of neuroactive substances in the dorsal vagal complex of the medulla oblongata. *Neurochemistry International* 7, 213–219.

Price, J. L., Russchen, F. T., and Amaral, D. G. (1987). The limbic region. II: The amygdaloid complex. In: *Chemical Neuroanatomy,* Vol. 5. *Integrated Systems of the CNS,* Part I, A. Björklund, T. Hokfelt, and L. W. Swanson (eds.), Elsevier, Amsterdam, pp. 279–388.

Schramm, L. P. (1986). Spinal factors in sympathetic regulation. In: *Central and Peripheral Mechanisms of Cardiovascular Regulation,* A. Magro, W. Osswald, D. Reis, and P. Vanhoutte, (eds.), Plenum, New York, pp. 303–352.

Swanson, L. W. (1987). The hypothalamus. In: *Chemical Neuroanatomy,* Vol. 5. *Integrated Systems of the CNS,* Part I, A. Björklund, T. Hokfelt, and L. W. Swanson (eds.), Elsevier, Amsterdam, pp. 1–124.

Widdicombe, J. G. (1982). Pulmonary and respiratory tract receptors. *Journal of Experimental Biology* 100, 41–57.

Research Articles

Altschuler, S. M., Bao, X., Bieger, D., Hopkins, D. A., and Miselis, R. R. (1989). Viscerotopic representation of the upper alimentary tract in the rat: Sensory ganglia and nuclei of the solitary and spinal trigeminal tracts. *Journal of Comparative Neurology* 283, 248–268.

Aston-Jones, G., Ennis, M., Pieribone, V. A., Nickell, W. T., and Shipley, M. T. (1986). The brain nucleus locus coeruleus: Restricted afferent control of a broad efferent network. *Science* 234, 734–737.

Azuma, S., Yamamoto, T., and Kawamura, Y. (1984). Studies on gustatory responses of amygdaloid neurons in rats. *Experimental Brain Research* 56, 12–22.

Backman, S. B., Anders, C., Ballantyne, D., Rohrig, N., Camerer, H., Mifflin, S., Jordan, D., Dickhaus, H., Spyer, K. M., and Richter, D. W. (1984). Evidence for a monosynaptic connection between slowly adapting pulmonary stretch receptor afferents and inspiratory beta neurones. *Pflugers Archives* 402, 129–136.

Beckstead, R. M., Morse, J. R., and Norgren, R. (1980). The nucleus of the solitary tract in the monkey: Projections to the thalamus and brain stem nuclei. *Journal of Comparative Neurology* 190, 259–282.

Berger, A. J., and Dick, T. E. (1987). Connectivity of slowly adapting pulmonary stretch receptors with dorsal medullary respiratory neurons. *Journal of Neurophysiology* 58, 1259–1274.

Cassell, M. D., and Gray, T. S. (1989). The amygdala directly innervates adrenergic (C1) neurons in the ventrolateral medulla in the rat. *Neuroscience Letters* 97, 163–168.

Caille, D., Vibert, J. F., and Hugelin, A. (1981). Apneusis and apnea after parabrachial or Kölliker-Fuse N. lesion; influence of wakefulness. *Respiration Physiology* 45, 79–95.

Cechetto, D. F., and Calaresu, F. R. (1985). Central pathways relaying cardiovascular afferent information to amygdala. *American Journal of Physiology* 248, R38–R45.

Ciriello, J., and Calaresu, F. R. (1980). Role of paraventricular and supraoptic nuclei in central cardiovascular regulation in the cat. *American Journal of Physiology* 239, R137–R142.

Contreras, R. J., and Kosten, T. (1981). Changes in salt intake after abdominal vagotomy: Evidence for hepatic sodium receptors. *Physiology and Behavior* 26, 575–582.

Czachurski, J., Dembowsky, K., Seller, H., Nobling, R., and Taugner, R. (1988). Morphology of electrophysiologically identified baroreceptor afferents and second order neurones in the brainstem of the cat. *Archives Italiennes de Biologie* 126, 129–144.

Davies, R. O., and Kubin, L. (1986). Projection of pulmonary rapidly adapting receptors to the medulla of the cat: An antidromic mapping study. *Journal of Physiology (London)* 373, 63–86.

Elam, M., Yao, T., Svensson, T. H., and Thoren, P. (1984). Regulation of locus coeruleus neurons and splanchnic sympathetic nerves by cardiovascular afferents. *Brain Research* 390, 281–287.

Elam, M., Thoren, P., and Svensson, T. H. (1986). Locus coeruleus neurons and sympathetic nerves. Activation by visceral afferents. *Brain Research* 375, 117–125.

Ennis, M., and Aston-Jones, G. (1986). A potent excitatory input to the nucleus locus coeruleus from the ventrolateral medulla. *Neuroscience Letters* 71, 299–305.

Ennis, M., and Aston-Jones, G. (1987). Two physiologically distinct populations of neurons in the ventrolateral medulla innervate the locus coeruleus. *Brain Research* 425, 257–282.

Fulwiler, C. E., and Saper, C. B. (1984). Subnuclear organization of the efferent connections of the parabrachial nucleus in the rat. *Brain Research Reviews* 7, 229–259.

Fulwiler, C. E., and Saper, C. B. (1985). Cholecystokinin-immunoreactive innervation of the ventromedial hypothalamus in the rat: Possible substrate for autonomic regulation of feeding. *Neuroscience Letters* 53, 289–296.

Grill, H. J. (1980). Production and regulation of ingestive consummatory behavior in the chronic decerebrate rat. *Brain Research Bulletin* 5, Suppl. 4, 79–87.

Gwyn, D. G., Leslie, R. A., and Hopkins, D. A. (1985). Observations on the afferent and efferent organization of the vagus nerve and the innervation of the stomach in the squirrel monkey. *Journal of Comparative Neurology* 239, 163–175.

Hamilton, R. B., and Norgren, R. (1984). Central projections of gustatory nerves in the rat. *Journal of Comparative Neurology* 222, 560–577.

Herbert, H., Moga, M. M., and Saper, C. B. (1990). Connections of the parabrachial nucleus with the nucleus of the solitary tract and the medullary reticular formation in the rat. *Journal of Comparative Neurology* (in press).

Holstege, G., Meiners, L., and Tan, K. (1985). Projections of the bed nucleus of the stria terminalis to the mesencephalon, pons, and medulla oblongata in the cat. *Experimental Brain Research* 58, 370–391.

Hopkins, D. A., and Holstege, G. (1978). Amygdaloid projections to the mesencephalon, pons and medulla oblongata in the cat. *Experimental Brain Research* 32, 529–547.

Housley, G. D., Martin-Body, R. L., Dawson, N. J., and Sinclair, J. D. (1987). Brain stem projections of the glossopharyngeal nerve and its carotid sinus branch in the rat. *Neuroscience* 22, 237–250.

Jones, B. E., and Yang, T. Z. (1985). The efferent projections from the reticular formation and the locus coeruleus studied by anterograde and retrograde axonal transport in the rat. *Journal of Comparative Neurology* 242, 56–92.

Kalia, M., and Mesulam, M. M. (1980). Brain stem projections of sensory and motor components of the vagus complex in the cat. II. Laryngeal, tracheobronchial, pulmonary, cardiac, and gastrointestinal branches. *Journal of Comparative Neurology* 193, 467–508.

Katafuchi, T., Oɔ nura, Y., and Kurosawa, M. (1988). Effects of chemical stimulation of paraventricular nucleus on adrenal and renal nerve activity in rats. *Neuroscience Letters* 86, 195–200.

Kobashi, M., and Adachi, A. (1988). A direct hepatic osmoreceptive afferent projection from nucleus tractus solitarius to dorsal hypothalamus. *Brain Research Bulletin* 20, 487–492.

Krettek, J. E., and Price, J. L. (1978). Amygdaloid projections to subcortical structures within the basal forebrain and brainstem in the rat and cat. *Journal of Comparative Neurology* 178, 225–254.

Leibowitz, S. F., Hammer, N. J., and Chang, L. (1981). Hypothalamic paraventricular nucleus lesions produce overeating and obesity in the rat. *Physiology and Behavior* 27, 1031–1040.

Leslie, R. A., Gwyn, D. G., and Hopkins, D. A. (1982). The central distribution of the cervical vagus nerve and gastric afferent and efferent projections in the rat. *Brain Research Bulletin* 8, 37–43.

Loewy, A. D., and Burton, H. (1978). Nuclei of the solitary tract: Efferent projections ot the lower brain stem and spinal cord of the cat. *Journal of Comparative Neurology* 181, 421–450.

Loewy, A. D., McKellar, S., and Saper, C. B. (1979). Direct projections from the A5 catecholamine cell group to the intermediolateral cell column. *Brain Research* 174, 309–314.

Loewy, A. D., Marson, L., Parkinson, D., Perry, M. A., and

Sawyer, W. B. (1986). Descending noradrenergic pathways involved in the A5 depressor response. *Brain Research* 386, 313–324.

Luiten, P. G. M., ter Horst, G. J., Karst, H., and Steffens, A. B. (1985). The course of paraventricular hypothalamic efferents to autonomic structures in medulla and spinal cord. *Brain Research* 329, 374–378.

Mantyh, P. W., and Hunt, S. P. (1984). Neuropeptides are present in projection neurones at all levels in visceral and taste pathways: From periphery to sensory cortex. *Brain Research* 299, 297–311.

Menetrey, D., and Basbaum, A. I. (1987). Spinal and trigeminal projections to the nucleus of the solitary tract: A possible substrate for somatovisceral and viscerovisceral reflex activation. *Journal of Comparative Neurology* 255, 439–450.

Moga, M. M., and Gray, T. S. (1985). Evidence for corticotropin-releasing factor, neurotensin, and somatostatin in the neural pathway from the central nucleus of the amygdala to the parabrachial nucleus. *Journal of Comparative Neurology* 241, 275–284.

Norgren, R. (1978). Projections from the nucleus of the solitary tract in the rat. *Neuroscience* 3, 207–218.

Price, J. L., and Amaral, D. G. (1981). An autoradiographic study of the projections of the central nucleus of the monkey amygdala. *Journal of Neuroscience* 1, 1242–1259.

Ricardo, J. A., and Koh, E. T. (1978). Anatomical evidence of direct projections from the nucleus of the solitary tract to the hypothalamus, amygdala, and other forebrain structures in the rat. *Brain Research* 153, 1–26.

Rogers, R. C., and Hermann, G. E. (1980). Central connections of the hepatic branch of the vagus nerve: a horseradish peroxidase study. *Journal of the Autonomic Nervous System* 7, 165–174.

Russchen, F. T. (1982). Amygdalopetal projections in the cat. II. Subcortical afferent connections. A study with retrograde tracing techniques. *Journal of Comparative Neurology* 207, 157–176.

Saper, C. B., and Loewy, A. D. (1980). Efferent connections of the parabrachial nucleus in the rat. *Brain Research* 197, 291–317.

Shapiro, R. E., and Miselis, R. R. (1985). The central organization of the vagus nerve innervating the stomach of the rat. *Journal of Comparative Neurology* 238, 473–488.

Shimada, S., Shiosaka, S., Emson, P. C., Hillyard, C. J., Girgis, S., MacIntyre, I., and Tohyama, M. (1985). Calcitonin gene-related peptidergic projection from the parabrachial area to the forebrain and diencephalon in the rat: An immunohistochemical analysis. *Neuroscience* 16, 607–616.

Shimizu, N., Oomura, Y., Plata-Salaman, C. R., and Morimoto, M. (1987). Hyperphagia and obesity in rats with bilateral ibotenic acid-induced lesions of the ventromedial hypothalamic nucleus. *Brain Research* 416, 153–156.

Spencer, S. E., Sawyer, W. B., and Loewy, A. D. (1989). Cardiovascular effects produced by L-glutamate stimulation of the lateral hypothalamic area. *American Journal of Physiology* 257, H540–H552.

Strack, A. M., Sawyer, W. B., Hughes, J. H., Platt, K. B., and Loewy, A. D. (1989a). A general pattern of CNS innervation of the sympathetic outflow demonstrated by transneuronal pseudorabies viral infections. *Brain Research* 491, 156–162.

Strack, A. M., Sawyer, W. B., Platt, K. B., and Loewy, A. D. (1989b). CNS cell groups regulating the sympathetic nervous outflow to adrenal gland as revealed by transneuronal cell body labeling with pseudorabies virus. *Brain Research* 491, 276–296.

Sved, A., and Felsten, G. (1987). Stimulation of the locus coeruleus decreases arterial pressure. *Brain Research* 414, 119–132.

Svensson, T. H., and Thoren, P. (1979). Brain noradrenergic neurons in the locus coeruleus: Inhibition by blood volume load through vagal afferents. *Brain Research* 172, 174–178.

Thompson, R. L., and Cassell, M. D. (1989). Differential distribution and noncollateralization of the central amygdaloid neurons projecting to different medullary regions. *Neuroscience Letters* 97, 245–251.

Thor, K. B., and Helke, C. J. (1987). Serotonin- and substance P-containing projections to the nucleus tractus solitarii of the rat. *Journal of Comparative Neurology* 265, 275–293.

Thor, K. B., and Helke, C. J. (1988). Catecholamine-synthesizing neuronal projections to the nucleus tractus solitarii of the rat. *Journal of Compartive Neurology* 264, 265–280.

Travers, J. B. (1988). Efferent projections from the anterior nucleus of the solitary tract of the hamster. *Brain Research* 457, 1–11.

Travers, J. B., and Norgren, R. (1983). Afferent projections to the oral motor nuclei in the rat. *Journal of Comparative Neurology* 220, 280–298.

Wallace, D. M., Magnuson, D. J., and Gray, T. S. (1989). The amygdalo-brainstem pathway: Selective innervation of dopaminergic, noradrenergic and adrenergic cells in the rat. *Neuroscience Letters* 97, 252–258.

Weller, K. L., and Smith, D. A. (1982). Afferent connections to the bed nucleus of the stria terminalis. *Brain Research* 232, 255–270.

7

Sensory Innervation of the Viscera

F. CERVERO AND R. D. FOREMAN

The autonomic nervous system has been regarded traditionally as a motor system with the specific responsibility of regulating the internal environment. Visceral afferent fibers are also an integral part of this system, through they have not always been regarded as such because their anatomical and physiological properties were indistinguishable from those of somatic afferent fibers. Both were viewed as part of the sensory equipment of the body. It is impossible, however, to understand integrative autonomic functions without reference to the afferent signals that trigger and modulate autonomic reflexes and without knowledge of the peripheral and central sensory systems responsible for signaling visceral pain. Whether afferent fibers are part of the autonomic nervous system is largely a semantic debate that neither helps the newcomer to this field of neuroscience nor contributes to an integrated view of the nervous system. Therefore, due consideration will be given in this chapter to the role of the afferent component of the sympathetic nervous system. This will be done by examining the anatomical distribution of sympathetic afferents arising from different internal organs, their relative numbers, their peripheral pathways of projection to the central nervous system, and the mechansims of encoding of adequate visceral stimuli. These properties of sympathetic afferent fibers will be discussed within the context of their relevance to autonomic reflex control, to visceral sensation, and to the signaling of visceral pain.

VISCERAL AFFERENT FIBERS AND THE AUTONOMIC NERVOUS SYSTEM

Current thinking about the role of the autonomic nervous system in physiological regulation originates from the work of Langley, who in a 1921 monograph summarized his research work and his views about the autonomic nervous system. The opening paragraph of his monograph defines the autonomic nervous system as "the nerve cells and nerve fibers by means of which efferent impulses pass to tissues other than multinuclear striated muscle" (Langley, 1921). This statement has been interpreted as meaning that the autonomic nervous system is exclusively an efferent component of the nervous system, a view that is reflected in many contemporary textbooks of physiology. These texts customarily discuss the afferent innervation of internal organs not in the chapters on the autonomic nervous system, but rather in those on visceral and somatic sensation. Moreover, some neuroscientists not only exclude visceral afferent fibers from the autonomic nervous system but also oppose applying the terms *sympathetic* or *parasympathetic* to the afferent components of autonomic nerves.

Langley's approach to this question is stated clearly in his chapter on the autonomic nervous system in Schafer's *Textbook of Physiology* (Langley, 1900). He deals with visceral afferent fibers in a section of the chapter that includes general questions about the autonomic nervous system and repeatedly uses the term "afferent sympathetic fibers" when referring to visceral afferent fibers in sympathetic nerves. He then argues about the role of such fibers in visceral pain and in autonomic reflex action, leaving no doubt that he regarded visceral afferents as an important constituent of autonomic regulation. Thus, it is curious that so many accounts of the autonomic nervous system have left aside the afferent innervation of internal organs and claim to have done so "following Langley's approach."

The presence of visceral afferent fibers in autonomic nerves was first demonstrated anatomically by Langley and Anderson (1894), who estimated a ratio of efferent to afferent fibers in the hypogastric and splanchnic nerves of 10:1 and in the pelvic nerve of 3:1. They also showed that the cervical sympathetic trunk contained few afferent fibers and that all visceral afferent fibers in sympathetic nerve have their cell bodies in the spinal ganglia and not in the sympathetic ganglia. Subsequent histological and physiological examinations of sympathetic and parasympathetic nerves (see review by Ranson, 1921) confirmed the existence of afferent fibers in these nerves and their involvement in both autonomic regulation and visceral sensation, including visceral pain.

Afferent fibers of autonomic nerves subserve two main functions: (1) sensing of changes in the internal environment that will trigger or modulate reflex control of the viscera, and (2) signaling of certain events in internal organs that are perceived by the subject as painful sensations. This duality makes them fundamentally different from somatic afferents since sensory and regulatory properties of the latter cannot be separated. Afferent impulses from skin or from muscle trigger reflex and behavioral regulation as well as evoke a sensory experience. In the case of visceral afferent fibers, some of the signals generated by internal stimuli never evoke conscious sensations (i.e., blood pressure changes, lung inflation, chemical composition of chyme), whereas others result in the conscious perception of a sensation (gut distention, smooth muscle spasms, cardiac ischemia).

To which extent these functional roles are subserved by two different sets of visceral afferent fibers is still an open question. The functional properties of their receptor endings and, perhaps more importantly, the connections and actions of their central projections will determine the differential role of these afferent fibers in autonomic regulation and in visceral sensation.

TYPES OF AFFERENT FIBERS IN AUTONOMIC NERVES

Two different types of visceral afferent fibers are present in autonomic nerves: primary afferent fibers and enteric afferent fibers (Figure 7-1).

Primary Afferent Fibers

These afferent fibers are anatomically similar to somatic primary afferents and have their cell bodies in

the spinal and cranial ganglia. Their receptor endings are located in the walls or in the parenchyma of internal organs, in the vessels that supply the viscera, or in the serosal membranes that cover them. Visceral primary afferent fibers travel in sympathetic and parasympathetic nerves. Cell bodies of the sympathetic afferents lie in the dorsal root ganglia at the thoracic and upper lumbar spinal levels. Cell bodies for the sacral division of the parasympathetic nervous system lie in the S2–S4 dorsal root ganglia. Cell bodies for the cranial parasympathetic fibers lie in the geniculate ganglion (VIIth nerve), petrosal ganglion (IXth nerve), and nodose ganglion (Xth nerve). These nerve cells act as transmission lines between the internal environment and the central nervous system, carrying afferent information from the internal organs that will be used for integrated autonomic regulation or for the perception of visceral sensations. In addition, there is evidence to suggest that some of the sympathetic primary afferents have collateral branches that make contact with sympathetic preganglionic neurons in prevertebral ganglia (Matthews and Cuello, 1984) (Figure 7-1). This would indicate that, in addition to their central actions, visceral primary afferents may also play a role as part of peripheral regulatory reflexes. Whether the parasympathetic primary afferents are arranged in a similar way is unknown.

Enteric Afferent Neurons

These are nerve cells specifically associated with the innervation of the gut and of associated hollow viscera such as the gallbladder. They are part of the enteric nervous system—a system of neurons whose cell bodies are located in the walls of the gastrointestinal tract. Some of these enteric neurons subserve afferent functions in that their peripheral endings act as senory receptors capable of signaling changes in the motor or secretory activities of the gut. Their cell bodies are located inside the walls of the gut, and their axonal projections are also contained within the enteric nerve plexus. However, anatomical and physiological evidence suggests that some afferent enteric neurons send projections beyond the confines of the gastrointestinal tract (see review by Costa

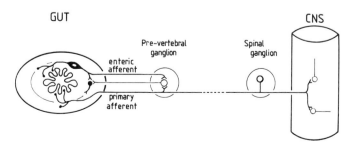

Figure 7-1 Schematic diagram of the two types of visceral afferent fibers present in sympathetic nerves: primary afferent fibers and enteric afferent fibers.

et al., 1987). These enteric afferent fibers run in mesenteric nerves and can reach the prevertebral ganglia
of the sympathetic nervous system (Figure 7-1),
where they make synaptic contacts with terminals or
axons of the sympathetic preganglionic neurons.
Their functional actions are thus contained within a
reflex arc that does not involve the central nervous
system. There is no anatomical evidence to suggest
that the central axonal projection of the enteric afferent neurons reach the spinal cord or have direct
influences on primary afferent neurons.

Although it seems clear that enteric afferent neurons cannot have a direct influence in the processing
of visceral sensation, there is still some argument
about the differential role of visceral primary afferents in autonomic regulation and sensation. This
question will be discussed in some detail later in this
chapter.

NUMBERS AND PERIPHERAL PATHWAYS OF VISCERAL PRIMARY AFFERENTS

Most internal organs have a dual visceral innervation. Both sympathetic and parasympathetic afferents innervate the major thoracic, abdominal, and
pelvic organs. For example, some of these afferents
join the sympathetic nerves, such as the splanchnic
nerves, whereas other afferent fibers from the same
viscera course in parasympathetic nerves such as the
vagus or the pelvic nerves (Figure 7-2). The functional significance of this dual innervation has been
the subject of considerable debate, particularly in relation to the question of whether afferent fibers in
sympathetic and parasympathetic nerves subserve
different functions (see review by Cervero and Tattersall, 1986).

The number of primary afferents in sympathetic
and parasympathetic nerves varies considerably.
The immediate consequence of this discrepancy is
that, for a given viscus, the density of innervation by
sympathetic and parasympathetic afferents may be
substantially different.

Quantitative estimates of the total number of visceral primary afferents are available for a number of
mammalian species and, in some cases, are broken
down by individual nerves and organs (see reviews
by Andrews, 1986; Jänig and Morrison, 1986; de
Groat, 1986). These accurate estimates have been
obtained by fiber counts in electron microscopic
studies of autonomic nerves or by the use of retrograde tracing methods using fluorescent tracers or
the enzyme horseradish peroxidase. Using retrograde cell body tracing methods, it is possible not

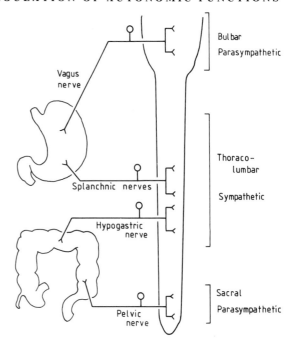

Figure 7-2 Most organs receive a dual visceral afferent innervation. Vagal-parasympathetic fibers innervate the thoracic and abdominal organs. This information is sent to the
nucleus tractus solitarius. The sacral parasympathetic fibers innervate the distal colon, rectum, and other pelvic organs and project to laminae I and V of the sacral dorsal
horn. Sympathetic visceral afferents provide an additional
sensory input to most organs.

only to obtain an estimate of the total number of afferent fibers in a given nerve or from a given viscus
but also to obtain information about the projection
pathway of the afferent fiber under study. Two main
findings have emerged from these studies: (1) the low
density of innervation of viscera compared to that of
the skin, and (2) the discrepancies between the numbers of visceral afferents in sympathetic and parasympathetic nerves.

The total number of visceral primary afferents in
all sympathetic nerves of the cat is approximately
16,000 fibers (for references see review by Jänig and
Morrison, 1986): some 1,000 fibers in the thoracic
sympathetic nerves, 6,000–7,000 fibers in the greater
splanchnic nerves, 3,000–4,000 fibers in the lesser
splanchnic nerve, and about 5,000 fibers in the lumbar splanchnic and colonic nerves. These numbers
indicate that afferent fibers constitute less than 20%
of all fibers in sympathetic nerves and about 2% of
the total number of afferent fibers in the thoracic
and lumbar dorsal roots.

The corresponding figures for parasympathetic
nerves are quite different. More than 80% of all fibers in the vagus nerve of the cat are afferent, as are

almost 50% of all fibers in the pelvic nerve. These proportions are considerably higher than those of their sympathetic counterparts. As for the actual numbers, it is estimated that some 40,000 vagal afferent fibers and about 7,500 pelvic afferents innervate the abdominal organs of the cat (see review by Andrews, 1986). The same viscera are innervated by only 15,000 afferents in sympathetic nerves, thus giving a ratio of more than 3:1 in favor of the parasympathetic innervation.

A common property of the sympathetic and parasympathetic afferent innervation is the overwhelming preponderance of unmyelinated fibers. More than 90% of all visceral afferents are unmyelinated or lose their myelin as they approach their target organs (Kuo et al., 1982). The mesenteric nerves, which constitute the terminal branches of the sympathetic and parasympathetic innervation of the small intestine, are made up entirely of unmyelinated nerve fibers (Cervero and Sharkey, 1988). There are only a handful of large myelinated afferent fibers in sympathetic nerves, and these are believed to be connected to mesenteric Pacinian corpuscles (see review by Leek, 1972).

The most commonly held view about the functional significance of this dual afferent innervation of internal organs is that visceral sensation, and particularly visceral pain, is mediated by afferent fibers in sympathetic nerves, whereas the reflex and regulatory functions evoked by visceral stimulation are triggered by activity in afferent fibers running in parasympathetic nerves (see review by Ruch, 1946).

There are notable exceptions to this generalization, particularly in some pelvic viscera such as the bladder and colon. This contention is supported by clinical evidence. It has been known for some time that stimulation of the splanchnic nerves in conscious humans under local anesthesia elicits severe pain. Also, clinical studies combining stimulation and blocking techniques have shown repeatedly that abdominal pain is evoked by stimulating sympathetic but not parasympathetic nerves, and that it is relieved by section or blockade of sympathetic but not parasympathetic nerve trunks (White, 1943). Splanchnic nerve blockade during major abdominal surgery under general anesthesia not only prevents endocrine-metabolic responses to the visceral surgical procedure such as increases in plasma cortisol, glucose, free fatty acids, and urinary adrenaline excretion but also helps postoperative recovery (Shirasaka et al., 1986). These clinical results show that the pseudoaffective components of the visceral nociceptive response are also mediated by afferent impulses in sympathetic nerves. Therefore, it can be concluded that many forms of visceral pain are signaled by sympathetic nerves and that the parasympathetic afferent innervation of some internal organs is mainly concerned with the regulatory functions of autonomic control.

ENCODING MECHANISMS OF VISCERAL SENSORY RECEPTORS

One of the fundamental questions of sensory physiology is, What is the encoding mechanism of sensory receptors? As far as cutaneous sensation is concerned, this problem seems to have been solved by demonstrating the existence of three separate categories of peripheral receptors that respond specifically to different stimulus modalities: (1) mechanoreceptors that are responsible for sending information about tactile events, (2) thermoreceptors that transmit temperature information, and (3) nociceptors that specifically signal noxious events and whose activation results in the perception of cutaneous pain.

This problem is considerably more complicated when examining the relationship between visceral sensory receptors and visceral sensation. The following peculiarities of visceral sensation must be taken into account. (1) There are many receptors in internal organs whose activation never evokes a conscious experience, and it is therefore very difficult to establish the nature of their adequate stimuli, other than by the reflex actions evoked by their stimulation. (2) The conscious sensations evoked from internal organs are very limited in range and are often only discomfort and pain. (3) Some forms of visceral sensation (e.g., gastric distension or bladder fullness) start as nonpainful experiences but can progress, if the stimulus persists, to become unpleasant and painful sensations without changing the quality of the sensation. (4) In some cases, the sensation of visceral pain starts as a unique and extremely painful sensory experience and is the only sensation that can be evoked from certain viscera (e.g., cardiac pain or gallbladder pain). (5) Most forms of visceral sensation are poorly localized or referred to somatic areas of the body away from the originating viscus.

It therefore seems appropriate to separate those visceral receptors that are never involved in the signaling of conscious sensory events from those that may or may not be concerned with visceral sensation. This requires the identification of the range of sensations that can be evoked from a given viscus prior to the discussion of the encoding mechanism of its sensory receptors. This approach also takes into account the fact that most visceral receptors are not concerned with sensation but with the signaling of changes in the internal environment for the purposes of reflex autonomic regulation. It is important not to lose sight of this elementary fact in order to extract some functional meaning from the known properties of visceral receptors.

Visceral Receptors Not Concerned with Conscious Sensation

There are receptor endings of visceral afferent fibers whose stimulation evokes no sensations. These afferent signals are used for reflex regulation of the internal environment, and their central actions do not include the activation of sensory pathways. Examples of these receptors are the arterial baroreceptors that signal changes in blood pressure, the carotid body chemoreceptors that are sensitive to changes in blood gases, the lung inflation and deflation receptors that transmit information about ventilation, and the atrial volume receptors whose signals help homeostatic control of body fluids.

All these receptors encode the nature, intensity, and time course of their adequate stimuli by being specifically sensitive to these stimuli and to no others. They are, therefore, specific visceral receptors in that they encode their responses for only one form of stimulation.

Visceral Receptors Concerned with Conscious Sensation

There are receptive endings of afferent fibers that innervate organs from which sensations can be evoked. These receptors must also be sensitive to the stimuli that elicit the sensation because not all forms of visceral stimulation are capable of evoking a sensory experience. Because the majority of these sensations are those of discomfort and pain, the central question is whether painful and nonpainful events are signaled by separate categories of visceral receptor.

There are three different neural encoding mechanisms that may function to distinguish between conscious sensation and reflex events in viscera: specificity of the receptor, pattern of neural discharge from the receptor, and central summation of the afferent response (Figure 7-3).

Specificity of the Receptor

This is the kind of encoding mechanism known to apply to cutaneous sensation or to visceral receptors not concerned with conscious sensation. According to this hypothesis, internal organs are innervated by two different categories of receptor: those whose stimulation does not evoke a sensation and those whose activation leads to the perception of visceral pain. Response properties of the latter (thresholds, adequate stimuli, time course of responses) must be consistent with the properties of the stimuli known to evoke pain. For instance, pain from the gallbladder and biliary ducts can be evoked only by large increases in the tension of their smooth muscle walls and, therefore, biliary nociceptors must respond to biliary distension only at intensities of stimulation above the normal range.

The main requirement for a separate category of visceral nociceptor is a close relationship between the parameters of the adequate stimulus for eliciting pain from the viscus and the parameters of the adequate stimulus encoded by the receptor. In addition, specific nociceptors must respond poorly or not at all to innocuous forms of stimulation that must be sensed by a separate category of sensory receptor.

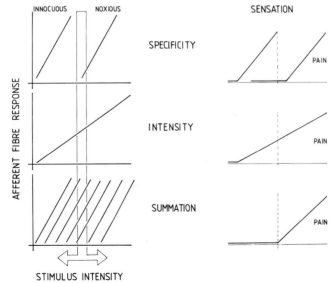

Figure 7-3 Diagrammatic representation of three possible encoding mechanisms of noxious events (Specificity, Intensity, and Summation) by visceral sensory receptors. The relation between stimulus intensity and afferent fiber response is represented for each of the three hypotheses and is correlated with the perception of pain sensations.

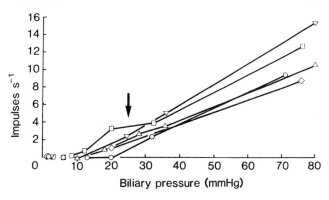

Figure 7-4 Stimulus–response relationship for five high threshold mechanoreceptors in the biliary system of the ferret. The arrow indicates the mean value of biliary pressure above which pseudoaffective reflexes occur. This level is considered to be the nociceptive threshold. (Reproduced from Cervero, 1982, with permission of the author and publisher.)

There is some experimental evidence for the existence of such a separate category of visceral nociceptor in the heart, lungs, gallbladder, biliary ducts (Figure 7-4), testes, and uterus (see Cervero, 1985 for review). The majority of these receptors have been found to be connected to afferent fibers running in sympathetic nerves, thus giving further support to the notion that afferent fibers in sympathetic nerves mediate visceral pain.

Pattern of Response of the Receptor

Goldscheider (1884) proposed that all forms of pain were encoded by the intensity of the response of the peripheral receptors. Low-intensity stimuli will generate low rates of response in the afferent fibers whereas high-intensity stimuli, such as those that can evoke pain, will evoke discharges of greater magnitude. The nature of the sensation will be dependent on the intensity of the afferent response and not on the activation of specific sets of afferent fibers.

This theory ignores the existence of separate categories of sensory receptors and postulates a single and functionally homogeneous population of receptors capable of encoding both innocuous and noxious stimulus intensities. The requirements of such a theory depend on a narrow range of thresholds for the sensory receptors, a threshold response of the afferent fibers compatible with the lowest stimulus intensity that can evoke a reflex action, and a stimulus–response curve for the receptor that encompasses low and high intensities of stimulation. Such a sensory receptor has not been found in the skin and other somatic structures. Indeed, all evidence from studies on the properties of somatic afferents demonstrates the specificity of cutaneous receptors and the lack of an "intensity" encoding mechanism for their afferent responses. However, the "intensity" interpretation for the encoding of visceral stimuli has been used to explain the receptor properties of some visceral afferent fibers from the colon and bladder (see Jänig and Morrison, 1986, for review). It must be noted that the experimental evidence points to a lack of homogeneity in the mechanical thresholds of visceral afferent fibers and this raises the possibility of an alternative version of the "intensity" interpretation as detailed below.

Central Summation of the Afferent Response

This is a modification of the "intensity" theory and proposes a central mechanism for encoding of the nature of the visceral sensation. According to this theory, some internal organs are innervated by a population of afferent fibers capable of responding to a wide range of stimulus intensities. However, the response thresholds of afferent fibers range from very low levels in some fibers at one end of the distribution to high levels in other fibers at the other end. The final sensation depends on a process of central summation as progressively higher intensities of stimulation recruit more and more afferent fibers. This implies that a given viscus is innervated by a series of afferent fibers whose wide-ranging thresholds form a continuum from the innocuous to the noxious level and do not fall into two distinct groups.

Some gastrointestinal sensations, such as those evoked by distension of the colon or rectum, begin as nonpainful feelings and evolve toward an uncomfortable and painful sensation as the distension progresses. These properties can be paralleled by the electrophysiological properties of some colonic receptors (Blumberg et al., 1983), which increase their discharge rate in a graded fashion with increasing distension of the colon. At a certain point, when the discharge reaches a certain critical level, pain is perceived. In contrast, other viscera such as the gallbladder and the biliary ducts from which pain is the only sensation that can be evoked appear to be innervated by specific visceral nociceptors (Cervero, 1982) (Figure 7-4).

It is important to point out that our understanding of the sensory innervation of viscera so far has been limited to studying only a few organs and that there are still many viscera from which we have few or no data. Thus, it is premature to make the generalization that visceral pain is mediated by a unique class of visceral receptor. Moreover, it is a gross oversimplification to relate the final perception of a visceral sensation to the properties of the peripheral sense organ. The final conscious perception of pain depends on the way in which the central nervous system integrates the afferent visceral inflow, regardless of the peripheral encoding mechanism.

CENTRAL PROJECTIONS OF VISCERAL AFFERENT FIBERS

Visceral pain is transmitted to the spinal cord by afferent fibers traveling in sympathetic nerves. These fibers arise from cell bodies in the dorsal root ganglia and terminate in laminae I and V of the thoracic or upper lumbar spinal cord (Figure 7-5A; Neuhuber, 1982; also see de Groat, 1986, for review).

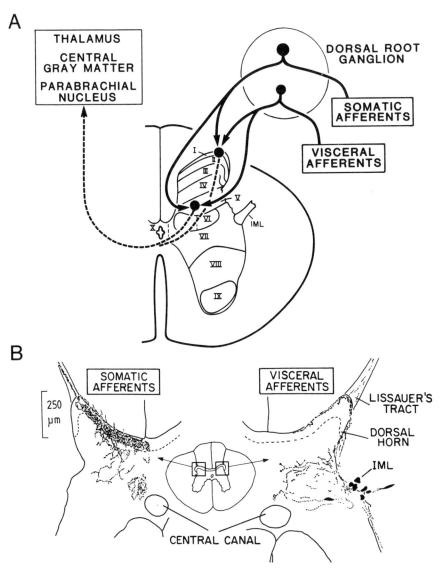

Figure 7-5 Termination of visceral and somatic afferents in the dorsal horn. (A) Schematic diagram showing visceral and somatic afferents converge on neurons in laminae I and V that project to specific regions of the brain. [Modified from Loewy, A. D. (1986). In: *Central Nervous System Control of the Heart,* T. Stober et al., (eds.), Nijhoff, Boston, with permission of the author and publisher.] (B)Reconstruction from three (left) and from seven (right) 80-μm transverse serial sections of the projections of somatic (left) and visceral (right) afferent fibers to the T9 segment of the spinal cord of the cat. Horseradish peroxidase was applied to the ventral ramus (intercostal nerve) of the T9 spinal nerve (left) and to the splanchnic nerve (right). Note the absence of a visceral afferent projection to the substantia gelatinosa, whose ventral border is indicated by the dotted line (Cervero and Connell, 1984).

When sympathetic afferent fibers reach the spinal cord, they enter Lissauer's tract where they may ascend or descend one or two spinal segments or terminate at the same spinal segment in which they enter the spinal cord. Here, the fibers curve around along the edges of the dorsal horn (Figure 7-5B) and terminate in lamina I and lamina V of the dorsal horn. The substantia gelatinosa (lamina II) does not receive a direct input from visceral afferent fibers. However, some neurons in lamina II send dendrites into lamina I, but it is uncertain if these neurons are involved in visceral afferent processing.

Neuroanatomical studies using the anterograde transport horseradish peroxidase method have shown that less that 10% of all afferent fibers in the thoracic and lumbar dorsal roots are of visceral origin (Cervero et al., 1984). This low proportion is also reflected in a relative scarcity of central visceral terminals in the spinal cord (Figure 7-5B). Thus, it is important to emphasize that only a relatively smaller number of sympathetic afferents mediate visceral pain from most thoracic and upper abdominal viscera, which includes the heart and the entire gastrointestinal tract, both of which can be the source of intense pain. In contrast, sensory innervation of the thoracic and abdominal skin, which involves more than 90% of the afferent dorsal root fibers projecting to the thoracic and upper lumbar spinal cord, subserves somatic sensations from the areas of the body with relatively poor spatial discrimination properties when compared to the face and fingers (Figure 7-5B). It is, therefore, no surprise that visceral sensations have similar properties; they are diffuse and difficult to precisely localize. This is a direct result of a relative sparsity in innervation of both the peripheral and central structures.

NEUROPEPTIDES IN VISCERAL SENSORY NEURONS

Many of the fine afferents that terminate in the deep dorsal horn (lamina V) contain immunoreactive substance P and have been shown to be largely of visceral afferent origin (Sharkey et al., 1987). In fact, other neuropeptides have been shown to be contained in visceral sensory dorsal root ganglion cells, including substance P, calcitonin gene-related peptide, and vasoactive intestinal polypeptide. Some of the visceral sensory neurons contain multiple neuropeptides such as calcitonin gene-related peptide and substance P (Molander et al., 1987). Other neuropeptides are present in dorsal root ganglion cells, but these have not yet been shown to be present in visceral dorsal root ganglion cells. It is important to stress that just because a neuropeptide has been identified at a particular site with an immunohistochemical method, this is not, by itself, definitive evidence that it is a neurotransmitter. Therefore, statements about the functional role of these peptides as central neurotransmitters or neuromodulators must be viewed as speculative.

Since these neuropeptides are present in the peripheral end of the afferent fiber, it has been hypothesized that they may modulate the sensory receptor (Figure 7-6). For instance, substance P can modulate the vascular, secretory, and motor functions of some abdominal viscera via a peripheral action on the target organ. These actions mediated by the release of substance P from the afferent terminals may function by a mechanism similar to the cutaneous axonal reflex (Delbro et al., 1986; see reviews by Lembeck, 1983 and Muramato, 1987). Also, some evidence exists for slow synaptic actions of some of

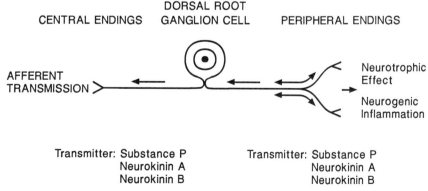

Figure 7-6 Putative neurotransmission of a cutaneous and possibly a visceral axonal reflex of a primary sensory neuron. Substance P or a related tachykinin is the most likely transmitter that is involved in neurogenic inflammation. The arrows indicate the direction in which action potentials are conducted. (Modified from Muramatsu, 1987.)

the neuropeptides contained in visceral afferent fibers on sympathetic postganglionic neurons in prevertebral ganglia (de Groat, 1986 for review). Although it is not possible to rule out a central action of the neuropeptides contained in visceral afferents, the bulk of the studies so far have concentrated on the peripheral site of action of these compounds through their release from the receptor endings of the afferent fibers.

SPINAL MECHANISMS OF VISCERAL SENSATION

Neurons in the thoracic spinal cord receive convergent inputs from viscera and from the skin (Figure 7-5A; see Cervero and Tattersall, 1986 for review). Since the actual number of visceral afferent fibers entering the spinal cord is very small (viz. 10%), this figure is an expression of the considerable amount of central divergence that must occur to the visceral sensory input in the spinal cord. Many of these viscerosomatic neurons are probably not concerned with the sensory components of visceral nociception but with the handling of the general increase in excitability produced by the arrival to the nervous system of a visceral nociceptive volley and that is expressed by motor and autonomic activity (Cervero and Tattersall, 1987).

Visceral nociceptive information must reach the brain to activate the systems that are responsible for producing the responses to the painful stimulus. These responses include sensory-discriminative perceptions, motivational-affective behavior (see review by Melzack and Casey, 1968), and autonomic adjustments. Several different ascending pathways originate in the gray matter of the spinal cord and are responsible for transmitting this information. Axons of these ascending pathways travel mainly in the ventrolateral quadrant of the spinal cord, although some neurons located in the superficial layers of the dorsal horn may also send their axons in the dorsolateral funiculi.

The following paragraphs will discuss the anatomical and electrophysiological characteristics of the ascending pathways that transmit visceral nociceptive information from the thoracic spinal cord to the brainstem and thalamus. Most of the experimental observations come from studies of the afferent projection of cardiopulmonary afferents to the central nervous system. Pathways originating from the lumbosacral segments of the spinal cord have been reviewed by Willis (1985).

Spinothalamic Tract

The spinothalamic tract is separated into two divisions: the lateral spinothalamic tract and the medial spinothalamic tract (Figure 7-7A). One division, the lateral spinothalamic tract system, ascends to the ventral and ventral posterior lateral regions of the thalamus, and neurons of this tract respond to a wide range of stimuli (Mehler et al., 1960; Dennis and Melzack, 1977; Price and Mayer, 1974). Lateral spinothalamic neurons mediate the sensory discriminative aspects of pain (see reviews by Melzack and Wall, 1982; Price and Dubner, 1977). Signals transmitted in this pathway may help an organism to locate precisely areas from which pain originates. The other division is the medial spinothalamic tract, a smaller pathway that projects directly to the medial and intralaminar nuclear complex of the thalamus (Mehler et al., 1960; Boivie, 1979). This second ascending pathway is thought to be involved with the transmission of tonic information about the state of the organism and may be partially responsible for the motivational affective components of pain, including autonomic adjustment (for further discussion, see reviews by Melzack and Casey, 1968; Melzack and Wall, 1982).

The spinothalamic tract originates from neurons found in the gray matter of the spinal cord. Cells of origin of the lateral spinothalamic tract have been located by using the retrograde cell body labeling method and the antidromic mapping technique. Injections of horseradish peroxidase into the lateral regions of the ventral posterior lateral thalamus of monkeys result in retrogradely labeled cells, primarily in laminae I and V of the dorsal horn in the thoracic spinal cord contralateral to the injection (Figure 7-7; see review by Trevino, 1976). Antidromic mapping studies confirm this observation (Figure 7-7; Ammons et al., 1985a; Giesler et al., 1979; Trevino et al., 1973). Cells of the origin of the lateral spinothalamic tract are found to be more concentrated in lamina I of the dorsal horn (marginal zone), whereas a higher proportion of medial spinothalamic cells originate from the intermediate spinal gray matter and the ventral horn (Ammons et al., 1985a; Carstens and Trevino, 1978; Giesler et al., 1979; Willis et al., 1979).

Visceral pain, such as angina pectoris and gastrointestinal pain, is usually referred to an overlying or nearby somatic structure (Figure 7-8). Ruch (1946) proposed the convergence-projection theory to explain this referral of pain. He wrote, "some visceral afferents converge with cutaneous pain afferents to end upon the same neuron at some point in the sensory pathway—spinal, thalamic, or cortical—this system of fibers is sufficiently organized topographically to provide the dermatomal reference." The spinothalamic tract can transmit this information because somatic and visceral afferent inputs converge onto laminae I and V neurons (Ammons et al., 1985a,b; Blair et al., 1981). All lateral spinothalamic

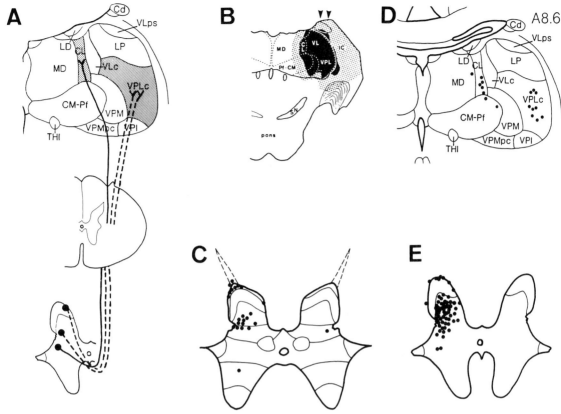

Figure 7-7 The spinothalamic tract system. A schematic drawing of the cells of origin and the course of the thoracic primate spinothalamic tract is shown in A. In the lateral-spinothalamic tract (1-STT), neurons of laminae I, IV, and V project (dashed lines represent axons) primarily to the lateral thalamus (hatched sections). In the medial spinothalamic tract (solid line) the cells of origin tend to be deeper in the spinal gray matter and project to the medial thalamus (dots). B and C show the results of an experimental study where horseradish peroxidase (HRP) was injected into the lateral thalamus of a monkey (B) and cells filled with HRP were distributed with gray matter (C) (Trevino, 1976). D shows the stimulation sites in the thalamus that antidromically activated cells of origin of the spinothalamic tract in the T3 gray matter of the spinal cord as shown in E. Abbreviations of thalamic nuclei: Cd, caudate nucleus; CL, nucleus centralis lateralis; CM, centrum medianum; LD, lateral dorsal nucleus; LP, lateral posterior nucleus; MD, dorsomedial nucleus; Pf, parafascicular nucleus; VLc, ventral lateral nucleus caudal part; VLps, ventral lateral nucleus, pars posterior; VPI, ventral posteroinferior nucleus; VPLc, ventral posterolateral nucleus, caudal part; VPM, ventral posteromedial nucleus; VPMpc, ventral posteromedial nucleus, parvocellular part; THl, habenulointerpeduncular tract; IC, internal capsule; SN, substantia nigra (Ammons et al., 1985a).

cells and about 90% of the medial spinothalamic cells have been found to receive both visceral and somatic input (Ammons et al., 1985a).

Spinothalamic tract cells usually respond to noxious stimuli and very rarely respond only to innocuous stimuli. These cells are generally classified as low threshold, wide dynamic range (or multireceptive), or high threshold (or nociceptive specific). Wide dynamic range cells are the most common. These neurons discharge at low frequency to hair movement or touching of the skin, but at a higher frequency when a pinch is applied to the skin or skin and muscle (Figure 7-9A). High threshold cells increase their discharge rate during the pinch of skin or skin and muscle, but are not affected by moving

hairs (Figure 7-9B). High threshold inhibitory cells markedly increase their discharge rate to noxious pinch, but spontaneous activity of cells is suppressed when hairs are moved.

Cells responding to electrical stimulation of A-delta (myelinated) and C (unmyelinated) cardiopulmonary afferent fibers excite the same spinothalamic neurons that receive somatic input (Ammons et al., 1985a,b; Blair et al., 1981). Cardiopulmonary afferent fibers contain only A-delta and C fibers (Emery et al., 1978; Seagard et al., 1978). At low stimulus strengths, an A-delta fiber volley was observed with a minimum afferent conduction velocity of approximately 9 m/sec (Figure 7-9C). When the intensity, and sometimes the duration, of the stimulus was in-

A.

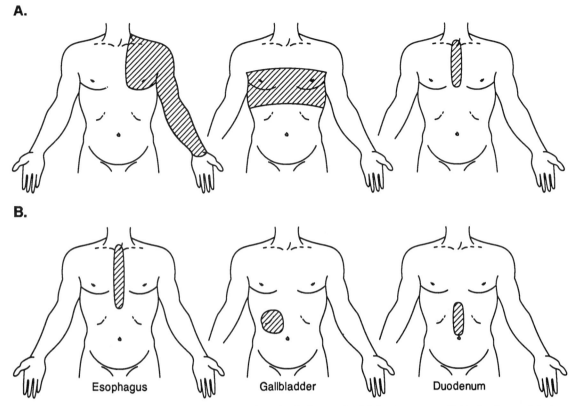

B.

Esophagus   Gallbladder   Duodenum

Figure 7-8 Location of somatic fields where deep referred pain is perceived following myocardial infarction and during angina pectoris originating from the heart (A) and is felt in visceral pain from the gastrointestinal tract (B). The figures in A illustrate the variable location of pain with angina pectoris. [These are based on data of Teodori and Galletti (1985), cited by Wall, P. D., and Melzack, R. (eds.). (1985). *Textbook of Pain,* Churchill, Livingstone, Edinburgh.] The esophageal and duodenal fields are modified from Jones (1938) and the gallbladder field was modified from Morley (1931).

creased, approximately 50% of the cells had a long latency volley that coincided with a C-fiber input of approximately 1 m/sec (Figure 7-9D).

Somatic receptive fields of the lateral spinothalamic cells are usually restricted to the ipsilateral chest and forelimb and do not cross the midline (Figure 7-10A; Ammons et al., 1985a). By contrast, medial spinothalamic cells have more complicated receptive fields. Often the receptive fields are bilateral or they have large unilateral fields (Figure 7-10B). A large number of thoracic cells respond most vigorously when skin and muscle are pinched together. The increased activity resulting from muscle input may contribute to understanding the sensations that are commonly associated with referred pain (see review by Lewis, 1942). Thus, spinothalamic cells receiving muscle input may produce a unique pattern of activity that is transmitted to higher pain centers.

Stimulation of sensory receptors using "natural" conditions is necessary to understanding how cells of the spinal cord respond to events occurring in visceral organs and, in particular, the cardiopulmonary region. Stimuli such as injection of the algesic chemical bradykinin, a peptide thought to be released during cardiac ischemia, into the heart or occlusion of a coronary artery are used to activate cardiac receptors. Injecting bradykinin into the left atrium activates receptors directly in the heart and/or throughout the coronary distribution (Blair et al., 1982, 1984a). Approximately 75% of the spinothalamic cells increase their activity approximately 15 seconds after injection of bradykinin (Figure 7-11A). The response time corresponds closely to the time required for bradykinin to activate receptors in studies of single units from sympathetic afferent fibers (see Malliani, 1982, for review). Spinothalamic tract cells also increase their discharge rate when myocardial ischemia results from coronary artery occlusion (Figure 7-11B). These studies reveal that referred pain associated with coronary artery disease most likely occurs because spinothalamic neurons increase their discharge rate as a result of myocardial ischemia. The viscerosomatic convergence onto the same spinothalamic cell forms the basis for the referred pain that occurs with angina pectoris.

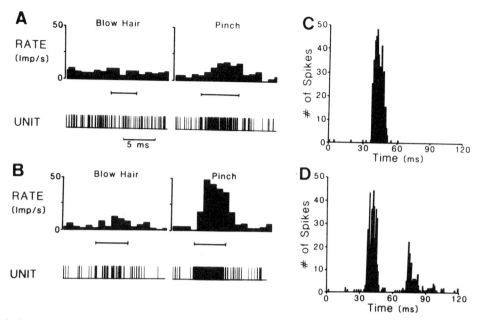

Figure 7-9 Convergence of somatic (A,B) and visceral (C,D) input on STT cells. A shows the responses of a nociceptive-specific or high threshold cell and B shows the responses of a wide dynamic range cell. In both A,B the top trace is the rate of discharge of the STT cell and the bottom tract is the individual action potentials after being processed in a window discriminator (unit). The horizontal bar is the period the stimulus was applied to the somatic receptive field. The peristimulus histograms in C and D are responses of an STT cell when the cardiopulmonary sympathetic afferents were stimulated 50 times at 1 Hz. The stimulus strengths were sufficient to activate A-delta fibers in C and A-delta and C fibers in D. The stimulus was applied at 30 msec (Foreman, 1986).

Many visceral disorders cause chest pain, which can be interpreted as angina pectoris. Esophageal or gastrointestinal disorders can produce similar symptoms (see Figure 7-8). This common pattern of referred pain suggests that there may be convergence of input from the upper part of the gastrointestinal tract, and from the heart, onto the same spinothalamic neurons in the upper thoracic segments. This has been documented by showing that some of the spinothalamic cells in the T1–T5 segments that respond to electrical stimulation of A-delta and C fibers in the splanchnic nerve are also activated by both electrical stimulation of the cardiopulmonary afferent fibers and activation of somatic fields (Ammons et al., 1984a). This implies that these neurons receive convergent information from multiple visceral as well as somatic structures. Transection of the lateral and ventrolateral funiculi on the ipsilateral side of the spinal cord at approximately the T6 segment abolished most of the spinothalamic cell responses to splanchnic input that enter the spinal cord in segments caudal to T5 (Ammons et al., 1984a). This projection may represent propriospinal connections between the upper and lower segments, but there is a possibility that this pathway may be part of an ascending limb of a supraspinal loop (Cervero, 1983; Cervero et al., 1985). Gallbladder distention also activates T2–T5 spinothalamic cells

(Ammons et al., 1984b). The presence of this population of neurons may explain why patients who have gallbladder disease are likely to experience angina-like pain during cholecystitis.

Spinoreticular Tract

The spinoreticular tract is another major pathway that ascends in the ventrolateral quadrant of the spinal cord (Figure 7-12A) (Bowsher, 1957, 1961; Mehler et al., 1960). Anatomical studies have shown that the spinoreticular tract projects primarily to the gigantocellular tegmental field (equivalent to paramedian reticular formation) and has lighter projections to the caudal raphe nuclei and the magnocellular tegmental field (equivalent to ventromedial reticular formation) (Abols and Basbaum, 1981; Gallagher and Pert, 1978). These medial regions of the brainstem reticular formation then project primarily to the intralaminar region of the thalamus (Bowsher, 1975). Electrophysiological studies agree with anatomical studies (Figure 7-12B; Blair et al., 1984a,b; Foreman et al., 1984; Kevetter et al., 1982; Maunz et al., 1978). Cells of origin of the spinoreticular tract have been mapped using retrograde cell body labeling and electrophysiological techniques (Figure 7-12C; cat: Abols and Basbaum, 1981; rat: Chaouch et al., 1983; Kevetter and Willis, 1983; monkey: Kev-

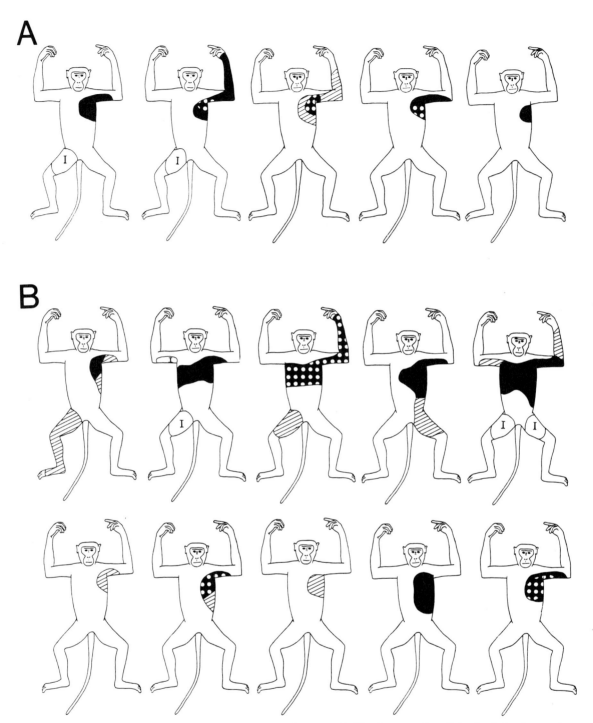

Figure 7-10 Somatic receptive fields of lateral spinothalamic tract (1-STT) cells (A) and medial spinothalamic tract (m-STT) cells (B) found in the T2–T5 spinal segments. Black areas are input from skin and muscle; white dots = excitatory hair field overlaying skin and muscle field; striped area = response to muscle only; white triangles are inhibitory input caused by hair movement; I = inhibitory receptive field from skin or muscle (Ammons et al., 1985).

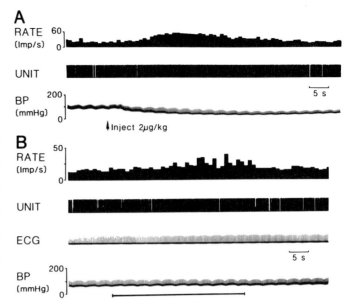

Figure 7-11 Effects of natural cardiac stimuli on STT cells. In A bradykinin (2 mg/kg) was injected into the left atrium and in B the left circumflex branch of the coronary artery was occluded. The upper tracing is the rate the cell discharged in impulses/second, the second tracing is individual action potentials after passing through a window discriminator (unit), and the bottom trace is blood pressure (BP) in mm Hg. In B, the third tracing is the electrocardiogram (ECG). The arrow in A marks the time of injection of bradykinin. The black horizontal bar in B marks the period of coronary artery occlusion (Foreman, 1986).

etter et al., 1982). These cells are concentrated in laminae VII and VIII of the intermediate spinal gray matter, although some are found in the dorsal horn (laminae I, IV, and V).

Electrophysiological characteristics of the spinoreticular cells have been studied in a variety of mammals, including monkeys, cats, and rats (Fields et al., 1975, 1977; Foreman et al., 1984; Haber et al., 1982; Maunz et al., 1978; Menetrey et al., 1980). Spinoreticular tract cells in the thoracic region of the spinal cord receive convergent input from visceral and somatic afferents (Foreman et al., 1984). Cells of the upper thoracic region respond to variable somatic inputs, and these can be subdivided into four categories: 86% of the cells had receptive fields classified as high threshold; 10% of the cells were classified as wide dynamic range; 3% were high threshold inhibitory; and only 1% were low threshold stimuli. The receptive somatic fields can also be classified into two groups: simple and complex. The simple fields (71%) were localized to the left forearm and left upper thorax. The remaining 29% of the cells were classified as complex because their receptive fields extended beyond the left forearm and chest.

These cells, just like spinothalamic neurons, respond to A-delta (myelinated) and C fiber (unmyelinated) inputs from the cardiopulmonary region (Foreman et al., 1984). In addition to responding to electrical stimulation of visceral afferents, the cells also increase their discharge rate when bradykinin is injected into the coronary circulation (Blair et al., 1984a). Based on the responsiveness of the cells, evidence indicates that many of these cells are nociceptive; therefore, it can be presumed that the cells account for the nociceptive response of neurons in the

medial reticular formation (Casey, 1969, 1971; Guilbaud et al., 1973).

In addition to the transmission of nociceptive information, spinoreticular neurons also respond to innocuous stimuli, such as premature ventricular contractions (Figure 7-13). Therefore, the medial reticular formation may not only be processing nociceptive information, but also is receiving innocuous information that may be important for central modulation of the peripheral cardiovascular system. Inputs arising from the spinoreticular pathway and collaterals of the spinothalamic tract are integrated with other inputs in the medial reticular formation (Blair, 1985). The medial reticular formation may mediate motor responses to cardiac pain as well as motor responses associated with escape and alerting behavior and, in addition, may modulate sympathetic function via collaterals to the intermediolateral cell column or to interneurons (Blair, 1987).

Spinomesencephalic Tract

The spinomesencephalic tract in the primate has major projections to the central periaqueductal gray matter and parabrachial nucleus (Wiberg et al., 1987; see Figure 7-14). Similar projections are found in the cat and rat (Menetrey et al., 1982; Wiberg and Blomqvist, 1984; Bjorkeland and Boivie, 1984; Cechetto et al., 1985). There may be a collateral projection to both the ventral posterior lateral nucleus of the thalamus and the central gray matter (Price et al., 1978). The largest concentration of projecting cells is found in lamina I, with a lesser concentration in lamina V (Wiberg et al., 1987). This distribution differs from the spinothalamic tract because cells are

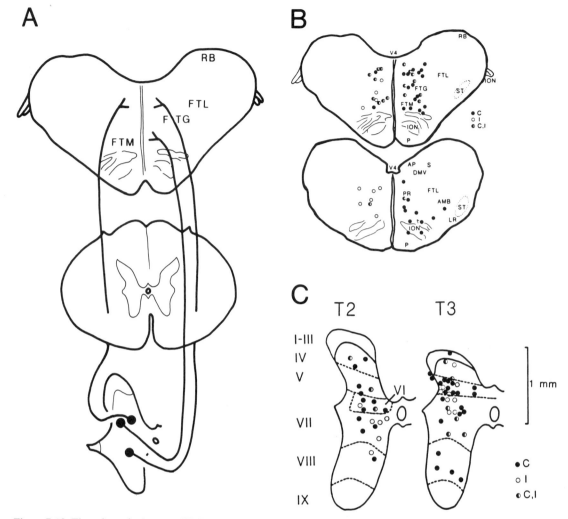

Figure 7-12 The spinoreticular tract (SRT). A schematic drawing of the cells of origin and the course of the spinoreticular tract is shown in A. The SRT neurons are found primarily in laminae V, VII, and VIII and course through the ipsilateral and contralateral ventrolateral funiculus to the medial regions of the medulla including the gigantocellular tegmental field (FTG), magnocellular tegmental field (FTM), and paramedian reticular nucleus (PR). Electrophysiological studies from the cat are shown in B and C. The stimulus sites for antidromically activating SRT cells are shown in B and the locations of the antidromically activated cells are marked by electrolytic lesions in C. Filled circles are cells projecting to the contralateral reticular formation (C); open circles are cells projecting to the ipsilateral reticular formation (I); half filled circles are cells projecting to both sides of the reticular formation (C,I). The Roman numerals are Rexed's laminae. The medullary sections in B are redrawn from the Berman atlas (1968) and are P8.5 (top) and P13 (bottom) (C). AMB, nucleus ambiguus; AP, area postrema; CI, inferior central nucleus; DMB, dorsal motor nucleus of the vagus; FTG, gigantocellular tegmental field; FTL, lateral tegmental field; FTM, magnocellular tegmental field; ION, inferior olivary nucleus; LR, lateral reticular nucleus; P, pyramidal tract; PPR, postpyramidal nucleus of the raphe; PR, paramedial reticular nucleus; RB, restiform body; S, solitary tract; ST, spinothalamic tract; V4, fourth ventricle; 10N, vagus nerve (Foreman et al., 1984).

more equally distributed in laminae IV, V, and VI (Willis et al., 1979). Electrophysiological studies done in the lumbosacral region in the rat (Menetrey et al., 1980) and cat (Yezierski and Schwartz, 1986) show that the spinomesencephalic tract may play an important role in somatic sensory mechanisms related to nociception. No electrophysiological studies have been done to examine the spinomesencephalic input arising from the thoracic segments of the spi-

nal cord. Visceral input may also be transmitted, but the evidence is lacking. Yezierski and Schwartz (1986) noted that a few cells responded exclusively to testicular stimulation.

Spinosolitary Tract

The spinosolitary tract has received little attention, but it may be part of a larger system that integrates

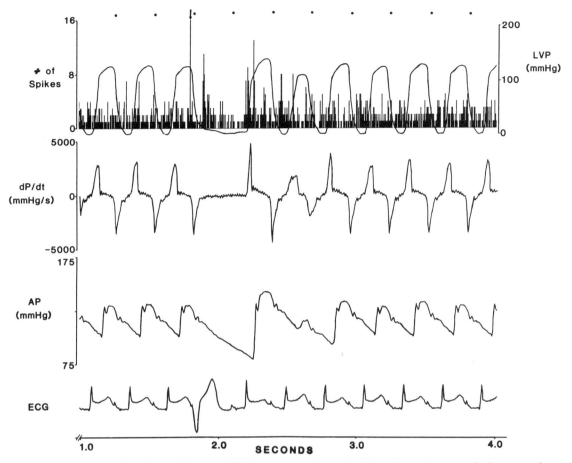

Figure 7-13 Responses of a spinoreticular tract (SRT) neuron to electrically induced premature ventricular contractions in the cat. The heart was paced at 205 beats/minute. (R–R interval of 290 msec.) The dots above the top panel indicate delivery of pacing stimuli and 25 repetitions of a 15 beat cycle were compiled for the figure. Only 11 cycles are shown in the figure. In the figure, cell activity was summed and the remainder of the traces were averaged. An extra stimulus was delivered at the arrow (top) 280 msec after the pacing stimulus and caused a premature ventricular contraction as noted in the VEG. In the top tracing the number (#) of spikes is a summation of extracellular action potentials recorded from the SRT neuron and LVP is left ventricular pressure. In the second trace *dP/dt* is a measure of heart contractility and is obtained by computer differentiation of the LVP. The third tract is aorta pressure (AP) and the fourth tract is the ventricular electrogram (ECG) obtained from a bipolar electrode inserted into the free wall of the left ventricle. The SRT cell responded with an early burst and late bursts just preceding, during, and following the compensatory contraction; first cardiac cycle after the compensatory pause. The early burst after the stimulus artifact (arrow) was not caused by direct electrical stimulation of cardiac afferent fibers (Blair and Foreman, 1988).

somatic and visceral afferent inputs from wide areas of the body. The terminal field of the spinal projection is bilateral and is concentrated in the caudal part of the nucleus tractus solitarius. The retrograde cell body labeling technique has been used to study this projection (Menetrey and Basbaum, 1987; Leah et al., 1988). It originates from cell bodies in lamina I, the lateral spinal nucleus of the dorsolateral funiculus, the lateral part of lamina V, and lamina X surrounding the central canal. Additional cells in the region of the thoracic and sacral autonomic cell columns project to the nucleus tractus solitarius. The spinosolitary cells in lamina I contain immunoreactive dynorphin, those in the lateral spinal nu-

cleus contain immunoreactive vasoactive intestinal polypeptide, and those in lamina X contain immunoreactive bombesin (Leah et al., 1988). The location of these cells resembles the locations seen for the cells of origin of the spinomesencephalic, spinoreticular, and spinothalamic tracts. Since the cells of the spinosolitary tract are clustered in lamina V and in areas where it has been demonstrated that these cells receive visceral and somatic input, there is a possibility that indeed these participate in viscerosomatic and viscerovisceral interactions.

Only limited information exists about the characteristics of lamina X neurons. They receive visceral afferent inputs (Neuhuber, 1982; Ciriello and

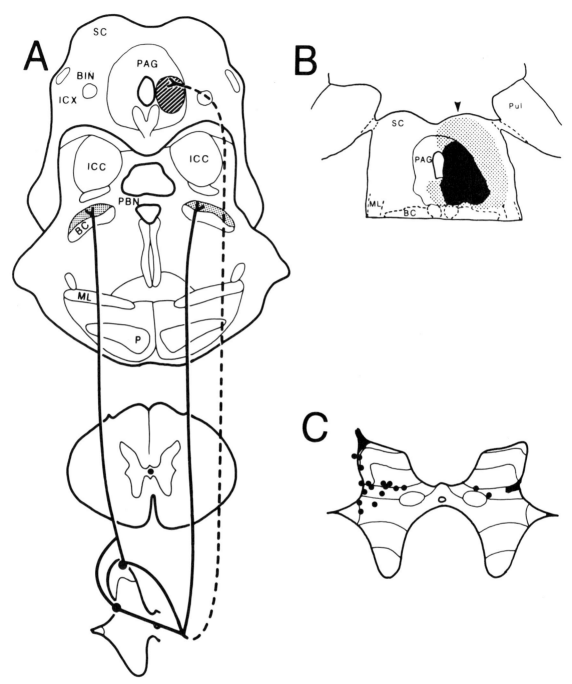

Figure 7-14 A schematic diagram of the cells of origin of the T3 spinal segment and course of the primate spinomesencephalic tract are shown in A. The neurons projecting to the mesencephalon are found primarily in laminae I and V. The spinoparabrachial tract (termination sites represented with dots are the parabrachial nuclei) has both ipsilateral and contralateral projections while the pathway projecting to the periaqueductal gray (termination sites represented with lines) has primarily contralateral projections (A is modified from Wiberg et al., 1987). To locate spinomesencephalic neurons in the primate thoracic T5 spinal cord (C) horseradish peroxidase was injected primarily in the periaqueductal gray and adjacent reticular formation. BC, brachium conjunctivum; BIN, nucleus of the brachium of the inferior colliculus; ICC, inferior colliculus; ICX, external nucleus of the inferior colliculus; ML, medial lemniscus; P, pyramidal tract; PAG, periaqueductal gray matter; PBN, parabrachial nucleus; PUL, pulvinar. The arrow indicates the position of the microsyringe needle track (Trevino, 1976).

Caleresu, 1983; Honda, 1985), and others receive somatosensory information (Honda and Perl, 1985). The cells that populate this region are quite heterogeneous in terms of their efferent projections. Some are preganglionic neurons (Petras and Cummings, 1972; Hancock and Peveto, 1979) and others project to the central gray matter (Menetrey et al., 1982). No information exists about the characteristics of these cells in the upper thoracic spinal cord.

Other Pathways

A number of other ascending spinal pathways may be involved in relaying visceral sensation to the brain. However, no study has systematically explored whether visceral information is carried by these pathways. For example, studies dealing with the spinocervical tract have not examined the question of whether visceral information is relayed in this pathway. In the lumbar and sacral spinal cord, spinocervical tract neurons are not involved in viscerosomatic convergence because neurons in the lumbosacral cord are not affected by activation of urinary bladder afferent fibers (Cervero and Iggo, 1978; McMahon and Morrison, 1982). Studies of the postsynaptic dorsal column pathway have not determined whether visceral information is conveyed in this system (Brown et al., 1983; Lu et al., 1983; Angaut-Petit, 1975). Although nociceptive somatic information is transmitted in the dorsal column postsynaptic and the spinohypothalamic pathways (Burstein et al., 1987), no evidence exists that this pathway transmits visceral information, and, in particular, no information has been obtained for the responses of neurons in the upper thoracic spinal cord.

SUMMARY

Afferents from thoracic, abdominal, and pelvic organs travel as part of the sympathetic nervous system. Receptors sense changes in the internal environment that will trigger or modulate the reflex perceived by the subject as conscious sensations. This chapter examines the anatomical distribution of visceral afferent fibers in different internal organs, relative numbers, peripheral pathways of projection to the central nervous system, mechanisms of encoding of adequate visceral stimuli, and pathways ascending in the spinal cord that transmit visceral afferent information.

Primary and enteric afferent fibers are present in the sympathetic nerves. Primary fibers act as transmission lines between the internal environment and the central nervous system and transmit afferent information that will be used for integrated autonomic regulated responses and for perception of visceral sensations. Enteric efferent neurons are specifically associated with innervation of the gut and of associated hollow viscera such as the gallbladder.

Visceral primary afferents of sympathetic and parasympathetic origin innervate most internal organs. The number of parasympathetic to sympathetic afferents is, in general, greater by a ratio of more than 3:1. Another common property of these afferents is that more than 90% of all visceral afferents are unmyelinated and of the remaining 10%, the majority are thinly myelinated or lose their myelin as they approach their target organs.

Encoding mechanisms of visceral sensory receptors must account for characteristics of visceral sensation that are more complicated than that of cutaneous sensation, because visceral receptors with and without sensation are activated with a stimulus. Visceral receptors not concerned with conscious sensation are endings whose stimulation evokes no sensations and are used for reflex regulation of internal environment. Visceral receptors concerned with conscious sensation are endings that innervate organs from which sensations can be evoked. Three possible encoding mechanisms that could distinguish between sensory and nonsensory events or between painful and nonpainful experiences are by specificity of the receptor, by the pattern of response of the receptor, and by central summation of the afferent response.

Visceral afferent fibers reach the dorsal horn of the spinal cord via Lissauer's tract and join medial and lateral bundles of fine fibers that course along the edges of the dorsal horn and terminate within laminae I and V of the dorsal horn gray matter. Less than 10% of all afferent fibers in the thoracolumbar dorsal roots are of visceral origin, yet more than 75% of all neurons in the thoracic spinal cord are viscerosomatic; that is, they receive convergent inputs from visceral organs and from somatic structures. Many of the visceral fine afferent fibers contain several neuropeptides, including substance P, calcitonin gene-related peptide (CGRP), and vasoactive intestinal polypeptide (VIP), among others.

Electrophysiological and anatomical characteristics of ascending pathways, including the spinothalamic tract, spinoreticular tract, spinomesencephalic tract, spinosolitary tract, and other pathways, are discussed as they relate to the transmission of visceral nociceptive information from the thoracic spinal cord to the brainstem and thalamus. Visceral nociceptive information must reach the brain to activate the systems that are responsible for producing the responses to the painful stimulus. These responses include sensory-discriminative perceptions and motivational-affective behavior.

REFERENCES

Reviews

Andrews, P. L. R. (1986). Vagal afferent innervation of the gastrointestinal tract. In: *Visceral Sensation. Progress in Brain Research,* Vol. 67, F. Cervero and J. F. B. Morrison (eds.), Elsevier, Amsterdam, pp. 65–86.

Cervero, F. (1985). Visceral nociception: Peripheral and central aspects of visceral nociceptive systems. *Philosophical Transactions of the Royal Society, Series B* 308, 325–337.

Cervero, F., and Tattersall, J. E. H. (1986). Somatic and visceral sensory integration in the thoracic spinal cord. In: *Visceral Sensation. Progress in Brain Research,* Vol. 67, F. Cervero and J. F. B. Morrison (eds.), Elsevier, Amsterdam, pp. 189–205.

Costa, M., Furness, J. B., and Llewellyn-Smith, I. J. (1987). Histochemistry of the enteric nervous system. In: *Physiology of the Gastrointestinal Tract,* 2nd ed. L. R. Johnson (ed.), Raven, New York, pp. 1–40.

De Groat, W. C. (1986). Spinal cord projections and neuropeptides in visceral afferent neurons. In: *Visceral Sensation. Progress in Brain Research,* Vol. 67, F. Cervero and J. F. B. Morrison (eds.), Elsevier, Amsterdam, pp. 165–187.

Foreman, R. D. (1986). Spinal substrates of visceral pain. In: *Spinal Afferent Processing,* T. L. Yaksh (ed.), Plenum, New York, pp. 217–242.

Goldscheider, A. (1884). The specific energies of the sensory nerves of the skin. (transl. from German). In: *Classical German Contributions to Brain Research,* H. O. Handwerker and K. Brune (eds.), (1987). Published by Gesellschaft zum Studium des Schmerzes für Deutschland, Österreich und die Schweiz, Prof. M. Zimmermann, II. Physiologisches Institut, Universität Heidelberg.

Jänig, W., and Morrison, J. F. B. (1986). Functional properties of spinal visceral afferents supplying abdominal and pelvic organs, with special emphasis on visceral nociception. In: *Visceral Sensation. Progress in Brain Research,* Vol. 67, F. Cervero and J. F. B. Morrison (eds.), Elsevier, Amsterdam, pp. 87–114.

Langley, J. N. (1900). The sympathetic and other related systems of nerves. In: *Text-Book of Physiology,* 2nd ed. E. A. Schafer (ed.), Young J. Pentland, Edinburgh and London, pp. 616–696.

Langley, J. N. (1921). *The Autonomic Nervous System.* W. Heffer, Cambridge.

Leek, B. R. (1972). Abdominal visceral receptors. In: *Handbook of Sensory Physiology,* Vol. III/I: *Enteroceptors,* E. Neil (ed.), Springer-Verlag, Berlin, pp. 113–160.

Lembeck, F. (1983). Sir Thomas Lewis's nocifensor system, histamine and substance P-containing primary afferent nerves. *Trends in Neuroscience* 6, 106–108.

Lewis, T. (1942). *Pain.* Macmillan, New York.

Malliani, A. (1982). Cardiovascular and sympathetic afferent fibers. *Reviews of Physiology, Biochemistry, and Pharmacology* 94, 11–74.

Melzack, R., and Casey, K. L. (1968). Sensory, motivational and central control determinants of pain. In: *The Skin Senses,* D. Kenshalo (ed.), Thomas, Springfield, pp. 423–443.

Melzack, R., and Wall, P. D. (1982). *The Challenge of Pain.* Basic Books, New York.

Muramoto, I. (1987). Peripheral transmission in primary sensory nerves. *Japanese Journal of Pharmacology* 43, 113–120.

Price, D. D., and Dubner, R. (1977). Neurons that subserve the sensory-discriminative aspects of pain. *Pain* 3, 307–338.

Ranson, S. W. (1921). Afferent paths for visceral reflexes. *Physiological Reviews* 1, 477–522.

Ruch, T. C. (1946). Visceral sensation and referred pain. In: *Howell's Textbook of Physiology,* 15th ed., J. F. Fulton (ed.), Saunders, Philadelphia, pp. 385–401.

Trevino, D. L. (1976). The origin and projections of a spinal nociceptive and thermoreceptive pathway. In: *Sensory Functions of the Skin in Primates, with Special Reference to Man,* Y. Zotterman (ed.), Pergamon, New York, pp. 367–376.

Willis, W. D., Jr. (1985). *The Pain System—The Neural Basis of Nociceptive Transmission in the Mammalian Nervous System.* Karger, Basel, pp. 145–212.

Research Papers

Abols, I. A., and Basbaum, A. I. (1981). Afferent connections of the rostral medulla of the cat: A neural substrate for midbrain-medullary interactions in the modulation of pain. *Journal of Comparative Neurology* 201, 285–297.

Ammons, W. S., Blair, R. W., and Foreman, R. D. (1984a). Responses of primate T1–T5 spinothalamic neurons to gallbladder distension. *American Journal of Physiology* 247, R995–R1002.

Ammons, W. S., Blair, R. W., and Foreman, R. D. (1984b). Greater splanchnic excitation of primate T1–T5 spinothalamic neurons. *Journal of Neurophysiology* 51, 592–603.

Ammons, W. S., Girardot, M.-N., and Foreman, R. D. (1985a). T2–T5 spinothalamic neurons projecting to medial thalamus with viscerosomatic input. *Journal of Neurophysiology* 54, 73–89.

Ammons, W. S., Girardot, M.-N., and Foreman, R. D. (1985b). Effects of intracardiac bradykinin on T2–T5 spinothalamic cells. *American Journal of Physiology* 249, R147–R152.

Angaut-Petit, D. (1975). The dorsal column system: II. Functional properties and bulbar relay of the postsynaptic fibres of the cat's fasciculus gracilis. *Experimental Brain Research* 22, 471–493.

Bjorkeland, M., and Boivie, J. (1984). The termination of spinomesencephalic fibres in cat. An experimental anatomical study. *Anatomy and Embryology* 170, 265–277.

Blair, R. W. (1985). Noxious cardiac input onto neurons in medullary reticular formation. *Brain Research* 326, 335–346.

Blair, R. W. (1987). Responses of feline medial medullary reticulospinal neurons to cardiac input. *Journal of Neurophysiology* 58, 1149–1167.

Blair, R. W., Weber, R. N., and Foreman, R. D. (1981). Characteristics of primate spinothalamic tract neurons receiving viscerosomatic convergent inputs in T3–T5 segments. *Journal of Neurophysiology* 46, 797–811.

Blair, R. W., Weber, R. N., and Foreman, R. D. (1982).

Responses of thoracic spinothalamic neurons to intra-cardiac injection of bradykinin in the monkey. *Circulation Research* 51, 83–94.

Blair, R. W., Weber, R. N., and Foreman, R. D. (1984a). Responses of spinoreticular and spinothalamic cells to intracardiac bradykinin. *American Journal of Physiology* 246, H500–H507.

Blair, R. W., Ammons, W. S., and Foreman, R. D. (1984b). Responses of thoracic spinothalamic and spinoreticular cells to coronary artery occlusion. *Journal of Neurophysiology* 51, 636–648.

Blumberg, H., Haupt, P., Jänig, W., and Kohler, W. (1983). Encoding of visceral noxious stimuli in the discharge patterns of visceral afferent fibres from the colon. *Pflugers Archives* 398, 33–40.

Boivie, J. (1979). An anatomical reinvestigation of the termination of the spinothalamic tract in the monkey. *Journal of Comparative Neurology* 186, 343–370.

Bowsher, D. (1957). Termination of the central pain pathway in man. The conscious appreciation of pain. *Brain* 80, 606–622.

Bowsher, D. (1961). The termination of secondary somatosensory neurons within the thalamus of *Macaca mulatta:* An experimental degeneration study. *Journal of Comparative Neurology* 117, 213–227.

Bowsher, D. (1975). Diencephalic projection from the midbrain reticular formation. *Brain Research* 94, 211–220.

Brown, A. G., Brown, P. B., Fyffe, R. E. W., and Pubols, L. M. (1983). Receptive field organization and response properties of spinal neurons with axons ascending the dorsal columns in the cat. *Journal of Physiology (London)* 337, 575–588.

Burstein, R., Cliffer, K. D., and Giesler, G. J., Jr. (1987). Direct somatosensory projections from the spinal cord to the hypothalamus and telencephalon. *Journal of Neuroscience* 7, 4159–4164.

Casey, K. L. (1969). Somatic stimuli, spinal pathways, and size of cutaneous fibres influencing unit activity in the medial medullary reticular formation. *Experimental Neurology* 25, 35–56.

Casey, K. L. (1971). Responses of bulboreticular units to somatic stimuli eliciting escape behavior in the cat. *International Journal of Neuroscience* 2, 15–28.

Carstens, E., and Trevino, D. L. (1978). Laminar origins of spinothalamic projections in the cat as determined by the retrograde transport of horseradish peroxidase. *Journal of Comparative Neurology* 182, 151–166.

Cechetto, D. F., Standaert, D. G., and Saper, C. B. (1985). Spinal and trigeminal dorsal horn projections to the parabrachial nucleus in the rat. *Journal of Comparative Neurology* 240, 153–160.

Cervero, F. (1982). Afferent activity evoked by natural stimulation of the biliary system in the ferret. *Pain* 13, 137–151.

Cervero, F. (1983). Supraspinal connections of neurones in the thoracic spinal cord of the cat: Ascending projections and effects of descending impulses. *Brain Research* 275, 251–261.

Cervero, F., and Connell, L. A. (1984). Distribution of somatic and visceral primary afferent fibres within the thoracic spinal cord of the cat. *Journal of Comparative Neurology* 230, 88–98.

Cervero, F., and Iggo, A. (1978). Natural stimulation of urinary bladder afferents does not affect transmission through lumbrosacral spinocervical tract neurones in the cat. *Brain Research* 156, 375–379.

Cervero, F., and Sharkey, K. A. (1988). An electrophysiological and anatomical study of intestinal afferent fibres in the rat. *Journal of Physiology (London)* 401, 361–380.

Cervero, F., and Tattersall, J. E. H. (1987). Somatic and visceral inputs to the thoracic spinal cord of the cat: Marginal zone (lamina I) of the dorsal horn. *Journal of Physiology (London)* 388, 383–395.

Cervero, F., Connell, L. A., and Lawson, S. N. (1984). Somatic and visceral primary afferents in the lower thoracic dorsal root ganglia of the cat. *Journal of Comparative Neurology* 228, 422–431.

Cervero, F., Lumb, B. M., and Tattersall, J. E. H. (1985). Supraspinal loops that mediate visceral inputs to thoracic spinal cord neurones in the cat: Involvement of descending pathways from raphe and reticular formation. *Neuroscience Letters* 56, 189–194.

Chaouch, A., Menetrey, D., Binder, D., and Besson, J. M. (1983). Neurons at the origin of the medial component of the bulbopontine spinorecticular tract in the rat: An anatomical study using horseradish peroxidase retrograde transport. *Journal of Comparative Neurology* 214, 309–320.

Ciriello, J., and Calaresu, F. R. (1983). Central projections of afferent renal fibres in the rat: An anterograde transport study of horseradish peroxidase. *Journal of the Autonomic Nervous System* 8, 273–285.

Delbro, D., Lisander, B., and Anderson, S. A. (1986). Bradykinin-induced atropine-sensitive gastric contractions. Activation of an intramural axon reflex? *Acta Physiologica Scandinavica* 127, 111–117.

Dennis, S. G., and Melzack, R. (1977). Pain-signalling systems in the dorsal and ventral spinal cord. *Pain* 4, 97–132.

Emery, D. G., Foreman, R. D., and Coggeshall, R. E. (1978). Categories of axons in the inferior cardiac nerve of the cat. *Journal of Comparative Neurology* 177, 301–310.

Fields, H. L., Clanton, C. H., and Anderson, S. D. (1977). Somatosensory properties of spinoreticular neurons in the cat. *Brain Research* 120, 49–66.

Fields, H. L., Wagner, G. M., and Anderson, S. D. (1975). Some properties of spinal neurons projecting to the medial brain-stem reticular formation. *Experimental Neurology* 47, 118–134.

Foreman, R. D., Blair, R. W., and Weber, R. N. (1984). Viscerosomatic convergence onto T-T spinoreticular, spinoreticular-spinothalamic and spinothalamic tract neurons in the cat. *Experimental Neurology* 85, 597–619.

Gallagher, D. W., and Pert, A. (1978). Afferents to brain stem nuclei (brain stem raphe, nucleus reticularis pontis caudalis and nucleus gigantocellularis) in the rat as demonstrated by microiontophoretically applied horseradish peroxidase. *Brain Research* 144, 257–275.

Giesler, G. J., Menetrey, D., and Basbaum, A. I. (1979). Differential origins of spinothalamic tract projections to medial and lateral thalamus in the rat. *Journal of Comparative Neurology* 184, 107–126.

Guilbaud, G., Besson, J. M., Oliveras, J. L., and Wyon-Maillard, M. C. (1973). Modification of the firing rate of bulbar reticular units (nucleus gigantocellularis) after intra-arterial injection of bradykinin into the limbs. *Brain Research* 63, 131–140.

Haber, L. H., Moore, B. D., and Willis, W. D. (1982). Electrophysiological response properties of spinoreticular neurons in the monkey. *Journal of Comparative Neurology* 207, 75–84.

Hancock, M. B., and Peveto, C. A. (1979). A preganglionic autonomic nucleus in the dorsal gray commissure of the lumbar sinal cord of the rat. *Journal of Comparative Neurology* 183, 65–72.

Honda, C. N. (1985). Visceral and somatic afferent convergence onto neurons near the central canal in the sacral spinal cord of the cat. *Journal of Neurophysiology* 53, 1059–1078.

Honda, C. N., and Perl, E. R. (1985). Functional and morphological features of neurons in the midline region of the caudal spinal cord of the cat. *Brain Research* 340, 285–295.

Jones, C. M. (1938). *Digestive Tract Pain. Diagnosis and Treatment.* Macmillan, New York, pp. 7–26.

Kevetter, G. A., and Willis, W. D. (1983). Collaterals of spinothalamic cells in the rat. *Journal of Comparative Neurology* 215, 453–464.

Kevetter, G. A., Haber, L. H., Yezierski, R. P., Chung, J. M., Martin, R. F., and Willis, W. D. (1982). Cells of origin of the spinoreticular tract in the monkey. *Journal of Comparative Neurology* 207, 61–74.

Kuo, D. C., Yang, G. C. H., Yamaskai, D. S., and Krauthamer, G. M. (1982). A wide field electron microscopic analysis of the fiber constituents of the major splanchnic nerve in the cat. *Journal of Comparative Neurology* 210, 49–58.

Langley, J. N., and Anderson, H. K. (1894). The constituents of the hypogastric nerves. *Journal of Physiology (London)* 17, 177–191.

Leah, J., Menetrey, D., and de Pommery, J. (1988). Neuropeptides in long ascending spinal tract cells in the rat: Evidence for parallel processing of ascending information. *Neuroscience* 24, 195–207.

Lu, G. W., Bennett, G. J., Nishikawa, N., Hoffert, M. J., and Dubner, R. (1983). Extra- and intracellular recordings from dorsal column postsynaptic spinomedullary neurons in the cat. *Experimental Neurology* 82, 456–477.

Matthews, M. R., and Cuello, A. C. (1984). The origin and possible significance of substance P immunoreactive networks in the prevertebral ganglia and related structures in the guinea-pig. *Philosophical Transactions of the Royal Society, Series B* 306, 247–276.

Maunz, R. A., Pitts, N. G., and Peterson, B. W. (1978). Cat spinoreticular neurons: Locations, responses and changes in responses during repetitive stimulation. *Brain Research* 148, 365–379.

McMahon, S. B., and Morrison, J. F. B. (1982). Spinal neurons with long projections activated from the abdominal viscera of the cat. *Journal of Physiology (London)* 322, 1–20.

Mehler, W. R., Feferman, M. E., and Nauta, W. J. H. (1960). Ascending axon degeneration following anterolateral cordotomy. An experimental study in the monkey. *Brain* 83, 718–751.

Menetrey, D., and Basbaum, A. I. (1987). Spinal and trigeminal projections to the nucleus of the solitary tract: A possible substrate for somatovisceral and viscerovisceral reflex activation. *Journal of Comparative Neurology* 255, 439–450.

Menetrey, D., Chaouch, A., and Besson, J. M. (1980). Location and properties of dorsal horn neurons at origin of spinoreticular tract in lumbar enlargement of the rat. *Journal of Neurophysiology* 44, 862–877.

Menetrey, D., Chaouch, A., Binder, D., and Besson, J. M. (1982). The origin of the spinomesencephalic tract in the rat: An anatomical study using the retrograde transport of horseradish peroxidase. *Journal of Comparative Neurology* 206, 193–207.

Molander, C., Ygge, J., and Dalsgaard, C. J. (1987). Substance P-, somatostatin- and calcitonin gene-related peptide-like immunoreactivity and fluoride resistant acid phosphatase-activity in relation to retrogradely labeled cutaneous, muscular and visceral primary sensory neurons in the rat. *Neuroscience Letters* 74, 37–42.

Morley, T. J. (1931). *Abdominal Pain.* Livingstone, Edinburgh, pp. 91–108.

Neuhuber, W. (1982). The central projections of visceral primary afferent neurons of the inferior mesenteric plexus and hypogastric nerve and the location of the related sensory and preganglionic sympathetic cell bodies in the rat. *Anatomy and Embryology* 164, 413–425.

Petras, J. M., and Cummings, J. F. (1972). Autonomic neurons in the spinal cord of the rhesus monkey: A correlation of the findings of cytoarchitectonics and sympathectomy with fibre degeneration following dorsal rhizotomy. *Journal of Comparative Neurology* 146, 189–218.

Price, D. D., and Mayer, D. J. (1974). Physiological laminar organization of the dorsal horn of *M. mulatta. Brain Research* 79, 321–325.

Price, D. D., Hayes, R. L., Ruda, M. A., and Dubner, R. (1978). Spatial and temporal transformations of input to spinothalamic tract neurons and their relation to somatic sensations. *Journal of Neurophysiology* 41, 933–947.

Seagard, J. L., Pederson, H. J., Kostreva, D. R., Van Horn, D. L., Cusik, J. F., and Kampine, J. P. (1978). Ultrastructural identification of afferent fibers of cardiac origin in thoracic sympathetic nerves in the dog. *American Journal of Anatomy* 153, 217–232.

Sharkey, K. A., Sobribo, J. A., and Cervero, F. (1987). Evidence for a visceral afferent origin of substance P-like immunoreactivity in lamina V of the rat thoracic spinal cord. *Neuroscience* 22, 1077–1083.

Shirasaka, C., Tsuji, H., Asoh, T., and Takeuchi, Y. (1986). Role of the splanchnic nerves in endocrine and metabolic responses to abdominal surgery. *British Journal of Surgery* 73, 142–145.

Tattersall, J. E. H., Cervero, F., and Lumb, B. M. (1986). Effects of reversible spinalization on the visceral input to viscerosomatic neurones in the lower thoracic spinal cord of the cat. *Journal of Neurophysiology* 56, 785–796.

Trevino, D. L., Coulter, J. D., and Willis, W. D. (1973). Location of cells of origin of spinothalamic tract in lumbar enlargement of the monkey. *Journal of Neurophysiology* 36, 750–761.

White, J. C. (1943). Sensory innervation of the viscera. *Research Publications—Association for Research in Nervous and Mental Disease* 23, 373–390.

Wiberg, M., and Blomqvist, A. (1984). The spinomesencephalic tract in the cat: Its cells of origin and termination pattern as demonstrated by the intraaxonal transport method. *Brain Research* 291, 1–18.

Wiberg, M., Westman, J., and Blomqvist, A. (1987). Somatosensory projection to the mesencephalon: An anatomical study in the monkey. *Journal of Comparative Neurology* 264, 92–117.

Willis, W. D., Kenshalo, D. R., Jr., and Leonard, R. B. (1979). The cells of origin of the primate spinothalamic tract. *Journal of Comparative Neurology* 188, 543–574.

Yezierski, R. P., and Schwartz, R. H. (1986). Response and receptive-field properties of spinomesencephalic tract cells in the cat. *Journal of Neurophysiology* 55, 76–96.

8

Central Determinants of Sympathetic Nerve Discharge

G. L. GEBBER

Sympathetic nerves innervating the heart, vasculature, and other visceral organs are tonically active under a variety of conditions in humans and animals. Such activity is critical for homeostasis, including the maintenance of blood pressure within normal limits. The level of activity in sympathetic nerves innervating different target organs can be nonuniformly changed, thus leading to complex visceral response patterns characteristic of such behavioral states as alerting, exercise, and sleep. The purpose of this chapter is to discuss how these functions of sympathetic nerves are controlled by the central nervous system.

Research in this field has centered on three issues. First, which cell groups in the central nervous system are responsible for sympathetic nerve discharge? Second, how do these neurons generate the basal (i.e., naturally occurring) activity of sympathetic nerves? Third, how does the central nervous system formulate complex visceral response patterns that include differential changes in regional blood flows? Moreover, what do these response patterns tell us about the organization of those central systems controlling sympathetic nerve activity? None of these issues has been resolved. Nevertheless, it is important to discuss them for several reasons. First, they are fundamental issues. Second, they are the subjects of considerable controversy and are likely to remain so in years to come. Finally, discussion of these issues provides a medium by which the student can be introduced to some of the contemporary experimental approaches used in this field. This is particularly true of electrophysiological methods used to test for a correlation between the discharges of single neurons in the brain and sympathetic nerve bundles. Since any given sympathetic nerve contains fibers controlling more than one target organ (e.g., vasculature, cardiac contractile and conductile tissue, gastrointestinal smooth muscle, renal tubules, sweat glands) data obtained by using the methods to be discussed must be viewed conservatively with regard to the control of a particular target organ. Rather, electrophysiological studies that characterize the relationships between the discharges of single neurons in the brain and sympathetic nerves best serve the purpose of revealing basic principles of the central control of sympathetic outflow.

EARLY STUDIES ON THE CENTRAL ORIGIN OF SYMPATHETIC NERVE DISCHARGE

Claude Bernard (1851) and Brown-Séquard (1852) are credited with the discovery that sympathetic nerves are tonically active. They demonstrated that sectioning of the cervical sympathetic nerve or removal of the superior cervical ganglion dilates the blood vessels of the rabbit ear. They also showed that electrical stimulation of the peripheral end of the sectioned cervical sympathetic nerve constricts the blood vessels of the ear. Thus, it became apparent that vascular tone is dependent, in part, on its sympathetic innervation.

Bernard (1863) focused attention on the role of supraspinal regions in generating sympathetic nerve activity. He demonstrated that transection of the neuraxis near the medullospinal junction is followed by an immediate and profound fall in blood pressure. Bernard's experiments led to the view that the tonic discharges of sympathetic vasoconstrictor nerves are generated primarily by supraspinal neuronal circuits. This view was reinforced when Sherrington (1906) reported that following recovery from spinal shock, neither blood pressure nor somatomotor reflexes were again depressed by a second spinal section performed caudal to the level of the first transection. Assuming that the trauma produced by the second transection is as severe as that following the first, Sherrington concluded that the fall in blood pressure accompanying the initial transection arises from the loss of tonically active supraspinal influences.

The search for the regions of the brain responsible for sympathetic nerve activity began in the laboratory of Carl Ludwig. One of his students, Oswjannikow (1871), found that serial transections of the rabbit or cat brain stem did not markedly affect blood pressure until a cut was made through the pons 1–2 mm behind the caudal border of the inferior colliculus (i.e., near level I in Figure 8-1D). Serial transections between this level and one somewhat rostral to the obex in the medulla (II in Figure 8-1D) progressively lowered blood pressure to a value near that observed after transection of the cervical spinal cord (III in Figure 8-1D). Alexander (1946) later demonstrated directly with nerve recordings that the fall in blood pressure was the consequence of a decrease in postganglionic sympathetic nerve activity. Thus, it became clear that the integrity of connections between the brain stem and spinal cord is essential for maintaining sympathetic nerve activity within normal limits. The view that regions rostral to the brain stem do not significantly contribute to sympathetic nerve discharge, however, has recently been questioned. This topic will be discussed later.

Dittmar (1873), also working in Ludwig's laboratory, more precisely localized a brain stem region involved in the control of blood pressure in the rabbit. Using knife cuts, he deduced that the maintenance of blood pressure within normal limits was dependent on the integrity of the ventral medulla at a level near the facial nucleus. Dittmar's region was rediscovered in 1967 when Schlaefke and Loeschcke found that local cooling of the rostral ventrolateral medulla caused a pronounced fall in blood pressure. That this region contains the cell bodies of neurons involved in controlling sympathetic outflow was established by Feldberg and his colleagues (see Feldberg, 1976). They showed that changes in blood pressure were produced by the local application to the ventral surface of the medulla of drugs that affect neuronal cell bodies, but not fibers of passage.

A different approach to the problem of localizing the central source of sympathetic nerve activity was developed in the laboratory of Ranson. Ranson and Billingsley (1916) stimulated electrically sites on the dorsal surface of the brain stem with the aim of identifying cardiovascular reactive sites. They found two circumscribed areas on the dorsal medullary surface from which blood pressure responses were consistently elicited by electrical stimulation. An increase in blood pressure was produced by stimulation of points somewhat rostral and lateral to the obex. A decrease in blood pressure (later shown to result from inhibition of sympathetic nerve activity) was elicited by stimulation of a small area near the obex just ventral to the area postrema. This response most likely resulted from stimulation of the nucleus of the tractus solitarius. The positions of the dorsal pressor and depressor areas are shown by the arrowheads in Figure 8-1D. Although Ranson and Billingsley were

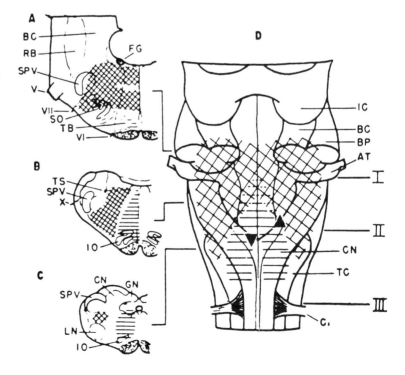

Figure 8-1 Pressor and depressor regions of cat brain stem. (A–C) Frontal sections of medulla at levels indicated by guide lines to D. The pressor region is denoted by crosshatching and the depressor region by horizontal ruling. (D) Pressor and depressor regions projected onto the dorsal surface of brain stem. I, II, and III are levels of transection discussed in the text. Dorsal pressor (▲) and depressor (▼) points of Ranson and Billingsley (1916) are also shown. AT, auditory tubercle; BC, brachium conjunctivum; BP, brachium pontis; C1, first cervical nerve; CN, cuneate nucleus; FG, facial genu; GN, gracilis nucleus; IC, inferior colliculus; IO, inferior olive; LN, lateral reticular nucleus; RB, restiform body; SO, superior olive; SPV, spinal trigeminal tract; TB, trapezoid body; TC, tuberculum cinereum; TS, tractus solitarius; V, VI, VII, corresponding cranial nerves. (Modified from Alexander, 1946.)

careful not to attribute their results to the activation of functionally discrete and anatomically circumscribed centers for cardiovascular control, others were not so cautious in their interpretation. Thus, between 1916 and 1939 it was generally assumed that the "vasomotor center," that is, the source of basal sympathetic nerve discharge to the vasculature, resided in the dorsal medulla. The work of Dittmar (1873) showing that the ventral medulla was essential for maintenance of blood pressure within normal limits was ignored during this period.

In 1939, Wang and Ranson used electrical stimulation to map the depths of the cat brain stem for cardiovascular reactive sites. They found that the pressor and depressor points on the dorsal medullary surface were not anatomically circumscribed centers. Rather, these points represent the dorsal limits of two large regions (pressor and depressor) that extend through the reticular formation to the ventral surface of the brain stem (Figure 8-1B). Decreases in blood pressure were produced most often by electrical stimulation of medial medullary sites, while pressor responses usually were elicited from sites in the lateral reticular formation. These observations ushered in yet another view on the central origin of the basal discharges of sympathetic nerves. Rather than being generated in an anatomically circumscribed center, the excitatory drive to sympathetic nerves was considered to arise from a diffuse network of brain stem neurons. Kumada et al. (1979) demonstrated that blood pressure in the rabbit is decreased by electrolytic lesions of the dorsal medullary reticular formation. Dampney and Moon (1980) found that electrolytic lesions of either the dorsal medullary reticular formation or the rostral ventrolateral medulla markedly lower blood pressure in the rabbit. They also observed that electrical stimulation of either of these regions increased blood pressure. Interpretation of these results is marred by the experimental technique used in these studies. For example, did the dorsal medullary lesions destroy the cell bodies of neurons involved in generating sympathetic nerve activity? Alternatively, as suggested by Dampney and Moon, did the dorsal medullary lesions destroy the axons of rostral ventrolateral medullary neurons? Clearly, additional experimental approaches are required to distinguish between these possibilities.

RESEARCH APPROACHES UTILIZING ANATOMICAL TRACING TECHNIQUES AND CHEMICAL STIMULATION

In the mid-1970s, a number of laboratories began to use an array of new anatomical and neurochemical techniques to locate those cell groups in the brain that project directly to the thoracolumbar intermediolateral cell column. The intermediolateral cell column contains most of the preganglionic neurons of the sympathetic system. The techniques employed included the anterograde transport of amino acids, retrograde transport of horseradish peroxidase, and immunocytochemical staining of putative neurotransmitters and their synthesizing enzymes. The results of these studies are briefly summarized here. (See Chapters 6, 9, and 16 for more detailed discussions.)

Direct projections to the intermediolateral cell column originate in the medulla, pons, and hypothalamus. Neurons in the medulla whose axons innervate the intermediolateral cell column are located in the ventral medulla and the caudal raphe nuclei. The former region is composed of two divisions, a rostral ventrolateral area and a ventromedial area. Some of the neurons in the rostral ventrolateral medulla that project to the intermediolateral cell column contain phenylethanolamine-N-methyltransferase, and others contain substance P. Several putative transmitters have been localized in caudal raphe neurons that innervate the sympathetic preganglionic neurons. These include serotonin, substance P, and thyrotropin releasing hormone (see Chapter 6). Pontine projections to the intermediolateral cell column arise from the Kölliker–Fuse nucleus. Noradrenaline-containing neurons of the A5 cell group also provide an input. The intermediolateral cell column also receives direct input from the paraventricular and lateral hypothalamic nuclei. Those neurons in the paraventricular hypothalamic nucleus projecting to the intermediolateral cell column contain an oxytocin-like substance. Thus, the intermediolateral cell column is innervated by parallel pathways originating in the brain stem and diencephalon. These pathways are depicted schematically in Figure 8-2. The degree to which these parallel pathways converge onto common pools of sympathetic preganglionic neurons and/or their antecedent spinal interneurons remains to be established.

Anatomical studies also revealed that many of the above-mentioned nuclei are reciprocally connected. This work has been summarized by Swanson and Sawchenko (1983) and Calaresu et al. (1984). The functional implications of these studies remain to be determined. Most importantly, it is not known whether the reciprocal connections form true neuronal loops and, if so, whether these loops are involved in the control of sympathetic nerve activity. These questions cannot be answered solely on the basis of neuroanatomical studies since the regions that are reciprocally connected are functionally heterogeneous.

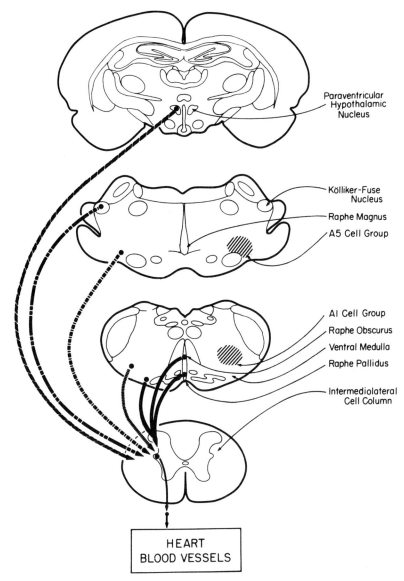

Paraventricular
Hypothalamic
Nucleus

Kölliker-Fuse
Nucleus

Raphe Magnus

A5 Cell Group

AI Cell Group

Raphe Obscurus

Ventral Medulla

Raphe Pallidus

Intermediolateral
Cell Column

HEART
BLOOD VESSELS

Figure 8-2 Brain stem and hypothalamic inputs to the intermediolateral cell column. See text for description. (Modified from Loewy, 1982.)

Microinjection of excitatory amino acids into the brain has yielded important information on the location and function of neurons controlling sympathetic nerve discharge. Whereas electrical stimuli activate neuronal cell bodies and axons of passage, excitatory amino acids such as L-glutamate are believed to activate selectively neuronal cell bodies (Fries and Zieglgansberger, 1974). The selective action of excitatory amino acids on neuronal cell bodies serves two purposes. The first is to determine whether the cell groups identified previously with anatomical techniques subserve sympathoexcitatory or sympathoinhibitory function. For example, microinjection of L-glutamate into the rostral ventro-

lateral medulla raises blood pressure (Ross et al., 1984) whereas injection into the A5 cell group lowers blood pressure (Loewy et al., 1986).

A second purpose of microinjecting excitatory amino acids is to determine whether neurons influencing sympathetic nerve activity are contained in regions of the brain that do not project directly to the intermediolateral cell column. It would be difficult to identify such neurons using anatomical technqiues, especially if they are located in and/or project to functionally heterogeneous regions. Goodchild and Dampney (1985) and Hilton and Redfern (1986) have identified three such neuronal groups that when chemically activated raise blood pressure. These neurons are located in the dorsal medullary reticular formation, and central gray matter and ventral tegmentum of the midbrain.

RHYTHMIC COMPONENTS OF SYMPATHETIC NERVE DISCHARGE

Whereas the studies using neuroanatomical tracing and chemical stimulation techniques have been enlightening, they have not dealt directly with the question of how and where sympathetic nerve discharge is generated. As a prelude to discussing these issues, it is necessary to describe the patterns of activity that are most commonly recorded from pre- and postganglionic sympathetic nerve bundles.

As first demonstrated by Adrian et al. (1932), the two most common patterns in sympathetic nerve discharge are the cardiac- and respiratory-related rhythms. In the example shown in Figure 8-3, the discharges of fibers comprising the postganglionic external carotid sympathetic nerve of a vagotomized cat took the form of bursts that were synchronized to the arterial pulse wave. These bursts were recorded as slow waves (i.e., envelopes of spikes) with a preamplifier bandpass of 1–1,000 Hz. The cardiac-related slow waves were most prominent during inspiration (as monitored from phrenic nerve), thus accounting for the respiratory-related rhythm. Respiratory-related sympathetic nerve discharge is re-

duced in parallel with phrenic nerve activity when the animal is made hypocapnic (Cohen and Gootman, 1970; Bachoo and Polosa, 1987). This had led to the idea that the slow rhythm in sympathetic nerve discharge reflects influences of respiratory neurons on central circuits controlling sympathetic activity (Bachoo and Polosa, 1987). This subject is comprehensively reviewed in Chapter 11. Elimination of respiratory-related sympathetic nerve discharge during hypocapnia occurs without loss of the cardiac-related rhythm (Barman and Gebber, 1976). The degree to which blood pressure is supported by the respiratory-related component of sympathetic nerve discharge has not yet been studied in a systematic fashion.

There are two hypotheses for generation of the cardiac-related rhythm in sympathetic nerve discharge. The classic view attributes this rhythm directly to the pulse synchronous activity of baroreceptor afferent nerves. More specifically, it has been proposed that baroreceptor nerve traffic during systole inhibits tonic central drive to sympathetic nerves, thus accounting for the cardiac-related rhythm. Although there is no doubt that such central inhibition occurs, the second hypothesis attributes the cardiac-related rhythm in sympathetic nerve discharge to a central oscillator that is entrained by pulse synchronous baroreceptor afferent nerve activity. Entrainment is of paramount importance in biology as it allows free-running oscillators to "latch

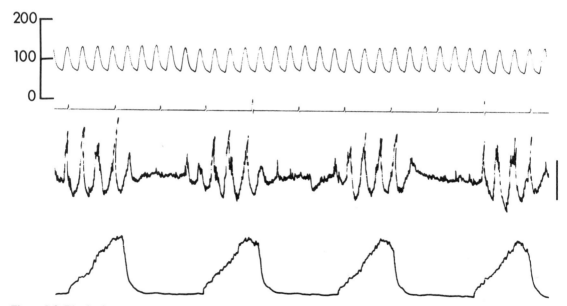

Figure 8-3 Rhythmic components in external carotid sympathetic postganglionic nerve discharge of a vagotomized cat. Top trace is blood pressure (mm Hg); the middle trace is sympathetic nerve discharge (negativity recorded as an upward deflection here and in subsequent figures); the bottom trace shows RC-integrated phrenic nerve discharge (inspiration recorded as upward deflection). Time base (below blood pressure) is 1 second/division. Vertical calibration is 40 μV and applies to sympathetic nerve discharge. (Reprinted from Barman and Gebber, 1976.)

on" to the environment. The entrainment of biological oscillators by extrinsic periodic input is discussed by Pavlidis (1973).

Two lines of evidence support the hypothesis that a central oscillator is responsible for the sympathetic nerve rhythm that normally is synchronized to the cardiac cycle (see review by Gebber, 1980). First, a rhythm with a frequency (2–6 Hz) that is close to the heart rate persists in sympathetic nerve discharge of the cat after complete surgical denervation of the arterial baroreceptors. This rhythm does not arise from cardiac-related activity in extra-baroreceptor afferent nerves since the temporal relations between the cardiac cycle and the 2- to 6-Hz sympathetic nerve slow wave are completely disrupted by baroreceptor denervation (Barman and Gebber, 1980). The second line of evidence is that the phase relations between baroreceptor nerve activity and sympathetic nerve discharge can be dramatically shifted by changing heart rate (Gebber, 1976). The traces in Figure 8-4 show averages of the femoral arteral pulse (top), carotid sinus nerve activity (middle), and renal sympathetic nerve discharge (bottom) at different heart rates in a cat in which the vagi and aortic depressor nerves were sectioned. These averages were constructed using the R wave of the electrocardiogram as a reference signal. As expected, slowing of the heart, accomplished in this experiment by electrically stimulating the peripheral end of a cut vagus nerve, did not alter the interval between the onset of the systolic phase of the femoral arterial pulse wave and the peak of carotid sinus nerve activity. The carotid pulse precedes that in the femoral artery, thus explaining why pulse synchronous carotid sinus nerve activity began before the onset of femoral systole. Most importantly, slowing of the heart markedly changed the interval between peak activity in the carotid sinus afferent and renal sympathetic nerves (Figure 8-4A,C). This interval should not have changed, provided that the cardiac-related rhythm in renal sympathetic nerve activity was the simple consequence of the waxing and waning of central inhibition of baroreceptor reflex origin. On the other hand, phase shifts should be expected when the duration of the cycle of afferent activity acting to entrain a central oscillator is changed. This is because a change in the periodicity of the input (pulse synchronous baroreceptor activity in this case) will cause that input to be received at a different point in the centrally generated cycle of rhythmic activity (Pavlidis, 1973). Thus, the change of the interval between peak activity in the carotid sinus and renal postganglionic nerves supports the view that the 2–6 Hz rhythm in sympathetic nerve discharge was generated centrally and then entrained to the cardiac cycle by pulse synchronous baroreceptor afferent nerve activity. The shifts in phase between

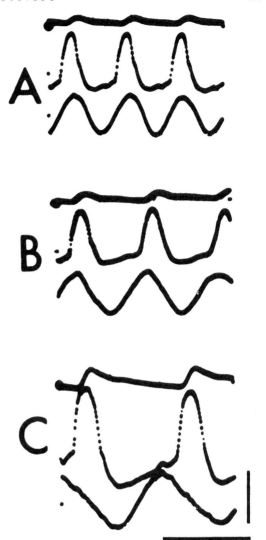

Figure 8-4 Phase relations between carotid sinus afferent nerve activity and renal sympathetic postganglionic nerve discharge at different heart rates in a cat with sectioned aortic depressor and vagus nerves. Records are averages of 64 trials, each triggered by the R wave of the electrocardiogram. The top trace in each panel is femoral blood pressure (mm Hg); the middle trace is carotid sinus nerve activity; the bottom trace is sympathetic nerve discharge. (A) Control heart rate; (B) during slowed heart rate produced by stimulation of the peripheral end of the cut right vagus nerve at 3 Hz; (C) during vagus stimulation at 5 Hz. Computer bin width for averages was 1 msec. Horizontal calibration is 500 msec; vertical calibration is 534 μV. (Reprinted from Gebber, 1980.)

carotid sinus nerve activity and sympathetic nerve discharge also strongly suggest that the cardiac-related rhythm in the baroreceptor-innervated cat and the 2–6 Hz rhythm in the baroreceptor-denervated cat monitor two states (entrained and free-running) of the same central oscillator.

The 2–6 Hz rhythm is present in sympathetic nerve discharge under a wide variety of experimental conditions, including extremes of arterial pCO_2, pO_2 and body temperature (see review by Gebber, 1984). This rhythm has been observed in all of those sympathetic nerves from which we have recorded. These include the splanchnic preganglionic and external carotid, inferior cardiac, and renal postganglionic nerves of the cat. As demonstrated with power density spectral analysis (Barman and Gebber, 1980), the 2–6 Hz rhythm accounts for most of the activity of these nerves before and after baroreceptor denervation and decerebration (i.e., surgical separation of the forebrain from remainder of neuraxis). Power density spectral analysis performed by fast Fourier transform (Bendat and Piersol, 1971) separates the frequency components in a signal and quantifies the proportion of total activity contained within designated frequency bands. Power (voltage^2) of the signal is plotted against frequency. The power density spectrum of inferior cardiac sympathetic nerve discharge obtained from a baroreceptor-denervated cat is shown in Figure 8-5.

Sympathetic postganglionic nerve bundles are functionally heterogeneous in composition. For example, the postganglionic fibers of the renal nerve innervate not only renal arterioles but also renal tubules and the juxtaglomerular apparatus; those of the inferior cardiac nerve innervate contractile and conductile tissue in the heart and the coronary and pulmonary blood vessels. Whether the 2–6 Hz rhythm is contained in the discharges of all the fibers of these nerves is not known. Nevertheless, it is likely that this rhythm is present in the activity of at least some of those fibers involved in the control of cardiovascular function. There are two reasons for suggesting this. First, the one function common to all of the nerve bundles studied in our laboratory is the control of vascular resistance. Second, the acute loss of this rhythm following transection of the cer-

vical spinal cord is accompanied by a profound decrease in blood pressure (McCall and Gebber, 1975).

Although the importance of rhythmic neural discharge is inherently clear for such motor acts as respiration and locomotion, such is not the case for the 2–6 Hz rhythm in sympathetic nerve discharge. Following baroreceptor denervation, the frequency of the rhythm is close to but not equal to the heart rate. Thus, the rhythm in sympathetic nerve discharge is not the major determinant of heart rate. There is no indication that vascular smooth muscle contracts at a rate that follows the 2–6 Hz rhythm. These facts, however, do not diminish the importance of the rhythm. First, it should be recognized that rhythm generation is a convenient means to ensure the appropriate timing and thus synchronization of the discharges of large numbers of central neurons. Regarding this point, it is likely that spatial and temporal summation are critical factors that govern the discharges of neurons (e.g., preganglionic sympathetic cells) that convey the influences of the generator to the target organ. Second, the rhythm can be viewed as the signature of those central circuits responsible for a significant component of sympathetic nerve discharge. Regarding this point, the 2–6 Hz sympathetic nerve rhythm persists in the cat after baroreceptor denervation and decerebration (Barman and Gebber, 1980), but is eliminated acutely by transection of the cervical spinal cord (McCall and Gebber, 1975). On this basis, it has been proposed that the brain stem is inherently capable of generating this pattern of sympathetic activity. Experimental approaches used to identify those brain stem neurons that generate the 2–6 Hz rhythm are reviewed in the next section.

ELECTROPHYSIOLOGICAL ANALYSIS OF CENTRAL CIRCUITS THAT CONTROL SYMPATHETIC NERVE DISCHARGE

Spike-triggered averaging is a method used to locate single neurons in the brain with naturally occurring (i.e., spontaneous) activity correlated to that in sympathetic nerve bundles. For this purpose, the extracellularly recorded action potentials (i.e., spikes) of the neurons (i.e., unit) serve as reference signals for computation of an average of accompanying changes in sympathetic nerve discharge. Sympathetic nerve activity occurring in a time window (e.g., $\pm$ 500 msec) surrounding each of the spikes in a series is digitized and subsequently averaged by a computer (see Barman and Gebber, 1981). An example of the results obtained with this method is shown in Figure 8-6D1. The spike-triggered average shows renal sympathetic nerve discharge that pre-

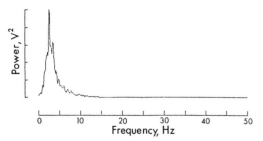

Figure 8-5 Power spectrum of inferior cardiac sympathetic postganglionic nerve discharge in a baroreceptor-denervated cat. Power (voltage^2) is plotted against frequency (Hz). Sympathetic nerve discharge was recorded with a preamplifier bandpass of 1–1000 Hz. The spectrum is the average of nine 20-second data blocks. Frequency resolution is 0.2 Hz.

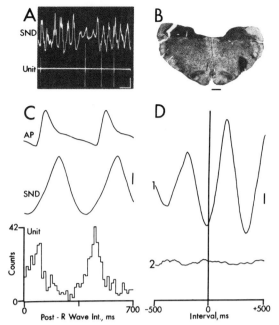

Figure 8-6 Cat ventrolateral medullary neuron with cardiac- and sympathetic nerve-related discharges. (A) Oscilloscopic records of renal sympathetic nerve discharge (SND) (top) and medullary unit spikes (bottom). Vertical calibration is 50 μV for SND and 200 μV for unit spikes; horizontal calibration is 500 msec. (B) Frontal section through the medulla approximately 2 mm posterior to the caudal border of trapezoid body. The arrow marks the site of unit recording. Calibration is 1 mm. (C) Post-R wave averages of arterial pulse (AP) wave (top) and SND (middle), and histogram of unit spikes (bottom). The number of trials was 1500. Mean blood pressure was 140 mm Hg. Bin width for averages was 1.4 msec and for unit histogram was 14 msec. Vertical calibration for SND is 20 μV. (D) Spike-triggered average of SND (trace 1) and "dummy" pulse-triggered average of SND (trace 2). Unit spikes and "dummy" pulses are at zero lag. The number of trials is 700. Bin width was 1 msec. Vertical calibration is 5 μV. (Reprinted from Barman and Gebber, 1983.)

ceded (left of zero lag) and followed (right of zero lag) the action potential of a neuron in the cat rostral ventrolateral medulla. The average of renal nerve activity contains a rhythmic component whose period was 340 msec. Thus, the activity of the rostral ventrolateral medullary neuron was correlated to a rhythm in renal sympathetic nerve discharge with a frequency in the 2–6 Hz range. A randomly generated series of pulses (same number and frequency as for the unit spike train) also was used to compute an average of renal nerve activity. Such averages are termed "dummy" averages and the one shown in Figure 8-6D2 was basically flat. Single neurons in the brain are considered to have sympathetic nerve-related activity when the amplitude of the first peak to the right of zero lag in the spike-triggerd average

exceeds that of the largest deflection in the "dummy" average by at least a factor of three.

The 2–6 Hz rhythm in sympathetic nerve discharge normally is synchronized to the cardiac cycle in baroreceptor-innervated cats. It follows that single unit activity correlated to 2–6 Hz sympathetic nerve discharge should also be cardiac related. That such is the case can be demonstrated with the method of post-R wave analysis. Averages of the arterial pulse wave and sympathetic nerve discharge, and a histogram of the occurrences of the spikes of a single neuron are constructed using the R wave of the electrocardiogram as the reference signal. As shown in Figure 8-6C, sympathetic nerve activity and the discharges of the rostral ventrolateral medullary neuron contained a prominent cardiac-related rhythm whose period was that of the rhythm in the spike-triggered average of sympathetic nerve discharge (Figure 8-6D1). At least some brain stem neurons with sympathetic nerve- and cardiac-related activity also have respiratory-related discharges (Barman and Gebber, 1981).

Central neurons with cardiac-related activity might be contained in circuits directly involved in generating sympathetic nerve discharge. Alternatively, they might be interneurons in the afferent limb of the baroreceptor reflex arc. These two neuronal types can be distinguished by comparing the relationship between unit activity and sympathetic nerve discharge at control blood pressure with that after blood pressure is lowered to a level at which synchronization of the 2–6 Hz sympathetic nerve rhythm to the cardiac cycle is disrupted due to reduced baroreceptor nerve activity (see Gebber and Barman, 1985). The discharges of neurons directly responsible for sympathetic nerve discharge should remain correlated to the 2–6 Hz rhythm when blood pressure is lowered while those of baroreceptor interneurons should not. In the case shown in Figure 8-7, the action potentials of a single neuron located in the lateral tegmental field of the cat medullary reticular formation was recorded. The spike-triggered average in 8-7IA1 shows that unit activity is correlated to a 2–6 Hz rhythm in inferior cardiac sympathetic nerve discharge. As demonstrated with post-R wave analysis, this rhythm had the period of the cardiac cycle when mean blood pressure was 135 mm Hg (8-7IB). Blood pressure was then lowered to disrupt the synchronization of sympathetic nerve discharge and unit activity to the cardiac cycle. This is indicated by the flat post-R wave average of sympathetic nerve discharge and histogram of unit spike occurences shown in 8-7IIB. As demonstrated with spike-triggered averaging (8-7IIA1), the discharges of the lateral tegmental field neuron remained correlated to sympathetic nerve activity. Thus, the naturally occurring discharges of this neuron were more

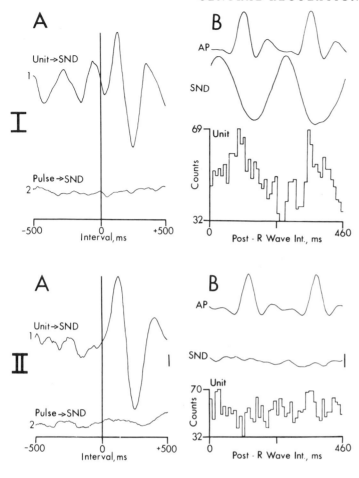

Figure 8-7 Sympathetic nerve-related activity of a neuron in lateral tegmental field of cat medulla at two levels of mean blood pressure. Mean blood pressure was 135 mm Hg in I and 90 mm Hg in II. (IA, IIA) Spike-triggered (trace 1) and "dummy" pulse-triggered (trace 2) averages of inferior cardiac sympathetic nerve discharge (SND). Unit spikes and "dummy" pulses are at zero lag. The number of trials was 340 (IA) and 363 (IIA). Bin width was 1 msec. Vertical calibration is 10 μV. (IB, IIB) Post-R wave averages of arterial pulse (AP, top) and SND (middle), and histogram of unit spikes. The number of trials was 653 (IB) and 725 (IIB). Bin width was 920 μsec for averages and 9.2 msec for histogram. Vertical calibration for SND is 20 μV. (Reprinted from Gebber and Barman, 1985.)

closely associated with sympathetic nerve discharge than with baroreceptor afferent nerve activity. It should also be noted that the interval (132 msec) between unit spike occurence and the peak of the next sympathetic nerve slow wave was unchanged when blood pressure was lowered from 135 to 90 mm Hg (see spike-triggered averages in 8-7IA1 and 8-7IIA1). This observation supports the view that unit activity was correlated to the same component in sympathetic nerve discharge at the two levels of blood pressure.

Neurons with the properties illustrated in Figure 8-7 are presumed to comprise central circuits responsible for the 2–6 Hz rhythm in sympathetic nerve discharge. The distribution of such neurons in the cat medulla is shown in Figure 8-8. They were located in three regions—the lateral tegmental field, rostral ventrolateral medulla, and caudal raphe nuclei. Lateral tegmental field neurons with sympathetic nerve-related activity were found in nucleus reticularis parvocellularis and nucleus reticularis ventralis 10.0–14.7 mm posterior to the interaural line (stereotaxic planes P10 and P14.7). Rostral ven-

trolateral medullary neurons were located caudal to the facial nucleus (stereotaxic planes P8.5–P10) in a region ventral to the nucleus reticularis parvocellularis and ventrolateral to the nucleus reticularis gigantocellularis. Medullary neurons with sympathetic nerve-related activity located on or near the midline (stereotaxic planes P9.2–P12.1) were located in nuclei raphe magnus, pallidus, and obscurus.

Forty-five percent of the neurons sampled in the cat rostral ventrolateral medulla had activity correlated to the 2–6 Hz rhythm in sympathetic nerve discharge (Barman and Gebber, 1983). The corresponding values for lateral tegmental field (Barman and Gebber, 1981) and caudal raphe (Morrison and Gebber, 1982) neurons were 28 and 24%, respectively. Neurons with and those without sympathetic nerve-related activity were intermingled in each of these three regions. The discharges of both types of neurons often were recorded simultaneously (Gebber et al., 1987). Thus, the brain stem regions containing neurons with sympathetic nerve-related activity are functionally heterogeneous in nature. The importance of electrophysiological techniques that

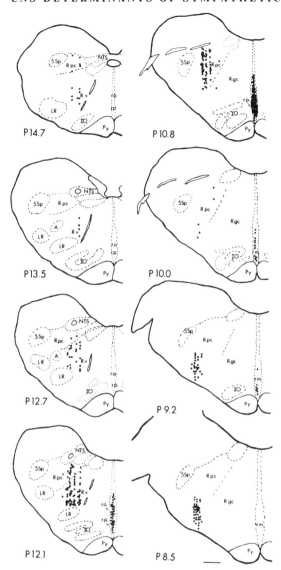

Figure 8-8 Anatomical distribution of cat medullary neurons with sympathetic nerve-related activity. Frontal sections 8.5–14.7 mm posterior to the interaural line are shown. A, nucleus ambiguus; IO, inferior olive; LR, lateral reticular nucleus; NTS, nucleus of tractus solitarius; Py, pyramid; R.gc., nucleus reticularis gigantocellularis; R.pc., nucleus reticularis parvocellularis; R.v., nucleus reticularis ventralis; r.m., nucleus raphe magnus; r.o., nucleus raphe obscurus; r.p., nucleus raphe pallidus; 5Sp, spinal nucleus of trigeminal nerve. Calibration is 1 mm. (Reprinted from Gebber and Barman, 1985.)

allow the investigator to characterize the relationships between the activity of single brain neurons and sympathetic nerves becomes clearer in this light.

Baroreceptor reflex activation can be used to determine which brain stem neurons with sympathetic nerve-related activity subserve excitatory function and which subserve inhibitory function. For this purpose, changes in the firing rate of the brain stem neuron are monitored when baroreceptor afferent nerve traffic is increased. Neurons mediating sympathoexcitatory effects should be inhibited by baroreceptor reflex activation. Neurons exerting sympathoinhibitory actions should be excited by baroreceptor reflex activation. In the case shown in Figure 8-9C, baroreceptor reflex activation was accomplished by raising pressure in a carotid sinus that had been reversibly isolated from the systemic circulation. The discharges of the inferior cardiac nerve

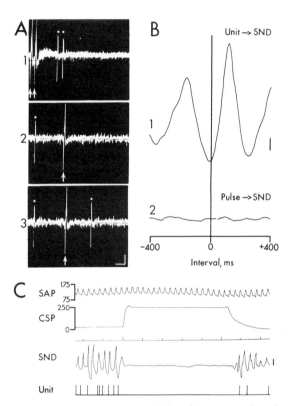

Figure 8-9 Discharge characteristics of a cat ventrolateral medullospinal sympathoexcitatory neuron. (A) Antidromic responses initiated by stimulation in gray matter of second thoracic spinal segment. Four superimposed traces appear in each panel. Dots mark spontaneous and stimulus-induced action potentials; arrows mark spinal stimuli. (1) Estimation of axonal refractory period with paired stimuli. (2 and 3) Time-controlled collision test for antidromic activation (see text for details). Stimulus current was 1.5 × threshold. Horizontal calibration is 10 msec; vertical calibration is 50 μV. (B) Spike-triggered (trace 1) and "dummy" pulse-triggered (trace 2) averages of inferior cardiac sympathetic nerve discharge (SND) each based on 700 trials. Unit spikes and "dummy" pulses are at zero lag. Bin width is 0.8 msec and vertical calibration is 30 μV. (C) Baroreceptor reflex response. Traces show (top to bottom) systemic arterial pressure (SAP; mm Hg), carotid sinus pressure (CSP; mm Hg), time base (1 second/division) SND, and standardized pulses derived from action potentials of the neuron. Vertical calibration is 100 μV. (Reprinted from Barman and Gebber, 1985.)

and of a neuron in the rostral ventrolateral medulla were inhibited in parallel during the rise in carotid sinus pressure. Thus, this rostral ventrolateral medullary neuron likely subserved a sympathoexcitatory function.

The identification and characterization of brain stem neurons with sympathetic nerve-related activity is only the first step in understanding how the central nervous system controls sympathetic nerve discharge. The second step, which is much more arduous, is to define the connections made by these neurons. This serves two purposes: the first, is the construction of a wiring diagram of those circuits responsible for sympathetic nerve discharge; the second is to verify that the temporal relationship between brain stem unit activity and sympathetic nerve discharge revealed by correlational techniques (e.g., spike-triggered averaging) is functionally relevant. One can be confident of this if the neuron is shown to project to a known sympathetic nucleus or region (e.g., spinal intermediolateral nucleus).

Antidromic mapping can be used to define the connections made by individual central neurons. An electrical stimulus is applied through a microelectrode placed in a region suspected to contain the axon or terminal field of the neuron. When the electrical stimulus excites the axon or a terminal, the action potential travels antidromically to the cell body (i.e., the neuron is backfired). Such responses are proven to be antidromic in nature by colliding them with spontaneously occurring action potentials of the same cell traveling in the orthodromic direction. When the electrical stimulus is applied too soon after occurrence of a spontaneous spike, the antidromic and orthodromic spike collide somewhere along the axon. As a consequence, the antidromic response fails to reach the cell body. The antidromic spike can again be recorded at the cell body when the interval between the spontaneous spike and the electrical stimulus is lengthened to a value equal to the sum of the latency of the antidromic spike (L) and the refractory period of the axon (R). This is the critical delay (CD) for antidromic activation: $CD = L + R$. R is defined as the period of reduced excitability following an action potential and is estimated by determining the minimum interval between paired electrical stimuli producing two action potentials. The refractory period of the cell body normally exceeds that of the axon. Thus, the interval determined experimentally overestimates R when the action potential is recorded near the cell body. The error in the critical delay, however, is small when the antidromic response latency far exceeds the estimated value of R. A more detailed discussion of the collision test has been provided by Lipski (1981).

The collision test for antidromic activation of a rostral ventrolateral medullary sympathoexcitatory

neuron by microstimulation in the second thoracic (T2) spinal segment is shown in Figure 8-9A. This neuron was activated with a constant onset latency (26 msec) and faithfully followed paired T2 stimuli separated by 3.8 msec (Figure 8-9A1). The response to electrical stimulation failed to occur (8-9A2) when the interval (28 msec) between a spontaneous spike and the spinal stimulus was less than the critical delay for antidromic activation (29.8 msec), but a response was recorded when the interval was 30 msec (8-9A3). Thus, the response elicited by spinal stimulation was antidromic in nature. It follows that the axon of this neuron projected to the T2 spinal segment.

The use of the antidromic mapping technique to locate the terminal field of a rostral ventrolateral medullospinal sympathoexcitatory neuron is illustrated in Figure 8-10. In this case, the neuron was antidromically activated by microstimulation in the T2 spinal segment. The stimulating microelectrode was moved vertically in 200-μm steps through a series of tracks separated by 500–1,000 μm in the mediolateral and rostrocaudal directions. Twelve tracks (four in each of three rostrocaudal planes) were made in this experiment. One of these planes is shown on the left side of Figure 8-10. Threshold current for antidromic activation of the neuron, response onset latency, and depth of the electrode tip below the dorsal surface of the T2 spinal segment were recorded at each site of stimulation. Depth–threshold curves were constructed from these data. The main axon of the rostral ventrolateral medullary

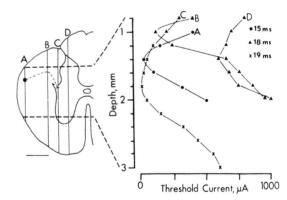

Figure 8-10 Dorsolateral funicular axon (filled circle) of a cat ventrolateral medullospinal sympathoexcitatory neuron projecting to the ipsilateral intermediolateral nucleus of the second thoracic (T2) spinal segment. The presumed path of a branch from the main axon to the intermediolateral cell column is shown as a dashed line. T2 cross section with electrode tracks (A–D) is on the left. Calibration is 1 mm. Corresponding depth–threshold curves for antidromic activation of the neuron are on the right. Dashed lines show extent of ordinate relative to the cross section. Depth below dorsal surface on the ordinate relates to track C. (Reprinted from Barman and Gebber, 1985.)

neuron was assumed to be near the site in the white matter (track A) from which the shortest latency (15 msec) antidromic response was initiated with the lowest threshold current (28 μA). The site (track C) from which the longest latency (19 msec) antidromic resonse was elicited with the lowest stimulus current (10 μA) was in the intermediolateral nucleus. This site presumably was near the terminal field of either the main axon or one of its branches. Antidromic mapping was continued until it was demonstrated that this point was surrounded by sites requiring the application of higher current to elicit an antidromic response with the same latency. The antidromic response of intermediate onset latency (18 msec) likely monitored activation of the main axon or one of its branches en route to the intermediolateral cell column. It can be noted that the stimulus currents needed to antidromically activate the neuron from sites in track D were higher than those needed in track C. This indicates that the axon did not cross the midline at this level.

Antidromic mapping can also be used to determine the extent over which individual bulbospinal neurons influence sympathetic outflow. Many rostral ventrolateral medullary and caudal raphe neurons with sympathetic nerve-related activity send their spinal axons at least as far caudally as the T11 segment (Barman and Gebber, 1985; Morrison and Gebber, 1985). These neurons might innervate a restricted portion of the lower thoracic intermediolateral cell column. Alternatively, the long axons of these neurons might branch to innervate the intermediolateral cell column at many levels of the thoracic spinal cord. Collision of the unit action potentials elicited by stimulation in the intermediolateral cell column at different thoracic levels can be used to distinguish between these possbilities. Specifically, one measures the maximum interval (collision interval, CI) after a threshold stimulus applied to the intermediolateral nucleus at a rostral level (e.g., T2) at which stimulation at a more caudal level (Tc) fails to elicit an antidromic response at the recording site in the medulla. If stimulation in the T2 intermediolateral cell column activates the main axon (en route to a lower level) via current spread to the white matter (case I in Figure 8-11), then CI equals the difference between the latencies of the antidromic responses elicited by stimulation in Tc and T2 plus the axonal refractory period (R_c) in Tc: $CI = L_c - L_2 + R_c$. If, on the other hand, stimulation in T2 activates an axonal branch (case II in Figure 8-11), then $CI > L_c - L_2 + R_c$. Conduction time (t_B) from the branch point on the main axon to the site of activation of the collateral in the spinal gray matter is calculated using the formula: $t_B = \frac{1}{2}(CI - L_c + L_2 - R_c)$. The derivations of these formulas are contained in a paper by Shinoda et al. (1976).

The results obtained with the above-described collision test indicate that the majority of rostral ventrolateral medullospinal and caudal raphespinal neurons with sympathetic nerve-related activity branch to innervate the intermediolateral cell column at upper, middle, and lower thoracic levels (Barman and Gebber, 1985; Morrison and Gebber, 1985). The role played by these neurons in the control of sympathetic nerve discharge remains to be determined. They may comprise a system involved in the global control of spinal sympathetic outflow. Alternatively, these neurons may be involved in formulating complex cardiovascular response patterns. Neurons with widespread axonal projections might coordinate the activity of selected groups of sympathetic preganglionic neurons located at different spinal levels, thus producing a specific pattern of spinal sympathetic outflow.

The axonal projections of other rostral ventrolat-

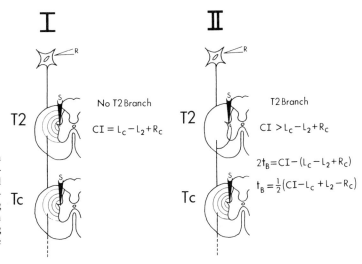

Figure 8-11 Schematic depicting collision test for axonal branching. T2 is second thoracic spinal segment. Tc is a more caudal thoracic spinal segment. R is recording microelectrode in medulla. S is stimulating microelectrode. Case I shows a no branch situation. Case II shows axonal branching in T2. Terms in formulas are defined in the text.

eral medullary and caudal raphe neurons with sympathetic nerve-related activity were restricted to the intermediolateral cell column of upper thoracic segments (Barman and Gebber, 1985; Morrison and Gebber, 1985). These neurons could be antidromically activated by stimulation in the T1 and T2 spinal segments, but not by stimulation at more caudal levels of the thoracic spinal cord. Such neurons undoubtedly are involved in the regional control of spinal sympathetic outflow. Whether analogous groups of rostral ventrolateral medullary and caudal raphe neurons exist that innervate restricted portions of the intermediolateral cell column at lower thoracic levels remains to be determined.

THEORIES ON THE CENTRAL GENERATION OF SYMPATHETIC NERVE DISCHARGE

The long-term goal of studies on brain stem neurons with sympathetic nerve-related activity is to understand how the various components of sympathetic nerve discharge are generated. Since only some of these neurons have been identified and their properties are incompletely defined, we are far from attaining this goal. Nevertheless, available information permits some discussion of the potential source(s) and mechanisms of generation of one of the major components of sympathetic nerve discharge—the 2–6 Hz rhythm. To begin, a synthesis of existing knowledge of the properties and connections of central neurons with activity correlated to this sympathetic nerve rhythm is required. Four groups of brain stem neurons with naturally occurring activity correlated to the 2–6 Hz rhythm in sympathetic nerve discharge have been identified. These are sympathoexcitatory neurons of the medullary lateral tegmental field and rostral ventrolateral medulla, and sympathoinhibitory neurons of the lateral tegmental field and caudal medullary raphe nuclei (Figure 8-12A). The axons of rostral ventrolateral medullary sympathoexcitatory and raphe sympathoinhibitory neurons innervate the thoracic intermediolateral nucleus (Barman and Gebber, 1985; Morrison and Gebber, 1985). Their axonal conduction velocities are 3.5 ± 0.3 and 2.1 ± 0.1 m/second, respectively. The lateral tegmental field neurons do not project to the spinal cord. Rather, those that are sympathoexcitatory project to the region of the rostral ventrolateral medulla containing sympathoexcitatory neurons with spinal axons (Barman and Gebber, 1987), whereas those that are sympathoinhibitory project to the region of the medullary raphe containing sympathoinhibitory neurons with spinal axons (Barman and Gebber, 1988). It has also been established that the axons of rostral ventrolateral medullospinal

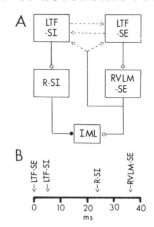

Figure 8-12 Connections made by cat medullary neurons with activity correlated to 2- to 6-Hz sympathetic nerve discharge. (A) Circuit diagram. LTF-SE, sympathoexcitatory neuron in lateral tegmental field; LTF-SI, sympathoinhibitory neuron in lateral tegmental field; RVLM-SE, sympathoexcitatory neuron in rostral ventrolateral medulla; R-SI, sympathoinhibitory neuron in medullary raphe; IML, intermediolateral cell column. Solid lines are established pathways. Dashed lines are hypothetical pathways. Unfilled circle is excitatory connection. Filled circle is inhibitory connection. Arrowhead is connection of unknown sign. See text for details. (B) Time line depicting the sequence of firing of medullary neurons relative to the peak of the next inferior cardiac sympathetic nerve slow wave. LTF-SE neurons fired earliest, on the average 118 ± 10 msec before the peak of sympathetic nerve slow wave.

sympathoexcitatory neurons emit branches in the vicinity of the lateral tegmental field (Barman and Gebber, 1987).

It is now logical to ask whether the cooperative properties of neurons comprising the circuits in Figure 8-12A account for generation of the 2–6 Hz sympathetic nerve rhythm. That is, is the 2–6 Hz rhythm a property of a network oscillator, i.e., an ensemble of neurons interconnected in such a way as to generate rhythmic activity? Alternatively, does one of the identified neuronal types act as a pacemaker? The rhythmic activity (i.e., near constant interspike or interburst intervals) of a pacemaker neuron can be attributed to the intrinsic properties (activation and/or inactivation of specific ionic currents) of its membrane rather than to periodic synaptic input. Distinguishing between an endogenous pacemaker and a network oscillator is not an easy task (see review by Feldman and Cleland, 1982). Theoretically, pacemaker neurons should continue to fire rhythmically after blockade of their synaptic input. Blockade of synaptic transmission in *in vitro* preparations (e.g., brain slices, isolated brain stem) can be accomplished by manipulation of the extracellular concentrations of divalent cations (calcium and magnesium) that regulate transmitter release. The disappearance of rhythmic activity after blocking transmitter release, however, does not necessarily disprove a pacemaker function of the neuron under study. First, tonic synaptic input might be required to activate the membrane currents responsible for pacemaker activity. Second, altered divalent cation concentrations might interfere with pacemaker membrane conductance mechanisms. A second test for pacemaker activity involves the intracellular injection of a short pulse of depolarizing current of sufficient intensity to elicit an action potential or burst of action potentials. If properly timed, the stimulus will reset the rhythm of a pacemaker cell. That is, the electrically evoked response will either advance or delay the onset of the next cycle of rhythmic activity. The pacemaker then resumes its normal periodicity (i.e., natural period between action potentials or bursts). A detailed discussion of the resetting of pacemakers is provided by Winfree (1983). Whereas this test appears straightforward, interpretation of the results obtained requires a complete understanding of the network containing the cell under study. If, for instance, a pacemaker neuron is entrained by phasic input, current injection into the pacemaker might not reset its rhythmic discharge pattern. Furthermore, resetting might not reflect the existence of pacemaker activity, but rather feedback from the cell to its antecedent phasic inputs. The antecedent neurons might themselves comprise a network oscillator or they might be endogenous pacemakers.

Under certain conditions, Sun et al. (1988) observed that some rat rostral ventrolateral medullospinal neurons exhibit pacemaker-like activity. They believe that these neurons are responsible for a component of sympathetic nerve discharge. Pacemaker-like activity in the rostral ventrolateral medulla is manifested *in vivo* after blockade of synaptic transmission mediated by excitatory amino acids and also in brain stem slices. These experiments are summarized in Chapter 9. In contrast, our *in vivo* experiments on cats have not revealed signs of pacemaker activity for rostral ventrolateral medullary, lateral tegmental field, or caudal raphe neurons whose discharges are correlated to the 2–6 Hz rhythm in sympathetic nerve discharge. The naturally occurring firing rates of these neurons generally are lower than the frequency of occurrence of 2–6 Hz slow waves in sympathetic nerve discharge. It is because of the low firing rates of these cells that averaging techniques must be used to demonstrate their sympathetic nerve-related activity. A representative example of the discharge pattern of a cat brain stem neuron with sympathetic nerve-related activity is shown in Figure 8-6A. This rostral ventrolateral medullospinal sympathoexcitatory neuron failed to fire during the majority of 2–6 Hz sympathetic nerve slow waves, and the number of cycles missed varied.

These are not the properties of endogenous pacemaker neurons. Thus, the available information favors the hypothesis that a network oscillator is responsible for the 2–6 Hz sympathetic nerve rhythm of the cat. Furthermore, only a small and continuously changing segment of the population of neurons comprising the network oscillator accounts for each 2–6 Hz sympathetic nerve slow wave. This is evident since the individual brain stem neuron does not participate in every cycle of sympathetic nerve discharge.

Detailed models of network oscillators have been presented by Kristan (1980) and Selverston and Moulins (1985). Although it would be premature to relate our data to these models, some information is available concerning the potential central source(s) of the 2–6 Hz rhythm. One approach to the problem of identifying the region(s) of origin of the 2–6 Hz rhythm in sympathetic nerve discharge is to compare the firing times of different groups of brain stem neurons with this activity pattern (Gebber and Barman, 1985). Those neurons that fire earliest during the 2–6 Hz sympathetic nerve slow wave should be the source of such activity. The reference point used to compare the firing times of the four groups of medullary neurons was the lag between unit spike occurrence and the peak of the next 2–6 Hz slow wave in the postganglionic inferior cardiac sympathetic nerve. This interval, measured from spike-triggered averages, is unchanged when synchronization of the 2–6 Hz sympathetic nerve slow wave to the cardiac cycle is disrupted by lowering blood pressure (see Figure 8-7) or when the period of the cardiac cycle and, thus the slow wave in sympathetic nerve discharge, is changed by pacing the heart (Morrison and Gebber, 1982; Barman and Gebber, 1983).

The time line in Figure 8-12B shows the sequence of firing of the four groups of medullary neurons. The earliest firing neurons were lateral tegmental field sympathoexcitatory neurons. On average, they fired 118 ± 10 msec before the peak of the accompanying slow wave in the inferior cardiac nerve. The naturally occurring discharges of these neurons were followed in sequence by those of lateral tegmental field sympathoinhibitory, raphespinal sympathoinhibitory, and rostral ventrolateral medullospinal sympathoexcitatory neurons. Rostral ventrolateral medullary and raphe neurons fired significantly later than lateral tegmental field neurons during the 2–6 Hz sympathetic nerve slow wave (Gebber and Barman, 1985). These data support the view that the 2–6 Hz rhythm in sympathetic nerve discharge is generated not by bulbospinal neurons, but rather by their antecedent inputs. Regarding this possibility, Barman and Gebber (1987) found that the difference in the firing times of sympathoexcitatory neurons of the lateral tegmental field and rostral ventrolateral medulla relative to the peak of the 2–6 Hz sympathetic nerve slow wave was close to the modal onset latency of synaptic activation of the latter neurons by microstimulation in the lateral tegmental field. This observation implies that sympathoexcitatory neurons in the lateral tegmental field are an important source of the basal activity of rostral ventrolateral medullary sympathoexcitatory neurons that innervate the intermediolateral nucleus. Whether local circuits of lateral tegmental field neurons comprise a generator of the 2–6 Hz sympathetic nerve rhythm remains to be tested. Alternatively, lateral tegmental field neurons might be driven by inputs from a 2–6 ythm generator located elsewhere. It is also possible that lateral tegmental field neurons are part of a network oscillator that is anatomically distributed in the brain stem. Regarding this possibility, it is worth reiterating that the axons of rostral ventrolateral medullospinal sympathoexcitatory neurons emit branches in the vicinity of the lateral tegmental field (Figure 8-12A). Feedback from the rostral ventrolateral medulla to the lateral tegmental field is consistent with the possibility that the 2–6 Hz rhythm is an emergent property of an anatomically distributed system of reciprocally connected neurons.

MULTIPLICITY OF CENTRAL CIRCUITS CONTROLLING SYMPATHETIC NERVE DISCHARGE

At one time, the sympathetic nervous system was considered a functionally homogeneous system, i.e., one whose components exhibit uniform increases or decreases in activity in response to a changing environment. That is, the sympathetic nervous system was thought always to act "en masse" (Cannon, 1929). This view is no longer accepted. It is now clear that central circuits controlling sympathetic nerve discharge are capable of formulating complex and highly differentiated response patterns. The cardiovascular components of the so-called defense reaction provide an excellent example of one of these response patterns. The behavioral, somatic, and visceral responses accompanying alerting, fear, or rage are collectively termed the *defense reaction* (Hilton, 1982; see also Chapter 19). The cardiovascular components of the defense reaction include sympathetic nerve-mediated tachycardia, increased cardiac contractile force, and vasoconstriction in the splanchnic region, kidneys, and skin. Concurrently, blood flow to skeletal muscle is increased due to inhibition of sympathetic vasoconstrictor outflow and activation, in some species, of a sympathetic cholinergic vasodilator system. The net result is increased cardiac output directed chiefly to skeletal muscle.

The cardiovascular pattern described above is mimicked in anesthetized animals by electrical stimulation of the perifornical hypothalamic area or chemical stimulation of the central gray matter of the midbrain (Hilton and Redfern, 1986). It is not known how neurons in these regions engage the central program leading to this complex response pattern. At least two possibilities are worthy of future investigation. First, direct projections from the hypothalamus and midbrain to the spinal cord might differentially affect the activity of the selected pools of sympathetic preganglionic neurons. Second, hypothalamic and midbrain neurons might differentially act on subsets of lower brain stem neurons, each in turn related to a functionally distinct pool of sympathetic preganglionic cells.

Barman et al. (1984) have provided evidence for the differential control of sympathetic nerves by brain stem circuits in anesthetized, baroreceptor-denervated cats. They used autocorrelation analysis to compare the frequencies of the 2–6 Hz rhythm in the simultaneously recorded discharges of pairs of sympathetic postganglionic nerves whose members receive inputs from sympathetic preganglionic neurons located at different levels of the thoracolumbar spinal cord. Autocorrelation analysis extracts the rhythmic components in a noisy signal by analyzing the dependence of the amplitude of the signal sampled at regular intervals on that of the same signal at a specified point in time (Lee, 1960). Barman et al. (1984) found that the average frequency of the 2–6 Hz rhythm (presumed to be of brain stem origin) in one postganglionic nerve was not always the same as that in the second member of a pair. A summary of their results is presented in Figure 8-13. The frequency of the rhythm in the autocorrelogram of inferior cardiac (A) or external carc d sympathetic nerve discharge (B) is plotted against .hat in the autocorrelogram of renal sympathetic nerve discharge. The diagonal line in each plot runs through points of equal frequency (identity line). It can be noted that many of the data points fell far from the identity line. Data points that deviated from the identity line fell either above or below it. Thus, the predominant rhythm in renal nerve activity could be slower or faster than that in inferior cardiac or external carotid sympathetic nerve discharge. These data support the view that the basal discharges of sympathetic nerves arising from different spinal segments are controlled in a nonuniform manner by the brain stem. The data also raise the possibility that multiple circuits of brain stem neurons generate a 2–6 Hz rhythm, the period of which can be different in each circuit. Each of these circuits might be dedicated to a particular portion of the spinal sympathetic outflow.

Alternatively, each circuit might exert differential actions on sympathetic nerves arising from different

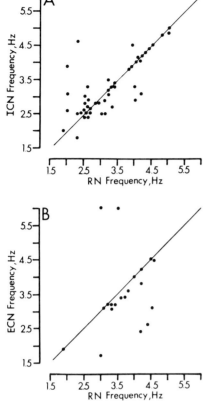

Figure 8-13 Comparison of frequencies of the rhythms in autocorrelograms of simultaneously recorded discharges of sympathetic nerve pairs. (A) Frequency of rhythm in inferior cardiac nerve (ICN) activity is plotted against that in renal nerve (RN) activity. (B) Frequency of rhythm in external carotid nerve (ECN) activity is plotted against that in RN activity. Sixty-seven data points were obtained in 22 cats. (Reprinted in Barman et al., 1984.)

spinal levels. The latter possibility seems more likely since the axons of many rostral ventrolateral medullary sympathoexcitatory and caudal raphe sympathoinhibitory neurons innervate the intermediolateral cell column of widely separated spinal segments. Thus, the 2- to 6-Hz activity pattern in any given sympathetic postganglionic nerve might reflect superimposition of the rhythms arising from multiple circuits of brain stem neurons.

More than one level of the neuraxis is involved in generating the background discharges of sympathetic nerves. The fact that brain stem circuits are inherently capable of generating sympathetic nerve activity has already been discussed. Studies indicating that sympathetic nerve discharge can also be generated by forebrain and spinal circuits are briefly reviewed below.

The hypothalamus participates in the expression of various forms of experimental hypertension in unanesthetized rats that arise, at least in part, from increased sympathetic nerve discharge. For example, destruction either of the region surrounding the anteroventral portion of the third ventricle (AV3V region) (Brody et al., 1984) or of the paraventricular hypothalamic nucleus (Zhang and Ciriello, 1985) prevents or reverses the hypertension produced by sinoaortic or aortic baroreceptor denervation.

Huang et al. (1987, 1988) have proposed that forebrain regions, including the hypothalamus, contribute to sympathetic nerve discharge in anesthetized cats. They studied the effects of midbrain transection (i.e., decerebration) on blood pressure and inferior cardiac and renal sympathetic nerve discharge. Sympathetic nerve discharge and blood pressure fell transiently but significantly after decerebration. The decreases in sympathetic activity (38%) and blood pressure (34 mm Hg) were most prominent in baroreceptor-denervated cats. Three observations led Huang and his colleagues to conclude that these effects monitored the loss of a forebrain-dependent component of sympathetic nerve discharge rather than a nonspecific phenomenon such as generalized trauma or the mechanical stimulation of a descending sympathoinhibitory system. First, following recovery from the effects of decerebration, a second transection performed more caudally in the midbrain failed to affect sympathetic nerve activity and blood pressure. The first and second transections should have produced similar effects if trauma and/or the mechanical stimulation of a descending sympathoinhibitory system were responsible for the reductions in sympathetic nerve discharge and blood pressure. Second, a component of sympathetic nerve discharge was synchronized to frontal-parietal cortical activity in those experiments in which subsequent midbrain transection reduced inferior cardiac and renal nerve activity ≥ 30%. Third, the effects of midbrain transection were prevented by prior lesioning of either the posterior or lateral hypothalamus. The possibility that the hypothalamic lesions involved the cell bodies of neurons that generate a component of sympathetic nerve discharge is supported by the results obtained with single cell recording techniques (Barman and Gebber, 1982; Varner et al., 1988). These investigators located posterior and lateral hypothalamic neurons in anesthetized cats whose naturally occurring activity was synchronized to inferior cardiac sympathetic nerve discharge.

The evidence pointing to a role of spinal circuits in generating sympathetic tone has been reviewed by Schramm (1986). Although there is agreement that arterial pressure is reduced by spinal transection, activity in sympathetic nerves supplying different organs is not uniformly affected. For example, Meckler and Weaver (1985) found that acute transection of the cervical spinal cord in the cat significantly reduced cardiac and renal sympathetic nerve activity, but not splenic sympathetic nerve activity. Section of the dorsal roots betwen the T4 and L5 spinal segments failed to reduce splenic sympathetic activity in spinal preparations when blood gases were within normal limits. Thus, splenic nerve activity was dependent on intrinsic spinal mechanisms, at least after interrupting bulbospinal pathways. The results of Taylor and Schramm (1987) are generally supportive of Meckler and Weaver's results, although some species-related differences were observed. They noted an increase in renal sympathetic nerve discharge upon acute spinal transection in the rat.

SUMMARY

The genesis of the basal (i.e., naturally occurring) discharges of sympathetic nerves has fascinated investigators for over a hundred years. This chapter focuses on the neural substrates and mechanisms that account for one of the major components of sympathetic nerve discharge, the 2–6 Hz rhythm. Because bursts of sympathetic nerve discharge are normally locked 1:1 to the cardiac cycle, the 2–6 Hz rhythm was initially thought to arise as the direct consequence of the waxing and waning of central inhibition attendant on pulse synchronous baroreceptor afferent nerve activity. This view has given way to one of a centrally generated rhythm that is entrained to the cardiac cycle by the baroreceptor reflexes.

Brain stem circuits are inherently capable of generating the 2–6 Hz rhythm in sympathetic nerve discharge. Some of the components of these circuits have been identified by using averaging techniques to study the temporal relationships between the discharges of single brain stem neurons and sympathetic nerves. Moreover, the interconnections of these neurons have been defined by using electrical stimulation to map their axonal projections and terminal fields.

The data available from experiments on cats have led to two hypotheses. The first hypothesis is that the 2–6 Hz rhythm in sympathetic nerve discharge is generated not by medullospinal neurons that innervate the intermediolateral cell column, but rather by their antecedent inputs. Neurons in the lateral tegmental field of the medullary reticular formation are candidates for this role since they discharge earlier during the 2–6 Hz burst of sympathetic nerve discharge than neurons with axons projecting to the spinal intermediolateral nucleus. The latter neurons are located in the rostral ventrolateral medulla and medullary raphe nuclei. The second hypothesis is that the 2–6 Hz rhythm is a property of a network oscillator, that is, an ensemble of sympathoexcita-

tory and sympathoinhibitory neurons interconnected in such a way as to generate rhythmic activity. There is not yet evidence to suggest that the network oscillator is driven by intrinsic pacemaker neurons under normal conditions. This point deserves further study since some rat rostral ventrolateral medullary neurons develop pacemaker-like activity (i.e., near constant interspike intervals) after glutamate-receptor blockade. It remains to be determined whether these pacemakers are generators of sympathetic nerve discharge in the normal physiological state.

ACKNOWLEDGMENTS

I am indebted to those who helped design and perform the experiments from my laboratory. They are Drs. Susan M. Barman, Zhong-Sun Huang, Shaun F. Morrison, and Kurt J. Varner. Special thanks are due to Dr. Barman who critically reviewed the manuscript. Ms. Diane Hummel's secretarial assistance is greatly appreciated. The studies from my laboratory were sponsored by the National Heart, Lung and Blood Institute (grants HL13187 and HL33266).

REFERENCES

Reviews

Bendat, J. S., and Piersol, A. G., (1971). *Random Data: Analysis and Measurement Procedures.* Wiley, New York.

Brody, M. J., Faber, J. E., Mangiapane, M. L., and Porter, J. P. (1984). The central nervous system and prevention of hypertension. In: *Handbook of Hypertension, Vol. 4: Experimental and Genetic Models of Hypertension,* W. de Jong, (ed.), Elsevier Biomedical Press, New York, pp. 474–497.

Calaresu, F. R., Ciriello, J., Caverson, M. M., Cechetto, D. F., and Krukoff, T. L., (1984). Functional neuroanatomy of central pathways controlling the circulation. In: *Hypertension and the Brain,* T. A. Kotchen and C. P. Guthrie (eds.), Futura, Mount Kisco, NY, pp. 3–21.

Cannon, W. B. (1929). *Bodily Changes in Pain, Hunger, Fear and Rage,* 2nd ed. Appleton, New York.

Feldberg, W. (1976). The ventral surface of the brain stem: A scarcely explored region of pharmacological sensitivity. *Neuroscience* 1, 427–441.

Feldman, J. L., and Cleland, C. L. (1982). Possible roles of pacemaker neurons in mammalian respiratory rhythmogenesis. In: *Cellular Pacemakers, Vol. 2: Function in Normal and Disease States,* D. O. Carpenter (ed.), Wiley, New York, pp. 101–119.

Gebber, G. L., (1980). Central oscillators responsible for sympathetic nerve discharge. *American Journal of Physiology* 239, H143–H155.

Gebber, G. L., (1984). Brainstem systems involved in cardiovascular regulation. In: *Nervous Control of Cardio-*

vascular Function, W. C. Randall (ed.), Oxford University Press, New York, pp. 346–368.

Hilton, S. M. (1982). The defence-arousal system and its relevance for circulatory and respiratory control. *Journal of Experimental Biology* 100, 159–174.

Kristan, W. B. (1980). Generation of rhythmic motor patterns. In: *Information Processing in the Nervous System,* H. M. Pinsker, W. D. Willis (eds), Raven, New York, pp. 241–261.

Lee, Y. W. (1960). *Statistical Theory of Communication.* Wiley, New York.

Lipski, J. (1981). Antidromic activation of neurones as an analytic tool in the study of the central nervous system. *Journal of Neuroscience Methods* 4, 1–32.

Loewy, A. D. (1982). Descending pathways to the sympathetic preganglionic neurons. In: *Progress in Brain Research, Vol. 57: Descending Pathways to the Spinal Cord,* H. G. J. M. Kuypers and G. F. Martin (eds.), Elsevier Biomedical Press, Amsterdam, pp. 267–277.

Pavlidis, T. (1973). *Biological Oscillators: Their Mathematical Analysis.* Academic Press, New York.

Schramm, L. P. (1986). Spinal factors in sympathetic regulation. In: *Central and Peripheral Mechanisms of Cardiovascular Regulation,* A. Magro, W. Osswald, D. Reis, and P. Vanhoutte (eds.), Plenum, New York, pp. 303–352.

Selverston, A. I., and Moulins, M. (1985). Oscillatory neural networks. *Annual Review of Physiology* 47, 29–48.

Sherrington, C. (1906). *The Integrative Action of the Nervous System.* Yale University Press, New Haven.

Swanson, L. W., and Sawchenko, P. E. (1983). Hypothalamic integration: Organization of the paraventricular and supraoptic nuclei. *Annual Review of Neuroscience* 6, 269–324.

Winfree, A. T. (1983). Sudden cardiac death: A problem in topology. *Scientific American* 248, 144–161.

Research Articles

Adrian, E. D., Bronk, D. W., Phillips, G. (1932). Discharges in mammalian sympathetic nerves. *Journal of Physiology* (London) 74, 115–133.

Alexander, R. S. (1946). Tonic and reflex functions of medullary sympathetic cardiovascular centers. *Journal of Neurophysiology* 53, 1551–1566.

Bachoo, M., and Polosa, C. (1987). Properties of the inspiration-related activity of sympathetic preganglionic neurones of the cervical trunk in the cat. *Journal of Physiology* (London) 385, 545–564.

Barman, S. M., and Gebber, G. L. (1976). Basis for synchronization of sympathetic and phrenic nerve discharges. *American Journal of Physiology* 231, 1601–1607.

Barman, S. M., and Gebber, G. L. (1980). Sympathetic nerve rhythm of brain stem origin. *American Journal of Physiology* 239, R42–R47.

Barman, S. M., and Gebber, G. L. (1981). Brain stem neuronal types with activity patterns related to sympathetic nerve discharge. *American Journal of Physiology* 240, R335–R347.

Barman, S. M., and Gebber, G. L. (1982). Hypothalamic neurons with activity patterns related to sympathetic nerve discharge. *American Journal of Physiology* 242, R34–R43.

Barman, S. M., and Gebber, G. L. (1983). Sequence of activation of ventrolateral and dorsal medullary sympathetic neurons. *American Journal of Physiology* 245, R438–R447.

Barman, S. M., and Gebber, G. L., (1985). Axonal projection patterns of ventrolateral medullospinal sympathoexcitatory neurons. *Journal of Neurophysiology* 53, 1551–1566.

Barman, S. M., and Gebber, G. L. (1987). Lateral tegmental field neurons of cat medulla: A source of basal activity of ventrolateral medullospinal sympathoexcitatory neurons. *Journal of Neurophysiology* 57, 1410–1424.

Barman, S. M., and Gebber, G. L. (1989). Lateral tegmental neurons of cat medulla: A source of basal activity of raphespinal sympathoinhibitory neurons. *Journal of Neurophysiology* 61, 1011–1024.

Barman, S. M., Gebber, G. L., and Calaresu, F. R. (1984). Differential control of sympathetic nerve discharge by the brain stem. *American Journal of Physiology* 247, R513–R519.

Bernard, C. (1851). Influence de grand sympathetique sur la sensibilité et sur la calorification, *C. R. Soc. Biol. Paris* 3, 163–164.

Bernard, C. (1863). Leçons sur la physiologie et la pathologie du système nerveux, Vol. 1. Baillière, Paris, p. 381.

Brown-Séquard, C.-E. (1852) Recherches sur l'influence du système nerveux sur les fonctions de la vie organique. *Med. Exam. Philad.,* p. 486.

Brown-Séquard, C.-E. (1852). Recherches sur l'influence du système nerveux sur les fonctions de la vie organique. *Med. Exam. Philad., p. 486.*

Cohen, M. I., and Gootman, P. M. (1970). Periodicities in efferent discharge of splanchnic nerve of the cat. *American Journal of Physiology* 218, 1092–1101.

Dampney, R. A. L., and Moon, E. A. (1980). Role of ventrolateral medulla in vasomotor response to cerebral ischemia. *American Journal of Physiology* 239, H349–H358.

Dittmar, C. (1873). Uber die Lage des sogenannten Gefasscentrums in der Medulla oblongata. *Ber. Verh. Saechs. Wiss. Leipzig Math Phys.* Kl 25, 449–469.

Fries, W., and Zieglgansberger, W. (1974). A method to discriminate axonal from cell body activity and to analyze 'silent' cells. *Experimental Brain Research* 21, 441–445.

Gebber, G. L. (1976). Basis for phase relations between baroreceptor and sympathetic nervous discharge. *American Journal of Physiology* 230, 263–270.

Gebber, G. L., and Barman, S. M. (1985). Lateral tegmental field neurons of cat medulla: A potential source of basal sympathetic nerve discharge. *Journal of Neurophysiology* 54, 1498–1512.

Gebber, G. L., Barman, S. M., and Morrison, S. F. (1987). Electrophysiological evidence for the modular organization of the reticular formation: Sympathetic controlling circuits. *Brain Research* 410, 106–110.

Goodchild, A. K., and Dampney, R. A. L. (1985). A vasopressor cell group in the rostral dorsomedial medulla of the rabbit. *Brain Research* 360, 24–32.

Hilton, S. M., and Redfern, W. S. (1986). A search for

brain stem cell groups integrating the defence reaction in the rat. *Journal of Physiology* (London) 378, 213–228.

Huang, Z.-S., Gebber, G. L., Barman, S. M., and Varner, K. J., (1987). Forebrain contribution to sympathetic nerve discharge in anesthetized cats. *American Journal of Physiology* 252, R645–R652.

Huang, Z.-S., Varner, K. J., Barman, S. M., and Gebber, G. L. (1988). Diencephalic regions contributing to sympathetic nerve discharge in anesthetized cats. *American Journal of Physiology* 254, R249–R256.

Kumada, M., Dampney, R. A. L., and Reis, D. J. (1979). Profound hypotension and abolition of the vasomotor component of the cerebral ischemic response produced by restricted lesions of medulla oblongata in rabbit. *Circulation Research* 45, 63–70.

Loewy, A. D., Marson, L., Parkinson, D., Perry, M. A., and Sawyer, W. B. (1986). Descending noradrenergic pathways involved in the A5 depressor response. *Brain Research* 388, 313–324.

McCall, R. B., and Gebber, G. L. (1975). Brain stem and spinal synchronization of sympathetic nervous discharge. *Brain Research* 89, 139–143.

Meckler, R. L., and Weaver, L. C., (1985). Splenic, renal and cardiac nerves have unequal dependence upon tonic supraspinal inputs. *Brain Research* 338, 123–135.

Morrison, S. F., and Gebber, G. L. (1982). Classification of raphe neurons with cardiac-related activity. *American Journal of Physiology* 243, R49–R59.

Morrison, S. F., and Gebber, G. L. (1985). Axonal branching patterns and funicular trajectories of raphespinal sympathoinhibitory neurons. *Journal of Neurophysiology* 53, 759–772.

Owsjannikow, P. (1871). Die tonischen und reflectorischen Centren der Gefassnerven. *Ber. Verh. Saechs. Wiss. Leipzig Math Phys. Kl.* 23, 135–143.

Ranson, S. W., and Billingsley, P. R. (1916). Vasomotor reactions from stimulation of the floor of the fourth ventricle. *American Journal of Physiology* 41, 85–90.

Ross, C. A., Ruggiero, D. A., Park, D. H., Joh, T. H., Sved, A. F., Fernandez-Pardal, J., Saavedra, J. M., and Reis, D. J. (1984). Tonic vasomotor control by the rostral ventrolateral medulla: Effect of electrical or chemical stimulation of the area containing C1 adrenaline neurons on arterial pressure, heart rate, and plasma catecholamines and vasopressin. *Journal of Neuroscience* 4, 474–494.

Schlafke, M. E. and Loeschcke, H. H. (1967). Lokalisation eines an der Regulation von Atmung und Kreislauf bewilligen Gebietes an der ventralen Oberflache der Medulla oblongata durch Kalteblockade. *Pflugers Archiv Ges. Physiol.* 297, 201–220.

Shinoda, Y., Arnold, A. P., and Asanuma, H. (1976). Spinal branching of corticospinal axons in the cat. *Experimental Brain Research* 26, 215–234.

Sun, M.-K., Hackett, J. T., and Guyenet, P. G. (1988). Sympathoexcitatory neurons of rostral ventrolateral medulla exhibit pacemaker properties in the presence of a glutamate-receptor antagonist. *Brain Research* 438, 23–40.

Taylor, R. F., and Schramm, L. P. (1987). Differential effects of spinal transection on sympathetic nerve activities in rats. *American Journal of Physiology* 253, R611–R618.

Varner, K. J., Barman, S. M., and Gebber, G. L. (1988). Cat diencephalic neurons with sympathetic nerve-related activity. *American Journal of Physiology* 254, R257–R267.

Wang, S. C., and Ranson, S. W. (1939). Autonomic responses to electrical stimulation of the lower brain stem. *Journal of Comparative Neurology* 71, 437–455.

Zhang, T.-X., and Ciriello, J. (1985). Effect of paraventricular nucleus lesions on arterial pressure and heart rate after aortic baroreceptor denervation in the rat. *Brain Research* 34, 101–109.

9

Role of the Ventral Medulla Oblongata in Blood Pressure Regulation

P. G. GUYENET

The sympathetic vasomotor outflow is composed of a series of parallel and differentially regulated efferent pathways that control the cardiac output and the vascular tone of somatic and visceral structures. These pathways are thought to be organized in a highly specific fashion. For example, it is currently believed that specific sets of sympathetic preganglionic neurons may regulate the activity of muscle vasoconstrictor sympathetic postganglionic fibers and other sympathetic preganglionic neurons may control cutaneous vasoconstrictor postganglionic neurons (see Chapter 18). One of the general aims of research in this area of neuroscience has been to identify the central networks that regulate the activity of each of these sympathetic efferent pathways and to determine the neurotransmitters used by these central pathways. Sympathetic vasomotor preganglionic neurons receive synaptic inputs from both spinal and supraspinal sources. In this chapter the main focus will be on the role of one of these supraspinal areas, the ventral medulla oblongata, in regulating the vasomotor sympathetic outflow.

A characteristic feature of the vasomotor sympathetic outflow is its tonic activity, which persists under anesthesia. However, it is important to recognize that this tonic activity is probably restricted to sympathetic neurons with cardioaccelerator or vasoconstrictor function. In contrast, sudomotor, piloerector, and pupillomotor sympathetic fibers discharge only under very specific circumstances in the anesthetized mammal. Thus, an additional aim of research in this area has been to determine the central mechanisms responsible for the continuous excitatory drive of these sympathetic preganglionic vasomotor neurons.

ANATOMICAL CONSIDERATIONS

Brain Nuclei Involved in Cardiovascular Regulation

Several interconnected brain stem networks regulate the sympathetic outflow. Reciprocal pathways between the nucleus tractus solitarius, the ventrolateral medulla, the A5 cell group, the parabrachial nucleus, and several forebrain areas, including the paraventricular hypothalamic nucleus, the bed nucleus of the stria terminalis, and the central nucleus of the amygdala, provide the anatomical substrate for cardiovascular regulation. These interconnected systems provide inputs to or are part of several key areas of the brain that project directly to the sympathetic preganglionic neurons. Direct projections to the intermediolateral cell column originate from only seven areas of the brain: (1) the rostral ventrolateral medulla, (2) the caudal raphe nuclei (raphe pallidus and raphe obscurus), (3) the A5 noradrenergic cell group, (4) the Kölliker–Fuse nucleus, (5) the paraventricular hypothalamic nucleus, (6) the lateral hypothalamic area, and (7) the central gray matter (see Loewy and Neil, 1981 and Luiten et al., 1987 for reviews). It has not been demonstrated that each of these projections has a vasomotor role, however.

The possibility that additional afferents of supraspinal origin might influence the activity of vasomotor preganglionic neurons by way of projections to interneurons located in other laminae of the spinal gray matter should not be overlooked. To identify these hypothetical neurons, however, will require a knowledge of the intrinsic spinal circuits governing the activity of sympathetic preganglionic neurons.

The Ventrolateral Medulla

The ventrolateral quadrant of the medullary reticular formation has been termed loosely the *ventrolateral medulla.* In this section, various rostrocaudal portions of the ventrolateral medulla will be discussed. These areas will be largely defined by their proximity to rostrocaudal subdivisions of the nucleus ambiguus. For this reason, a brief summary of the cytoarchitecture of the nucleus ambiguus will be given. According to Bieger and Hopkins (1987), the nucleus ambiguus of the rat consists of two major divisions (Figure 9-1). The first division, or nucleus ambiguus of classical anatomy, includes three serially arranged subdivisions, which contain motor neurons innervating the striated muscles of the esophagus, pharynx, and larynx. These subdivisions consist of (1) a rostral compact portion sometimes, but inappropriately, called the retrofacial nucleus (see Berman, 1968), containing mostly motor neurons that innervate the esophagus; (2) a semicompact portion located ventral and posterior to the compact region and composed of motor neurons that innervate the pharyngeal muscles and the cricothyroid muscle of the larynx; and (3) a disperse set of neurons called the loose formation, which projects to the rest of the intrinsic laryngeal musculature. The second major division or "external formation" is not identifiable as a distinct nucleus on architectonic grounds. It is located ventrolateral to the nucleus ambiguus at rostral levels and surrounds it at caudal levels. This area contains preganglionic parasympathetic neurons projecting to the heart, trachea, bronchi, and mucus membranes of the larynx (Bieger and Hopkins, 1987). Cardiac preganglionic motor neurons are concentrated predominantly in the external formation at the level of the obex and extend rostrally (see Chapter 5). The external formation also contains bulbospinal respiratory premotoneurons organized in three rostrocaudally arranged groups of cells (for review see Von Euler, 1986). The caudalmost third, the nucleus retroambigualis, contains a predominance of expiratory neurons. The intermediate part centered around the obex level, termed the nucleus paraambigualis, involves a concentration of inspiratory neurons. The rostral segment contains a group of reticulospinal expiratory neurons that has been termed the *Bötzinger complex* (see Feldman, 1986 for review).

The "rostral ventrolateral medulla" of the rat lies rostral to the lateral reticular nucleus, caudal to the facial nucleus, and extends to the ventral medullary surface (RVL in Figure 9-1). This area overlaps dorsally with the rostral subcompact and external subdivisions of the nucleus ambiguus, and its lateral aspect may actually represent the rodent equivalent of the rostral subtrigeminal subnucleus of the lateral reticular nucleus. The medial two-thirds of this area contains a particularly dense concentration of reticulospinal cells with projections to the intermediolateral cell column (for references see Guyenet and Young, 1987). This projection consists of roughly an equal proportion of adrenergic (called C1 neurons) and nonaminergic neurons (Tucker et al., 1987) that are involved in vasomotor function (see below). The rostral ventrolateral medulla has occasionally been called the *pressor area* of the ventrolateral medulla because of the large elevations in arterial pressure triggered by the application of excitatory drugs or putative transmitters. It is important to note that this area contains a variety of different cells that project to the intermediolateral cell column and elsewhere and is not rigidly defined by clear cytoarchitectonic borders. For example, many C1 adrenergic cells are also scattered medially in the neighboring gigantocellular reticular formation.

The external formation of the nucleus ambiguus at the level of the obex should be clearly separated from the rostral ventrolateral medulla. In rats, this zone contains, among many other cells, A1 noradrenergic neurons. This general area is also occasionally referred to as the ventrolateral medullary *depressor area* because hypotension is produced by local microinjections of neuronal depolarizing chemicals (e.g., glutamate) in this site. To avoid the parochial connotation of the terms *A1 area* or *depressor area,* and the unwieldy term of external formation of nucleus ambiguus at the obex level (Bieger and Hopkins, 1987), this area will henceforth be called the *caudal periambigual area* (Figure 9-1).

It must be noted that in Taber's atlas of the cat brain (1961), the rostral ventrolateral medulla caudal to the facial nucleus is subdivided into two nuclei, a lateral one called the retrofacial nucleus and a medial part, the nucleus paragigantocellularis, which also extends in a rostral direction to the pontomedullary junction. A similar mediolateral subdivision of the rostral ventrolateral medulla has been proposed by Kalia and Fuxe (1985) in the rat (Figure 9-2), but the dividing line appears arbitrary since it bisects the area containing reticulospinal neurons with vasomotor function. Since the rostral extension of the paragigantocellular nucleus is probably involved in pain control and not in cardiovascular regulation (see Chapter 7), it also seems preferable not to use this terminology. The definition of the paragigantocellular nucleus provided by Andrezik and colleagues (1981a) has also become too broad in view of physiological data that will be discussed later. In this review, the term *rostral ventrolateral medulla*

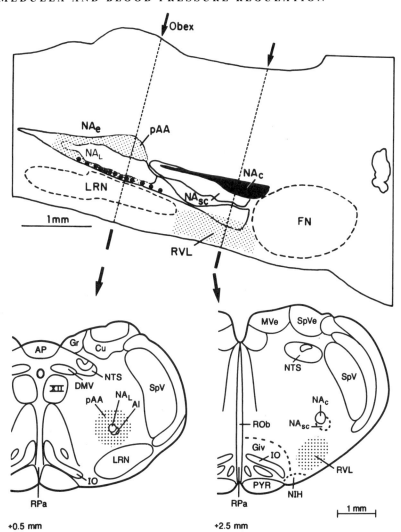

Figure 9-1 Major subdivisions of the ventrolateral medulla and nucleus ambiguus of the rat. Top: Schematic drawing of a parasagittal section of the rat medulla oblongata illustrating the major subdivisions of nucleus ambiguus according to Bieger and Hopkins (1987). Bottom: Two transverse sections of the medulla at the levels +0.5 and +2.5 mm rostral to the calamus scriptorius are presented. The periambigual area (pAA) represents the immediate vicinity of the "loose" subdivision of the nucleus ambiguus at the obex level. This general area contains A1 noradrenergic and C1 adrenergic neurons, cardiac parasympathetic preganglionic neurons, bulbospinal inspiratory neurons, and noncatecholamine bulbospinal neurons involved in the control of the sympathetic outflow. All other nuclei except RVL are defined according to the atlas entitled *The Rat Brain in Stereotaxic Coordinates,* 2nd ed., by G. Paxinos and C. Watson (Academic Press, Syndey, 1986). The two lower drawings are modifications of drawings that appear in this atlas (with permission of the authors and publishers). A1, area of the A1 cell group; AP, area postrema; Cu, cuneate nucleus; DMV, dorsal motor nucleus of vagus nerve; FN, facial nucleus; Giv, gigantocellular reticular nucleus, ventral part; Gr, gracile nucleus; IO, inferior olive; LRN, lateral reticular nucleus; MVe, medial vestibular nucleus; NA$_c$, compact rostral end of nucleus ambiguus; NA$_L$, loose formation of nucleus ambiguous; NA$_e$, external formation of nucleus ambiguus; NA$_{sc}$, subcompact region of nucleus ambiguus; NIH, nucleus interfascicularis hypoglossi; NTS, nucleus tractus solitarius; pAA, periambigual area; PYR, pyramidal tract; ROb, nucleus raphe obscurus; RPa, nucleus raphe pallidus; RVL, rostral ventrolateral medulla; SpV, spinal trigeminal nucleus; SpVe, spinal vestibular nucleus; XII, hypoglossal nucleus.

will be used as a synonym for the area defined by Ross et al. (1984a) as the "nucleus reticularis rostroventrolateralis." The area thus defined excludes the rostral-most portion of the ventrolateral medullary reticular formation in which A5 noradrenergic neurons are located. It seems to be approximately

equivalent to the "retrofacial nucleus" of Berman in cats or to the "nucleus reticularis lateralis" of Mcesen and Olszewski in rabbits (for references see Berman, 1968).

The rostral ventrolateral medulla receives inputs from a number of areas in the brain and spinal cord

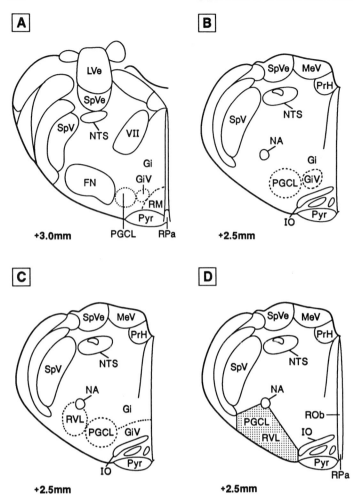

Figure 9-2 Various anatomical cytoarchitectonic classifications of the rostral medulla oblongata. The drawings are modified from illustrations in Paxinos and Watson (1986) with permission of the authors and publisher. The number in the left-hand corner indicates the distance from the calamus scriptorius. The difficulty of defining nuclear aggregates on cytoarchitectonic grounds within the rostral ventrolateral medulla is illustrated by the diverging terms applied by various investigators. These figures represent the various interpretations of the cytoarchitectonic subdivisions in the rat. A and B illustrate one classification presented by Kalia and Fuxe (1985). Note their parcellation of the ventral part of the gigantocellular reticular nucleus (GiV) is different from the scheme used by Paxinos and Watson (1986), which is illustrated in C and D, the PGCL area described by Andrezik et al. (1981a) is compared to the same area termed RVL by Ross et al. (1984a). PGCL, nucleus paragigantocellularis lateralis. For other abbreviations, see Figure 9-1.

(Andrezik et al., 1981b) and sends fibers throughout the CNS (Loewy et al., 1981). It is heavily innervated by the nucleus tractus solitarius (Loewy and Burton, 1978; Ross et al., 1985). There are reciprocal connections between the two areas. Fibers take the shortest route between the two areas and are highly concentrated within a triangular wedge of the medulla inserted between the nuclei reticularis ventralis or gigantocellularis and nucleus reticularis parvocellularis (Ross et al., 1985). In addition, the rostral ventrolateral medulla receives inputs from the area postrema (Shapiro and Miselis, 1985; Ross et al., 1985). These two medullary afferents serve to relay two general classes of cardiovascular information. The region of the nucleus tractus solitarius (medial part) that projects to this area probably relays mainly cardiopulmonary information. The area postrema presumably functions to convey information regarding various hormones in the plasma. In addition, reciprocal longitudinal connections possibly link the rostrocaudal segments of the ventrolateral medulla, although a detailed understanding of these proprio-

bulbar circuits is lacking. The ventrolateral medulla is also heavily interconnected with specific subnuclei of the parabrachial complex (Fulwiler and Saper, 1984; Loewy et al., 1981; Guyenet and Young, 1987). Moreover, a number of reciprocal connections also exist between the rostral ventrolateral medulla and the central gray matter, lateral hypothalamic area, zona incerta, and paraventricular hypothalamic nucleus. The function of these interactions is unknown.

IDENTIFICATION OF CNS NEURONS INVOLVED IN GENERATING THE VASOMOTOR OUTPUT: GENERAL PRINCIPLES

From 1920 to 1980, electrical stimulation was the method of choice to locate neurons involved in cardiovascular regulation. This is exemplified by the frequently cited study of Alexander (1946), which indicated that the entire reticular formation is involved in vasomotor function and consists of a diffuse lateral pressor area and a midline depressor one. This view has been widely abandoned because of its complete reliance on the results of electrical stimulation. Indeed, unless they can be reproduced by microinjections of chemicals that excite or inhibit neuronal cell bodies or their dendrites, the effects of electrical stimulation are likely to result from the activation of remote neurons that merely send an axonal process in the vicinity of the site of stimulation.

Until the early 1980s, an equally vague picture of the role of the reticular formation in vasomotor control had emerged from single-unit recording experiments. The fact that to that time reticular formation neurons were randomly sampled and characterized largely by their response to electrical stimulation of baroreceptor nerves with little regard for their anatomical location and axonal projections probably explains this (Koepchen et al., 1975). These experiments, however, have illustrated the general difficulty of characterizing the function of a reticular neuron solely on the basis of its responsiveness to a limited set of sensory afferents. The shortcomings of this approach have also served as an impetus for the development of the circuit-analysis approach, which consists of identifying small groups of neurons homologous from the standpoint of connectivity and immunohistochemical properties and systematically studying their information processing (input–output relationships).

Three approaches have been used to identify the medullary neurons involved in generating the sympathetic vasomotor output. The first approach involves the identification of medullary neurons that discharge in a pattern that correlates mathematically with sympathetic fiber discharge. Investigators using this approach have postulated that central neurons with an activity pattern exhibiting a significant correlation with the 2–6 Hz rhythm of the sympathetic discharge may directly or indirectly (via polysynaptic pathways) contribute to the generation of the sympathetic outflow (see Chapter 8). The disadvantage of this method is that it is likely to also identify large populations of neurons sharing common inputs with central sympathetic networks but not directly contributing to the autonomic outflow.

The second approach is to locate neurons with electrophysiological recording techniques that respond to the electrical stimulation of baroreceptor afferent nerves (generally the aortic depressor nerve or the carotid sinus nerve). Used alone, without other identifying criteria, this approach has been of marginal significance because of the overwhelmingly large number of responsive neurons (Koepchen et al., 1975). This is probably due to several factors. First, neurons may receive baroreceptor information via multisynaptic inputs and not be involved in the generation of the sympathetic vasomotor outflow and vice versa. Second, the synchronous stimulation of all baroreceptor afferents may be an inappropriate stimulus because it may recruit pathways that are not activated by physiological stimuli (McAllen and Spyer, 1978). Third, electrical stimulation of baroreceptor nerves may, under certain conditions, fail to excite unmyelinated C fibers, and, thus, this may introduce a sampling bias, which would exclude many cardiovascular neurons.

The third approach to the identification of central neurons involved in generating the sympathetic outflow has been achieved through the combined use of neuroanatomical tract-tracing techniques, chemical and electrical stimulation methods, and single-unit electrophysiological analysis. This multidisciplinary approach has provided the most complete knowledge, which is summarized in this chapter.

VASOMOTOR NEURONS OF THE ROSTRAL VENTROLATERAL MEDULLA AND CAUDAL RAPHE NUCLEI

Historical Background

A major source of excitatory input to sympathetic preganglionic neurons lies within the rostral ventrolateral medulla. The identification of this structure resulted from investigations dating back to Dittmar (1873) (see Chapter 8 for historical perspective). Dittmar observed that sequential rostral-to-caudal transections of the brain stem produced relatively minimal effects on arterial pressure until the transection encroached on the rostral medulla. By also destroying the dorsal half of the medulla oblongata along with medullary transections, Dittmar deduced that the critical area for maintaining normal blood pressure was just caudal to the facial nucleus. Destruction of this ventral area produced a drop in arterial pressure comparable to that seen after transection of the spinal cord at the first cervical segment. Hence, the concept of a vasomotor center lying somewhere in the ventral medulla oblongata was formulated (Dittmar 1873).

The second major step in identifying the critical site was the observation that bilateral cooling of the surface of the rostral ventrolateral medulla, or bilateral topical application of chemicals on this restricted region, produces equally drastic falls in arterial pressure (Schläfke and Loeschke, 1967; Guertzenstein and Silver, 1974). Subsequently, the anatomical location of the "pressor area" was more precisely defined in the rat and the rabbit using intraparenchymal microinjections of glycine or GABA. When these inhibitory amino acids were microinjected into the rostral ventrolateral medulla, they produced a fall in arterial pressure; opposite effects were produced by excitatory amino acids such as glutamate (Ross et al., 1984b).

These experiments, along with anatomical evidence for direct projections from the rostral ventrolateral medulla to the intermediolateral cell column (Loewy et al., 1981; Ross et al., 1984a), led to the hypothesis that the rostral ventrolateral medulla contains reticulospinal cells that provide an essential excitatory drive to vasomotor preganglionic neurons.

Electrophysiological Identification of Rostral Medullary Neurons with Vasomotor Function

Exploration of the rostral ventrolateral medulla with single-unit extracellular recording techniques in the rat has revealed the presence of a cluster of barosensitive reticulospinal cells with a high rate of discharge in a location corresponding to the rostral ventrolateral nucleus (Brown and Guyenet, 1985, Figure 9-3). These neurons belong to at least two main classes of units that can be distinguished by the conduction velocity of their spinal axons, their sen-

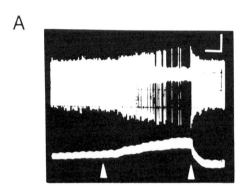

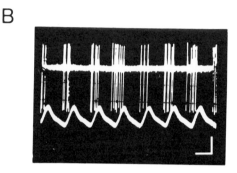

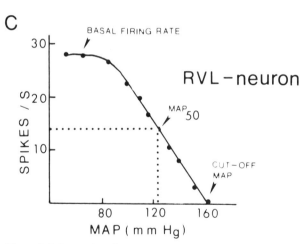

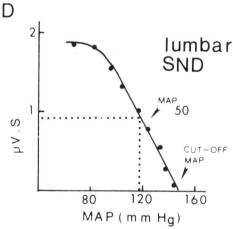

Figure 9-3 Properties of rostral ventrolateral medullary vasomotor neurons. Unit recordings of neuron identified as reticulospinal by antidromic stimulation from the thoracic spinal cord (conduction velocity: 4 m/second). (A) Baroreflex inhibition of neuronal discharges. Arterial pressure (lower trace) was gradually increased by restricting flow through descending aorta (between arrows) resulting in baroreceptor activation and time-locked inhibition of unit discharge (calibration: 0.2 mV, 2 seconds). (B) When examined at a faster time scale, the unit activity is distinctly pulse synchronous due to the phasic nature of arterial baroreceptor discharges relayed multisynaptically to the rostral medulla (calibration: 0.5 mV, 120 msec). (C) Relationship between mean discharge rate of vasomotor neuron and mean arterial pressure (MAP). Note the high basal firing rate below the baroreceptor threshold, linear reduction thereafter, and abrupt well-defined cutoff pressure beyond which the cell is silent. This cutoff does not represent the saturation of baroreceptor inputs but the point at which this input hyperpolarizes the cell below firing threshold. The cutoff MAP thus depends on the presence or absence of excitatory inputs to these neurons and can be raised by hypothalamic stimulation for example. (D) The lumbar sympathetic nerve discharge in the same preparation exhibits the same relationship to mean arterial pressure as that of rostral medullary neurons. [Reproduced from Sun and Guyenet (1986) *American Journal of Physiology* 250, R910–R917, with permission of the authors and publisher.]

sitivity to intravenous or iontophoretic application of the α_2-adrenergic agonist clonidine, and their average discharge rate (Sun and Guyenet, 1986b). Similar observations were later made by Morrison et al. (1988), who also demonstrated that these cells project specifically to the lateral horn. The first class of units consists of clonidine-insensitive cells with axonal conduction velocity of 2.5–8 m/second and a maximum discharge rate of 15–35 spikes/second measured below baroreceptor threshold. The second class is characterized by a much slower conduction velocity (0.4–0.8 m/sec), a slower discharge rate, and the fact that they are inhibited by clonidine. These two populations of cells are also probably present in the rabbit (Terui et al, 1986). In the rat, both cell types are intermingled within 500 μm of the ventral medullary surface in the area defined above as the rostral ventrolateral nucleus. This zone coincides with the middle third of the nucleus paragigantocellularis lateralis as defined in the rat by Andrezik et al., (1981a), hence the name paragigantocellularis neurons was used to describe these cells in earlier publications (Sun and Guyenet, 1986a, b, 1987). However, for reasons detailed above, these neurons will be called the vasomotor neurons of the rostral ventrolateral medulla. Their superficial location, spontaneous activity, and spinal projection are characteristics that support the hypothesis that they represent the neurons that may regulate vasomotor sympathetic tone. This view is further reinforced by the fact that the only other type of tonically active cells recorded in this area in rats is related to respiration and thought to be largely devoid of baroreceptor input and cardiac modulation (Brown and Guyenet, 1985). In both rats and cats, a powerful baroreceptor input imparts rostral ventrolateral medullary vasomotor neurons with a strongly pulse-synchronous pattern of discharge, related to the phasic nature of the baroreceptor afferent traffic (Brown and Guyenet, 1985; Barman and Gebber, 1985; Mc Allen, 1987, Figure 9-3B). In rats, these cells exhibit their lowest probability of firing 65–70 msec after the R wave of the electrocardiogram and around 25 msec after the discharge of presumed second-order baroreceptor neurons of the dorsomedial nucleus of the nucleus tractus solitarius (Moore and Guyenet, 1983). These long delays indicate that intramedullary baroreceptor pathways have a very low conduction velocity ($\leq$0.4 m/second), an observation already made in the case of the cardiac limb of the reflex (McAllen and Spyer, 1978).

The average discharge rate of the fast-conducting rostral medullary vasomotor neurons exhibits the same relationship with regard to mean arterial pressure as the lumbar sympathetic nerve discharge (Sun and Guyenet, 1986b, Figure 9-3C and D). The neural discharge of putative homologs in cat seems to correlate with the 2- to 6-Hz rhythm of the sympathetic nerve discharge even in the absence of baroreceptor input (Barman and Gebber, 1985). Taken together, the above evidence leaves little doubt that these cells belong to the tonically active neurons of the rostral ventrolateral medulla that regulate ongoing vasomotor sympathetic activity. However, final proof that the electrophysiologically identified rostral ventrolateral medullary vasomotor neurons make monosynaptic contact with sympathetic preganglionic neurons is still lacking. In addition, it has not been finally determined whether their projection to the sympathetic preganglionic neurons is solely responsible for their vasomotor function. Some of these cells may form collaterals in the medulla oblongata (Barman and Gebber, 1985) and, therefore, could activate or inhibit subsidiary sets of descending vasomotor neurons.

Vasomotor Neurons with Intrinsic Pacemaker Properties

Some of the vasomotor neurons of the rostral ventrolateral medulla exhibit intrinsic pacemaker properties, but before reviewing these findings, some general background information on pacemaker cells will be provided. Many neurons are capable of generating a rhythmic pattern of discharge when appropriately depolarized (for review see Connor, 1985). Neurons with intrinsic pacemaker activity are characterized by the unique ability to generate a tonic rhythmic discharge even in the absence of any synaptic input. These cells fall into two classes: bursting and nonbursting. In both cases, action potentials result from a gradual membrane depolarization caused by the sequential closing or opening of specific ionic channels. In nonbursting neurons, each spike triggers an after-hyperpolarization of a magnitude that precludes repetitive firing and reinitiates a cycle of slow membrane depolarization. The following four criteria need to be fulfilled to ascertain that a rhythmically firing nonbursting neuron has intrinsic pacemaker properties:

1. Each spike should result from a gradual interspike membrane depolarization as opposed to regularly occurring excitatory postsynaptic potentials (EPSPs).
2. When hyperpolarized by injection of small negative current, the pacemaker activity should stop and regularly occurring EPSPs should still not be observed despite the increase in driving force.
3. The pacemaking activity should be reset by brief periods of hyperpolarizing current or by the untimely occurrence of an action potential produced by a brief depolarizing pulse.
4. The pacemaking activity should not depend on the synaptic release of a neuromodulator.

Although rostral ventrolateral medullary vasomotor neurons receive a large number of excitatory
synaptic inputs, all of those examined so far are
blocked by kynurenic acid, a glutamate-receptor antagonist (Sun and Guyenet, 1986a, 1987; Sun et al.,
1988a). Since this agent does not influence the resting level of discharge of these cells (see Mayer and
Westbrook, 1987 and Stone and Burton, 1988 for

reviews on glutamate transmission), this provides
the first hint that their tonic activity might be in part
generated by a nonsynaptic mechanism such as intrinsic pacemaker discharges. Moreover, if kynurenic acid is injected into the cisterna magna but
prevented from migrating to the spinal cord, arterial
pressure is well maintained and virtually all sympathetic reflexes are blocked (Sun et al., 1988a). Under

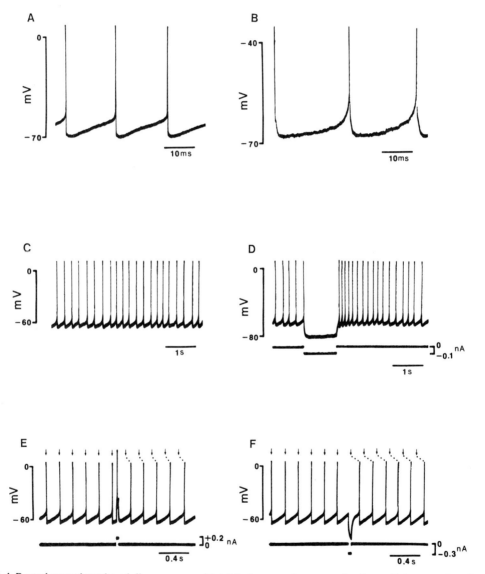

Figure 9-4 Rostral ventrolateral medullary neurons with intrinsic pacemaker properties. Intracellular recordings from cells
located in the ventral part of the rostral ventrolateral area and identified as reticulospinal neurons. Note typical pacemaker
potentials reset after a single spike (A,B). Hyperpolarizing the neurons by passing small negative currents intracellularly
eliminates pacemaking activity and does not uncover any rhythmic EPSPs (C,D). Resetting of pacemaking activity by
depolarizing (E) or hyperpolarizing current pulse (F) applied through recording microelectrode. The discharge rate of these
neurons at 37°C *in vitro* is on average 21 spikes/second, which is identical to that of the fast-conducting, clonidine-insensitive vasomotor neurons of the rostral ventrolateral medulla. The pacemaker neurons are not adrenergic but possibly
glutamatergic. [A–D reprinted from Sun and Guyenet (1988b) with permission from *Brain Research* 442, 229–239, E-F
unpublished data of Sun and Guyenet.]

these conditions of reduced reflex activity, the rostral ventrolateral medullary vasomotor neurons with fast conduction velocity adopt a very regular pacemaker-like discharge that can be reset by antidromic activation (Sun et al., 1988a). Cells with identical characteristics with respect to location, action potential configuration, and rate and pattern of discharge can be recorded *in vitro* in a vascularly perfused medulla oblongata or in tissue slices (Sun et al., 1988a). Intracellular recordings from these characteristic cells (rate: 22 spikes/sec at 37°C) in tissue slices reveal the presence of typical pacemaker potentials and a complete absence of detectable EPSPs even when the neurons are hyperpolarized to increase the driving force of hypothetical EPSPs (Sun et al., 1988b, Figure 9-4). These cells have been labeled with intracellular injections of the fluorescent dye lucifer yellow and the tissue subsequently processed for the immunocytochemical detection of either phenylethanolamine *N*-methyltransferase (PNMT), the enzyme marker for C1 adrenergic cells, or tyrosine hydroxylase, an enzyme marker for all catecholaminergic cells. This procedure has revealed that the pacemaker neurons of the rostral ventrolateral medulla are not C1 adrenergic cells (Sun et al., 1988b).

Many neurons display rhythmic pacemaker activity only in the presence of a neuromodulator such as a neuropeptide or a catecholamine. The effect is probably mediated by receptors coupled to one of several G proteins, which modulate ion channels either directly or via a second messenger system (e.g., cyclic AMP). Receptor activation usually results in long-lasting conductance changes that may not be associated with clear EPSPs or inhibitory postsynaptic potentials (IPSPs), or in the alteration of an ionic channel involved in generating the pacemaker potential. Cells that display a rhythmic discharge only in the presence of a modulator could be called "conditional" pacemaker neurons. This is the case of many dorsal raphe cells *in vitro* (Aghajanian, 1985). It has not yet been possible to determine if the rostral medullary pacemaker neurons are true or "conditional" pacemaker cells.

Intracellular staining of electrophysiologically identified pacemaker neurons was used to establish that these neurons belong to a class of nonadrenergic spinally projecting cells of the rostral medulla (Sun et al., 1988b; see Figure 9-5). This subgroup represents a maximum of 50% of the reticulospinal neurons of the rostral ventrolateral reticular nucleus (Tucker et al., 1987). It is probable that the pacemaker neurons belong to the subgroup of fast-conducting, clonidine-insensitive vasomotor neurons of the rostral ventrolateral reticular nucleus (Sun et al., 1988a).

Nonbursting neurons with similar intrinsic pacemaker properties are not unique to the vasomotor system. Other mammalian neurons such as the nor-

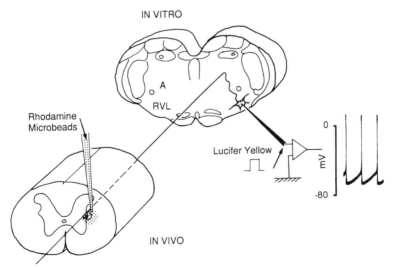

Figure 9-5 Rostral ventrolateral medullary pacemaker neurons project to the cord. Rhodamine-tagged microbeads were injected in the dorsolateral portion of the lateral funiculus of rats (third thoracic segment) 1 week before the electrophysiological experiments that were carried out in tissue slices of the medulla oblongata. These beads are taken up by terminals and damaged axons in the spinal cord and are retrogradely transported to the cell bodies located in the rostral ventrolateral medulla. *In vitro* intracellular recordings were made from these neurons. The fluorescent dye lucifer yellow was injected into neurons identified to have intrinsic pacemaker properties. At the end of the experiment, tissue sections were examined with a fluorescence microscope using two different excitation wavelengths and filters appropriate for observing rhodamine beads or lucifer yellow. Most lucifer yellow-stained pacemaker neurons contained fluorescent red beads, thus demonstrating that they were reticulospinal cells.

adrenergic locus coeruleus cells (Williams et al., 1984) and the serotonergic neurons of the raphe dorsalis (Vandermaelen and Aghajanian, 1983) exhibit similar properties.

Intracellular labeling of the rostral ventrolateral medullary pacemaker neurons with horseradish peroxidase or lucifer yellow reveals smooth dendrites with a 600- to 800-μm span in the coronal plane and limited rostrocaudal expansion (≤250 μm, Figure 9-6). The dendrites of these cells radiate in all directions but are confined within the limits of the rostral ventrolateral medulla as defined in this chapter. Some of the dendrites reach the ventral surface of the medulla oblongata and may belong to the cells responsible for the cardiovascular responses in experiments in which drugs are applied to the ventral medullary surface.

The transmitter released in the intermediolateral cell column by the pacemaker reticulospinal neurons is unknown, although there is pharmacological evidence to suggest that glutamate, or a closely related amino acid or small peptide, may be involved. First, intrathecal injections of kynurenic acid in the subarachnoid space of the thoracic spinal cord blocks the sympathetic outflow and the sympathoexcitation produced by electrical stimulation of the rostral ventrolateral nucleus. This is supportive but not definitive evidence, since it has yet to be proven that the pacemaker neurons make monosynaptic connections with sympathetic preganglionic neurons and the selectivity and the site of action of kynurenic acid cannot be fully ascertained by this mode of administration. Second, in most sympathetic preganglionic neurons recorded in tissue slices, Nishi et al. (1987) found that focal electrical stimulation produced fast EPSPs that were reversibly depressed by D-glutamylglycine—a glutamate antagonist with a slight preference for blocking kainate/quisqualate receptors (see Stone and Burton, 1988 for further discussion of excitatory amino acid receptors). More-

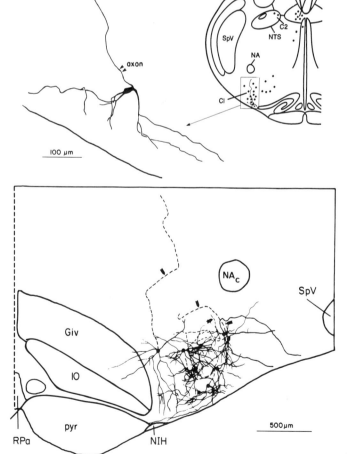

Figure 9-6 Morphology of pacemaker neuron in the rostral ventrolateral medulla. Top: An intracellularly labeled pacemaker neuron is shown in relationship to C1 neurons represented as dots. Recordings were made *in vitro* and the staining done by intracellular injection of lucifer yellow. This particular neuron (as shown in higher magnification on the left) exhibits features typical for this cell group, viz. three or four major dendrites that divide a maximum of three times, a limited dendrite span spreading 500–700 μm mediolaterally and 120–200 μm rostrocaudally, and an axon devoid of local collaterals (n = 14). Pacemaker neurons, like many reticular cells, have dendrites that spread out in a plane perpendicular to the long axis of the brain (unpublished data from Sun and Guyenet). Bottom: Nine intracellularly labeled pacemaker neurons are superimposed on a standardized section to show overall dendritic spread. Axons are indicated by dotted lines.

over, the conductance changes associated with these EPSPs are precisely reproduced by the application of glutamate but not aspartate or *N*-methyl D-aspartate (Nishi et al., 1987). A major problem in these studies is the inability to ascertain if the recordings were made from vasomotor sympathetic preganglionic neurons. Moreover, focal stimulation may also activate spinal interneurons. Thus, the identification of the neurotransmitter released by the pacemaker cells of the rostral ventrolateral medulla may have to await the use of an *in vitro* brain stem–spinal cord preparation. Under these conditions, the postsynaptic effect envoked in preganglionic neurons by stimulating the ventrolateral medulla could be studied with appropriate intracellular techniques. Another clue may result from by the use of immunocytochemical approaches designed to detect the presence in the pacemaker neurons, or their processes, of glutamate or of an enzyme involved in the synthesis of this amino acid. These techniques (see Wenthold et al., 1986 for additional references) rely on the premise, which has been verified in only a few cases, that neurons that seem on electrophysiological grounds to use glutamate as a neurotransmitter may have higher cytoplasmic levels of this amino acid and also contain high levels of the appropriate biosynthetic enzymes.

Other Ventral Medullary Reticulospinal Neurons with Putative Vasomotor Function

The C1 Adrenergic Group

At least 50% of the neurons of the rostral ventrolateral medulla that project to the intermediolateral cell column contain immunoreactive phenylethanolamine *N*-methyltransferase (PNMT) (C1 cells, Figure 9-7).

Some of the PNMT neurons appear to belong to the subgroup of neurons that receives baroreceptor information, have axonal conduction velocities below 0.8 m/second (Sun and Guyenet, 1986b), have predominantly fine unmyelinated axons that project to the spinal cord (Milner et al., 1987), and terminate on sympathetic preganglionic neurons (Milner et al., 1988). Whether these cells are responsible for maintaining vasomotor tone is still undetermined. C1 neurons also project massively ($\geq$ 85%) to rostral structures via the central tegmental tract (Sun and Guyenet, 1986b; Tucker et al., 1987). Since at least the same proportion project to the spinal cord, whatever information is conveyed by these cells to sympathetic preganglionic neurons also reaches other CNS sites as well.

A discussion of the putative actions of the C1 neurons on sympathetic preganglionic neurons is fraught with uncertainties. Apart from not knowing

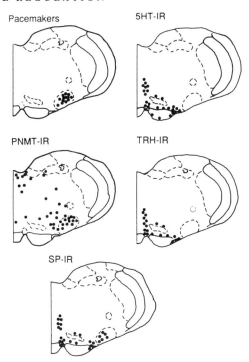

Figure 9-7 Location of reticulospinal neurons with projections to the intermediolateral cell column. The distribution of the nonmonoaminergic pacemaker cells is based on *in vitro* electrophysiological data and may therefore be artificially restricted. The location of the other cell group is based on immunocytochemical data. PMNT, phenylethanolamine *N*-methyltransferase; 5-HT, serotonin; SP, substance P; TRH, thyrotropin-releasing hormone.

the full axonal trajectory of these cells, there is no good understanding of the putative neurotransmitters used by these neurons. Basic facts such as whether these neurons actually release adrenaline have not been resolved. This issue needs to be considered in light of the report by Sved et al., (1988) who failed to show the presence of adrenaline in the spinal cord of the adult rat. Whether this failure is the result of a technical problem or represents an accurate negative finding needs further exploration. In addition, Connor and Drew (1987) reported that inhibition of phenylethanolamine *N*-methyltransferase did not modify tachycardic or pressor responses elicited by rostral ventrolateral medulla stimulation. Similarly, intrathecal administration of α- or β-adrenoreceptor antagonists did not affect tachycardia induced by stimulation of the rostral ventrolateral medulla. These investigators suggested that this pathway does not use adrenaline. Since some of the C1 cells stain with antibodies to PNMT and other putative neurotransmitters such as substance P and neuropeptide Y, the possibility remains that these cells contain multiple neurotransmitters. Although the presence of substance P-like immunoreactivity has been detected by some C1 neurons (Lorenz et al., 1985), definitive proof that these cells are capable of synthesizing this peptide will depend on the future demonstration of preprotachykinin mRNA in these cells by *in situ* hybridization histochemistry. The same comment applies to the finding that these cells contain neuropeptide Y. Thus, further studies will be needed for a more rigorous analysis of the putative transmitter(s) used by these C1 cells.

Investigators of the effects of catecholamines on sympathetic preganglionic neurons have produced conflicting findings. Iontophoretic studies in intact animals have shown that noradrenaline and adrenaline inhibit sympathetic preganglionic neurons (Coote, 1985), and *in vitro* studies suggest that noradrenaline can produce both excitatory and inhibitory effects (Yoshimura et al., 1987). Excitatory effects are mediated by a α_1-receptors and inhibitory ones by a α_2-receptors, the latter being probably linked to potassium channels as in other systems (for a review see Nishi et al., 1987). Since the intermediolateral cell column receives both a noradrenergic and an adrenergic input, the physiologically relevant endogenous agonist of each class of α-receptor remains unknown.

In summary, the C1 neurons probably represent a group of vasomotor reticulospinal neurons. These cells may contain multiple putative neurotransmitters. The reasons for this coexistence remain elusive. It is quite possible that these neurons are functionally heterogeneous and that they either excite or inhibit specific subsets of sympathetic preganglionic neurons depending on the type of receptors expressed by the latter (e.g., α_1-adrenergic, α_2-adrenergic, substance P, neuropeptide Y). The answers to these questions will have to await a better knowledge of the neurochemical properties of these cells and a clearer understanding of the significance of cotransmission.

Ventromedial Medulla and Caudal Raphe Nuclei

The intermediolateral cell column is innervated by various types of neurons that lie in the ventromedial medulla (nucleus interfascicularis hypoglossi) and the caudal raphe nuclei (raphe pallidus and raphe obscurus) (Loewy and McKellar, 1981). These projections originate from neurons that contain immunoreactive serotonin, substance P, thyrotropin-releasing hormone, and probably other neuropeptides (Charlton and Helke, 1987; Helke et al., 1986; Hirsch and Helke, 1988). Many of these cells appear to contain multiple transmitters such as substance P, thyrotropin-releasing hormone, and serotonin (see Helke et al., 1986, for review).

The idea that serotonin is a neurotransmitter in the intermediolateral cell column is supported by three lines of evidence:

1. The projection from the caudal medullary raphe nuclei and neighboring serotonergic neurons of the ventromedial medulla (which has been called the nucleus interfascicularis hypoglossi) is largely eliminated by the serotonin-selective toxin 5,7-dihydroxytryptamine (Loewy and McKellar, 1981).
2. Serotonin excites sympathetic preganglionic neurons via methysergide-sensitive receptors (the same are found on somatic motor neurons, see references in McCall, 1984).
3. Stimulation of the nuclei raphe pallidus or obscurus in cat can increase the sympathetic outflow and when a sympathoexcitatory response is produced, it can be blocked by systemic administrations of the serotonergic antagonist methysergide (McCall, 1984).

However, the following issues are still unresolved:

1. Do serotonergic fibers make monosynaptic contacts with sympathetic preganglionic neurons?
2. Do individual raphe neurons project to specific spinal nuclei such as the dorsal horn, intermediolateral cell column, or ventral horn and do they innervate multiple spinal cord nuclei?
3. Are the vasomotor effects produced by stimulating the raphe nuclei due to the spinal projections or to other CNS projections of these neurons such as the nucleus tractus solitarius?
4. What are the sources and functional role of the synaptic input that impinge on raphe neurons?
5. What is the physiological role of the vasomotor effects produced by stimulation of the cells of the raphe nuclei?

A discussion of the role of midline raphe serotonergic neurons in cardiovascular regulation cannot ignore the characteristics of the other raphe nuclei, especially the data on the dorsal raphe serotonergic neurons whose neural activity depends on the state of vigilance (for review see Fornal and Jacobs, 1987). Dorsal raphe neurons are silent during rapid eye movement (REM) sleep, exhibit a low level of discharge during slow wave sleep, and are most active in the awake state. In fact, this may be a general characteristic of raphe serotonergic neurons. Therefore, the cardiovascular functions ascribed to the medullary raphe nuclei on sympathetic networks may represent only a small aspect of a more general role of raphe serotonergic neurons in modulating CNS neuronal activity in relation to the states of vigilance. Since most of the studies have been performed under anesthesia, it is not possible to determine whether these cells could change autonomic functions in a differential way related to the sleep–wake cycle. Since the ongoing activity of medullary raphe serotonergic neurons appears to contribute to the vasomotor tone, it is legitimate to hypothesize that their inactivity during REM sleep could contribute to the reduction (or lability) in arterial pressure observed during this behavorial state (Futuro-Neto and Coote, 1982).

Immunoreactive thyrotropin-releasing hormone (TRH) is contained in raphe and reticulospinal neurons that project to the intermediolateral cell column. TRH-immunoreactive cells in the caudal ventral medulla of the rat are confined to raphe pallidus, raphe obscurus, raphe magnus, and the ventral medulla just lateral to the pyramidal tract (nucleus interfascicularis hypoglossi) (Figure 9-7) (Helke et al., 1986). TRH neurons are concentrated in the same areas that contain a large number of serotonin neurons. However, none of these neurons is present where either the pacemaker vasomotor neurons or the majority of the C1 cells are located. They are concentrated in areas more medial. TRH-like immunoreactivity is found in high concentrations in fibers within the intermediolateral cell column and other related autonomic areas of the spinal cord. It is also present in lower concentration in the ventral horn. Since the TRH content of the intermediolateral cell column is reduced substantially by intraventricular injections of the serotonergic neurotoxin 5,7-dihydroxytryptamine, it is likely that some of these neurons contain both serotonin and TRH (Helke et al., 1986). Three observations support the idea that the TRH neurons are likely to be involved in vasomotor control. First, TRH-binding sites are present in the intermediolateral cell column. Second, TRH causes excitation of sympathetic preganglionic neurons when applied by iontophoresis. Third, intrathecal administration of a TRH analog, MK-711, causes an increase in blood pressure that could play a role in vasomotor control (Helke et al., 1986; Helke and Phillips, 1988). Whether the site of action of MK-711 was the intermediolateral cell column remains unknown.

The same rostral medullary areas (nuclei raphe pallidus and obscurus, nucleus interfascicularis hypoglossi) also contain substance P-immunoreactive cells. Some of these neurons contain all three putative transmitters (Johansson et al., 1981). The possible role of substance P in vasomotor control has been already examined in the previous section. It is clear that the exact origin of the substance P input to the intermediolateral cell column will have to be clarified before any meaningful conclusion on the role of this peptide can be reached.

A5 Noradrenergic Neurons

The A5 cell group lies in the rostral-most portion of the ventrolateral medulla just lateral and dorsal to the superior olivary nucleus. The area in which A5 cells are scattered receives inputs from paraventricular hypothalamic nucleus, perifornical hypothalamic area, zona incerta, parabrachial nucleus, nucleus tractus solitarius, raphe obscurus, and caudal ventrolateral medulla (Byrum and Guyenet, 1987). A5 neurons project to multiple sites in the CNS involved with cardiovascular function including the nucleus tractus solitarius, dorsal vagal nucleus, parabrachial nucleus, lateral hypothalamic area, paraventricular thalamic nucleus, central gray matter, and central nucleus of the amygdala (Byrum and Guyenet, 1987). In addition, this cell group provides a dense input to the intermediolateral cell column (Loewy et al., 1979).

L-Glutamate stimulation of the A5 area in anesthetized rats produces a decrease in arterial pressure associated with a redistribution of blood flow. The arterial bed supplying the limb skeletal muscle dilates while the arterial system supplying the gastrointestinal tract constricts (Stanek et al., 1984). Whether this involves a direct sympathetic effect or also occurs with concomitant release of adrenal catecholamines has not been explored. The blood pressure effect can be eliminated by combined 6-hydroxydopamine lesions of noradrenergic terminals both in the spinal cord and in the dorsal medulla (Loewy et al., 1986). Although these suggest that single A5 noradrenergic neurons infuence multiple CNS vasomotor centers, a complete understanding of the anatomy of the A5 neurons is still lacking.

Destruction of A5 cell bodies by local microinjections of 6-hydroxydopamine causes no detectable alteration in resting arterial pressure in freely behaving rats. It does, however, induce modest changes in the vagal and sympathetic baroreflex control of heart rate (Stornetta et al., 1986).

Spinally projecting A5 neurons in the rat have conduction velocities of about 2.5 m/second and discharge at a mean rate of 4 spikes/second (Byrum et al., 1984). These cells show an inverse relationship to changes in peripheral blood pressure (Andrade and Aghajanian, 1982; Guyenet, 1984). Presumably, this is mediated via projections from the nucleus tractus solitarius to the A5 cell group.

Andrade and Aghajanian (1982) studied the effects of microiontophoresis of various α-adrenoceptor agonists on A5 neurons and found that they inhibited the neurons in a manner characteristic for the presence of an α_2-receptor. Surprisingly, little else is known about the functional and pharmacological characteristics of these cells.

In summary, it is still difficult to clearly assess the functions of A5 noradrenergic neurons. One possibility is that A5 neurons are to the "visceral brain" what the locus coeruleus is to the brain areas involved in somatosensory processing, that is, a widespread modulatory system with an activity linked to the process of behavioral arousal and the state of vigilance in general (for review see Jacobs, 1986). The redistribution of blood to muscle may be a small aspect of the function of A5 noradrenergic neurons.

Indeed, there is no evidence that A5 cells are specifically innervating neurons with a role in cardiovascular function and ignore cells that process other types of autonomic information within the same general brain areas.

Role of the Rostral Ventrolateral Medulla in Vasomotor Reflexes

This section will focus on the reflex control of the rostral medullary vasomotor neurons (i.e., exclusive of A5 noradrenergic cells). It should be recalled that one operational criterion used for the identification of vasomotor neurons in the rostral ventrolateral medulla is that they are inhibited by baroreceptor activation. The transmitter mediating this inhibitory effect is thought to be GABA because inotophoretically applied bicuculline blocks the inhibition of single vasomotor neurons induced by baroreceptor activation (Sun and Guyenet, 1985, Figure 9-8). However, the location of the GABA-releasing neurons that inhibit the vasomotor neurons is still unknown. Two ideas have emerged: one suggests that the cell bodies lie in the caudal aspect of the ventrolateral medulla (see next section) and the other suggests that these inhibitory neurons reside in the nucleus tractus solitarius.

A larger and still unanswered question is whether the baroreflex inhibition of the sympathetic discharge is simply due to a reduction of excitatory drive to spinal preganglionic neurons (disfacilitation) or involves the activation of reticulospinal in-

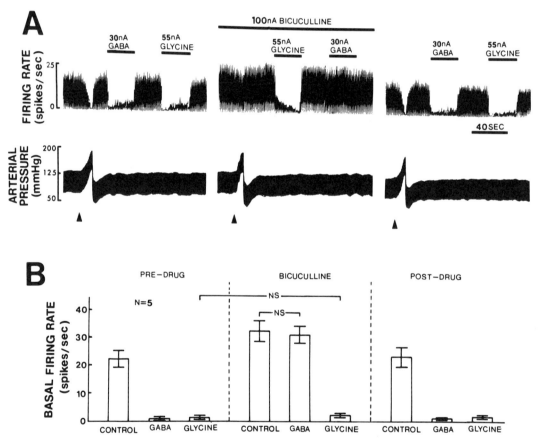

Figure 9-8 Baroreflex inhibition of rostral ventrolateral vasomotor neurons is mediated by GABA. (A) Neural activity of a single vasomotor neuron was recorded with a multibarrelled electrode allowing the iontophoretic ejection of glycine, GABA, and/or bicuculline (GABA receptor antagonist) within 40 μm of the cell. Iontophoretic currents for glycine and GABA were selected to produce the same degree of neuronal inhibition. The discharge rate of the cell is presented as an integrated rate histogram with a bin size of 1 second. Raising arterial pressure (at arrows) inhibits cellular discharges in the absence (control period of left, recovery from drug on right) but not in the presence (center panel) of bicuculline. The selectivity of the GABA-receptor antagonist is demonstrated by its effectiveness in blocking neuronal inhibition mediated by GABA and its inability to modify the effect of glycine (A and B). The success of this experiment is probably due to the limited dendritic span of rostral ventrolateral reticular neurons in rats (Figure 9-7), which allows effective bicuculline concentrations to reach most GABAergic synapses on a given cell despite point-source delivery of the drug. [From Sun and Guyenet (1985) with permission from the *American Journal of Physiology.*]

hibitory inputs to these cells as well. The evidence available at present suggests that the withdrawal of the excitatory drive contributed by rostral medullary vasomotor neurons is the predominant factor, at least under specific anesthetic conditions, since the baroreflex inhibition of the sympathetic outflow and its pulse-synchrony can be totally abolished by microinjections of the GABA receptor antagonist bicuculline restricted to the rostral ventrolateral medulla (Sun and Guyenet, 1987). However, this issue will be resolved only by intracellular recordings of sympathetic preganglionic neurons during baroreflex activation.

High-frequency, low-intensity electrical stimulation of the central end of the vagus nerve with short-duration pulses activates myelinated fibers and produces sympathoexcitation, while low-frequency, high-intensity stimulation with longer pulses activates predominantly unmyelinated fibers and results in sympathoinhibition and hypotension. These fibers convey afferent information from both cardiopulmonary and gastrointestinal receptors. In the rat, both effects appear to be mediated in large part by changes in the activity of rostral ventrolateral medullary vasomotor neurons. These cells are uniformly excited by high-frequency stimulation of the vagus nerve and inhibited by low-frequency stimulation (Sun and Guyenet, 1987). Moreover, the vagally mediated excitation of the lumbar sympathetic outflow can be selectively blocked by microinjection of kynurenic acid in the region of the rostral ventrolateral medulla while the vagally mediated sympathoinhibition can be blocked by microinjection of a GABA receptor antagonist in the same site (Sun and Guyenet, 1987). This sort of evidence indicates that the rostral ventrolateral medullary vasomotor neurons represent a crucial site of convergence and integration for a variety of vagally driven inputs from the nucleus tractus solitarius that affect the vasomotor sympathetic outflow. The precise nature of the vagal afferent inputs that leads to inhibition or excitation of the vasomotor neurons has not yet been determined. Those responsible for the excitation of these cells could represent visceral nociceptive afferents, chemoreceptors, or medullated low-threshold pulmonary afferents (Bachoo and Polosa, 1986).

Cardiovascular changes can also be caused by activation of a variety of somatosensory afferents. These reflexive changes appear to be mediated in part by reticulospinal neurons of the rostral ventrolateral medulla (Morrison and Reis, 1988; Stornetta et al., 1989).

The reticulospinal vasomotor neurons of the rostral ventrolateral medulla of both rat and cat also supply some of the respiratory-related drive to sympathetic preganglionic cells (McAllen, 1987; Haselton and Guyenet, unpublished results). This view relies on the observation that in vagotomized debuffered animals with pneumothorax, both sympathetic preganglionic (e.g., Gilbey et al., 1986) and rostral medullary vasomotor neurons (McAllen, 1987) display one of three basic activity patterns: (1) inspiratory excitation, (2) inspiratory depression, or (3) no respiratory modulation. However, these observations are still insufficient to conclude that the respiratory-related drive to sympathetic preganglionic neurons originates entirely from these reticulospinal neurons. An overview of the mechanisms responsible for integrating the vasomotor and respiratory outflows is presented elsewhere in this volume (see Chapter 11).

Caudal Periambigual Area and Lateral Tegmental Field

Electrolytic lesions of an area of the caudal ventrolateral medulla more or less centered on the A1 group of noradrenergic cell group result in increases in arterial pressure (Blessing et al., 1981). In contrast, microinjections of L-glutamate in this area cause depressor effects resulting in large part from sympathoinhibition and perhaps also from direct activation of cardiac vagal motoneurons located nearby in the nucleus ambiguus (Willette et al., 1983). Microinjections of the inhibitory GABA agonist muscimol at this site causes pressor and sympathoexcitatory effects (Willette et al., 1983). As is the case in all experimental studies based on drug microinjections into the brain parenchyma, the exact location of the neurons responsible for the observed effect remains imprecise and on the basis of additional data it seems probable that the A1 noradrenergic cells are slightly or not involved, contrary to initial beliefs.

A clue to the potential significance of the caudal periambigual area was provided by Sapru and collaborators who demonstrated that sympathetic baroreflexes as well as the depressor effect caused by activation of pulmonary J receptors could be blocked by injecting the GABA-mimetic agent muscimol into this area (Willette et al., 1983). Since this agent silences neurons without interfering with passing axonal traffic, these investigators proposed that this area, which they termed the ventrolateral depressor area, contains inhibitory interneurons relaying baroreceptor and pulmonary afferent information to the rostral ventrolateral vasomotor neurons. Direct evidence that rostral ventrolateral medullary vasomotor neurons receive an inhibitory input from the caudal ventrolateral medulla is still lacking, however. Injections of D-2-amino-5-phosphonovaleric acid—an N-methyl-D-aspartate receptor antagonist—into this area also block the baroreceptor reflex (Gordon, 1987). Similarly, both sympathetic and vagal baroreflexes can be blocked by microinjections of kynurenic acid into the caudal periambigual area (Guyenet, et al., 1987).

One interpretation of these results is that second-order baroreceptor neurons in the nucleus tractus solitarius project to the caudal periambigual area and release a glutamate-like substance responsible for the activation of both vagal cardiac motoneurons and GABAergic medullary interneurons, which then project to the rostral ventrolateral medulla. The latter would finally be responsible for the inhibition of rostral ventrolateral medullary vasomotor neurons (Figure 9-9). This hypothetical scheme appears compatible with existing anatomical data. The caudal periambigual area projects heavily to the rostral ventrolateral medulla, but this projection does not seem

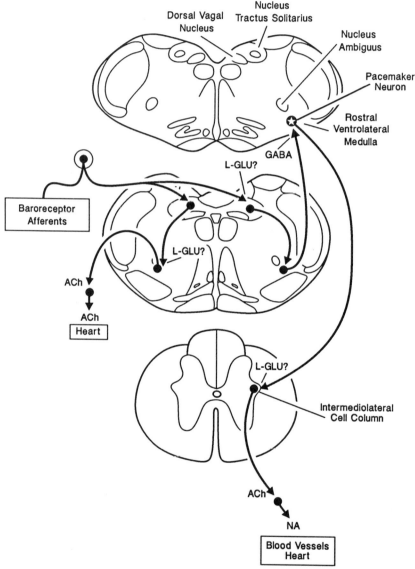

Figure 9-9 A model of the neural circuitry involved in the baroreflex. Incoming baroreceptor afferents terminate in the nucleus tractus solitarius. These first-order neurons have their cell bodies in the ganglia of the IXth and Xth cranial nerves. The transmitter involved is unknown, but may be L-glutamate or a related chemical. Second-order neurons in the nucleus tractus solitarius project to two sites in the medulla oblongata: cardiac preganglionic neurons (shown on left) and GABA-containing neurons in the region near the nucleus ambiguus (shown on right). The latter are thought to project to pacemaker neurons in the rostral ventrolateral medulla. The pacemaker neurons may project directly to the sympathetic preganglionic neurons and use a L-glutamate or a related chemical as a transmitter. The transmitters used at each central synapse remain speculative because the full requirements needed for proof that a particular chemical is acting as a transmitter have not been fulfilled.

to involve A1 noradrenergic neurons (Ross et al., 1985; Sun and Guyenet, 1986b). However, this hypothesis requires better anatomical and neurophysiological documentation.

The presence in the caudal periambigual area of inhibitory interneurons mediating sympathetic baroreflexes does not account for all the observations. For instance, the injection of GABA-mimetic agents or glutamate receptor antagonists in the caudal periambigual area raises the sympathetic discharge even when pressure is maintained below the threshold for arterial baroreceptor activation. This observation can perhaps be explained by the presence in this area of neurons that are discharging as a result of an additional "glutamatergic" input that is not driven by the activity of baroreceptors. It is possible, but still unproven, that these neurons could also exert their tonic sympathoinhibitory effect by releasing GABA in the vicinity of rostral ventrolateral medullary vasomotor neurons since the latter do receive a tonic GABAergic inhibitory input even at arterial pressures below the threshold for baroreceptor activation (Sun and Guyenet, 1985). The caudal periambigual area also contains neurons involved in the release of vasopressin during hypotension (Blessing and Willoughby, 1985). Although it has been proposed that these neurons could belong to the A1 noradrenergic group, this has not been satisfactorily established.

Some portion of the cat lateral tegmental field (nucleus medullae oblongatae centralis, Cv, Taber, 1961) contains units (including spontaneously active ones) that can be antidromically activated from the rostral ventrolateral medulla. Microstimulation of the lateral tegmental field in the cat often excites rostral medullary vasomotor neurons. Additionally, the discharges of these lateral tegmental neurons is correlated to the 2- to 6-Hz rhythm of the sympathetic nerve discharge and occurs earlier in the cycle than that of the rostral medullary vasomotor neurons (Barman and Gebber, 1987). Taken together, this evidence suggests that some portion of the lateral tegmental field may contain the cell bodies or the axons of neurons that contribute a tonic excitatory drive to the reticulospinal neurons of the rostral ventrolateral medulla and may synchronize their discharges. However, to be fully accepted, this theory remains to be backed by evidence that the sympathetic outflow and its synchronization are affected when lateral tegmental field neurons are inhibited by microinjections of a neuronal-hypolarizing substance such as GABA or glycine.

Differential Regulation of Peripheral Vascular Beds: Role of the Rostral Ventrolateral Medulla

The sympathetic vasomotor output to peripheral vascular beds is differentially regulated. Various activities such as standing, exercise, fear, and food intake result in specific patterns of sympathetic activity. These affect blood flow in these different vascular beds. A key area of interest has been to determine the neuronal networks responsible for this diversity and the levels of the neuraxis at which circuits become committed to control of specific vascular beds. For example, are complex sympathetic responses programmed within spinal networks like their somatic counterparts or fully elaborated at the medullary level and then simply relayed to the spinal cord by brain stem projection neurons without further spinal processing? It is quite likely that the brain stem imposes two general control patterns on the sympathetic outflow. One may be a general modulation like what would be expected under different conditions such as sleep, wakefulness, or in emergency conditions. The other would subserve to fine tune responses. Just how these conditions can be regulated is unknown.

The rostral ventrolateral nucleus seems to contain clusters of sympathoexcitatory neurons whose activation results in a selective increase in discharge of either cutaneous or muscular sympathetic fibers innervating the hindlimb (Dampney and McAllen, 1988; Figure 9-10). A possible interpretation of these data is that the sympathetic outflow to the separate vascular beds could be already compartmentalized within specific rostral medullary cell groups.

ACTION OF CENTRALLY ACTING HYPOTENSIVE AGENTS IN THE MEDULLA

Several antihypertensive drugs, such as clonidine and α-methyldopa, cause a reduction in vasoconstrictor and cardioaccelerator sympathetic outflow by acting in the CNS. Clonidine acts by an α_2-adrenergic receptor agonist mechanism at specific sites in the brain, whereas α-methyldopa acts as a prodrug; it must be metabolized into α-methylnoradrenaline or α-methyladrenaline within nerve terminals of the central noradrenergic or adrenergic neurons (see Langer et al., 1980 for review). These metabolites are false transmitters that appear to exert their sympathoinhibitory effect by virtue of the fact that their affinity for central α_2-adrenergic receptors is higher than that of the endogenous transmitters (noradrenaline or adrenaline). This type of receptor is found on both the terminals and somatodendritic portion of central noradrenergic neurons. Central noradrenergic neurons (such as in the locus coeruleus, the subcoeruleus nucleus, A5, and A2 cell groups) are silenced by low hypotensive doses of clonidine. In the case of the locus coeruleus, this effect is due to the coupling of these α_2-receptors to potassium channels (Williams et al., 1985). Although a tiny

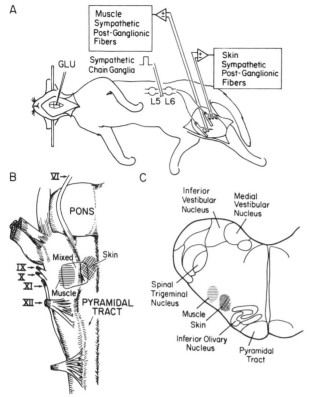

A

Muscle
Sympathetic
Post-Ganglionic
Fibers

GLU   Sympathetic
Chain Ganglia

Skin
Sympathetic
Post-Ganglionic
Fibers

L5 L6

B

VI→

PONS

Mixed   Skin

IX→
X→
XI→   Muscle

XII→   PYRAMIDAL
            TRACT

C

Inferior   Medial
Vestibular   Vestibular
Nucleus   Nucleus

Spinal
Trigeminal
Nucleus
              Muscle
              Skin

Inferior Olivary
Nucleus   Pyramidal
              Tract

Figure 9-10 Differential control of vascular beds: role of medulla. (A) The activity of sympathetic postganglionic neurons innervating either the skin or skeletal muscles was recorded in anesthetized cats and the effect produced by microinjections of L-glutamate in the rostral ventrolateral medulla were assessed. (B) Two distinct regions of the ventral surface of the medulla oblongata can be stimulated with L-glutamate to elicit excitation in sympathetic nerves innervating specific target tissues of the hindlimb. (C) Transverse section showing the sites where L-glutamate microinjections cause selective excitation of either skin or muscle sympathetic nerves. Their spatial separation suggests that subgroups of neurons in the rostral ventrolateral medulla regulate specific target tissues. [Redrawn and modified from Dampney and McAllen (1988) with permission from *Neuroscience* and the authors.]

fraction of central α_2-receptors is in fact located on central noradrenergic neurons, their activation is of considerable pharmacological significance since it leads to widespread reductions in noradrenaline release throughout the brain. This effect, in turn, must reduce the degree of activation of central α_1- and β-adrenergic receptors that are normal postsynaptic targets for neurally released noradrenaline.

The sites of action of clonidine in the brain are not known with certainty. Three main approaches have been used. First, the *in vivo* autoradiographic technique was used by Unnerstall et al. (1984) to map of α_2-adrenergic binding sites in the rat and human CNS. *p*-[³H]Aminoclonidine was used as a ligand, and high densities of binding sites were found in a number of CNS regions associated with autonomic function, including the intermediolateral cell column, the nucleus tractus solitarius, and the rostral ventrolateral medulla. The latter region has a lower number of binding sites than the two former areas. A second method used to identify sites of action has been the microinjection method. A major problem with this approach is that the local drug concentration may greatly exceed the CNS concentrations that occur after systemic administration of the relevant hypotensive doses. For example, a standard hypotensive dose of 10 μg/kg iv of clonidine should result in less than 50 n*M* concentration in the brain. In-

vestigators have uniformly used concentrations much greater than this for parenchyma injections. This is a significant problem because high concentrations of clonidine could modify local blood flow, produce local anesthetic effects, or activate α_1-adrenergic and histamine H2 receptors. Moreover, local injections may activate receptors located at considerable distances from the injection site. Third, the hypotensive action of clonidine has been tested following medullary lesions of the nucleus tractus solitarius and medial reticular formation (see Rockhold and Caldwell, 1980 and Punnen et al., 1987 for references). This approach has a number of inherent problems associated with CNS lesion studies. Since lesions destroy both cell bodies and nerve fibers, the exact critical site of action cannot be determined.

Microinjections of clonidine in the nucleus tractus solitarius result in dose-dependent (1.25–40 nmol) depressor and bradycardic changes that can be blocked by prior microinjections of the α_2-adrenoreceptor antagonist, yohimbine (10 nmol) (Rockhold and Caldwell, 1980; cf. Zandberg et al., 1979). Baroreceptors themselves are insensitive to low doses of clonidine and "sensitized" only by a α_1-adrenergic agonists including noradrenaline released from sympathetic fibers (Goldman and Saum, 1984). Although hypotension occurs on microinjection of clonidine and other α_2-adrenergic agonists into the nucleus tractus solitarius (Kubo et al., 1987), the baroreflex inhibition of most rostral ventrolateral medullary vasomotor neurons is unaffected by systemic doses of clonidine, thus providing no support to the hypothesis that the nucleus tractus solitarius is the critical site (Sun and Guyenet, 1986b).

Moreover, injections of lidocaine in the nucleus tractus solitarius at doses sufficient to block local L-glutamate-induced hypotensive and bradycardic responses did not abolish or attenuate the hypotensive actions of intravenously administered clonidine (Punnen et al., 1987). The rostral ventrolateral medulla and the spinal cord itself are more likely sites of action of clonidine. Microinjections of clonidine into the rostral ventrolateral medulla cause hypotension and bradycardia; these responses can be attenuated by microinjections of idazoxan, a specific α_2-adrenergic receptor antagonist, in the same area (Punnen et al., 1987). Similarly, localized injections of this drug in the rostral ventrolateral medulla reverse the hypotension and bradycardia caused by intravenous clonidine. Finally, systemic hypotensive doses of clonidine inhibit the slow-conducting reticulospinal neurons of the rostral ventrolateral medulla, which may be the C1 adrenergic cells (Sun and Guyenet, 1986b).

Since clonidine mimics some of the actions of noradrenaline, it becomes necessary to understand the actual role of central catecholaminergic neurons in central autonomic regulation. It is fair to say that despite the considerable amount of research devoted to this problem, no definitive answer can be provided (see review by Loewy and Neil, 1981). The depletion of up to 95% of central noradrenaline stores in the CNS by reserpine does not perceptibly change the basal sympathetic tone and baroreflexes (Iggo and Vogt, 1960). As indicated before, the integrity of the A5 cell cluster does not appear essential to the maintenance of arterial pressure and baroreflexes (Stornetta et al., 1986). In both cases, however, the rapid development of supersensitivity may compensate for the reduction in the presynaptic level of the amine. The precise role of the A1 noradrenergic cell cluster of the caudal ventrolateral medulla is difficult to determine in the absence of definitive anatomical electrophysiological data regarding local connections that these neurons may make with other neurons of the rostral ventrolateral medulla. It has been argued that clonidine mimics the postsynaptic inhibitory effect of noradrenaline released by the A1 noradrenergic neurons that were theorized to terminate on the C1 adrenergic neurons (Granata et al., 1986). However, this interpretation has to be tempered by the lack of supporting connectional data. Similarly, a very confusing picture emerges from studies in which lesions of this cell group have been attempted.

For instance, hypertension and vasopressin release are attributed to the lesion of A1 noradrenergic neurons (for references see Blessing and Willoughby, 1985). In apparent contradiction to such results, inhibition of these cells or damage to their axons is believed to prevent the release of this hormone during hypotension or hemorrhage (Blessing and Willoughby, 1985) and their stimulation to produce its release. Although all these experiments underline the importance of the periambigual region of the ventrolateral medulla, none of them clearly implicates the noradrenergic neurons because even the most selective agents used to destroy these neurons inevitably produce some amount of nonspecific lesion in an area that is critically involved in baroreflexes, respiration, and cardiac vagal control.

SUMMARY

Several key components of the medullary networks involved in controlling the activity of spinal preganglionic vasomotor neurons have now been identified. A major component of the vasomotor center of the rostral ventrolateral medulla can be equated with a cluster of reticulospinal neurons, including cells with intrinsic pacemaker properties, which provide a tonic excitatory drive to vasoconstrictor spinal preganglionic neurons. The discharge of these neurons is up- or down-regulated by a number of inputs that are only partially identified and include polysynaptic pathways activated by a variety of visceral and somatic sensory afferents, the hypothalamus, and probably many additional structures. There is good evidence that many of the sympathetic cardiovascular reflexes (somatosympathetic, baroreceptor reflex, vagosympathetic) elicited in anesthetized animals are in large part mediated by an increase or decrease in the activity of these vasomotor neurons. Although the contribution of these cells is probably critical in depolarizing vasoconstrictor sympathetic preganglionic neurons beyond their firing threshold, it is probable that other tonically active bulbospinal pathways also influence the discharge rate of these neurons. Two of them, the A5 noradrenergic input and the serotonergic input from the raphe obscurus, the raphe pallidus, or the outlying cells of the B1–B3 groups, have been identified. A third one, the C1 group of the rostral ventrolateral medulla, is also certainly involved in vasomotor function, although its exact role is still unknown.

The central mechanisms involved in the differential control of the sympathetic outflow to the various peripheral beds (muscular, splanchnic, renal, cutaneous) are still also virtually unknown, although some of the subgroups of rostral ventrolateral medullary neurons might be at least partially specialized in the control of separate peripheral beds. It is also conceivable that these cells produce a background excitatory input to many types of vasoconstrictor sympathetic preganglionic neurons irrespective of which vascular bed these spinal neurons regulate and that the fine, differential control of subpopulations of preganglionic neurons largely operates via other circuits (including spinal ones) that may or may not be under baroreceptor control.

The persistence of a low degree of sympathetic nerve discharge in spinal animals suggests that circuits endogenous to the spinal cord or activated by sensory afferent information may generate enough excitatory drive to sympathetic preganglionic neurons to make them discharge. These spinal mechanisms may even predominate in the control of certain sympathetic outflows such as to the kidney and spleen.

ACKNOWLEDGMENTS

My warmest thanks are extended to my current collaborators, Drs. James Haselton and Miao-Kun Sun, for their help in preparing this review and for their enthusiastic research contribution.

REFERENCES

Reviews

Connor, J. A. (1985). Neural pacemakers and rhythmicity. *Annual Review of Physiology* 47, 17–28.

Feldman, J. L. (1986). Neurophysiology of breathing in mammals. In: *Handbook of Physiology—The Nervous System IV—Intrinsic Regulatory Systems of the Brain,* F. E. Bloom (ed.), American Physiological Society, Bethesda, Md, pp. 463–524.

Fornal, C. A., and Jacobs, B. L. (1987). Physiological and behavioral correlates of serotonergic single-unit activity. In: *Neuronal Serotonin,* N. N. Osborne and M. Hamon (eds.), Wiley, Chichester, UK (in press).

Helke, C. J., Charlton, C. G., and Keeler, J. R. (1985). Bulbospinal substance P and sympathetic regulation of the cardiovascular system: a review. *Peptides* 6: Suppl. 2, 69–74.

Jacobs, B. L. (1986). Single-unit activity of locus coeruleus neurons in behaving animals. *Progress in Neurobiology* 27, 183–194.

Langer, S. Z., Cavero, I., and Massingham, R. (1980). Recent developments in noradrenergic neurotransmission and its relevance to the mechanism of action of certain antihypertensive agents. *Hypertension* 2, 372–382.

Loewy, A. D., and Neil, J. J. (1981). The role of descending monoaminergic systems in central control of blood pressure. *Federation Proceedings* 40(13), 56–63.

Loewy, A. D. (1987). Substance P neurons of the ventral medulla: Their role in the control of vasomotor tone. In: *Cardiogenic Reflexes,* R. Hainsworth, R. J. Linden, P. N. McWilliam, and D. A. S. G. Mary (eds.), Oxford University Press, Oxford, England, pp. 269–284.

Luiten, P. G. M., ter Horst, G. J., and Steffens, A. B.

(1987). The hypothalamus, intrinsic connections and outflow pathways to the endocrine system in relation to the control of feeding and metabolism. *Progress in Neurobiology* 28, 1–54.

Mayer, M. L., and Westbrook, G. L. (1987). The physiology of excitatory amino acids in the vertebrate central nervous system. *Progress in Neurobiology* 28, 197–276.

Nishi, S., Yoshimura, M., and Polosa, C. (1987). Synaptic potentials and putative transmitter actions in sympathetic preganglionic neurons. In: *Organization of the Autonomic Nervous System: Central and Peripheral Mechanisms,* J. Ciriello, F. R. Calaresu, L. P. Renaud, C. Polosa (eds.), Liss, New York, pp. 15–26.

Stone, T. W., and Burton, N. R. (1988). NMDA receptors and ligands in the vertebrate CNS. *Progress in Neurobiology* 30, 333–368.

Von Euler, C. (1986). Brain stem mechanisms for generation and control of breathing pattern. *Handbook of Physiology* Vol. 2, Part 1. American Physiological Society, Bethesda, Md, pp. 1–67.

Research Papers

Aghajanian, G. K. (1985). Modulation of a transient outward current in serotonergic neruons by α_1-adrenoceptors. *Nature* 315, 501–503.

Alexander, R. S. (1946). Tonic and reflex functions of medullary sympathetic cardiovascular centers. *Journal of Neurophysiology* 9, 205–217.

Andrade, R., and Aghajanian, G. K. (1982). Single cell activity in the noradrenergic A5 region: Response to drugs and peripheral manipulations of blood pressure. *Brain Research* 242, 125–213.

Andrezik, T. A., Chan-Palay, V., and Palay, S. L. (1981a). The nucleus paragigantocellularis lateralis in the rat: Conformation and cytology. *Anatomy and Embryology* 161, 355–371.

Andrezik, J. A., Chan-Palay, V., and Palay, S. L. (1981b). The nucleus paragigantocellularis lateralis in the rat: Demonstration of afferents by the retrograde transport of HRP. *Anatomy and Embryology* 161, 373–390.

Bachoo, M., and Polosa, C. (1986). The pattern of sympathetic neurone activity during expiration in the cat. *Journal of Physiology (London)* 378, 375–390.

Barman, S. M., and Gebber, G. L. (1985). Axonal projection patterns of ventrolateral medullospinal sympathoexcitatory neurons. *Journal of Neurophysiology* 53, 1567–1582.

Barman, S. M., and Gebber, G. L. (1987). Lateral tegmental field neurones of cat medulla: A source of basal activity of ventrolateral medullospinal sympathoexcitatory neurons. *Journal of Neurophysiology* 57, 1410–1425.

Berman, A. L. (1968). *The Brain Stem of the Cat: A Cytoarchitectonic Atlas with Stereotaxic Coordinates.* University of Wisconsin Press, Madison, WI.

Bieger, D., and Hopkins, D. A. (1987). Viscerotopic representation of the upper alimentary tract in the medulla oblongata in the rat: The nucleus ambiguus. *Journal of Comparative Neurology* 262, 546–562.

Blessing, W. W., and Willoughby, J. O. (1985). Inhibiting the rabbit caudal ventrolateral medulla prevents baroreceptor-initiated secretion of vasopressin. *Journal of Physiology (London)* 367, 253–266.

Blessing, W. W., West, M. J., and Chalmers, J. P. (1981). Hypertension, bradycardia and pulmonary oedema in the conscious rabbit after brain stem lesions coinciding with the A1 group of catecholamine neruons. *Circulation Research* 49, 949–958.

Brown, D. L., and Guyenet, P. G. (1985). Electrophysiological study of cardiovascular neurons in the rostral ventrolateral medulla. *Circulation Research* 56, 359–369.

Byrum, C. E., Stornetta, R. L., and Guyenet, P. G. (1984). Electrophysiological properties of spinally projecting A5 noradrenergic neurons. *Brain Research* 303, 15–29.

Byrum, C. E., and Guyenet, P. G. (1987). The afferent and efferent connections of the A5 noradrenergic cell group in the rat. *Journal of Comparative Neurology* 261, 529–542.

Charlton, C. G., and Helke, C. J. (1987). Substance P-containing medullary projections to the intermediolateral cell column: Identification with retrogradely transported rhodamine-labelled latex microspheres and immunohistochemistry. *Brain Research* 418, 245–254.

Connor, H. E., and Drew, G. M. (1987). Do adrenaline-containing neurones from the rostral ventrolateral medulla excite preganglionic sympathetic cell bodies? *Journal of Autonomic Pharmacology* 7, 87–96.

Coote, J. H. (1985). Noradrenergic projections to the spinal cord and their role in cardiovascular control. *Journal of the Autonomic Nervous System* 14, 255–262.

Dampney, R. A. L., and McAllen, R. M. (1988). Differential control of sympathetic fibers supplying hindlimb, skin, and muscle by subretrofacial neurones in the cat. *Journal of Physiology (London)* 395, 41–56.

Dittmar, C. (1873). Uber die Lage des sogenannten Gefässcentrums in der Medulla oblongata. *Bericht uber die Verhandlungen der Sachischen* 25, 449–469.

Fulwiler, C. E., and Saper, C. B. (1984). Subnuclear organization of the efferent connections of the parabrachial nucleus in the rat. *Brain Research Reviews* 7, 229–259.

Futuro-Neto, H. A., and Coote, J. H. (1982). Changes in sympathetic activity to heart and blood vessels during desynchronized sleep. *Brain Research* 225, 259–268.

Gilbey, M. P., Numao, Y., and Spyer, K. M. (1986). Discharge patterns of cervical sympathetic preganglionic neurones related to central respiratory drive in the rat. *Journal of Physiology (London)* 378, 253–265.

Goldman, W. F., and Saum, W. R. (1984). A direct excitatory effect of catecholamines on rat aortic baroreceptors *in vitro. Circulation Research* 55, 18–30.

Gordon, F. J. (1987). Aortic baroreceptor reflexes are mediated by NMDA receptors in caudal ventrolateral medulla. *American Journal of Physiology* 252, R628–R633.

Granata, A. R., Numao, Y., Kumada, M., and Reis, D. J. (1986). A1 noradrenergic neurons tonically inhibit sympathoexcitatory neurons of C1 area in rat brain stem. *Brain Research* 377, 127–146.

Guertzenstein, P. G., and Silver, A. (1974). Fall in blood pressure produced from discrete regions of the ventral surface of the medulla by glycine and lesions. *Journal of Physiology (London)* 242, 489–503.

Guyenet, P. G. (1984). Baroreceptor-mediated inhibition of A5 noradrenergic neurons. *Brain Research* 303, 31–40.

Guyenet, P. G., and Brown, D. L. (1986). Nucleus para-gigantocellularis lateralis and lumbar sympathetic discharge in the rat. *American Journal of Physiology* 250, R1081–R1094.

Guyenet, P. G., and Young, B. S. (1987). Projections of nucleus paragigantocellularis lateralis to locus coeruleus and other structures in rat. *Brain Research* 406, 171–184.

Guyenet, P. G., Filtz, T. M., and Donaldson, S. R. (1987). Role of excitatory aminoacids in rat vagal and sympathetic baroreflexes. *Brain Research* 407, 272–284.

Helke, C. J., and Phillips, E. T. (1988). Thyrotropin-releasing hormone receptor activation in the spinal cord increase blood pressure and sympathetic tone to the vasculature and the adrenals. *Journal of Pharmacology and Experimental Therapeutics* 245, 41–46.

Helke, C. J., Sayson, S. C., Keeler, J. R., and Charlton, C. G. (1986). Thyrotropin-releasing hormone-immunoreactive neurons project from the ventral medulla to the intermediolateral cell column: Partial coexistence with serotonin. *Brain Research* 381, 1–7.

Hirsch, M. D., and Helke, C. J. (1988). Bulbospinal thyrotropin-releasing hormone projections to the intermediolateral cell column: A double fluorescence immunohistochemical-retrograde tracing study in the rat. *Neuroscience* 25, 625–637.

Iggo, A., and Vogt, M. (1960). Preganglionic sympathetic activity in normal and in reserpine-treated cats. *Journal of Physiology (London)* 150, 114–133.

Johansson, O., Hokfelt, T., Pernow, B., Jeffcoate, S. L., White, N., Steinbusch, H. W. M., Verhofstad, A. A. J., Emson, P. C., and Spindel, E. (1981). Immunohistochemical support for three putative transmitters in one neuron: Coexistence of 5-hydroxytryptamine, substance P, and thyrotropin-releasing hormone-like immunoreactivity in medullary neurons projecting to the spinal cord. *Neuroscience* 6, 1857–1881.

Kalia, M., and Fuxe, K. (1985). Rat medulla oblongata I. Cytoarchitectonic considerations. *Journal of Comparative Neurology* 233, 285–307.

Koepchen, H. P., Langhorst, P., and Seller, H. (1975). The problem of identification of autonomic neurons in the lower brain stem. *Brain Research* 87, 375–393.

Kubo, T., Nihara, M., Hata, H., and Misu, Y. (1987). Cardiovascular effects in rats of α1 and α2 adrenergic agents injected into the nucleus tractus solitarii. *Naunyn-Schmiedeberg's Archives Pharmacology* 335(3), 274–277.

Loewy, A. D. (1981). Raphe pallidus and raphe obscurus projections to the intermediolateral cell column in the rat. *Brain Research* 222, 129–133.

Loewy, A. D. and Burton, H. (1978). Nuclei of the solitary tract: Efferent projections to the lower brain stem and spinal cord of the cat. *Journal of Comparative Neurology* 181, 421–450.

Loewy, A. D., and McKellar, S. (1981). Serotonergic projections from the ventral medulla to the intermediolateral cell column in the rat. *Brain Research* 211, 146–152.

Loewy, A. D., McKellar, S., and Saper, C. B. (1979). Direct projections from the A5 catecholamine cell group to the intermediolateral cell column. *Brain Research* 174, 309–314.

Loewy, A. D., Wallach, J. H., and McKellar, S. (1981). Efferent connections of the ventral medulla oblongata in the rat. *Brain Research Reviews* 3, 63–80.

Loewy, A. D., Marson, L., Parkinson, D., Perry, M. A., and Sawyer, W. B. (1986). Descending noradrenergic pathways involved in the A5 depressor response. *Brain Research* 386, 313–324.

Lorenz, R. G., Saper, C. B., Wong, D. L., Cianarello, R. D., and Loewy, A. D. (1985). Co-localization of substance P- and phenylethanolamine N-methyltransferase-like immunoreactivity in neurons of ventrolateral medulla that project to the spinal cord: Potential role in control of vasomotor tone. *Neuroscience Letters* 55, 255–260.

McAllen, R. M. (1986). Location of neurones with cardiovascular and respiratory function at the ventral surface of the cat's medulla. *Neuroscience* 18, 43–49.

McAllen, R. M. (1987). Central respiratory modulation of subretrofacial bulbospinal neurones in the cat. *Journal of Physiology (London)* 388, 533–545.

McAllen, R. M., and Spyer, K. M. (1978). The baroreceptor input to cardiac vagal motorneurons. *Journal of Physiology (London)* 282, 365–374.

McCall, R. B. (1984). Evidence for a serotonergically-mediated sympathoexcitatory response to stimulation of medullary raphe nuclei. *Brain Research* 311, 131–140.

Milner, T. A., Pickel, V. M., Park, D. H., Joh, T. H., and Reis, D. J. (1987). Phenylethanolamine N-methyltransferase-containing neurons in the rostral ventrolateral medulla of the rat. I. Normal ultrastructure. *Brain Research* 411, 28–45.

Milner, T. A. Morrison, S. F., Abate, C., and Reis, D. J. (1988). Phenylethanolamine N-methyltransferase containing terminals synapse directly on sympathetic preganglionic neurons in the rat. *Brain Research* 448, 205–222.

Moore, S. D., and Guyenet, P. G. (1983). α-Receptor mediated inhibition of A2 noradrenergic neurons. *Brain Research* 276, 188–191.

Morrison, S. F., and Reis, D. J. (1989). Reticulospinal vasomotor neurons in the RVL mediate the somatosympathetic reflex. *American Journal of Physiology* 256, R1084–R1097.

Morrison, S. F., Milner, T.A., Pickel, V. M., and Reis, D. J. (1988). Retinospinal vasomotor neurons of the rat rostral ventrolateral medulla (RVL): Relationship to sympathetic nerve activity and the C1 adrenergic cell group. *Journal of Neuroscience* 8, 1286–1301.

Paxinos, G., and Watson, C. (1986). *The Rat Brain in Stereotaxic Coordinates,* 2nd ed. Academic Press, Sydney.

Punnen, S., Urbanski, R., Krieger, A. J., and Sapru, H. N. (1987). Ventrolateral medullary pressor area: Site of hypotensive action of clonidine. *Brain Research* 422, 336–346.

Rockhold, R. W., and Caldwell, R. W. (1980). Cardiovascular effects following clonidine microinjection into the nucleus tractus solitarii of the rat. *Neuropharmacology* 19, 919–922.

Ross, C. A., Ruggiero, D. A. Joh, T. H., Park, D. H., and Reis, D. J. (1984a). Rostral ventrolateral medulla: Selective projections to the thoracic autonomic cell column from the region containing C1 adrenaline neurons. *Journal of Comparative Neurology* 228, 168–185.

Ross, C. A., Ruggiero, D. A., Park, D. H., Joh, T. H., Sved,

A. F., Fernandez-Pardal, J., Saavedra, J. M., and Reis, D. J. (1984b). Tonic vasomotor control by the rostral ventrolateral medulla: Effect of electrical or chemical stimulation of the area containing C1 adrenaline neurons on arterial pressure, heart rate, and plasma catecholamines and vasopressin. *Journal of Neuroscience* 4, 474–494.

Ross, C. A., Ruggiero, D. A., and Reis, D. J. (1985). Projections from the nucleus tractus solitarii to the rostral ventrolateral medulla. *Journal of Comparative Neurology* 242, 511–534.

Schläfke, M. E., and Loeschcke, H. H. (1967). Lokalisation eines an der Regulation von Atmung und Kreislauf beteiligten Gebietes an der Ventralen Oberflaeche des Medulla oblongata durch Kaelteblockade. *Pflügers Archives European Journal of Physiology* 297, 201–220.

Shapiro, R. E., and Miselis, R. R. (1985). The central connections of the area postrema of the rat. *Journal of Comparative Neurology* 234, 344–364.

Stanek, K. A., Neil, J. J., Sawyer, W. B., and Loewy, A. D. (1984). Changes in regional blood flow and cardiac output after glutamate stimulation of the A5 cell group. *American Journal of Physiology* 246, H44–H51.

Stornetta, R. L., Guyenet, P. G., and McCarty, R. (1986). Modulation of autonomic outflow by pontine A5 noradrenergic neurons. In: *Brain and Blood Pressure Control,* K. Nakamura (ed.), Elsevier Science Publishers, Amsterdam, pp. 23–28.

Stornetta, R. L., Morrison, S. F., Ruggiero, D. A., and Reis, D. J. (1989). Neurons of the rostral ventrolateral medulla mediate the somatic pressor reflex. *American Journal of Physiology,* 256, R448–R462.

Sun, M.-K., and Guyenet, P. G. (1985). GABA-mediated baroreceptor inhibition of reticulospinal neurons. *American Journal of Physiology* 249, R672–R680.

Sun, M.-K., and Guyenet, P. G. (1986a). Medulospinal sympathoexcitatory neurons in normotensive and spontaneously hypertensive rats. *American Journal of Physiology* 250, R910–R917.

Sun, M.-K., and Guyenet, P. G. (1986b). Effect of clonidine and GABA on the discharges of medullospinal sympathoexcitatory neurons in the rat. *Brain Research* 368, 1–19.

Sun, M.-K., and Guyenet, P. G. (1987). Arterial baroreceptor and vagal inputs to sympathoexcitatory neurons in rat medulla. *American Journal of Physiology* 252, R699–R709.

Sun, M.-K., Hackett, J. T., and Guyenet, P. G. (1988a). Sympathoexcitatory neurons of rostral ventrolateral medulla exhibit pacemaker properties in presence of a glutamate-receptor antagonist. *Brain Research* 438, 23–40.

Sun, M.-K., Young, B. S., Hackett, J. T., and Guyenet, P. G. (1988b). Reticulospinal pacemaker neurons of the rat rostral ventrolateral medulla with putative sympathoexcitatory function: An intracellular study *in vitro. Brain Research* 442, 229–239.

Sved, A. F. (1989). PNMT-containing catecholaminergic neurons are not necessarily adrenergic. *Brain Research* 481, 113–118.

Taber, E. (1961). The cytoarchitecture of the brain stem of the cat I. Brain stem nuclei of cat. *Journal of Comparative Neurology* 116, 27–69.

Terui, N., Saeki, Y., and Kumada, M. (1986). Barosensory

neurons in the ventrolateral medulla in rabbits and their responses to various afferent inputs from peripheral and central sources. *Japanese Journal of Physiology* 36, 1141–1164.

Tucker, D. C., Saper, C. B., Ruggiero, D. A., and Reis, D. J. (1987). Organization of central adrenergic pathways: 1. Relationships of ventrolateral medullary projections to the hypothalamus and spinal cord. *Journal of Comparative Neurology* 259, 591–603.

Unnerstall, J. M., Kopajtic, T. A., and Kuhar, M. J. (1984). Distributions of α_2 agonist binding sites in the rat and human central nervous system: Analysis of some functional, anatomic correlates of the pharmacologic effects of clonidine and related adernergic agents. *Brain Research Reviews* 7, 69–101.

VanderMaelen, C. P., and Aghajanian, G. K. (1983). Electrophysiological and pharmacological characterization of serotonergic dorsal raphe neurons recorded extracellularly and intracellularly in rat brain slices. *Brain Research* 289, 109–119.

Wenthold, R. J., Skaggs, K. K., and Altschuler, R. A. (1986). Immunocytochemical localization of aspartate aminotransferase and glutaminase immunoreactivities in the cerebellum. *Brain Research* 363, 371–375.

Werman, R. (1966). Criteria for identification of a central nervous system transmitter. *Comparative Biochemistry and Physiology* 18, 745–766.

Willette, R. N., Krieger, A. J., Barcas, P. P., and Sapru, H. N. (1983). Medullary-aminobutyric acid (GABA) receptors and the regulation of blood pressure in the rat. *Journal of Pharmacology and Experimental Therapeutics,* 266, 893–899.

Williams, J. T., North, R. A., Shefner, S. A., Nishi, S., and Egan, T. M. (1984). Membrane properties of rat locus coeruleus neurones. *Neuroscience* 13, 136–156.

Williams, J. T., Henderson, G., and North, R. A. (1985). Characterization of α-2 adrenoceptors which increase potassium conductance in rat locus coeruleus neurones. *Neuroscience* 14, 95–101.

Yoshimura, M., Polosa, C., and Nishi, S. (1987). Noradrenaline-induced afterdepolarization in cat sympathetic preganglionic neurons in vitro. *Journal of Neurophysiology* 57, 1314–1324.

Zandberg, D., DeJong, W., and De Wied, D. (1979). Effect of catecholamine-receptor stimulating agents on blood pressure after local application in the nucleus tractus solitarii of the medulla oblongata. *European Journal of Pharmacology* 55, 43–56.

10

The Central Nervous Organization of Reflex Circulatory Control

K. M. SPYER

The cardiovascular system plays an essential role in maintaining the constancy of the internal environment (homeostasis) during the life of the individual. As indicated in Chapter 11, there are close similarities between the central organization of the nervous control of cardiovascular and respiratory activities as their fundamental role is the supply of oxygen to the tissues. This strong interrelationship extends even further to the reflex regulation of the two systems (see Daly, 1985 for review). Regulation of the cardiovascular system invariably involves the activation of several groups of receptors whose inputs to the CNS result in negative feedback reflex loops (see Heymans and Neil, 1958). In the case of the cardiovascular system, the variables that are regulated are arterial blood pressure, cardiac output, circulating blood volume, and arterial blood gas tensions. To achieve and maintain homeostasis, the ongoing levels of these variables are monitored by the various peripheral receptors, and their afferent input to the CNS modifies the autonomic outflows to the cardiovascular system, the pattern of respiratory activity, and the release of humoral agents to produce appropriate physiological responses.

The major reflex control of the circulation is mediated by receptors located within the cardiovascular system itself. They fall into two main categories: mechanoreceptors and chemoreceptors. Mechanoreceptors are located in both the main systemic arteries and within the heart. Those localized in the aortic arch and the carotid sinuses are known as arterial baroreceptors and they monitor arterial blood pressure. These have the properties of high-pressure receptors and each individual receptor has a threshold for activation in the range 30–150 mm Hg. They relay to the CNS via the aortic nerve, a branch of the vagus, for those with endings in the aortic arch. Receptors in the carotid sinus relay mechanoreceptor information through the sinus nerve, which is itself a branch of the glossopharyngeal nerve. The receptors have axons ranging from unmyelinated to those with small to large myelinated axons and properties that indicate that they are most sensitive to a change of pressure since they show rapid adaptation to prolonged and maintained elevations of pressure. The basic properties of these receptors have been detailed elsewhere (see Kirchheim, 1976, for a more detailed exposition). There had been some controversy as to whether basic differences existed between the properties of aortic and carotid baroreceptors, but recent studies have shown convincingly that their fundamental properties are equivalent (Samodelov et al., 1979).

Additional evidence has now been obtained that shows that the receptors themselves are subject to a degree of resetting when they are subjected to maintained alterations of arterial pressure for both short and long periods of time. The chemical and physical properties of the receptor and arterial wall contribute to this process(es) and this mechanism has often been believed to play a role in the etiology of hypertension. This has been the subject of several reviews and remains controversial (Brown, 1980; Chapleau et al., 1988).

The second major group of mechanoreceptors is collectively known as cardiac receptors. These have endings in either the great veins close to their entry to the heart or within the walls of the atria, the atrial apendange, or the walls of the ventricles (Heymans and Neil, 1958). Those that do not end in the ventricles are low-pressure receptors and provide information via the vagus on the magnitude of venous return, and hence circulating blood volume. These relay via both myelinated and nonmyelinated axons, with those having small myelinated axons termed the classical atrial receptors. In addition to those receptors with well-defined mechanoreceptor properties, there are numerous receptors within the heart, many in close association with the coronary circulation, that have ill-defined receptive properties, although many appear to subserve a chemosensitive function. These relay to the CNS with small myelinated or unmyelinated afferent fibers via both the vagus and the sympathetic nerves that innervate the heart. The role of sympathetic innervation is reviewed by Cervero and Foreman (Chapter 7).

There are also receptors with either mechanoreceptor or chemosensitive function in the arterial supply to the kidney, and perhaps other organs, that contribute to cardiovascular control. The major set of receptors with a chemosensitive function is, however, the arterial chemoreceptors located within the carotid bodies and the aortic arch. These, which are innervated by the sinus nerve and the aortic nerve, respectively, monitor the blood gas composition of arterial blood. They are specifically oxygen sensors but are also sensitive to carbon dioxide tension and pH. By means of their central connections these receptors participate in the regulation of both respiratory minute volume and cardiac output and its distribution to peripheral vascular beds. Their reflex role, and basic receptor properties, have been the subject of numerous reviews, the most recent being that of Ribiero and Pallot (1987). The influence they exert over the cardiovascular system has also received detailed attention (Daly, 1983). In these functions the peripheral chemoreceptors play an integrative role in association with central chemosensitive elements that have been identified on the ventral surface of the medulla oblongata that have a specific sensitivity for p_{CO_2}. Together these chemosensitive mechanisms act to maintain arterial p_{O_2}, p_{CO_2}, and pH within physiological limits.

Within skeletal muscle there is also evidence of the presence of a degree of chemoreceptor function. This chemosensitivity is mediated by receptors with afferent fibers in the group III and IV category. These provide information on the metabolic state of the muscle (Kniffke et al., 1981) and appear to exert influences over both the cardiovascular and respiratory systems in a manner that indicates that they promote the responses to exercise. There are claims that whereas the chemosensitive elements in muscle relay over group IV fibers, group III fibers innervate mechanoreceptor endings (see Kaufman et al., 1983). In this there is also evidence that joint receptors with undifferentiated endings, and presumed mechanoreceptive function, are similarly important in maintaining the cardiovascular and respiratory responses to exercise.

These varied and widely dispersed reflex inputs, together with other visceral afferent inputs (see Chapter 7) and those arising from receptors in the airways and the pulmonary vascular bed (see Daly, 1985 for review), contribute to the background afferent information that is used by the CNS in elaborating the discharge of the autonomic outflow to heart and blood vessels that patterns cardiac performance and peripheral blood flow. This chapter will concentrate on identifying the CNS mechanisms that are responsible for integrating these afferent inputs and will attempt to explain the interactions between these regulatory processes and the control that is exerted by those regions of the CNS concerned with the expression of behavior. In providing such an account it will be necessary to concentrate on the organization and control of the baroreceptor reflex since this is the particular reflex mechanism for which the most detailed information is available in the literature. Neurophysiological studies have largely been concerned with the central nervous organization of baroreceptor, chemoreceptor, and pulmonary reflex inputs, and this material will provide the basis on which a contemporary account of reflex control will be based. An attempt will also be made to correlate physiological information with neuroanatomical considerations and so establish what is known of the CNS pathways that link these afferent inputs to the vagal motor neurons that innervate the heart and the sympathetic preganglionic supply to the heart and blood vessels. Wherever possible the interactions between these specific reflex inputs and other reflex inputs will be stressed, since in most physiological situations several afferent systems are activated simultaneously, or secondary reflexes are elicited as a consequence of the elaboration of the initial response to a variation of one physiological variable. Finally the interactions that take place between reflex inputs and the neural drives that are developed during behavioral activity will be assessed. Several other chapters in this volume are of particular relevance to these discussions and should be read in conjunction with this one (see Chapters 8, 9, 11, and 19).

THE CENTRAL PROJECTIONS OF IXth AND Xth AFFERENTS

Until the last decade relatively little was known of the organization of the reflex inputs that arose from those receptors that relayed to the CNS via the IXth and Xth cranial nerves. With regard to the baroreceptor reflex the input–output relationships of the reflex were well established (see Figure 10-1), but other than a belief that a center in the medulla oblongata was responsible for its integration, nothing else of its neural organization was defined (Chapter 8). The application of a wide range of anatomical techniques had shown that baroreceptor afferents, among other IXth and Xth afferents, relayed primarily within the dorsomedial medulla in the vicinity of the nucleus of the solitary tract (NTS) (see Spyer, 1981 and Jordan and Spyer, 1986 for detailed reviews). The many advances in neuroanatomical technique, mainly through the use of the antero-

CAROTID SINUS REFLEXES

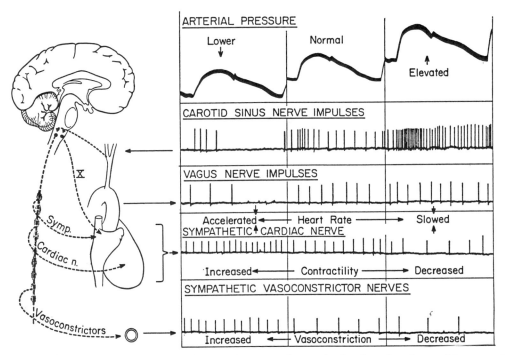

Figure 10-1 Single stretch receptors in the carotid sinus discharge at frequencies that depend on the arterial pressure. When the arterial pressure is lower, the pressoreceptor impulse frequency diminishes, the vagus nerve impulses diminish, sympathetic cardiac nerve impulses increase (accelerating the heart), and the sympathetic vasoconstrictor fibers become more active and increase peripheral resistance. The net effect is to raise the blood pressure. If the arterial pressure rises above the normal set value, the impulse frequency increases in carotid sinus nerves, reducing the sympathetic discharge and increasing the vagal discharge. Slowing of heart rate and peripheral vasodilation restore blood pressure to normal. (Reproduced with permission from Rushmer, 1965).

grade transport of ³H-labeled amino acids and horse-radish peroxidase (HRP) from either peripheral nerve endings or cut nerve branches, have provided a more coherent picture of the central projections of the sinus and aortic nerves. Similarly, the projections of the cervical vagus and the intrathoracic vagal branches have been identified in several species. The problem remains, however, that each of these nerves contains a heterogeneous mixture of afferents of different function so that even the sinus and aortic nerves contain baroreceptor and chemo-receptor afferents, each with axons in myelinated and unmyelinated classes. Vagal intrathoracic branches contain a mixture of both pulmonary and cardiac afferents arising from a large array of different receptor types. The alternative approach of placing HRP onto specific organs is hampered by the same heterogeneity of receptor type but also the added danger of vascularly mediated spread of the applied enzyme (see Kalia and Mesulum, 1980a,b).

Notwithstanding these problems it is now reasonably clear that all these afferents project into the immediate vicinity of the NTS. There may be a topo-graphical organization of the innervation provided by visceral organs (see Kalia and Mesulum, 1980a,b; Chapter 6), but the most striking feature of the available data is that although different nerves appear to project to the NTS in a reproducible manner (see Figure 10-2, the different subnuclei of the NTS receive input from several different sources (see Jordan and Spyer, 1987). The possibility that the NTS has an anatomically defined functional organization can be resolved only with use of neurophysiological studies. However, the early attempts at determining the pattern of projection of sinus, aortic, and vagal inputs using electrical stimulation and recording techniques were no more satisfactory than the anatomical approaches in providing unequivocal information. Indeed, in many cases they further complicated an already confused picture through their relatively crude application (see Spyer, 1981, for critical comments). These deficits have, in part, been redressed with the application of antidromic mapping techniques to the projection of baroreceptor, chemoreceptor, and pulmonary afferents. These studies have involved the recording of the ongoing discharge

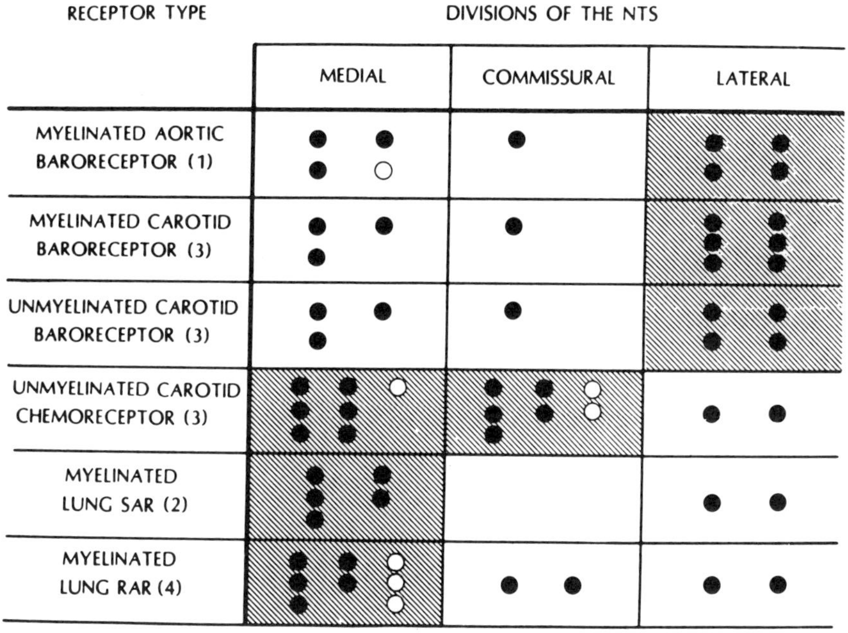

RECEPTOR TYPE	DIVISIONS OF THE NTS		
	MEDIAL	COMMISSURAL	LATERAL
MYELINATED AORTIC BARORECEPTOR (1)	● ● ● ○	●	(shaded) ● ● ● ●
MYELINATED CAROTID BARORECEPTOR (3)	● ● ●	●	(shaded) ● ● ● ● ● ●
UNMYELINATED CAROTID BARORECEPTOR (3)	● ● ●	●	(shaded) ● ● ● ●
UNMYELINATED CAROTID CHEMORECEPTOR (3)	(shaded) ● ● ○ ● ● ● ● ●	(shaded) ● ● ○ ● ● ○	● ●
MYELINATED LUNG SAR (2)	(shaded) ● ● ● ● ●		● ●
MYELINATED LUNG RAR (4)	(shaded) ● ● ○ ● ● ○ ○	● ●	● ●

Figure 10-2 Terminations within the cat NTS of cardiovascular and pulmonary afferents. A summary of the relative density of ipsilateral (●) and contralateral (○) regions of termination based on antidromic mapping studies. (1) Donoghue et al. (1982a); (2) Donoghue et al. (1982b); (3) Donoghue et al. (1984); (4) Kubin and Davies (1985). Shading represents the major projection for each afferent. SAR, slowly adapting vagal lung stretch afferent; RAR, rapidly adapting lung stretch afferent. (Reproduced with permission from Jordan and Spyer, 1986.)

of individual afferent with microelectrodes inserted into the extracranial ganglia of either the vagus (nodose ganglion) or the glossopharyngeal nerve (petrosal ganglion) (see Figure 10-3). The afferent is then characterized on the basis of its pattern of discharge, and its response to perturbations of its natural stimulus can be assessed. The intramedullary course of its axon and its points of branching and termination can then be traced by making serial penetrations through the medulla, noting the characteristics of the current necessary to evoke an antidromic response, its latency, and the depth–threshold profile for its activation over a number of penetrations (see Lipski, 1981 for detailed technical information on the method and analysis).

The available details of the projections of arterial baroreceptors, chemoreceptors, and slowly and rapidly adapting pulmonary receptors will now be summarized together with relevant information from other neurophysiological studies on afferent projections. A brief review of the literature concerning the projections of cardiac receptors will also be given.

Arterial Baroreceptors

In studies conducted in both the cat and rabbit, the pattern of projection of individual aortic baroreceptors has been determined (Donoghue et al., 1982a). To date, only those with myelinated axons have

been investigated (conduction velocity of these fibers was calculated as 12.5–22 m/second in the cat on the basis of antidromic latency and conduction distance and 14–23 m/second in the rabbit). In general, the pattern of projection in the two species was similar. There was a marked innervation of the lateral and medial divisions of the NTS, particularly to the more dorsal regions at levels rostral to the obex on the ipsilateral side. More caudally, the projections were restricted to medial and commissural divisions of the nucleus, continuing across the midline into equivalent areas of the contralateral NTS in a single case in the cat. Interestingly, at more rostral levels within the medulla these afferents were shown to project also into the ventrolateral region of the NTS. In previous studies in which the antidromic response of the complete aortic nerve was mapped in an equivalent manner a very similar pattern of projection had been revealed (Jordan and Spyer, 1980).

The central projections of the carotid sinus baroreceptors have since been mapped in this way (see Figure 10-4). Both myelinated and unmyelinated baroreceptor afferents were shown to project in a similar manner to the NTS. Their projections were restricted to the ipsilateral NTS, with the densest innervation being to dorsal regions of both the lateral and medial subnuclei at levels rostral to the obex (Donoghue et al., 1984). There was also evidence of a significant innervation of the ventrolateral NTS.

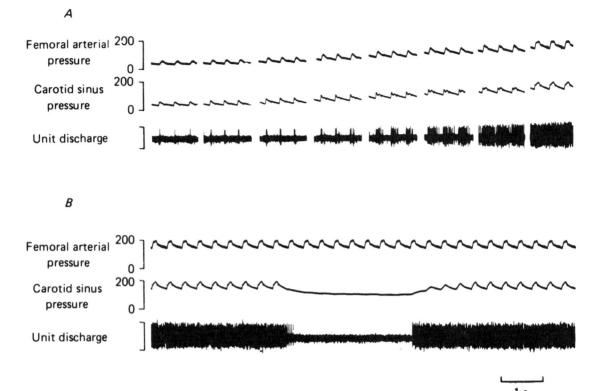

Figure 10-3 From above, original records of femoral arterial pressure, external carotid arterial pressure, and ongoing discharge of a carotid sinus baroreceptor afferent that was subsequently shown to have a myelinated axon (conduction velocity 7.5 m/second). (A) The fourth column shows the resting situation; columns to the left were taken at periods during controlled hemorrhage and columns to the right after reinfusion of blood and extracellular fluid expansion with an intravenous infusion of dextran saline. (B) The influence of occluding the ipsilateral common artery below the carotid sinus. This recording was made immediately after the one illustrated in A. The period of occlusion is indicated by the static pressure trace from the carotid artery. (Reproduced with permission from Donoghue et al., 1984.)

The commissural NTS was also innervated in the case of 7 of 12 afferents investigated, but this was never continued into the contralateral NTS. This pattern of afferent connection falls within the general description that was provided by studying the projection of sinus nerve using the antidromic mapping approach (Lipski et al., 1975).

These data are complemented by the results of neurophysiological studies that have been designed to record the activity of NTS neurons while stimulating electrically the sinus and/or the aortic nerves, and providing natural activation of the carotid sinus baroreceptors using a blind sac preparation (Lipski et al., 1975). Neurons receiving excitatory input from both the sinus nerve and the baroreceptors were found throughout the NTS at levels rostral to the obex, with a preponderance in more dorsal regions of lateral and medial divisions. There was also a significant population of neurons in the ventrolateral NTS, which was distinct physiologically from the respiratory neurons of this region (dorsal respiratory group—see Chapter 11). The responses were evoked at latencies compatible with the acti-

vation of myelinated afferents. These observations have been replicated in other similar studies (Miura and Reis, 1972) and most notably in a recent intracellular recording study (Mifflin et al., 1988a). In this most recent study neurons were identified in several of the expected regions of the NTS, many showing postsynaptic potentials (PSPs) to sinus nerve stimulation that indicated that they were activated monosynaptically. The majority of PSPs were, however, more characteristic of those to be expected if the cell were receiving both mono- and polysynaptic excitatory input (see Figure 10-5).

Indeed the influence of the sinus nerve, and specifically baroreceptor, input to the NTS is diverse as three distinct patterns of PSP are evoked—an excitatory postsynaptic potential (epsp) (Figure 10-5B), and EPSP–IPSP sequence (Figure 10-5A), and an inhibitory postsynaptic potential (IPSP) in different neurons. All three types of response were observed in neurons that were also influenced by inflation of a balloon-tipped catheter placed within the ipsilateral carotid sinus, which specifically activates baroreceptor afferent endings. In the case of the first two

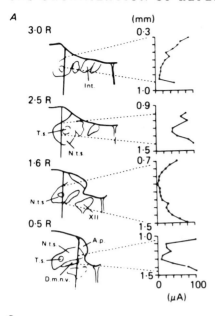

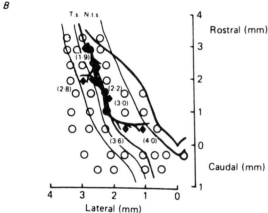

Figure 10-4 Myelinated baroreceptor afferent (conduction velocity 7.0 m/second). (A) Cross sections of the dorsomedial region of the medulla oblongata. Each of the thick vertical lines represents a stimulating electrode position. On the right are shown the depth–threshold profiles corresponding to these penetrations. (B) A schematic view of the dorsal surface of the medulla oblongata showing the fourth ventricle. Superimposed on this is the medial and lateral extent of the tractus solitarius and its nucleus. Scales indicate distances (in millimeters rostral (R), caudal (C), and lateral to the obex (O). Sites of stimulating electrode penetrations are indicated according to the type of depth–threshold profile obtained, that is, point (●), field (♦), or no response (○). Figures in parentheses indicate the antidromic latency. A possible course of the main axon is shown by the thick line connecting point types, and regions of branching or termination by the thin lines. Area postrema (A.p.), dorsal motor nucleus of vagus (D.m.n.v.), tractus solitarius (T.s.), nucleus tractus solitarius (N.t.s.), nucleus intercalatus (Int.), and hypoglossal nucleus (XII). (Reproduced with permission from Donoghue et al., 1984.)

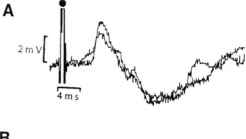

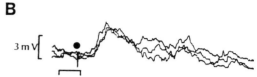

Figure 10-5 Postsynaptic potentials evoked by sinus nerve stimulation in two NTS neurons. In (A) an EPSP–IPSP is evoked, while in (B) an EPSP alone is evoked. Resting membrane potential, -52 mV in (A) and -56 mV in (B). Stimulus marked by (●). Results taken from the study of Mifflin et al. (1988b).

response patterns balloon inflation, when effective, excited the cell, whereas in the case of neurons receiving an IPSP, balloon inflation was inhibitory. These data indicate the existence of a pool of NTS neurons that is at least partially responsible for processing the baroreceptor afferent input (see Mifflin et al., 1988b, for discussion). Since many of these neurons also receive input from other peripheral afferent inputs (Mifflin et al, 1988a), excitatory or inhibitory, and are influenced by stimulation within the diencephalon (Mifflin et al., 1988b), it is reasonable to suggest that they may perform an integrative role in cardiovascular control. The detailed localization, morphology, and chemistry of the different categories of NTS neuron involved in these processes remain to be established, although some preliminary data are now available (Mifflin et al., 1987; Izzo et al., 1988).

Arterial Chemoreceptors

As yet the only arterial chemoreceptors subjected to detailed investigation are those of the carotid body. In the cat, a small number of such neurons with cell bodies in the petrosal ganglion have been mapped using antidromic stimulation. All showed an irregular ongoing discharge that was enhanced either by occlusion of the ipsilateral carotid artery or by raising the arterial pCO_2 (Donoghue et al., 1984). All had unmyelinated axons on the basis of their calculated conduction velocities, and these descended through the ipsilateral tractus solitarius. At levels rostral to the obex they sent branches into the lateral subnucleus, but at, and caudal, to the obex their major projection was to the medial and commissural subnuclei. There was also evidence of a contralateral projection into the medial and commissural nuclei at this level. These data may reveal, however, only a limited picture of the chemoreceptor innervation of the NTS, as it is believed that a large number of chemoreceptor afferents have myelinated axons (Fidone and Sato, 1969).

Further there are very few indications in the literature of the postsynaptic actions of specific chemoreceptor inputs onto individual NTS neurons. It is well documented that such inputs excite medullary inspiratory neurons (see Richter and Spyer, Chapter 11), of which a number are located within the ventrolateral subnucleus of the NTS. However, there is controversy as to whether the direct monosynaptic effect is excitatory, as Lipski et al., (1976) were unable to verify a direct excitatory action, believing that this was fed onto the neuron by whatever was elaborating its central respiratory drive input. When observed in situations where this input was absent and the cell was made excitable by either physiological or pharmacological means, the direct effect of chemoreceptor stimulation appeared to be inhibitory. Contrary conclusions were drawn by Kirkwood et al. (1979), who used spike-triggered averaging of NTS respiratory neuronal activity in relation to a trigger signal derived from the discharge of individual chemoreceptor afferents recorded in the petrosal ganglion. They observed sharp peaks in the spike-triggered histogram at short latency that were suggestive of a monosynaptic input from myelinated chemoreceptor afferents. The peaks were small, however, even over the long sampling periods. In contrast, unmyelinated chemoreceptor afferents failed to show any projections to the ventrolateral NTS when studied with antidromic mapping techniques (Donoghue et al., 1984). Aside from these mapping data, evidence has been obtained that shows that neurons within the commissural NTS receive an input from unmyelinated, and probably also small myelinated, carotid body chemoreceptor fibers (Izzo et al., 1988). The cells receiving these inputs have been labeled intracellularly with HRP and appear as a compact group of cells just dorsal to the tractus solitarius. They have dendrites distributed in a mediolateral direction extending beyond the confines of the NTS into the reticular formation. Interestingly, their excitatory influence from the chemoreceptors is unaffected by the timing of the stimulus in the respiratory cycle (this will be discussed later).

Using extracellular recordings other investigators have described chemoreceptor-evoked excitatory responses in cells distributed over a wide area of the NTS (Lipski et al., 1976; Miura and Reis, 1972). Lipski et al. (1976) even suggest a convergence of baroreceptor and chemoreceptor inputs onto individual nonrespiratory NTS neurons, particularly in the vicinity of the ventrolateral subnucleus and the neighboring reticular formation.

Slowly Adapting Pulmonary Stretch Afferents

Vagal afferent fibers with endings in the airways and lungs are known to exert potent influences on both the cardiovascular and respiratory systems. Of these, the pulmonary stretch afferents that adapt slowly to lung inflation are considered to have marked influences on the cardiovascular system. In particular they influence the performance of other reflex inputs that are known to regulate the cardiovascular system, especially those that are concerned with the regulation of heart rate (Daly, 1985). Their central projections have been analyzed in some detail using the antidromic mapping technique. In both the cat and rabbit their major projection is to the medial subnucleus at levels of the NTS rostral to the obex (Donoghue et al. 1982b). A weaker yet significant input is to the lateral and ventrolateral subnuclei. This relatively sparse projection to the ventrolateral NTS was unexpected, given that one group of inspiratory neuron is localized to the ventrolateral NTS—the R_β neurons that have been described as monosynaptically activated by pulmonary afferents (see Baumgarten and Kanzow, 1958; Averill et al., 1984; Backman et al., 1984; Berger and Dick, 1987). The apparent paucity of input to the ventrolateral NTS was also evident in a spike-triggered averaging study undertaken by Averill et al. (1984). Here the major projection of slowly adapting afferents was to the medial subnucleus. There is, however, evidence of a more widely dispersed monosynaptic input to NTS neurons termed *pump cells,* which are excited on lung inflation but have no central respiratory rhythm in their discharge (Averill et al., 1984; Berger and Dick, 1987).

This apparent discrepancy between the pattern of projection revealed by antidromic mapping and the physiological responses of NTS neurons may be a consequence of the morphology of NTS neurons. Although their cell bodies may be restricted to a particular division of the NTS, their dendrites may extend into adjacent subnuclei or beyond. Accordingly, connections may be made on distally located dendrites. Equally, intracellular labeling of individual slowly adapting vagal fibers within the medulla using HRP has shown terminal boutons within the ventrolateral, ventral, and allied areas of the NTS (Kalia and Richter, 1985a,b).

Rapidly Adapting Pulmonary Afferents

Rapidly adapting pulmonary receptors respond to lung inflation and deflation with an irregular discharge. As with slowly adapting afferents, they relay in the vagus with small myelinated fibers. Using the antidromic mapping technique, Davies and Kubin (1986) have shown that these afferents have a pattern of projection distinctly different from that of the slowly adapting fibers. They tend to provide a widespread innervation of more caudal regions of the NTS at, and just rostral to, the obex, but have their most conspicuous projections into the area caudal to the obex (Figure 10-6). Specifically, it is to the medial and commissural subnuclei that they project, with a sparser innervation into the lateral and ventrolateral subnuclei. They also have a marked contralateral projection into the medial subnucleus.

There are also numerous receptors in the airways that relay to the CNS in the vagus with unmyelinated axons. These mediate protective reflexes and are considered to be irritant receptors. As yet nothing is known of their pattern of central projection. Similarly, there are numerous largyngeal receptors with both myelinated and unmyelinated axons that function in a similar manner. These are known to influence the activity of NTS neurons (see Mifflin et al., 1988a) and interact in cardiovascular control (see later).

Cardiac Afferent Projections

As yet there are no major studies that describe the central projections of cardiac afferent fibers. The information that exists, other than simple descriptions of the projection of vagal afferents, derives from studies of the responses of NTS neurons to electrical stimulation of the cardiac vagal branches. In general, neurons that responded to stimulation at intensities effective enough to activate myelinated afferent were not excited when the intensity was raised to a level high enough to excite unmyelinated afferents. This information has been reviewed in a recent monograph by Kidd (1987). It would appear that atrial receptors are likely to activate neurons within the medial subnucleus of the NTS, which confirms evidence from a brief report that showed that such afferents could be antidromically activated from that region of the NTS (Donoghue and Jordan, 1980). But recent anatomical evidence from the anterograde transport of choleratoxin HRP indicates that the main focus of projection of cardiac afferents is the medial NTS at levels caudal to the obex in the rat (Miselis, Schwaber, and Spyer, unpublished data).

PATTERNS OF AUTONOMIC RESPONSE TO REFLEX ACTIVATION

In studying the central organization of reflex control of the cardiovascular system, it is essential to keep in mind how the reflexes under consideration influence the autonomic outflows, and, consequently, cardiovascular variables. Only a brief review will be provided here, concentrating on issues of specific rele-

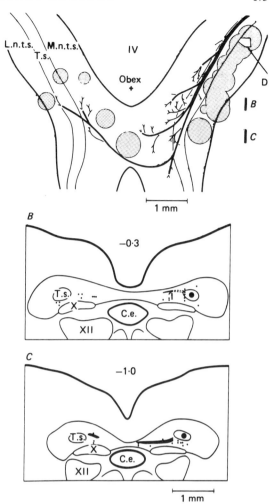

Figure 10-6 Schematic distribution (see text) within the NTS of fine branches of the same RAR cell as in Figures 10-2 and 10-5. In A, the branching pattern is shown in a dorsal view. The stippled circles cover the regions in which the presence of branches was excluded on the basis of current spread analysis. The white area in the upper portion of the shading indicates the region in which inspiratory cells (dorsal respiratory group) were recorded. B and C show two coronal sections on which the location of fine branches is indicated by small dots. Each drawing shows branches contained in a 0.3-mm-thick medullary segment located at the level indicated by heavy bars in A. The main axon is shown as a heavy filled circle within the T.s. on the right side. The continuous lines correspond to portions of major collaterals that course within the plane of the section. The small dots are located at the depth of the minimum threshold current to activate the fine branches. Most fine branches were located in the intermediate, medial, and commissural subnuclei of the NTS. C.e., central canal; T.s., solitary tract; X, dorsal motor nucleus of the vagus nerve; XII, hypoglossal nucleus. (Reproduced with permission from Davies and Kubin, 1986.)

vance to our discussions. There are several excellent reviews in the literature to which the reader is directed (Heymans and Neil, 1958; Jänig, 1985; Abboud and Thames, 1983; Daly, 1985).

Baroreceptor Reflex

Activation of the arterial baroreceptors leads to an increase in the discharge of vagal cardioinhibitory neurons and a decrease in the discharge of sympathetic pre- and postganglionic neurons both to the peripheral blood vessels and to the heart (see Figure 10-1). This results in bradycardia, decreased cardiac contractility, and decreased peripheral vascular resistance. Accordingly, blood pressure falls since both cardiac output and vascular resistance have fallen. Conversely, a decrease in arterial pressure is compensated by a decrease in baroreceptor afferent discharge, resulting in the appropriate changes in autonomic activity. The reflex is operating continuously, providing for short-term adjustments to arterial blood pressure, and it is likely that its major ongoing role is to prevent a decrease in pressure response to the demands imposed by activity-related metabolic drives.

The reflex also functions on a beat-by-beat basis to regulate heart rate so that baroreceptor inputs are crucial in maintaining a regulation of cardiac output. Indeed, the sensitivity of the reflex is often assessed by its ability to modify pulse intervals. Altering this sensitivity may provide the CNS with a powerful mechanism for adjusting the cardiovascular system in relation to behavioral activities. The significance of this will be discussed at length later.

The baroreceptor control of the sympathetic outflow is not uniform. Postganglionic sympathetic fibers supplying the blood vessels in skeletal muscle are particularly sensitive to baroreceptor inputs, whereas cutaneous vasoconstrictor fibers are less affected (see Chapter 18). In addition, the postganglionic innervation of blood vessels supplying visceral organs, including the kidney, seems highly sensitive to baroreceptor inputs, whereas those to the brain and heart are relatively insensitive.

Chemoreceptor Reflex

The main physiological role of the arterial chemoreceptors is the regulation of blood gas composition. This is achieved by modifying respiratory minute volume and cardiac output, particularly in relationship to variations in arterial pO_2. There are also changes produced in peripheral vascular resistance that are largely determined by the need to conserve O_2 and are brought about by appropriate changes in sympathetic vasoconstrictor activity. Sympathetic fibers innervating blood vessels to both the skin and

the skeletal muscle are affected by increased chemoreceptor drive, and the same applies to the sympathetic drive to the heart and kidney but not to the brain. This conservatory function is particularly marked in situations in which the respiratory effects of the chemoreceptor input are prevented, for example, during breath-holding in diving. The diving response is characterized by circulatory adjustments to conserve oxygen followed by a marked bradycardia through increased vagal drive and a reduced sympathetic drive to the heart (see also Chapter 11). Indeed, the normal tachycardia that accompanies chemoreceptor stimulation appears to be a secondary response that is dependent on the evoked increase in inspiratory drive. This clear influence of respiration on the performance of a reflex that has importance in cardiovascular regulation is not unique, and equivalent effects are seen in modifying the efficacy of the baroreceptor reflex. Central chemosensory drives, largely determined by arterial pCO_2, similarly affect sympathetic discharge by influencing the bulbospinal respiratory pathways (Millhorn, 1986).

Atrial Receptor Reflexes

The atrial receptors are believed to play an important role in monitoring venous return and providing the CNS with information specifically related to atrial distention and contraction. The reflex response to increased activity appears to involve a tachycardia that is sympathetically mediated and a reduction in sympathetic discharge to the kidney. There is no evidence that these receptors are able to modify the activity of the efferent vagal supply to the heart (Linden, 1987). This pattern of response indicates that they play an important role in the regulation of extracellular fluid volume. As yet there is no indication of other specific vascular actions of this reflex, although the control that it exerts over vasopressin release from the posterior pituitary (see Chapter 13) will add to this function.

The role of vagal afferent fibers with unmyelinated axons remains to be resolved. The ventricular receptors that relay to the CNS through the vagus and those unmyelinated atrial afferents, when stimulated electrically, evoke a profound bradycardia and systemic hypotension that is known as the Bezold–Jarisch reflex. Its physiological significance is still a matter for debate, and the specific roles of many of these as yet ill-defined cardiac afferents remain unknown. The sympathetic afferent fibers that innervate the heart are believed to signal cardiac pain, and there is evidence for sympathosympathetic reflexes that are considered to have a positive feedback role in evoking increases in heart rate and cardiac contractility (Malliani, 1986; and see Chapter 7).

Orthostatic Reflexes

So far the results of activating individual groups of receptors have been considered. In physiological situations this is unusual, as alterations invariably affect several classes of receptor simultaneously. In orthostasis arterial baroreceptors, chemoreceptors, and atrial receptors will all change their afferent discharge in proportion to the magnitude of the change in posture and the resulting shifts of blood. In addition, there may well be the interplay of these inputs with those resulting from the changes that are evoked in vestibular afferent information. The net response is thus the summation of all these various inputs to the CNS, and the challenge is to determine how these are integrated to provide the optimum autonomic pattern of activity to generate the necessary cardiovascular response to maintain homeostasis. It has often been supposed that the cerebellum might play an important role in organizing the orthostatic cardiovascular response (see Doba and Reis, 1974), but recent studies on cerebellar actions on the circulation, and particularly the role of the fastigial nucleus (see Bradley et al., 1987), have indicated that this may not be so. Additional studies are required to resolve this issue.

INTERACTION OF AFFERENT INPUTS WITHIN THE NTS

The studies reported above indicate that although individual classes of afferent have distinctive patterns of projection to the NTS, the various subnuclei receive input from several different classes of afferent mediating different reflex responses. The studies that have been reviewed are limited largely to those few classes of afferent whose receptors are most accessible to appropriate natural stimulation under experimental conditions so that the overlap of input may well be considerably greater as more becomes known of the central projections of these other afferent systems. This suggestion of apparent convergence at once raises the question of whether individual NTS neurons act to integrate these afferent inputs and so perhaps play a role in cardiorespiratory homeostasis. A range of specific questions can be posed for experimental study. Do afferent fibers interact presynaptically, as has been proposed in some other afferent systems? Is there a developed interneuronal system within the NTS that controls transmission through the various reflex pathways initiated there? To place these questions in a physiological context it is necessary to provide an indication of situations in which there is evidence that reflex inputs interact to develop appropriate responses. Mention has already been made of orthostatic reflexes in which such interactions occur. Further, on several occasions the influence of respiration on the performance of cardiovascular and respiratory reflexes has been described (see Daly, 1985).

This latter influence can perhaps be best appreciated when dealing with the baroreceptor reflex control of the vagal outflow to the heart and consequently heart rate (see Figure 10-7). In Figure 10-7, a recording taken from an anesthetized dog, a stimulus to the carotid sinus evokes vagal discharge only when the stimulus is timed to occur during expiration; the identical stimulus is ineffective when applied in inspiration (Davidson et al., 1976). The same would apply to a stimulus delivered to the carotid body chemoreceptors, although these will excite inspiratory neurons and phrenic nerve activity when the stimulus is applied during inspiration (see above). From the evidence presented in this study the effect could have been due to an influence of inputs related to lung inflation or phasic changes related to the central respiratory rhythm (see Chapter 11 for a fuller discussion). In a wide range of investigations, Daly (1985) has shown that inputs related specifically to lung inflation, and independent of central respiratory activity, modify both the cardiac and the vascular responses to numerous reflex inputs. These include the baroreceptor, chemoreceptor, cardiac, bladder, and both vascular and pulmonary vascular afferent inputs. It has been suggested that although central respiratory activity controls the tonic excitability of vagal activity to the heart, lung

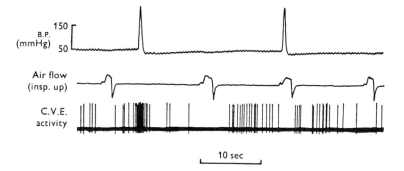

Figure 10-7 Dog. Chloralose and morphine. Records of carotid sinus blood pressure, respiratory air flow, and the activity of single cardiac vagal efferent nerve (C.V.E.) are shown. A burst of firing in the cardiac efferent nerve was evoked by a baroreceptor stimulus timed so as to occur in the expiratory pause. No firing was evoked when a similar stimulus was given during inspiration (Davidson et al. 1976).

B.P. (mmHg) 150 50

Air flow (insp. up)

C.V.E. activity

10 sec

inflation exerts its effects through a control of re-flexly evoked vagal activity (Potter, 1981). This is presumably through an action at the level of the NTS, or at a stage between it and the vagal pregan-glionic motoneurons (see later).

In addition to these interactions, and the many other instances of reflex summation (see Spyer, 1981 for detailed discussion), there is a growing literature that indicates a central modification of cardiovas-cular reflexes. In particular, there is evidence that areas of the forebrain and diencephalon involved in the expression of the behavioral and autonomic fea-tures of emotion modulate the baroreceptor reflex (see Chapter 19). In this chapter we will concentrate on the hypothalamic and amygdaloid influences on neuronal activity in the lower brain stem, and spe-cifically on the effects that are related to the control of the baroreceptor reflex. These may, however, pro-vide some more general indications of the synaptic mechanisms whereby the CNS modifies cardiovas-cular activity in relation to behavior.

Presynaptic Interactions of Afferents within the NTS

There is a body of information in the literature that indicates that there is a degree of presynaptic inter-action between afferent fibers that terminate within the NTS. This appears to be restricted to various cat-egories of vagal afferent and does not involve either aortic or sinus nerve afferent fibers (see Jordan and Spyer, 1986 for review). Anatomically axoaxonal synapses are prevalent in the NTS, and both lung stretch afferents and superior laryngeal afferents have been shown to exert reciprocal presynaptic ac-tions on each other. The absence of such influences on sinus and aortic nerve afferents inferred from electrophysiological evidence (Richter et al., 1986) may be taken as an indication that physiologically these connections play a minor, or insignificant, role in cardiovascular control. There are suggestions that some interactions between the sinus nerves of the two sides could involve a polysynaptic control of af-ferent transmission acting presynaptically on sinus afferent endings, or interneurons, in the NTS (Miff-lin and Felder, 1988).

Postsynaptic Interactions within the NTS

It has been mentioned that the NTS contains neu-rons that are excited by sinus nerve inputs, many of which are also excited by the arterial baroreceptors. Several of these neurons also receive input from other afferents such as those contained in the aortic nerve, superior laryngeal nerve, and vagus (see Cir-iello and Calaresu, 1981; Biscoe and Sampson, 1970; Mifflin et al., 1988a among others; Figure 10-8).

These neurons may offer the substrate for the inte-gration of these afferent inputs and, accordingly, their pattern of response to various inputs may pro-vide some indication of the functional role exerted by the NTS. The nature of PSPs evoked in individ-ual NTS neurons on sinus nerve stimulation and the convergent influences of other inputs onto these neurons may indicate how the efficacy of a particu-lar reflex is modified under different experimental conditions. For example, the variations in PSPs evoked at different times in the respiratory cycle might provide insight into the site of integration of cardiorespiratory control.

This has been tested in anesthetized, paralyzed, and artificially ventilated cats, in which it is possible to separate influences of lung inflation from those of central respiratory activity (Mifflin et al., 1988a). Neither form of ventilatory input modified the PSPs evoked in a range of NTS neurons (see Figure 10-8), including several that were shown to receive baro-receptor inputs. Since neurons demonstrating all three types of PSPs to sinus nerve stimulation were unaffected, it is unlikely that at normal levels of ven-tilation, with appropriate lung stretch afferent in-puts, this reflex (and probably others too) is in any way modified at this level of their processing.

Where might the powerful effects of respiration be exerted? Chapter 11 draws attention to the attractive possibility that there is a common central mecha-nism for the generation of the basic neural drives for cardiovascular and respiratory homeostasis. Much of this hypothesis rests on evidence derived from studies on the properties of vagal preganglionic neu-rons that control heart rate. In neurophysiological studies it became clear that these neurons had pow-erful respiratory-related patterns of activity. From recordings taken from vagal fibers it was known that they had a marked expiratory rhythm in their dis-charge (see Kunze, 1972, among others). In intracel-lular recordings from the cell bodies of these neurons it became apparent that this pattern was determined by a synaptic action involving a chloride-dependent IPSP during inspiration (Gilbey, et al., 1984). This leads to a marked fall in membrane input resistance through an increased membrane conductance, and this was sufficient to shunt the normal excitatory in-puts from the arterial baroreceptors (see Figure 10-9).

The effect of this is to maintain the baroreceptor influence at a subliminal level during inspiration; it is equally effective in suppressing other excitatory in-puts such as those arising from the arterial chemo-receptors as described earlier. It should be noted that in the study illustrated in Figure 10-9 the animal was ventilated artificially at a rate that was greater than that of the central respiratory rhythm, as shown in the simultaneous recording of phrenic nerve activ-

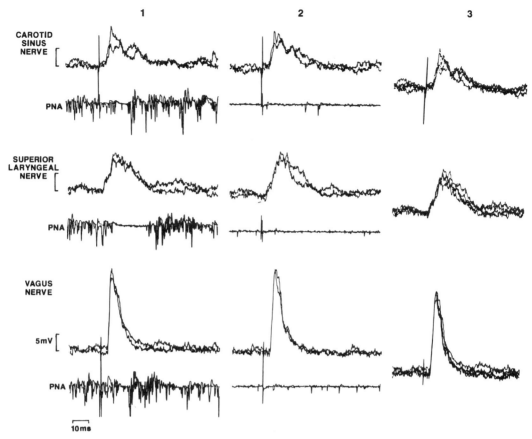

Figure 10-8 EPSPs evoked by carotid sinus nerve and vagal and superior laryngeal nerve stimulation in a cell depolarized during activation of the baroreceptors. Membrane potential was hyperpolarized with 4-nA dc current and the stimulus intensities adjusted so that EPSPs were subthreshold for action potential generation. Two sweeps during inspiration (1) and expiration (2), one with the lungs inflated and the other with the lungs deflated, are superimposed. Phrenic nerve activity (PNA) is displayed below. (3) Two sweeps superimposed from columns (1) and (2); resting membrane potential −56 mV. HRP-filled electrode. (Modified, with permission, from Mifflin et al., 1988a.)

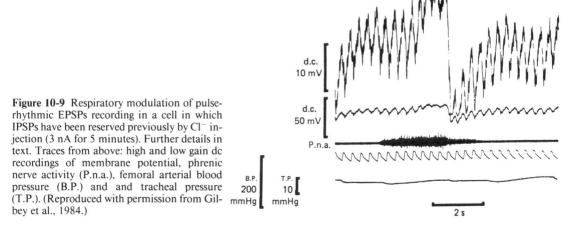

Figure 10-9 Respiratory modulation of pulse-rhythmic EPSPs recording in a cell in which IPSPs have been reserved previously by Cl⁻ injection (3 nA for 5 minutes). Further details in text. Traces from above: high and low gain dc recordings of membrane potential, phrenic nerve activity (P.n.a.), femoral arterial blood pressure (B.P.) and and tracheal pressure (T.P.). (Reproduced with permission from Gilbey et al., 1984.)

ity. No influence of lung inflation, measured as tracheal pressure, on the membrane potential of the vagal neuron is seen. This contrasts with observations reported in the literature that indicate powerful effects of lung inflation on vagally mediated reflex changes in heart rate (see Daly, 1985; Potter, 1981). There may be species-related differences in the effectiveness of lung inflation inputs in evoking these changes, but based on the evidence presented in this review it is unlikely that lung inflation inputs are exerting their effects at the level of the NTS or the vagal preganglionic neurons themselves. This would imply that lung stretch inputs exert their inhibitory action on vagal neurons indirectly, as illustrated diagrammatically in Figure 10-10. This indirect inhibitory action may involve control of a tonic excitatory input to cardiac vagal neurons so that their influence is an example of disfacilitation. This contrasts with the conclusion of Potter (1981), but is consistent with the hypothesis summarized in Chapter 11.

In regard to sympathetic reflexes there is also considerable variability in the effectiveness of lung inflation inputs in modifying regional discharge or vascular resistance changes. This makes it likely that the action of vagal afferent inputs must be at a site, or sites, between the NTS and the preganglionic vagal and sympathetic neurons. Potentially such sites should be within the brain stem, and their localization may be a matter of some significance in determining respiratory cardiovascular coupling. One possibility that needs to be considered is the suggestion that different pools of ventrolateral medullary "sympathoexcitatory" neurons are coded for projection to different populations of sympathetic preganglionic neurons and that these may have different susceptibilities to lung stretch inputs (see later).

Descending Inputs to the NTS

Aside from receiving a marked innervation from peripheral afferents, the NTS receives a powerful innervation from several levels of the CNS (see Figure 10-11). Many of these sites are known to be concerned with the generation of cardiovascular responses (see Chapters 12, 13, and 19). In part, the elaboration of these cardiovascular responses may involve a modification of the performance of basic cardiovascular reflexes, a possibility that is well established with regard to affective behavior (see Chapter 19).

Recent experimental studies involving intracellular recording have helped to resolve this issue. Continuing the studies indicated earlier, Mifflin et al. (1988b) demonstrated that electrical stimulation at sites within the hypothalamus that elicit the defense reaction was able to produce some quite marked influences on the activity of NTS neurons. In particular, when stimulation evoked a suppression of the baroreceptor reflex, NTS neurons that were normally excited on baroreceptor activation were inhibited from the hypothalamus, and the influences of the baroreceptor input were effectively shunted (Figure 10-12). The inhibitory action of the hypothalamus was not restricted to neurons that were excited by baroreceptor inputs, but every neuron that was activated by sinus inflation was routinely inhibited. This inhibitory action involved a chloride-dependent IPSP and was mediated by a GABAergic synapse, since it could be blocked by the iontophoretic application of bicuculline, a specific antagonist of GABA (see Jordan et al., 1988). Interestingly, these same neurons were often inhibited by the application of glycine, and this effect was antag-

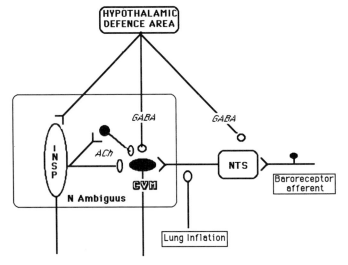

Figure 10-10 Diagrams illustrating the control exerted on vagal cardioinhibitory neurons by baroreceptor afferent input, inspiratory neurons (INSP), and the hypothalamic defense area. The influence of lung stretch inputs is also illustrated. Excitatory inputs are shown as <, inhibitory inputs as ○. ACh, acetylcholine; GABA, γ-aminobutyric acid. Further details are in the text. (Reproduced with permission from Spyer, 1989.)

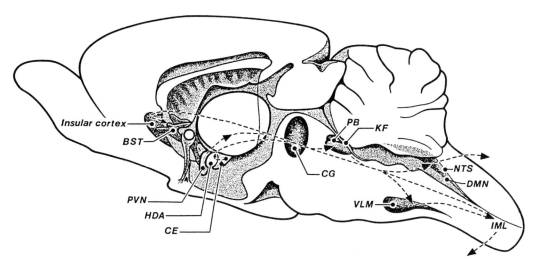

Figure 10-11 Diagrammatic representation of the descending pathways in the rat that are responsible for the cardiovascular component of affective behavior. For simplicity, the dorsal vagal nucleus (DVN) is used for the source of cardioinhibitory output, although the nucleus ambiguus is in many species the source. BST, bed nucleus of the stria terminals; CE, central nucleus of amygdala; CG, central gray; DMN, dorsal vagal nucleus; HDA, hypothalamic defense area; IML, intermediolateral cell column of thoracic spinal cord; KF; Kölliker–Fuse nucleus; NTS, nucleus tractus solitarius; PVN, paraventricular nucleus; VLM, ventrolateral medulla (see text for additional information). (Reproduced with permission from Spyer, 1988.)

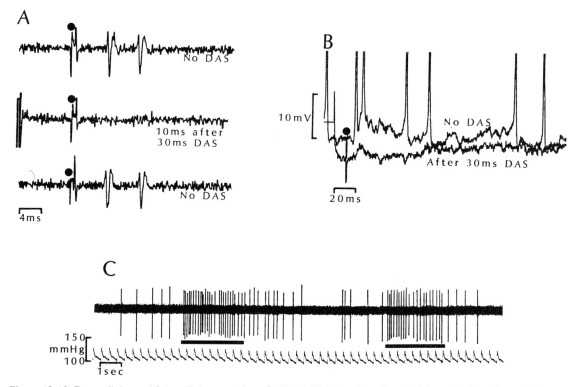

Figure 10-12 Extracellular and intracellular recording of HDA inhibition of a cell excited by activation of carotid sinus baroreceptors. (A) Extracellular responses to SN stimulation (stimulus artifact indicated by ●) in top and bottom traces. Between the two SN stimuli the SN stimulus was preceded by 10 msec by a 30-msec burst of HDA stimulation (middle trace) that abolished the SN-evoked discharge. (B) Intracellular recording from the same cell. SN stimulation alone (top trace, no defense area stimulation, no DAS) evoked a comparable number of action potentials (truncated) at the same latency as recorded extracellularly. At the end of HDA stimulation (lower trace, after 30 msec DAS) membrane potential was hyperpolarized (for approximately 150 msec) and SN stimulation (10 msec after the end of DAS) did not evoke discharge. (C) Extracellular recording of response to baroreceptor activation (during period indicated by the bars). Membrane potential: −53 mV. Potassium citrate-filled electrode. (Reproduced with permission from Mifflin et al., 1988b.)

onized by the application of strychnine, although strychnine alone failed to affect the inhibitory action of hypothalamic stimulation.

On occasions when the inhibitory action of hypothalamic stimulation had been blocked in this direct pharmacological manner using the iontophoretic application of bicuculline, stimulation then elicited a short latency excitation that was otherwise unobserved. This is consistent with other results obtained when recording from NTS neurons on stimulation in the hypothalamus and the amygdaloid central nucleus in the cat (see Spyer et al., 1985). In that study, stimulation at sites in these two areas was seen under different circumstances to either excite or inhibit NTS neurons that received excitatory input from the sinus nerve. Such observations may have particular importance in the expression of the overall responses that may be evoked from these areas. In Chapter 19, Jordan has drawn attention to the possible existence of two distinct patterns of affective behavior that can be evoked from the diencephalon. These contrasting influences on NTS activity may be an expression of these behaviors. Interestingly, in the rabbit the most consistent effect that can be evoked from the central nucleus is a bradycardia, systemic hypotension, and rapid shallow breathing in the anesthetized animal, which forms a part of the "playing dead response" that is seen in the conscious animal. In a series of experiments it has been shown that neurons in the NTS of the rabbit that are excited by electrical stimulation of the aortic nerve—which is considered to be solely barosensory in this species—are also excited by stimulation of the central nucleus (Cox et al., 1986). Subsequently studies have indicated that the amygdaloid stimulus facilitates the baroreceptor reflex (Pascoe et al., 1989), and the neuronal recordings appear to have provided the substrate for this facilitatory interaction. In addition, there is growing evidence that these same regions of the diencephalon, as well as midbrain areas that are involved in cardiovascular regulation, have marked connections, both directly and indirectly, with the preganglionic autonomic neurons (see Chapter 6).

In regard to the defense area, there are indications that stimulation can exert a direct inhibitory action on vagal cardioinhibitory neurons located in the nucleus ambiguus (Spyer, 1984; Jordan and Spyer, 1987). This implies that the activity of the neural outflows to the cardiovascular system are controlled in two rather general ways by regions of the CNS: first by control of the performance of reflex inputs that is largely achieved at the level of the NTS and second by control of excitability at the level of the preganglionic sympathetic and vagal neurons. Such an organization would appear to be designed to offer the opportunity of modifying both the *gain* and the *set point* of cardiovascular reflexes (see Figure 10-10). Accordingly, a growing understanding of the neural mechanisms that are concerned with the expression of emotion may provide greater understanding of the generation of cardiovascular responses in a full range of behavioral circumstances. Further, these observations may also suggest sites, and mechanisms, that underlie pathological changes in cardiovascular control and that may, in certain circumstances, culminate in the development of neurogenic hypertension.

Aside from the patterns of interaction that have been specified in this account, additional patterns within the NTS have been revealed (Ciriello and Calaresu, 1981; Mifflin et al., 1988a,b,). The NTS receives a profound innervation from numerous regions of the neuraxis, many of which are concerned with cardiovascular control. Unfortunately, the physiological consequences of activating these have not yet been analyzed but may provide a field of some challenge to investigators in the future.

THE OUTPUT FROM THE NTS

The discussion so far has indicated that baroreceptor afferent inputs, among other reflex inputs, undergo a degree of integration within the NTS, but that inputs related to lung inflation and central respiratory activity are not involved in these integrative processes. Conversely, baroreceptor-sensitive NTS neurons, and others, are powerfully influenced by descending inputs from the hypothalamus and amygdala, which in the cat usually seem to initiate a predominantly inhibitory action. The effectiveness of the output from the NTS in influencing vagal cardioinhibitory neurons has been assessed and has been shown to have interesting physiological properties. Thus, the general question of how, and by what routes, different reflex inputs affect sympathetic and vagal neurons appears to be of some physiological importance.

With regard to cardiac vagal neurons, there is plentiful evidence from neuroanatomical studies of an innervation of both the dorsal vagal nucleus and the nucleus ambiguus from the NTS (see Chapter 5; Figure 10-13). The physiological actions of these connections are as yet unresolved. For instance, although it is known that the nucleus ambiguus receives direct output from the NTS, it is not known whether vagal cardiomotor neurons receive monosynaptic input or whether a local interneuron(s) is interposed between the NTS projection neuron and the vagal neuron. To account for known properties of cardioinhibitory neurons in the nucleus ambiguus such connections will need to account for the fact that McAllen and Spyer (1978) found a variation in

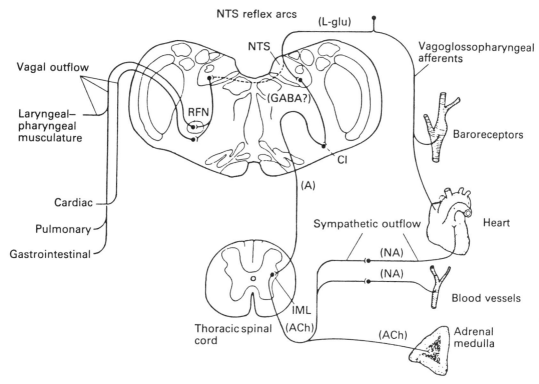

Figure 10-13 Summary of the proposed substrates for baroreceptor and other visceral reflexes. Afferent projections in the vagal and glossopharyngeal nerves terminate in the NTS. The NTS projects (right side of the figure) to the CI region, which in turn projects to the intermediolateral cell column (IML) of the spinal cord, controlling the sympathetic outflow. The NTS also projects (left side of the figure) to the vagal complex controlling the parasympathetic outflow. RFN, retrofacial nucleus; ACh, acetylcholine. (Reproduced with permission from Ross et al., 1985.)

the central delay of the baroreceptor–vagal reflex when comparing a naturally evoked response to that elicited when the sinus nerve was stimulated electrically. The timing between the sinus nerve volley to the natural pulse and the discharge of the vagal neuron was always longer than the measured latency to sinus nerve stimulation. Yet even the latency to sinus nerve stimulation was longer than would have been expected of a virtual segmental reflex involving only the medulla and as few as three synapses. On the basis of the latency there was a hint that indeed two pathways were involved—one relatively direct with a latency of around 20 msec and a second with a latency of 70–80 msec, with the effects of both often being seen in an individual neuron. Similar conclusions have been drawn by others in recordings made from vagal fibers (McCloskey and Potter, 1981). They have further suggested that the short latency pathway is the component blocked by respiratory-related influences and so accounts for respiratory arrhythmias.

The lateralization of the output of the NTS within the medulla would appear to be of major significance (see Figure 10-13). In close proximity of the nucleus ambiguus in the ventrolateral medulla are

groups of bulbospinal neurons that are considered of particular significance in the generation of vasomotor tone (see Guyenet, this volume). Whether the baroreceptor and chemoreceptor pathways involve direct connections with these neurons or whether they are relayed through the A1 cell group or the periambigual area as discussed in Chapter 9 is a matter of speculation. There is, however, a considerable literature that indicates that baroreceptor and chemoreceptor inputs have access to several cell groups within the medulla that have either inhibitory or excitatory connections through bulbospinal pathways with sympathetic preganglionic neurons (see Chapters 8 and 9 and Coote, 1988 for discussion). Many of these may be independent of those pathways that originate in the ventrolateral medulla, and this suggests that the baroreceptor input is widely distributed both at the medullary and at the supramedullary level (see later). This would seem to indicate that for both vagal and sympathetic arms of the baroreceptor reflex and other reflexes, the preganglionic elements are essential integrative units.

Although reflex inputs may be widely distributed and exhibit interactions at several levels with other inputs, it may well be the case that some preferential pathways exist for each particular input. For example, the powerful, relatively direct effects of chemoreceptor inputs on vagal discharge are exerted through connections resembling their baroreceptor inputs. However, the inhibitory actions of this input are mediated by the chemoreceptor control of respiratory drive. These will activate the inspiratory-evoked inhibition of vagal activity (see earlier) but may also have the potential to activate them during postinspiration (see Chapter 11 for discussion).

Atrial vagal afferent inputs are directed specifically to sympathetic outflows to the heart and renal vascular beds and their influences are not modified by baroreceptor inputs (Linden, 1987). They do not have any influence on the vagal control of heart rate and may affect sympathetic outflow through an action on a selected population of ventrolateral medullary neurons (McAllen, 1986; Dampney and McAllen, 1988), but this has yet to be proved. They thus represent an extreme case of specialization, although they may also contribute a weak generalized input to ventrolateral medullary sympathetic pathways (see Guyenet, this volume).

The NTS also communicates with the spinal cord directly (see Loewy and Burton, 1978). The major function of these descending connections is concerned with the control of respiratory motor neurons (Duffin and Lipski, 1987 among others) either through monosynaptic contacts or spinal interneurons. They may also contain elements that influence sympathetic activity through actions on spinal interneurons or propriospinal pathways (see Schramm, 1986). Further, the respiratory pathways themselves may play an important role in regulating sympathetic discharge (Chapter 11).

Elsewhere in this volume Harris and Loewy (Chapter 13) have reviewed the ascending connections of the NTS involved in the regulation of the release of vasopressin. It is reasonable to suppose that these connections are important in the integration of cardiovascular control. It would, however, seem inappropriate at this junction to spend time detailing these anatomical connections since so little is known of their physiological actions. This will, however, become an area of considerable interest in the future and may provide important insight into the mode of action of the CNS. It is clear from both results obtained using anatomical and physiological approaches that cell groups in the hypothalamus, amygdala, midbrain, and forebrain are affected and that both baroreceptor and chemoreceptor influences on circulation are mediated in part by these pathways (see Calaresu 1987). The pontine parabrachial and Kölliker–Fuse nuclei are also strongly implicated, as are the ascending monoaminergic pathways. These same general areas appear to have reciprocal connections with the NTS and

also often have profound connections with the vagal motoneurons. In many cases there are also indications that these areas communicate with the intermediolateral cell column of the spinal cord (see Chapter 6). Such connections demonstrate the richness of the opportunities that exist for the CNS to modify autonomic activity and emphasize the paucity of our existing physiological knowledge of their organization.

ADDITIONAL PATTERNS OF CARDIOVASCULAR ACTIVITY—EXERCISE

The preceding account has indicated the range of potential pathways over which the CNS may elaborate patterns of cardiovascular activity. With regard to affective behavior, a degree of information exists on the specific neural connections that are involved. For other activities this is not so. In the case of exercise, there is evidence that certain subthalamic and probably posterior hypothalamic "centers" regulate, or pattern, both the motor and cardiorespiratory components of the exercise response (Marshall and Timms, 1980; Eldridge et al., 1985). On the basis of the figures presented in published reports, the area probably corresponds to the dorsomedial nucleus of the hypothalamus that has the appropriate brain stem connections (see Saper et al., 1976). Electrical stimulation in these areas in both decorticate and althesin-anesthetized cats evokes both cardiovascular and respiratory changes that are typical of those seen during exercise. Presumably the descending autonomic pathways that have been described above (and Figure 10-11) are used to express these changes in autonomic activity. Unfortunately, there is as yet no specific information regarding the anatomical substrate of this "exercise" center. Some authors are skeptical of its origin, being in the hypothalamus (see Armstrong, 1986 for discussion). Indeed it has been suggested that stimulation involves activation of descending axons of passage that arise from cell bodies in the basal ganglia (Garcia-Rill, 1986). There is an absence of evidence that excitant amino acids injected into the area can evoke similar responses (see Tan and Dampney, 1983). Recent studies have shown, however, that both large and discrete injections of GABA antagonists into the posterior hypothalamus can evoke cardiovascular and respiratory responses (Eldridge et al., 1985; Wardrop et al., 1988). At present these data are not wholly convincing since the techniques employed have been relatively gross. Without additional anatomical information and detailed pharmacological control it is premature to conclude that evidence has been obtained for an exercise program setting substrate. Regardless, the responses evoked by stimulation in these areas are not dependent on baroreceptor or muscle afferent inputs. If indeed either the subthalamic area or basal ganglia are programming the cardiovascular features of exercise it is interesting to see that the functional link with respiration is included so that the descending connections presumably function through brain stem neural mechanisms of the sort described in Chapter 11.

In light of earlier suggestions that a fundamental feature of the CNS control of vagal motoneurons is achieved through a control of the gain and set point of cardiovascular reflexes, it is interesting to note that the set point of the baroreceptor reflex appears to be reset during exercise, although its effectiveness is not markedly influenced. Presumably this indicates that descending signals influence the excitability of vagal cardiomotor neurons, and sympathetic preganglionic neurons, but do not have access to the NTS. This contrasts with the action of descending connections in expressing affective behavior and may be important in maintaining baroreceptor control of sympathetic outflow to ensure appropriate redistribution of peripheral blood flow to prevent precipitous falls in blood pressure. In what manner the different bulbospinal pathways are recruited to provide this control remains a matter of conjecture.

SUMMARY

This chapter has concentrated on providing information about the basic reflex mechanisms that are responsible for the moment-by-moment regulation of the cardiovascular system. This control is provided largely by the action of reflex inputs arising from a range of receptors located in the cardiovascular system itself and in the airways and lungs and within the skeletal muscle. Afferents have been characterized as either mechanoreceptors or chemoreceptors. In relation to the role of the CNS in the integration of these various inputs to the autonomic outflows, consideration has largely been restricted to the arterial baroreceptors, the arterial chemoreceptors, and the slowly adapting pulmonary stretch afferents, since these are reflex inputs for which a reasonable data base is available. In particular, the reflex organization, and control, of the baroreceptor reflex has been a major concern since this may form an adequate model for cardiovascular regulation.

The importance of the nucleus tractus solitarius in the integration of these inputs has been shown, and it is clear that many levels of processing are occurring within this nucleus. Areas of the diencephalon and forebrain that are intimately involved in affec-

tive behavior have access to this nucleus, and there is striking evidence that through both inhibitory and excitatory actions these descending pathways can act to modify the performance of basic cardiovascular and respiratory reflexes. In particular, activating the region of the hypothalamus that is considered to play a role in the expression of affective behavior in the cat leads to a suppression of the baroreceptor reflex, largely through a powerful inhibitory input that is mediated by a local GABAergic interneuron. This is directed to those NTS neurons that are excited by stimulation of the arterial baroreceptors. There is also evidence that these same areas of the brain can exert control of the activity of vagal cardioinhibitory neurons and preganglionic sympathetic neurons by independent descending pathways through the neuraxis. In regard to cardioinhibitory vagal neurons this may result in part by initiating the inspiratory control of their excitability, which is the mechanism responsible for the appearance of respiratory arrhythmias also. In this way regions of the neuraxis concerned with behavioral activities appear to have the opportunity to express cardiovascular responses through a direct control of autonomic preganglionic neurons and also through regulation of both the *gain* and *set points* of reflexes such as the baroreceptor reflex, which is tonically controlling some components of autonomic discharge.

The importance of the interaction between the CNS control of the cardiovascular and respiratory systems has been highlighted in this chapter as indicated above. The neurophysiological basis of these interactions has been summarized, at least with regard to those resulting from the generation of respiratory activity. As yet the actions of inputs related to lung inflation and mediated by vagal afferent discharge have to be identified. However, the interplay of these varied processes and their integration with centrally patterned drives in eliciting behaviorally significant cardiovascular responses have been considered in regard to both orthostasis and exercise, in addition to the responses that accompany affective behavior as already mentioned. The central representation of the control for the former two responses is poorly understood, but some general mechanisms appear to have been identified that contribute to their expression. First, there is the interaction of several reflex inputs, and second the CNS components are able to control the activity of autonomic preganglionic neurons through parallel ascending and descending pathways that are influenced by the various reflex inputs to different extents.

ACKNOWLEDGMENTS

The financial support of the Medical Research Council and British Heart Foundation is gratefully acknowledged. Many present and past colleagues have contributed to the views expressed in this chapter.

REFERENCES

Reviews

Brown, A. M. (1980). Receptors under pressure an update on baroreceptors. *Circulation Research* 46, 1–10.

Chapleau, M. W., Hajduczok, G., and Abboud, F. M. (1988). Mechanisms of resetting of arterial baroreceptors: An overview. *The American Journal of Medical Sciences* 295, 327–334

Coote, J. H. (1988). The organisation of cardiovascular neurons in the spinal cord. *Reviews of Physiology, Biochemistry and Pharmacology* 110, 148–285.

Daly, M. de B. (1983). Peripheral arterial chemoreceptors and the cardiovascular system. In: *Physiology of the Peripheral Arterial Chemoreceptors,* H. Acker and R. G. O'Regan (eds), Elsevier/North-Holland, Amsterdam, pp. 325–393.

Daly, M. de B. (1985). Interactions between respiration and circulation. In: *Handbook of Physiology, The Respiratory System II.* American Physiological Society, Bethesda, MD, pp. 529–594.

Heymans, C., and Neil, E. (1958). *Reflexogenic Areas of the Cardiovascular System.* Churchill, London.

Jänig, W. (1985) Organisation of lumbar sympathetic outflow to skeletal muscle and skin of the cat hindlimb and tail. *Reviews of Physiology, Biochemistry and Pharmacology* 102, 121–213.

Jordan, D., and Spyer, K. M. (1986). Brainstem integration of cardiovascular and pulmonary afferent activity. In: *Progress in Brain Research,* Vol. 67. *Visceral Sensation,* F. Cerevero and J. F. B. Morrison (eds), Elsevier Science Publishers, Amsterdam, pp. 295–314.

Jordan, D., and Spyer, K. M. (1987). Central neural mechanisms mediating respiratory–cardiovascular interactions. In: *Neurobiology of the Cardio-Respiratory System,* E. W. Taylor (ed.), Studies in Neuroscience, University of Manchester Press, Manchester, UK, pp. 342–368.

Kidd, C. (1987). Central nervous pathways of cardiac and pulmonary reflexes. In: *Cardiogenic Reflexes,* R. Hainsworth, P. N. McWilliam, and D. A. S. G. Mary (eds.), Oxford University Press, Oxford, pp. 204–223.

Kirchheim, H. R. (1976). Systemic arterial baroreceptor reflexes. *Physiological Reviews* 56, 100–116.

Ribiero, J. A., and Pallot, D. J. (1987). *Chemoreceptors in Respiratory Control.* Croom Helm, London, Sydney.

Spyer, K. M. (1981). Neural organisation and control of the baroreceptor reflex. *Reviews of Physiology, Biochemistry and Pharmacology* 88, 23–24.

Spyer, K. M. (1988). Central nervous system control of the cardiovascular system. In: *Autonomic Failure,* 2nd ed., Sir R. Bannister (ed.), Oxford University Press, Oxford, pp. 56–79.

Spyer, K. M. (1989). Neural mechanisms involved in cardiovascular control during affective behavior. *Trends in Neuroscience* 12, 506–513.

Research Papers

Abboud, F. M., and Thames, M. D. (1983). Interaction of cardiovascular reflexes in circulatory control. In: *Handbook of Physiology, Section 2—The Cardiovascular System,* Volume III. *Peripheral Circulation and Organ Blood Flow.* Shepherd, J. T., and Abboud, F. M. (eds.). American Physiological Society, Bethesda, MD, pp. 675–753.

Armstrong, D. M. (1986). Supraspinal contributions to the initiation and control of locomotion in the cat. *Progress in Neurobiology* 26, 273–361.

Averill, D. B., Cameron, W. E., and Berger, A. J. (1984). Monosynaptic excitation of dorsal medullary respiratory neurones by slow adapting pulmonary stretch receptors. *Journal of Neurophysiology* 52, 771–785.

Backman, S. B., Anders, C., Ballantyne, D., Rohrig, N., Camerer, H., Mifflin, S., Jordan, D., Dickhaus, H., Spyer, K. M., and Richter, D. W. (1984). Evidence for a monosynaptic connection between slowly adapting pulmonary stretch receptor afferents and inspiratory beta neurones. Pflugers Archiv 402, 129–136.

Baumgarten, R. von, and Kanzow, E. (1958). The interaction of two types of inspiratory neurons in the region of the tractus solitarius. Archieves Italienne de Biologie 96, 361–373.

Berger, A. J., and Dick, T. E. (1987). Connectivity of slowly adapting pulmonary stretch receptors with dorsal medullary respiratory neurons. *Journal of Neurophysiology* 58, 1255–1274.

Biscoe, T. J., and Sampson, S. R. (1970). Response of cells in the brainstem of the cat to stimulation of the sinus, glossopharyngeal, aortic and superior laryngeal nerves. *Journal of Physiology (London)* 209, 359–373.

Bradley, D. J., Paton, J. F. R., and Spyer, K. M. (1987). Cardiovascular responses evoked from the fastigial region of the cerebellum in anaesthetized and decerebrate rabbits. *Journal of Physiology* 392, 475–491.

Calaresu, F. R. (1987). Cardiovascular afferent inputs to limbic neurons. In: *Organisation of the Autonomic Nervous System: Central and Peripheral Mechanisms. Neurology and Neurobiology,* Vol. 31, J. Ciriello, F. R. Calaresu, L. P. Renaud, and C. Polosa (eds.), Liss, New York, pp. 363–375.

Ciriello, J., and Calaresu, F. R. (1981). Projections from buffer nerves to the nucleus of the solitary tract: An anatomical and electrophysiological study in the cat. *Journal of the Autonomic Nervous System* 3, 299–310.

Cox, G. E., Jordan, D., Moruzzi, P., Schwaber, J. S., Spyer, K. M., and Turner, S. A. (1986). Amygdaloid influences on brainstem neurones in the rabbit. *Journal of Physiology (London)* 381, 135–148.

Dampney, R. A. L., and McAllen, R. M. (1988). Differential control of sympathetic fibres supplying hindlimb skin and muscle by subretrofacial neurones in the cat. *Journal of Physiology (London)* 395, 41–56.

Davidson, N. S., Goldner, A., and McCloskey, D. I. (1976). Respiratory modulation of baroreceptor and chemoreceptor reflexes affecting heart rate and cardiac vagal efferent nerve activity. *Journal of Physiology (London)* 259, 523–530.

Davies, R. D., and Kubin, L. (1986). Projection of pulmonary rapidly adapting receptors to the medulla of the cat: An antidromic mapping study. *Journal of Physiology (London)* 373, 63–86.

Doba, N., and Reis, D. J. (1974). Role of the cerebellum and the vestibular apparatus in regulation of orthostatic reflexes in the cat. *Circulation Research* 34, 9–18.

Donoghue, S., and Jordan, D. (1980). The location of cardiac vagal afferent neurones in cat nodose ganglion. *Journal of Physiology (London)* 307, 49P.

Donoghue, S., Garcia, M., Jordan, D., and Spyer, K. M. (1982a). Identification and brain-stem projections of aortic baroreceptor afferent neurones in nodose ganglia of cats and rabbits. *Journal of Physiology (London)* 322, 337–352.

Donoghue, S., Garcia, M., Jordan, D., and Spyer, K. M. (1982b). The brain-stem projections of pulmonary stretch afferent neurones in cats and rabbits. *Journal of Physiology (London)* 322, 353–363.

Donoghue, S., Felder, R. B., Jordan, D., and Spyer, K. M. (1984). The central projections of carotid baroreceptors and chemoreceptors in the cat: A neurophysiological study. *Journal of Physiology (London)* 347, 397–410.

Duffin, J., and Lipski, J. (1987). Monosynaptic excitation of thoracic motoneurones by inspiratory neurones of the nucleus tractus solitarius in the cat. *Journal of Physiology (London)* 390, 415–431.

Eldridge, F. L., Millhorn, D. E., Kiley, J. P., and Waldrop, T. G. (1985). Stimulation by central command of locomotion, respiration and circulation during exercise. *Respiratory Physiology* 59, 313–337.

Fidone, S. J., and Sato, A. (1969). A study of chemoreceptor and baroreceptor A & C fibres in the cat carotid nerve. *Journal of Physiology (London)* 205, 527–548.

Garcia-Rill, E. (1986). The basal ganglia and the locomotor regions. *Brain Research Reviews* 11, 47–63.

Gilbey, M. P., Jordan, D., Richter, D. W., and Spyer, K. M. (1984). Synaptic mechanisms involved in the inspiratory modulation of vagal cardio-inhibitory neurones in the cat. *Journal of Physiology (London)* 356, 65–78.

Izzo, P. N., Lin, R. J., Richter, D. W., and Spyer, K. M. (1988). Physiological and morphological identification of neurones receiving arterial chemoreceptive afferent input in the nucleus tractus solitarius of the cat. *Journal of Physiology (London)* 399, 31P.

Jordan, D., and Spyer, K. M. (1980). Observations on the termination of sinus and aortic nerve afferents. In: *Arterial Baroreceptors and Hypertension,* P. Sleight (ed.), Oxford University Press, Oxford, pp. 227–232.

Jordan, D., Mifflin, S. W., and Spyer, K. M. (1988). Hypothalamic inhibitions of neurones in the nucleus tractus solitarius of the cat is GABA mediated. *Journal of Physiology (London)* 399, 389–404.

Kalia, M., and Mesulam, M.-M. (1980a). Brain stem projections of sensory and motor component of the vagus complex in the cat. I. The cervical vagus and nodose ganglion. *Journal of Comparative Neurology* 193, 435–465.

Kalia, M., and Mesulam, M.-M. (1980b). Brain stem projections of sensory and motor components of the vagus complex in the cat. II. Laryngeal, tracheobronchial, pulmonary, cardiac and gastrointestinal branches. *Journal of Comparative Neurology* 193, 467–508.

Kalia, M., and Richter, D. W. (1985a). Morphology of physiologically identified slowly adapting lung stretch afferents stained with intra-axonal horseradish peroxidase

in the nucleus of the tractus solitarius of the cat. 1. A light microscopic analysis. *Journal of Comparative Neurology* 193, 467–508.

Kalia, M., and Richter, D. W. (1985b). Morphology of physiologically identified slowly adapting lung stretch afferents stained with intra-axonal horseradish peroxidase in the nucleus of the tractus solitarius of the cat. II. An unltrastructural analysis. *Journal of Comparative Neurology* 241, 521–535.

Kaufman, M. P., Longhurst, J. C., Rybicki, K. J., Wallach, J. H., Mitchell, J. H. (1983). Effects of static muscular contraction on impulse activity of groups III and IV afferents in cats. *Journal of Applied Physiology* 55, 105–112.

Kirkwood, P. A., Nisimaru, N., and Sears, T. A. (1979). Monosynaptic excitation of bulbospinal respiratory neurones by chemoreceptor afferents in the carotid sinus nerve. *Journal of Physiology* 293, 35P.

Kniffki, K.-D., Mense, S. L., and Schmidt, R. F. (1981). Muscle receptors with fine afferent fibers which may evoke circulatory reflexes. *Circulation Research* 48, 1-25–31.

Kunze, D. L. (1972). Reflex discharge patterns of cardiac vagal efferent fibres. *Journal of Physiology (London)* 222, 1–15.

Linden, R. J. (1987). The function of arterial receptors. In: *Cardiogenic Reflexes.* Hainsworth, R., McWilliams, P. N., and Mary, D. A. S. G. (eds.). Oxford Science Publications, Oxford, pp. 18–39.

Lipski, J. (1981). Antidromic activation of neurones as an analytic tool in the study of the central nervous system. *Journal of Neuroscience Methods* 4, 1–32.

Lipski, J., McAllen, R. M., and Spyer, K. M. (1975). The sinus nerve and baroreceptor input to the medulla of the cat. *Journal of Physiology (London)* 251, 61–78.

Lipski, J., McAllen, R. M., and Trzebski, A. (1976). Carotid baroreceptor and chemoreceptor inputs onto single medullary neurons. *Brain Research* 107, 132–136.

Loewy, A. D., and Burton, H. (1978). Nuclei of the solitary tract; efferent projection to the lower brainstem and spinal cord of the cat. *Journal of Comparative Neurology* 181, 421–450.

Malliani, A. (1986). Homeostasis and instability: The hypothesis of tonic interaction in the cardiovascular regulation of negative and positive feedback mechanisms. In: *Neural Mechanisms and Cardiovascular Disease,* B. Lown, A. Malliani, and M. Prosdocimi (eds.), Fidia Research Series Vol. 5, Livinia Press, Padova, pp. 1–11.

Marshall, J. M., and Timms, R. J. (1980). Experiments on the role of the subthalamus in the generation of the cardiovascular changes during locomotion in the cat. *Journal of Physiology (London)* 301, 92–93P.

McAllen, R. M. (1986). Action and specificity of ventral medullary vasopressor neurones in the cat. *Neuroscience* 18, 51–59.

McAllen, R. M., and Spyer, K. M. (1978). The baroreceptor input to cardiac vagal motoneurones. *Journal of Physiology (London)* 282, 365–374.

McCloskey, D. I., and Potter, E. K. (1981). Excitation and inhibition of cardiac vagal motoneurones by electrical stimulation of the carotid sinus nerves. *Journal of Physiology (London)* 316, 163–175.

Mifflin, S. W., and Felder, R. B. (1988). An intracellular

study of time-dependant cardiovascular afferent interactions in nucleus tractus solitarius. *Journal of Neurophysiology* 59, 1798–1813.

Mifflin, S. W., Spyer, K. M., and Withington-Wray, D. J. (1987). Intracellular labelling of neurones receiving carotid sinus nerve inputs in the cat. *Journal of Physiology (London)* 387, 60P.

Mifflin, S. W., Spyer, K. M., and Withington-Wray, D. J. (1988a). Baroreceptor inputs to the nucleus tractus solitarius in the cat: Postsynaptic actions and the influence of respiration. *Journal of Physiology (London)* 399, 349–367.

Mifflin, S. W., Spyer, K. M., and Withington-Wray, D. J. (1988b). Baroreceptor inputs to the nucleus tractus solitarius in the cat: Modulation by the hypothalamus. *Journal of Physiology (London)* 399, 369–387.

Millhorn, D. E. (1986). Neural respiratory and circulatory interaction during chemoreceptor stimulation and cooling of ventral medulla in cats. *Journal of Physiology (London)* 370, 217–231.

Miselis, R. S., Rogers, W. T., Schwaber, J. S., and Spyer, K. M. (1989). Localisation of cardiomotor neurons in the anaesthetised rat; choleratoxin HRP conjugate and pseudorabies labelling. *Journal of Physiology (London)* 416, 63P.

Miura, M., and Reis, D. J. (1972). The role of the solitary and paramedian reticular nuclei in mediating cardiovascular reflex responses from carotid baro- and chemoreceptors. *Journal of Physiology (London)* 225, 525–548.

Pascoe, J., Bradley, D. J., and Spyer, K. M. (1989). Interactive responses to stimulation of the amygdaloid central nucleus and baroreceptor afferents in the rabbit. *Journal of the Autonomic Nervous System* 26, 157–167.

Potter, E. K. (1981). Inspiratory inhibition of vagal responses to baroreceptor and chemoreceptor stimuli in the dog. *Journal of Physiology (London)* 316, 177–190.

Richter, D. W., Jordan, D., Ballantyne, D., Meesmann, M., and Spyer, K. M. (1986). Presynaptic depolarization in myelinated vagal afferent fibres terminating in the nucleus of the tractus solitarius in the cat. *Pflugers Archiv* 406, 12–19.

Ross, C. A., Ruggiero, D. A., and Reis, D. J. (1985). Projections from the nucleus tractus solitarii to the rostral vertrolateral medulla. *Journal of Comparative Neurology* 242, 511–534.

Samodelov, L. F., Godehard, E., and Arndt, J. D. (1979). A comparison of the stimulus-response curves of aortic and carotid sinus baroreceptors in decerebrate cats. *Pflugers Archiv* 383, 47–53.

Saper, C. B., Loewy, A. D., Swanson, L. W., and Cowan, W. M. (1976). Direct hypothalamo-autonomic connections. *Brain Research* 117, 305–312.

Schramm, L. P. (1986). Spinal factors in sympathetic regulation. In: *Central and Peripheral Mechanisms of Cardiovascular Regulation,* A. Magro, W. Osswald, D. Reis, and P. Vanhoutte (eds.), Plenum, New York, pp. 303–352.

Spyer, K. M. (1984). Central control of the cardiovascular system. In: *Recent Advances in Physiology,* 10, P. F. Baker (ed.), Churchill Livingstone, Edinburgh, pp. 163–200.

Spyer, K. M., Jordan, D., and Wood, L. M. (1985). Central organisation of cardiovascular reflex mechanisms. In: *Proceedings of an International Symposium of the Neural Mechanisms and Cardiovascular Disease.* Santa Marghcrita Ligure, Genova. Liviana Press, Padova, pp. 145–156.

Tan, E., and Dampney, R. A. L. (1983). Cardiovascular effects of stimulation of neurones within the 'defence area' of the hypothalamus and midbrain of the rabbit. *Clinical Experimental Pharmacology and Physiology* 10, 299–303.

Waldrop, T. G., Bauer, R. M., and Iwamoto, G. A. (1988). Microinjection of GABA antagonists into the posterior hypothalamus, locomotor activity and a cardiorespiratory activation. *Brain Research* 444, 84–94.

11

Cardiorespiratory Control

D. W. RICHTER AND K. M. SPYER

The primary role of both the cardiovascular and the respiratory systems in vertebrates is the exchange of respiratory gases between the external environment and the tissues. The respiratory system, involving either gills or lungs, has evolved together with the cardiovascular system, and only in cooperation can the two systems ensure maintenance of the appropriate diffusion gradients for oxygen and carbon dioxide between air (or water) and blood, and between arterial blood and the tissues. Tissue respiration thus depends on the physiological adjustments of both respiratory and cardiovascular functions. With regard to lung breathing in vertebrates, this is represented by a closely linked nervous control of alveolar ventilation, cardiac output, and peripheral blood flow. In this chapter we indicate why this makes it inappropriate to consider the control of either system separately. Our thesis is that there is a direct coupling between the neuronal structures involved in their regulation, which we term "cardiorespiratory regulation."

In this particular respect our description represents a return to a conceptual model that had been the basis of much of the nineteenth- and early twentieth-century attitudes toward this area of physiology (Anrep et al., 1936a,b; Hering, 1869; Traube, 1865). This reversion from the contemporary consideration of separate control systems for each function seems justified, as a number of recent studies of various peripheral and central inputs to these reticular networks have demonstrated that, rather than affecting either respiratory or cardiovascular functions, they influence both systems simultaneously in a manner that appears to have considerable physiological significance. Such close interaction rules against considering any one sensory system, for example, arterial baroreceptors or peripheral and central chemoreceptors, as having a specific role dedicated to the regulation of either the cardiovascular or respiratory function alone.

The powerful reflex interactions involving the nervous structures that control respiratory and cardiovascular functions have been reviewed in detail elsewhere (Daly, 1972; Koepchen, 1962; Schlaefke, 1981; Spyer, 1981, 1982; among others), and the central projections of these afferents and the organization of their central reflex pathways are described in Chapters 6, 9, and 10). Here we will concentrate on the synaptic interactions between those brain stem neurons that generate the discharge patterns displayed by the autonomic innervation of the heart, blood vessels, pupil, and kidney on the one hand and the respiratory (i.e., diaphragm, intercostal, abdominal, and laryngeal) muscles on the other. We will indicate how "cardiorespiratory" function may be controlled by a group of "cardiorespiratory" interneurons and both respiratory and cardiovascular premotor neurons, and we will attempt to demonstrate the ways in which physiologically relevant changes in the cardiovascular and respiratory control are organized to support behavioral activities that can be summarized as essentially matching respiratory minute volume to cardiac output.

DISCHARGE CHARACTERISTICS OF EFFERENT OUTFLOWS

In considering the neural basis of the interactions between the cardiovascular and respiratory systems, it is necessary to review the patterns of discharge that are characteristic of their respective neuronal outflows.

The central nervous output to respiratory muscles is largely rhythmic and is to some extent independent of peripheral feedback for its patterning (for review see von Euler, 1986; Feldman, 1987). The rhythmic discharge in sympathetic and vagal outflows to the heart, vascular beds, pupil, and kidney, although obviously more sensitively affected by reflex inputs from the periphery, and a variety of higher central nervous structures (for review see

Jänig, 1985; Spyer, 1981, among others), is also rhythmic and strongly modified in synchrony with the central respiratory activity (Cohen and Gootman, 1969, 1970; for review see Jänig, 1985; Koepchen, 1983). This respiratory modulation is seen in various recordings of mass and unitary sympathetic activities, although its pattern differs between animal species (Numao et al., 1987). Interestingly, both neuronal systems are particularly resistant to the effects of anesthetics when compared to other neuronal systems controlling motor activity. Central respiratory activity has the ability to influence the performance of basic cardiovascular and respiratory reflexes, and, by altering their efficacy, to

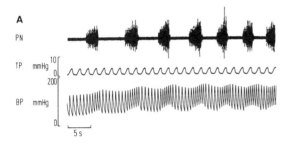

A

PN

TP mmHg

BP mmHg

5 s

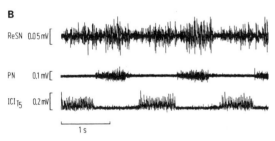

B

ReSN 0.05 mV

PN 0.1 mV

ICI T5 0.2 mV

1 s

Figure 11-1 Respiratory modulation of cardiovascular activities. (A) Sinus arrhythmia and blood pressure (BP) waves indicating modulation of vagal cardiomotor activity related to the central respiratory activity. The tracheal pressure (TP) was measured as an index for artificial ventilation of the anesthetized cat occurring independently from the central respiratory rhythm indicated by the phrenic nerve discharge (PN). (B) Respiratory modulation of sympathetic activity measured in an anesthetized and artificially ventilated cat with denervated baroreceptors. The recording from the renal nerve (ReSN) shows respiration-related modulations of sympathetic activity. The respiration-related fluctuations in activity become evident by correlating this activity with the inspiratory discharge of the phrenic nerve (PN) and the expiratory discharge of the internal branch of the fifth intercostal nerve (ICI$_{T5}$). The respiratory modulation has a biphasic pattern as sympathetic activity peaks during the late period of inspiration and expiration. Sympathetic activity is minimal during the early period of inspiration and during postinspiration, which approximately corresponds with the phase of phrenic nerve afterdischarge occurring in the period between the end of inspiration (after peak phrenic nerve discharge) and the onset of stage 2 expiration (discharge in the intercostal nerve). (From Bainton et al., 1985.)

affect the discharge of the respective autonomic and ventilatory outputs (Barillot, 1970; Davidson et al., 1976; Koepchen et al., 1981; Richter and Seller, 1975; Richter et al., 1986c). This action was first recognized by Anrep and his colleagues (1936a,b) who showed that sinus arrhythmia, the respiratory related variations in heart rate, resulted from two distinct mechanisms: one involving the central nervous system alone and the second depending on pulmonary afferent activity. In Figure 11-1A the first of these is shown to occur within the central nervous system as a change in heart rate is associated with the central respiratory rhythm, shown as phrenic nerve activity, while the lungs are inflated independently at a different rate in the paralyzed and artificially ventilated cat. The fall in heart rate during the expiratory interval in the rhythmic phrenic neurogram, whether or not the lungs are inflated, is a consequence of an expiratory discharge of the vagal nerves innervating the heart (Iriuchijima and Kumada, 1964; Kunze, 1972; McAllen and Spyer, 1978). The synaptic mechanisms underlying this phenomenon will be described more fully subsequently. Reflex inputs associated with lung inflation—Anrep's second mechanism—can similarly produce an acceleration of heart rate during inspiration and so contribute to sinus arrhythmia.

The sympathetic innervation of the heart and blood vessels, as well as the innervation of the kidney (Figure 11-1B), which may have a major vasomotor function, and the pupil show fluctuations of discharge related to respiration as well (Cohen and Gootman, 1969, 1970; Jänig, 1985; Numao et al., 1987; Seller et al., 1968). Several mechanisms have been shown to contribute to this modulation. First, the discharge of sympathetic nerves is strongly affected by baroreceptor inputs that evoke a pulse pressure-related inhibition of sympathetic activity, but the effectiveness of this inhibition varies within the respiratory cycle (Davidson et al., 1976; Seller et al., 1968). Another type of respiratory modulation of the sympathetic discharge, which becomes more obvious after denervation of arterial baroreceptors, occurs centrally and has been assumed to result from a close connection between the "vasomotor" and "respiratory centers" (Adrian et al., 1932). These assumptions provide effective explanations for the respiratory modulation of sympathetic activity, and together indicate that there must be synaptic interactions between the respiratory and the cardiovascular neurons within the brain stem or spinal networks (Cohen and Gootman, 1969, 1970; Connelly and Wurster, 1985a,b; Koepchen et al., 1981; Polosa et al., 1980).

Electrophysiological studies, however, have stressed the importance of propriobulbar subsystems of the respiratory network in eliciting respiratory influences on the sympathetic network (Bainton et al., 1985; Gilbey et al., 1986; McAllen, 1987; Numao et al., 1987). These imply that synaptic interaction between the respiratory and sympathetic systems largely, although not exclusively, occurs at the brain stem level. The strikingly similar discharge patterns in medullary respiratory neurons and the sympathetic outflows, which will be detailed later, and their disappearance after lesioning descending bulbospinal pathways (Connelly and Wurster, 1985a) suggest that an additional component of the respiratory imprinting of sympathetic discharge results from the actions of the respiratory network at the spinal level (Kirkwood et al., 1988; Sears, 1964b; Sears et al., 1982). This may imply an action of a common pool of thoracic interneurons (Gebber and McCall, 1976) or a divergent branching of bulbospinal respiratory neurons, or alternatively a mixture of both. The manner in which sympathetic activity is modulated during the respiratory cycle is varied within, and between, animal species. There is, however, a systematic pattern to this variation. Augmentation of activity occurs either during the inspiratory phase, that is, during early and/or late inspiration, and depression during postinspiration, or, alternatively, there is depression during inspiration and augmentation during postinspiration (compare Bainton et al., 1985; Jänig, 1985; Numao et al., 1987). During the second stage of expiration (see below) most sympathetic nerves discharge tonically (Figures 11-1B and 11-2).

Laryngeal muscles also reveal respiration-related activities (Barillot and Dussardier, 1976; Harding, 1984) and they control expiratory airflow during normal breathing (Harding, 1984; Remmers and Bartlett, 1977). In cooperation with them, respiratory muscles are also used in vocalization where their homeostatic rhythmic activity must be modified to meet the imposed demands of speech. Their rhythmic activity can similarly be entrained to locomotor rhythm, presumably involving vestibular and cerebellar control (or processing) (Bradley et al., 1987) and during locomotion (Feldman and Grillner, 1983; Sears, 1964a,b; Viala, 1986). Accordingly, the central respiratory rhythm is not the only pattern of discharge that may be displayed by the spinal motor outflow to the muscles controlling breathing movements. The same is true for the outflow in autonomic nerves that have tonic components of activity unrelated to ventilation (Barman and Gebber, 1976; Langhorst et al., 1981). For longer periods there is, however, the clear necessity of maintaining a close relationship between the cardiovascular and respiratory systems to achieve a "cardiorespiratory homeostasis," as outlined above.

These neuronal interactions can be analyzed by observing in both short (milliseconds) and long time frames (seconds–minutes) the occurrence of related rhythms in the central networks that generate the respective motor outputs. This parameter, a measurement of coincident neuronal discharge, reveals a close similarity between the patterns of discharge of various subgroups of medullary respiratory neurons and the pattern of discharge in sympathetic and cardiomotor vagal neurons (Figure 11-2), as well as in bronchomotor neurons and in laryngeal motoneurons. But it is important to note that the slow conduction in postganglionic sympathetic pathways imposes a considerable phase shift on coincident events

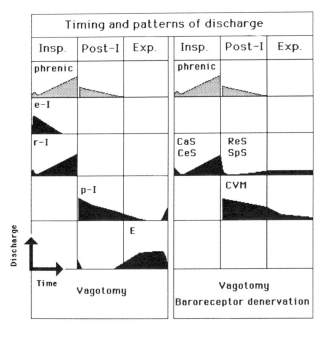

Figure 11-2 Timing and patterns of discharge of respiratory and cardiovascular neurons. The time frequency profile of the discharge of early (e-I), ramp (r-I), late (l-I), and postinspiratory (p-I) as well as stage 2 expiratory (E) neurons is illustrated schematically in the left panel and that of the cardiac (CaS), cervical (CeS), renal (ReS), and splanchnic (SpS) sympathetic neurons as well as vagal cardiomotor (CVM) neurons of the cat in the right panel. These activity patterns are related to the inspiratory, postinspiratory, and stage 2 expiratory phase of the respiratory cycle as indicated by the phrenic nerve discharge (PN). The illustration refers to the descriptions given by Bainton et al. (1985), Cohen and Gootman (1970), and Numao et al. (1987).

and complicates comparisons of the patterning of phrenic, intercostal, and sympathetic nerve discharges. Detailed analysis (see later) of the coincident activity in the two systems can justifiably be made only on neurons whose cell bodies are contained within the brain stem and spinal cord. Such a comparison, however, particularly when applied to the premotor brain stem neurons, allows a degree of functional correlation to be extracted that is not simply a measure of the connectivity between two individual neurons, as indicated by spike-triggered averaging of the postsynaptic effect of single afferent inputs, but contains the possibility of demonstrating the functional significance of synaptic coupling and integration of synaptic activity within a complex neuronal circuitry. This analysis of the synaptic activity produced by convergence of afferent inputs from different subsystems of the network onto a single cell can yield a potentially important, though complex, degree of functional information concerning the integration of various synaptic inputs. Such correlations also take note of the effects of nonsynaptic mechanisms, such as passive and active membrane properties of the individual neurons, that can determine temporal alterations in the responsiveness of a particular group of neurons and may also explain the occurrence of specific periods when the overall systems are perturbed (Champagnat et al., 1986; Hirst and McLachlan, 1986; McLachlan and Jänig, 1983; Richter, 1982; Richter et al., 1986b). This analysis, therefore, allows insight into the integrative neuronal mechanisms that control ventilatory and cardiovascular functions.

RESPIRATORY RHYTHM

In considering the rhythmic interrelationship between the cardiovascular and respiratory systems it is essential to define precisely the basic components of what is the dominant rhythm, namely, that of respiration. In an anesthetized, paralyzed, and artificially ventilated animal, this can be identified by recording the inspiratory, and postinspiratory, activity of the phrenic nerve, the expiratory activity of intercostal nerves, and/or the inspiratory, postinspiratory, and expiratory discharge of medullary neurons as illustrated in Figures 11-1 and 11-3. Central neural inspiratory discharge, like peripheral inspiratory movements, develops gradually as seen in the ramplike increase of the averaged phrenic nerve activity. This is followed by a sudden reduction in discharge that marks the end of inspiration and resets the activity to 30–50% of its maximum level. Phrenic

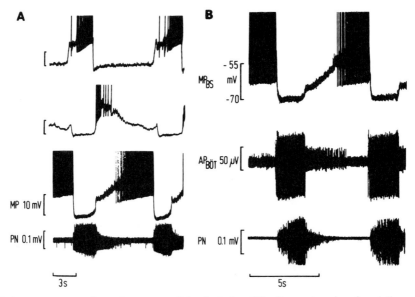

Figure 11-3 Discharge patterns and membrane potential trajectories of the three categories of medullary respiratory neurons. The normal respiratory rhythm is three phased, consisting of inspiratory, postinspiratory, and stage 2 expiratory phases. Each phase is represented within the brain stem by a corresponding population of respiratory neurons. The membrane potential (MP) trajectories underlying the discharge activity of these neurons are shown in A in three intracellular recordings performed independently in the anesthetized cat. The consecutive alternation of their discharge is shown in B in a simultaneous recording from all three types of neurons in addition to the phrenic nerve (PN). The bulbospinal neuron discharging during stage 2 of expiration was recorded intracellularly (MP$_{BS}$) from the ventral group of respiratory neurons within the lower brain stem, whereas the inspiratory (large spikes) and postinspiratory (small spikes) neurons were recorded extracellularly within the Bötzinger complex (AP$_{BöT}$). Action potentials are partly retouched in A.

nerve activity then declines at a variable rate in a period representing the first stage of expiration (stage 1 of expiration or postinspiration, synonymously). The magnitude of this "after-discharge" of phrenic motoneurons following inspiration (Gesell and White, 1938) actively controls the recoil action of lungs and thorax by regulating the intrathoracic pressure (Shee et al., 1985) and the flow resistance within the upper airways by modifying the movements of the vocal cords (Bartlett et al., 1973; Harding, 1984). During quiet breathing such "passive expiration" lasts for more than 70% of the total expiratory interval (Shee et al., 1985). At the time the phrenic nerve becomes silent there is a corresponding period of activity in expiratory muscles (Figure 11-1B) that represents the second phase of expiration (active expiration, stage 2 of expiration) and is the third phase of the respiratory cycle. All three phases—inspiration, postinspiration, and stage 2 expiration—are most clearly represented in the alternating discharge of medullary inspiratory, postinspiratory, and expiratory neurons (Figure 11-3).

There is a large body of evidence that the basic respiratory rhythm is dependent on the interaction of these groups of medullary neurons. These appear to be localized within two general areas of the medulla—the dorsal respiratory group in the nucleus of the tractus solitarius and the ventral group in the nucleus ambiguus–retroambigualis complex (see Figure 11-9). Many of the neurons contained within these groups have restricted patterns of axonal projection collateralizing only within the medulla, and these are termed *propriobulbar neurons.* Others are bulbar output neurons having axons running within the vagus nerve to the laryngeal muscles or descending axonal projections onto the respiratory motoneurons within the spinal cord, and onto spinal interneurons. The former are termed *laryngeal motoneurons* and the latter *bulbospinal neurons,* although they may well also send axon collaterals into other regions of the medulla (Merrill, 1974, for review).

Figure 11-3B provides a simultaneous recording of the discharge of all three types of medullary respiratory neuron. The discharge of each representative neuron is accompanied by a characteristic change in the excitability of the same and the other two classes of respiratory neurons. This can be demonstrated by cross-correlating their discharge (Feldman and Speck, 1983; Graham and Duffin, 1981a,b; Hilaire et al., 1984; Lindsay et al., 1987; Long and Duffin, 1984; Segers et al., 1985, 1987) and is seen in intracellular recordings from individual neurons in depolarized or hyperpolarizing "unitary" changes in the membrane potential (Merrill and Fedorko, 1984; Merrill et al., 1983) that by integration produce the respiration-related, slow fluctuations in the

membrane potential (see Ballantyne and Richter, 1984, 1986; Richter et al., 1979; among others). An essential control of the discharge of respiratory neurons in the adult as well as in the newborn animal is exerted by synaptic inhibition mostly producing voltage- and chloride-dependent membrane conductance changes (Lawson et al., 1988; Richter et al., 1979) that are sensitive to appropriate blocking substances (Champagnat et al., 1982; Haji et al., 1986). Figure 11-3B shows an example of the temporal correlation between the simultaneously recorded discharge of the three major categories of respiratory neurons (see also Figure 11-4). In the first instance, in a recording taken from a medullary "ramp inspiratory" neuron (Figures 11-3A and 11-4), there is a steep depolarization with the onset of inspiration, as measured by phrenic nerve discharge, that slowly augments and gives rise to a ramp-like pattern of action potential discharge (compare Figure 11-2). This is followed by a rapid repolarization extending to a maximal hyperpolarization during postinspiration (stage 1 expiration), the magnitude of which slowly declines during the remainder of the expiratory interval. The mechanism underlying this hyperpolarization is synaptic inhibition as verified by IPSP[1] reversal using intracellular chloride injection or passage of negative dc current (Richter, 1982). This wave of expiratory membrane hyperpolarization results from a summation of two inhibitory inputs, shown schematically in Figure 11-4 (right panel, second trace), which arises respectively, from the postinspiratory and the stage 2 expiratory network (see the white, vertically clipped areas).

Conversely, in Figure 11-3A (second trace), in a recording taken from another respiratory neuron, stage 1 expiration is accompanied by a distinct period of membrane depolarization with repolarization starting during this same phase of the cycle and continuing into stage 2 expiration. Marked hyper-

[1]Abbreviations: *Respiratory Phases:* Insp., inspiration; Post-I., postinspiration; Exp., stage 2 expiration. *Neurons/nerves:* e-I, early inspiratory neuron; r-I, ramp inspiratory neuron; l-I, late inspiratory neuron; p-I, postinspiratory neuron; E, stage 2 expiratory neuron; E_{bs}, expiratory bulbospinal neuron; I_{bs}, inspiratory bulbospinal neuron; CaS, cardiac sympathetic nerve; CeS, cervical sympathetic nerve; ReS, renal sympathetic nerve; SpS, splanchnic sympathetic nerve; CVM, vagal cardiomotor neuron; PN, phrenic nerve; ICI, internal intercostal nerve; AP, action potential; MP, membrane potential; BS, bulbospinal; EPSP, excitatory postsynaptic potential; IPSP, inhibitory postsynaptic potential. *Nervous Structures:* PH, nucleus praepositus hypoglosssi; ST5, spinal trigeminal tract; IO, inferior olive; RP, nucleus raphe magnus; P, pyramidal tract; RB, restiform body; AP, area postrema; Cl, lateral cuneate nucleus; TS, tractus solitarius; XII, hypoglossal nucleus; RVL, rostral ventrolateral medulla; CVL, caudal ventrolateral medulla; NA, nucleus ambiguus; DMV, dorsal vagal motor nucleus; SMP, spinal motoneuron pool; IML, intermediolateral nucleus; MLF, medial longitudinal fasciculus; BÖT, Bötzinger complex; VRG, ventral group of respiratory neurons; DRG, dorsal group of respiratory neurons.

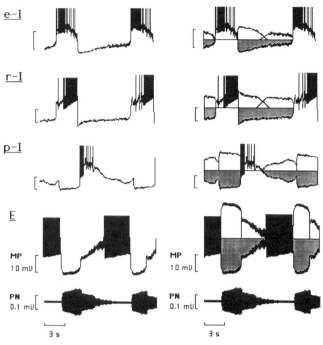

Figure 11-4 Action potential discharge, membrane potential trajectories, and underlying postsynaptic activities of medullary respiratory neurons. The membrane potential trajectories (MP) and action potential discharge of early inspiratory (e-I), ramp inspiratory (r-I), postinspiratory (p-I), and stage 2 expiratory (E) neurons recorded intracellularly within the ventral region of the brain stem are shown in temporal relation to phrenic nerve activity (PN) in the left panel. The same recordings are used in the right panel to indicate the patterns of postsynaptic inhibition modifying the activity of the neurons. Inhibitory synaptic potentials that are hyperpolarizing (gray areas) under control conditions can be reversed by chloride and/or current injection. The resulting waves of reversed inhibitory potentials are indicated by the vertically clipped (white) areas that are further split into various components and tentatively related to the different phases of the respiratory cycle to indicate the patterns of inhibitory inputs converging onto the neurons. The waves of "reversed" inhibitory synaptic potentials correspond with the discharge patterns of neurons that are active during that phase of the cycle.

polarization occurs during the following inspiration. This neuron is characterized as a "postinspiratory" neuron. Its membrane repolarization and hyperpolarization result from inspiratory and stage 2 expiratory synaptic inhibition as indicated in Figure 11-4 (third trace).

In the third group of neurons, maximal membrane depolarization is attained during stage 2 expiration (Figure 11-3A, third trace; Figure 11-3B, upper trace). Here, membrane depolarization starts with the end of inspiration, but further depolarization is delayed, and is often effectively suppressed during postinspiration, and develops fully only when postinspiration ceases, that is, at the time stage 2 expiration is initiated, as indicated in the neurograms of phrenic and intercostal nerves. Stage 2 expiratory neurons are strongly inhibited throughout inspiration because they receive both early inspiratory and continuous IPSPs throughout inspiration and subsequently postinspiratory IPSPs (Figure 11-4, fourth trace).

Another interneuron with inhibitory function, found within the dorsal and ventral part of the respiratory network, is the early inspiratory neuron (Figure 11-4, upper traces). This neuron depolarizes rapidly at the onset of inspiration, but this depolarization diminishes, partly as a consequence of intrinsic membrane properties (Merrill, 1974), and also as a result of synaptic inhibition during the second half of inspiration. It remains hyperpolarized throughout expiration, presumably as a result of postinspiratory and stage 2 expiratory synaptic inhibitory inputs

(Figure 11-4, right panel, first trace). Accordingly, the respiratory cycle can be subdivided into three distinct phases with each of the major subgroups of respiratory neurons becoming alternately active (see Figure 11-3B). These distinct periods of activity are seen in the motor outputs to the respiratory muscles, the accessory muscles of ventilation, and in other neural systems controlling the airways (and also in autonomic outflows, see below). Although these three distinct phases are apparent in the different categories of medullary respiratory neuron, their durations and form vary greatly in relation to the physiological state of the animal, including humans.

On the basis of the data presented, it is our belief that the overall respiratory pattern is largely determined by the postinspiratory phase. This is most obvious during conscious modifications of breathing, for example, during speaking or swallowing, but also during unconscious adjustments of breathing that accompany arousal. Under pathophysiological conditions this dominance of the postinspiratory activity produces disturbances to the respiratory rhythm (Richter et al., 1986a). The apnea resulting from protective reflexes, such as those evoked by activation of laryngeal afferents, is mediated largely through a prolonged activation of postinspiration (Remmers et al., 1986), whereas the hyperpnea associated with fever, or lung edema, involves a reduction, or absence, of stage 2 expiration leaving a two-phased central respiratory rhythm with a rapid alternation between inspiration and postinspiration (Richter, 1982). An example of the latter situation is

illustrated in Figure 11-5 where electrical stimulation of the vagus nerve at an intensity sufficient to
excite nonmyelinated pulmonary afferents evokes
rapid shallow breathing (Coleridge et al., 1983; Paintal, 1973). Here the membrane potential of an intracellularly recorded expiratory neuron shows an absence of stage 2 expiratory depolarization but a
persistence of inspiratory and postinspiratory inhibition (indicated by hatched areas in the middle
trace of Figure 11-5). This confirms that the central
respiratory rhythm can alternate between two phases
under such circumstances. Similar breathing patterns occur during the defense reaction in cats (Ballantyne et al., 1986) and in some species, such as the
dog, where temperature is controlled in part by ventilation. The absence of active expiratory movements allows rapid shallow ventilation (panting) at
an increased functional residual capacity that pro-
tects the organism from respiratory alkalosis and so
ensures cardiorespiratory homeostasis during thermoregulatory control.

In Figure 11-6, the most crucial patterns of excitatory and inhibitory postsynaptic activity are summarized for early, ramp, and postinspiratory neurons and stage 2 expiratory neurons that have been
seen in original recordings before (Figures 11-3 and
11-4) under situations of both quiet and rapid shallow breathing. This schema illustrates that inhibitory synaptic interactions dominate the sequence of
activity of the respiratory network. This involves
early inspiratory inhibition of postinspiratory, stage
2 expiratory and late inspiratory neurons (not illustrated here), late inspiratory inhibition of early inspiratory neurons, postinspiratory inhibition of early
inspiratory, ramp inspiratory and stage 2 expiratory

neurons, and stage 2 expiratory inhibition of early
inspiratory, ramp inspiratory, and postinspiratory
(and late inspiratory) neurons. This pattern of postsynaptic inhibition leads to the configurations of discharge of respiratory neurons that have been shown
in Figures 11-2 and 11-4.

The most significant recurrent excitatory synaptic
interactions are evident in ramp inspiratory neurons
whose pattern of discharge depends on incrementing
membrane depolarization. Such accumulation of
excitation is not seen in early inspiratory and postinspiratory neurons, although EPSPs become visible during their active periods. Intrinsic membrane properties such as low-threshold calcium currents (Richter et al., 1986b) are involved in the process of
rebound depolarization when these neurons are released from preceding synaptic inhibition. A similar
intrinsic mechanism appears to be involved in triggering the onset of ramp inspiratory neurons. A surprising result of analyzing the excitatory postsynaptic activity of expiratory neurons is the observation
that under quiet breathing conditions they do not
seem to receive a summated pattern of excitation, as
might be inferred from their augmenting discharge
pattern (see Figure 11-2). Rather, these neurons receive a tonic excitatory drive that is modified by a
declining pattern of synaptic inhibition. The resultant augmenting discharge is thus the consequence
of a decline of synaptic inhibition from inspiratory
and postinspiratory neurons that fades gradually
through postinspiration with some continuation
possibly also into stage 2 expiration (see the Figures
11-4 and 11-6). In periods of rapid shallow breathing, synaptic interactions remain largely as described
above, except that stage 2 expiratory neurons are not

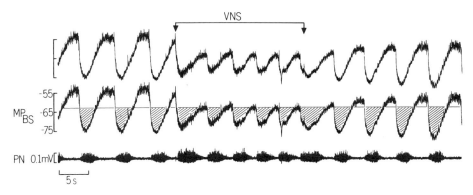

Figure 11-5 Respiratory phases during rapid shallow breathing. A bulbospinal expiratory neuron of the ventral respiratory group was recorded intracellularly while the proximal branch of the severed cervical vagus nerve was electrically stimulated (VNS) at high intensities (1.4 V, 0.05 msec, 80 cps) to excite pulmonary C-fibers. During stimulation phrenic nerve discharge (PN) revealed a pattern that would cause rapid shallow breathing movements if the anesthetized cat would not have been paralyzed and artifically ventilated. The membrane potential trajectories (MP$_{BS}$) of the expiratory neuron showed that stage 2 expiration failed during rapid shallow breathing while the inspiratory and postinspiratory phases persisted. The membrane potential is shown in two identical traces; inspiratory and postinspiratory synaptic inhibition is indicated in the lower trace by the hatched areas.

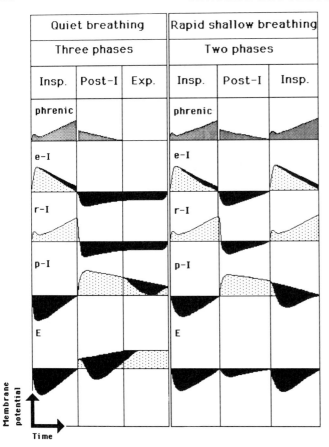

Quiet breathing			Rapid shallow breathing		
Three phases			Two phases		
Insp.	Post-I	Exp.	Insp.	Post-I	Insp.

Figure 11-6 Post synaptic activities in medullary respiratory neurons during quiet and rapid shallow breathing. The figure provides a schematic illustration of the postsynaptic activities measured in different types of medullary respiratory neurons during quiet, three-phase (left panel), and rapid shallow, two-phase (right panel) breathing patterns as seen in the phrenic nerve discharge (phrenic) of the anesthetized and artificially ventilated cat. Excitatory postsynaptic potentials (EPSPs) are shown as dotted areas and inhibitory postsynaptic potentials (IPSPs) as black areas. Abbreviations as for Figure 11-2.

activated and stage 2 expiratory inhibition is thus absent in inspiratory and postinspiratory neurons (Figure 11-6).

RESPIRATORY MODULATION OF CARDIAC VAGAL AND SPINAL SYMPATHETIC NEURONS

Similar variations in membrane potential and spike discharge associated with respiratory activity have been observed in the outflows that are concerned with cardiovascular control. This is particularly evident in those vagal neurons that innervate the heart that have a marked expiratory rhythm in their discharge (Iriuchijima and Kumada, 1964; Kunze, 1972; McAllen and Spyer, 1976, 1978). This activity is dependent on a tonic activation of an unknown origin, baroreceptor reflex activation, and synaptic inhibition that occurs during early inspiration. On the basis of their postsynaptic activity vagal cardioinhibitory neurons are very similar to postinspiratory neurons (Gilbey et al., 1984; see Figure 11-7). It is, however, still unclear whether the decline of the expiratory discharge of these neurons results from

stage 2 expiratory inhibition, as in the case of postinspiratory neurons, or from adaptation that is determined by intrinsic membrane properties of these neurons.

Various patterns of respiratory modulation have been observed in different sympathetic nerves of various species, demonstrating that sympathetic efferents are heterogeneous (Bainton et al., 1985; Cohen and Gootman, 1969, 1970; Jänig, 1985; Numao et al., 1987) and subserve numerous functions that vary from vasoconstrictor (and even these may have significantly different properties depending on the particular vascular bed they innervate), to pilomotor, sudomotor, pupillodilator, cardioaccelerator, and so on. It is hardly surprising that although the three phases of the respiratory rhythm can be seen in their activity, respiratory modulation varies greatly among classes. Indeed, in the anesthetized preparation many sympathetic neurons are silent, but when their activity is raised by application of excitatory pharmacological agents, subliminal respiratory modulation, of an equivalent form to that observed in neurons with ongoing activity, is revealed (Gilbey et al., 1986). This underlines the fundamental importance of the central respiratory rhythm. Although respiratory modulation of the discharge of various sympathetic nerves seems variable, and even for the same nerves seems to differ among animal species, there is usually a clear relation to one or the other of the three phases of the respiratory cycle. In the cat, augmenting activation during the late period of inspiration combined with depression during early inspiration and postinspiration is seen in the splanchnic, cardiac, cervical, and renal nerves (Bainton et al., 1985; Cohen and Gootman, 1969, 1970; Connely and Wurster, 1985a,b). The same sympathetic nerves reveal a different pattern of respiratory modulation in the rat (Numao et al., 1987). There is, however, a systematic pattern within this variation in discharge in that activation during one phase of respiration is accompanied by depression during an antagonistic phase. Thus, suppression occurs during postinspiration when sympathetic discharge is enhanced during inspiration, and early inspiratory depression occurs when the discharge is enhanced during postinspiration. Identified muscular vasoconstrictor nerves of the cat behave in a same manner (Jänig, 1985). If we convert activation of sympathetic discharge into postsynaptic excitation, and depression of discharge into postsynaptic inhibition, then we would expect a sequence of postsynaptic

events to occur in sympathetic neurons that is similar to that seen in respiratory neurons. This is illustrated schematically in Figure 11-7 for the cervical sympathetic neurons in the cat, but the consequences of phase shifts due to the different conduction times must be remembered.

Preliminary analysis of intracellular recordings from individual preganglionic sympathetic neurons within the thoracic spinal cord of the cat (Figure 11-8) reveals that under a normal central respiratory drive the neurons are not only controlled by tonic excitatory and inhibitory inputs from the reticular formation but also phasically driven by excitation related to medullary respiratory activity and possibly also modulated by phasic respiration-related inhibition (which in Figure 11-8 may partly derive from intact baroreceptor and pulmonary receptor afferents). Postsynaptic excitation becomes visible during inspiration and repolarization during postinspiration and stage 2 expiration (Figure 11-8B). There is some reduction of the synaptic noise occurring during early inspiration that could be taken as an index for the arrival of early inspiratory inhibition at the spinal level (or disfacilitation of bulbospinal sympathetic neurons) and might explain the late inspiratory onset of action potential discharge (Figure 11-8A). Thoracic sympathetic neurons that discharge in a manner similar to cervical sympathetic neurons, therefore, seem to behave as late inspiratory neurons in that they are inhibited or disfacilitated during early inspiration and receive inhibition or disfacilitation (K. Dembowsky, personal communication) of variable strength during postinspiration (Figure 11-7). Tonic excitatory drive, and mutual inhibition of early inspiratory neurons and postinspiratory neurons, may therefore produce the primary rhythm not only in the respiratory (Richter et al., 1986a) but also in the cardiovascular network within the brain stem.

LOCALIZATION OF NEURONS

There is an extensive literature indicating that the basic respiratory rhythm and tonic activity in the sympathetic nervous system remain intact in the decerebrate preparation (for review see Ciriello et al., 1986; Gebber, 1980; Hilton and Spyer, 1980). This suggests that the neural networks responsible for respiratory rhythm generation and the interactions between the central respiratory and cardiovascular networks are contained within the lower brain stem. There are certainly anatomical associations between those neurons that have been shown using a variety of techniques to be involved in the control of the circulation and respiration. Figure 11-9 provides a simple diagrammatic representation of the similar distributions of a proportion of these cell groups.

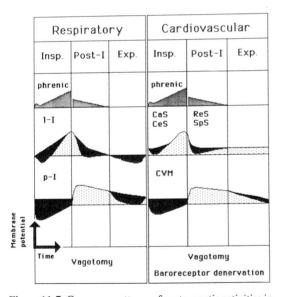

Figure 11-7 Common patterns of postsynaptic activities in respiratory and cardiovascular neurons. The scheme shows the membrane potential trajectories of intracellularly analyzed early inspiratory (e-I), late inspiratory (l-I), postinspiratory (p-I), and vagal cardiomotor (CVM) neurons of the cat. It also indicates which membrane potential changes could be inferred from the discharge pattern of respective nerves in cardiac (CaS), cervical (CeS), and splanchnic (SpS) sympathetic neurons of the cat. Excitatory postsynaptic potentials as dotted areas and inhibitory postsynaptic potentials as black areas.

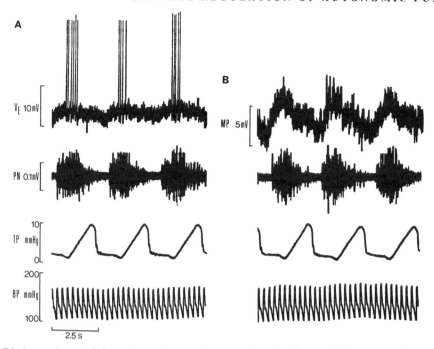

Figure 11-8 Discharge characteristics and membrane potential trajectories of sympathetic preganglionic neurons in the thoracic spinal cord. The discharge pattern of the neuron is illustrated in A in temporal relationship to the central respiratory rhythm as indicated by the phrenic nerve activity (PN) together with the tracheal pressure (TP) and arterial blood pressure (BP). The discharge pattern was determined in extracellular recordings before the neuron was further analyzed for the underlying postsynaptic activities in intracellular recording techniques, which are illustrated in B. The measurements were performed in the anesthetized and artificially ventilated cat with intact baroreceptors and pulmonary afferents. (From Gilbey, Numao, and Spyer, in preparation.)

Ignoring the pontine nuclei that have been shown to be involved in both cardiovascular and respiratory control (Bianchi and Barillot, 1982; Segers et al., 1985), the rostral ventrolateral medulla (Figure 11-9, RVL) seems to represent the most cranial medullary region that contains groups of neurons considered to be involved in the generation of sympathetic activity and the maintenance of arterial blood pressure (see Chapter 9). This part of the medulla is just caudal to the Bötzinger complex (Figure 11-9, BOT), a region believed to be involved in the initiation and timing of the respiratory rhythm (Bianchi and Barillot, 1982; Lipski and Merrill, 1980). These may be two separate groups of neurons or a single concentration whose pattern of axonal projection determines their multiple functional roles.

More caudally in the dorsomedial medulla oblongata, the nucleus of the solitary tract acts as the primary integrative station for the reflex inputs that regulate both the cardiovascular and respiratory systems (see Chapter 10). This complex of several subnuclei of the nucleus tractus solitarius contains a major population of dorsal groups of premotor respiratory neurons (Figure 11-9, DRG; see: Euler, 1986 and Feldman, 1987 for reviews) and interneu-

rons involved in the reflex control of the respiratory rhythm that receives afferent inputs from the lungs, airways, and larynx, called R-β or pump neurons (Anders and Richter, 1987; Averill et al., 1984; Backman et al., 1984; Davies and Kubin, 1986; Davies et al., 1987; McCrimmon et al., 1988; Panteleo and Corda, 1986), as well as from arterial chemoreceptors (chemoneurons; see Chapter 10). The area surrounding the solitary tract also contains interneurons receiving converging afferent inputs from the aortic and carotid sinus baroreceptors and other afferents and from rostral structures of the brain involved in cardiovascular control (see Chapter 10). Adjacent to this is the dorsal vagal motonucleus, which contains vagal preganglionic neurons including in some animal species a proportion of those that innervate the heart (Hopkins, 1987; Jordan and Spyer, 1987). In most species the major source of the vagal preganglionic innervation of the heart arises from, or near, the nucleus ambiguus in the ventrolateral medulla—the loose formation of the nucleus ambiguus (Hopkins 1987). These are located close to the caudal ventrolateral group of cardiovascular neurons (Figure 11-9, CVL) that seems to have direct projections to sympathetic preganglionic neu-

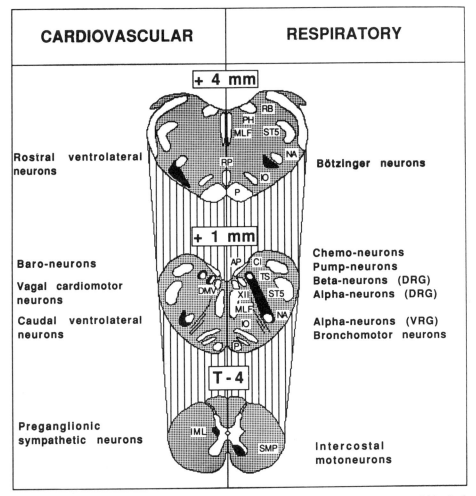

Figure 11-9 Schematic presentation of the localization of cardiovascular and respiratory neurons within the lower brain stem and the spinal cord. The localizations of cardiovascular neurons are indicated by black areas on the left side and those of respiratory neurons are indicated on the right side. Neighboring structures are shown as white areas for orientation. Pontine structures and those regions on the ventral surface of the medulla oblongata that might be involved in "central chemoreception" are not considered in this scheme. Note that the localizations of neurons reveal considerable overlap, which is even more extensive when the dimensions of the somatodendritic trees of these neurons are considered. The labels of various brain structures are explained in footnote 1.

rons (see Chapters 8 and 9). They are also in the vicinity of laryngeal motoneurons of the nucleus ambiguus, bronchomotor neurons in the ventroambigual region (Spyer, 1984; Spyer and Jordan, 1987), and ventral group respiratory neurons in the retroambigualis complex that extends from the rostral medulla to the first cervical segments of the spinal cord (Aoki et al., 1980; Lipski and Duffin, 1986; Merrill, 1974).

The innervation of the diaphragm arises from the phrenic motonucleus in segments C3–6 of the spinal cord (Berger et al., 1984; Duron et al., 1979; Lipski and Duffin, 1986). The intercostal muscles are innervated from the motoneurons of the thoracic spinal cord (T1–12) with the abdominal muscles that are involved in expiratory movements being inner-

vated by motoneurons of the thoracic and lumbar spinal cord (Hilaire and Monteau, 1976; Sears, 1964b). At thoracic levels, the dendrites of sympathetic preganglionic neurons are again in close proximity to respiratory motoneurons, though they are restricted to the intermediolateral nucleus (Dembowsky et al., 1985; McLachlan and Jänig, 1983).

It is conceivable that this close anatomical localization of these neurons may not be relevant to a functional coupling, but from a range of physiological evidence it appears likely to form the morphological basis for the direct axosomatic, axodendritic, or dendrodendritic synaptic interactions between respiratory and cardiovascular neurons that are responsible for three-phase synchronization (see Gilbey et al., 1984).

A MODEL FOR THE CARDIORESPIRATORY NETWORK

Extensive reviews have been published on the nature of the networks that are responsible for generating and maintaining respiratory (Long and Duffin, 1986; Euler, 1986; Feldman, 1987) and cardiovascular-related activities (see Chapter 8; Jänig, 1985; Spyer, 1981). It is not our intention to repeat that material. Rather we seek to establish the processes by which the different categories of respiratory and autonomic premotor neurons share common rhythms, to identify the physiological significance of these interactions, and then propose a model that integrates the cardiovascular and the respiratory control systems within the brain stem (Figure 11-10). This model represents a modification of that first proposed by Richter et al. (1986a) for the generation of respiratory rhythm and is expanded to include the principal control networks for sympathetic and vagal activity primarily related to circulatory regulation. Reflex inputs from peripheral receptors and afferent inflow from higher nervous structures are not considered in terms of the functioning of the

model, although it is reasonable to assume that they will act in modifying cardiorespiratory activity by accessing to this network at several sites. The model is based on the assumption that tonic excitatory drive inputs (not illustrated in the scheme) arise from the reticular formation (Hugelin and Cohen, 1963; Millhorn et al., 1980) including the structures responsible for central chemoreception (Schlaefke, 1981) or from tonically active pacemaker neurons (Champagnat et al., 1983; Chapter 9) and that phasic synaptic interactions that are either excitatory (white arrows) or inhibitory (black arrows) occur between neurons of different categories that are classified according to the phase within the respiratory cycle when the probability of their discharge is greatest (see footnote 1).

Tonic Drive

The model indicates synaptic interconnections within the network that ultimately evoke a rhythmic cardiorespiratory pattern of discharge in premotor neurons that relies on an extrinsic tonic excitatory input. The origin of this tonic drive is not known. Our thesis is that the cardiorespiratory output is dictated by a general reticular control of respiratory and autonomic neurons, the easiest analogy being the reticular "activating" and "deactivating" systems (Hugelin and Cohen, 1963; Magoun, 1950; Magoun and Rhines, 1946). The alternative is the existence of specific subsets of neuron in the medulla and upper cervical cord that could become endogenously active (Aoki et al., 1980; Suzue, 1984; see also Champagnat et al., 1983; Chapter 9) and that these neurons provide a tonic drive to the system. Whatever the nature of this input, its effectiveness is "gated" or "shunted" by intrinsic membrane conductances of the neurons of the network and by the synaptic interactions that include both tonic and phasic excitatory and inhibitory inputs (Camerer et al., 1979; Sears et al., 1982). Indeed the postinspiratory network that has been described earlier has an inhibitory feedback influence on the reticular formation (Richter, 1982) and may alter the degree of tonic activation of the cardiovascular and respiratory systems in this way. This postinspiratory network may also represent a major component of a tonic "deactivating" reticular system that is itself shaped by inhibitory (inspiratory) inputs. Its interaction with the tonic excitatory drive—a manifestation of the "reticular activating system"—would thus shape the patterns of respiratory and cardiovascular discharge in relation to behavior. Most certainly there is evidence that the postinspiratory network (and possibly also the early inspiratory network; see Figure 11-10) is functionally heterogeneous (Richter et al., 1987) since it may also exert excitatory influences on some

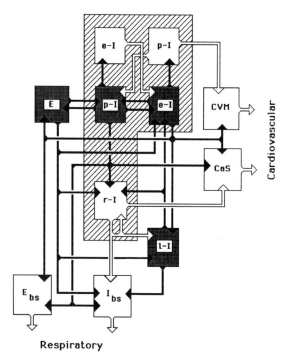

Figure 11-10 Scheme of a combined cardiorespiratory network. The scheme indicates a circuitry of synaptic interconnections between "respiratory" and "cardiovascular" neurons within the lower brain stem of cats. Excitatory connections are illustrated as white arrows and inhibitory connections as black arrows. A fuller description is provided in the text. The scheme is an expanded version of the descriptions first given by Richter et al. (1986a).

cardiovascular and respiratory premotor neurons. This activating postinspiratory network influences a range of motoneurons regulating the laryngeal (Barillot and Dussardier, 1976; Richter et al., 1987) and oropharyngeal muscles (Hwang et al., 1983; Mathew et al., 1982; Mifflin et al., 1986a), trigeminal activity (St. John and Bledsoe, 1985), and several other motor networks (Schmidt-Vanderheyden et al., 1970). It has an important behavioral role being prominent during vocalization, as in the cat, but is relatively less apparent in the rat, which uses vocalization to a lesser degree. Presumably in humans with their extensive use of speech, postinspiratory activity exerts an even more important function.

To assess the adequacy of our model, we should now move sequentially through the processes that occur within the network on it being brought to action through a tonic excitatory input.

Inspiration

The activating reticular formation excites, either directly or indirectly, all components of the cardiorespiratory network, but this is primarily a tonic and unpatterned influence. It will contribute a tonic yet variable input to ramp inspiratory, early inspiratory, stage 2 expiratory, expiratory bulbospinal, and components of the sympathetic network, and probably a weak input to vagal cardiomotor neurons. This tonic excitatory drive is thus analogous to the tonic expiratory drive described by Sears et al. (1982), which has been revealed in intracellular recordings (see earlier). Recycling excitation within the network of ramp inspiratory will initiate the incrementing inspiratory discharge ("inspiratory ramp generator") that is seen in inspiratory bulbospinal neurons, and in the phrenic nerve discharge, but not in late inspiratory neurons where early inspiratory inhibition shunts the excitatory input from ramp inspiratory neurons. Early inspiratory inhibition will also shunt the synaptic inputs to postinspiratory, stage 2 expiratory, sympathetic, and vagal cardiomotor neurons of the cat. The decline of early inspiratory discharge, which results partly from intrinsic membrane properties of these neurons such as an activity related (calcium- and voltage-dependent) increases in potassium conductances (Merrill, 1974, Champagnat et al., 1986; Mifflin and Richter, 1987; Richter et al., 1986b), reduces the shunting effect so that late inspiratory neurons gradually become active. There is suggestive evidence that these act to reduce and finally block early inspiratory discharge through their inhibitory synaptic connections. This initial decline and final block of early inspiratory activity is a key feature in the generation of rhythmic activity within the respiratory network. This progressive suppression of early inspiratory activity reduces inhibition

throughout the whole respiratory and sympathetic network of the cat. The augmenting inspiratory discharge is then able to develop fully and the excitatory inputs from the inspiratory ramp generator to the sympathetic neurons become marked with removal of the inhibitory "shunt." Disinhibition of late inspiratory neurons, however, occurs, which then limits the discharge of ramp inspiratory and inspiratory bulbospinal neurons leading to the "transient inspiratory off switch" (Euler, 1977; Richter et al., 1986a; Younes et al., 1978).

Early inspiratory and possibly also late inspiratory inhibition (not included into the scheme) of vagal cardiomotor neurons is pronounced and totally suppresses what must be a relatively weak tonic excitatory input from the reticular formation. Vagal cardiomotor neurons, therefore, remain silent during inspiration (Gilbey et al., 1984).

Postinspiration

Postinspiratory neurons, which in addition to early inspiratory neurons constitute a major group of inhibitory neurons of the "cardiorespiratory oscillator" (and probably also constitute an important component of the "deactivating reticular formation"), are progressively released from early inspiratory inhibition and depolarize to threshold as a consequence of a low-threshold Ca conductance, which is reactivated during the period of membrane hyperpolarization in early inspiration. Postinspiratory neurons then begin to discharge action potentials. The rapid onset of their firing "irreversibly" terminates the discharge of the inspiratory network, and this is reinforced by a concurrent disfacilitation through the removal of the excitatory drive to the network from the activating reticular formation, on which postinspiratory neurons exert an inhibitory influence. Tonic activation of stage 2 expiratory neurons within the Bötzinger complex and caudally located stage 2 expiratory bulbospinal neurons is further shunted by synaptic inhibition. Most sympathetic neurons in the cat are disfacilitated in a similar way and, in addition, many appear to receive a direct inhibition from postinspiratory neurons.

Vagal cardiomotor neurons in the cat are the only neurons in the model network released from inspiratory inhibition and, as a result of an increased excitability, which may be reinforced by direct postinspiratory excitation, discharge during postinspiration. This is consistent with the assumption that the early inspiratory and postinspiratory networks are not homogeneously inhibitory, but consist of excitatory and inhibitory subsystems. This is most clearly the case for the postinspiratory subsystem that partly is excitatory and widely distributes this pattern of activity to other brain stem structures modulating the discharge not only of inspiratory bulbospinal neurons and phrenic motoneurons (Gesell and White, 1938; Kirkwood et al., 1988; Shee et al., 1985) but also of the laryngeal (Harding, 1984), hypoglossal (Hwang et al., 1983; Mifflin et al., 1986b), and trigeminal neurons (St. John and Bledsoe, 1985). Such excitatory postinspiratory inputs may also directly activate the discharge of vagal cardiomotor neurons in the cat through synaptic excitation within the medulla.

Inactivation of postinspiratory discharge due to intrinsic membrane properties, which are similar to those acting in early inspiratory neurons, brings this phase to an end and enables stage 2 expiration (quiet breathing) or the next inspiration to start (rapid shallow breathing).

Stage II Expiration

Release from both early inspiratory and postinspiratory inhibition allows stage 2 expiratory neurons to respond to the tonic excitation they receive from the reticular formation. There is no evidence from electrophysiological studies that a pronounced recycling of excitation is needed within the stage 2 expiratory network to evoke an expiratory ramp discharge. The steady increase in stage 2 expiratory discharge results rather from a slowly declining pattern of inhibition by postinspiratory neurons that is superimposed on a tonic excitatory drive from the reticular formation. Incrementing discharge of stage 2 expiratory neurons thus seems to originate in a declining inhibition by postinspiratory neurons. Activation of the various types of sympathetic neuron that display a prominent discharge during stage 2 expiration is likely to be explained in a similar way.

Stage 2 expiratory activity exerts an inhibitory action on the inspiratory and postinspiratory network within the medulla, but its dependence on a tonic drive indicates that it will be highly modified by other events and indeed is very sensitive to the physiological state as we have stressed earlier. Activation of stage 2 expiratory neurons may well be totally suppressed if excitatory inputs to the inspiratory network dominate, and this may be sufficient for the production of rapid breathing patterns. Then muscular vasoconstrictor tone and vagal cardiomotor activity are increased in a reciprocal manner during such breathing patterns.

Respiratory Apnea

Activation of afferent inputs originating in the larynx, blockade of afferent activity from peripheral chemoreceptors by hyperoxic hyperventilation, or lesioning/cooling central chemoreceptive structures can produce respiratory arrest, which is accompanied by weak tonic discharges of inspiratory and expiratory motoneurons (Sears et al., 1982; Schlaefke, 1981) and superior laryngeal neurons (Fukuda and Honda, 1983). These effects are consistent with the concept that respiratory arrest is a result of tonic activation of postinspiration (Remmers et al., 1986). According to the model presented here, such tonic activation of the postinspiratory network should depress inspiratory and stage 2 expiratory activity and thus enhance the discharge of vagal cardiomotor neurons in the cat. Pronounced bradycardia is in fact the most evident effect on the cardiovascular system in many adult (Schlaefke, 1981) and neonatal mammals (Downing and Lee, 1975; Lee et al., 1977) under such conditions. Respiratory modulation of cardiac sympathetic activity of the cat disappears during such apneas (Connelly and Wurster, 1985b), and this can be explained by reduction of early inspiratory inhibition and ramp inspiratory activation and the continuing discharge of pI neurons, which would be predicted to have a tonic inhibitory effect on the reticular drive to these neurons. These observations are, therefore, consistent with the predictions of the model as presented. The complex cardiovascular responses that accompany respiratory changes evoked reflexly may well find their explanation in the patterns of connection made by these different inputs with the different components of the "cardiorespiratory" oscillator we have described.

IS THERE A COMMON CARDIORESPIRATORY OSCILLATOR?

The surprisingly close similarities between respiratory and cardiovascular neural activities indicate that parts of the respiratory and cardiovascular central neural networks are shared (Figure 11-10, hatched area), constituting a "common cardiorespiratory oscillator." The essential components of this oscillator seem to be 3-fold: the early inspiratory, ramp inspiratory, and postinspiratory activities (Figure 11-11). Stage 2 expiratory activity is not essential, as it may fail completely, as described above, while rhythmic behavior continues. This oscillator produces two components of rhythmic excitation superimposed on a tonic excitatory reticular drive, and these are seen in the efferent outflow, namely, in an augmenting inspiratory and a declining expiratory discharge. The oscillator would also produce two rhythmic components, namely, early inspiratory and postinspiratory activities that are mutually inhibitory and effectively modify the discharge of the outflows.

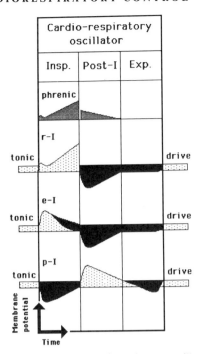

Figure 11-11 A common cardiorespiratory oscillator? The three—ramp (r-I), early (e-I), and postinspiratory (p-I)—subsystems of the cardiorespiratory network are suggested to constitute a common "cardiorespiratory oscillator." These components convert the excitatory, tonic drive from the activating reticular formation into rhythmic activity with alternating periods of rebound and synaptic excitation (dotted areas) and synaptic inhibition (black areas). For further explanation see text.

COMMENTS

There are important implications emerging from this model that are consistent with the suggestions of other laboratories (Koepchen, 1983; Koepchen et al., 1981). Primarily these concern the method of ascribing a functional role to medullary neurons whose ongoing discharge is modulated by respiration. Such neurons cannot be ascribed a function on the basis of their pattern of discharge alone because on the basis of our model they may belong to one or the other control system. To be truly provocative and to stimulate new experimental approaches, we would like to suggest that they belong to a "common cardiorespiratory network" within the lower brain stem. The cardiorespiratory network we describe consists of a limited number of (three, or at most five) subsystems with a fairly distinct pattern of activity that are common, namely, an excitatory ramp inspiratory and the two inhibitory, but possibly also excitatory early and postinspiratory networks. The

"respiratory movements of the vascular system" described by Hering in 1869 may be controlled by this cardiorespiratory network. However, the presence of respiratory-modulated discharge does not necessitate the functional dedication of the neuron to a cardiorespiratory role, since this rhythm can extend to other systems. The location, connections, and additional inputs to a particular neuron will add to its functional classification. The underlying rhythm may thus represent a basic tonic drive, that is state dependent, and attains a major functional significance only in a limited number of neurons.

SUMMARY

The cardiovascular and respiratory systems have had to develop in vertebrates for the exchange of respiratory gases between the external environment and the tissues. To maintain "cardiorespiratory homoeostasis" it is necessary to establish appropriate diffusion gradients for oxygen and carbon dioxide between air and blood and between blood and the tissue. Thus, the two effective pumps, the heart and the respiratory muscles, cannot work independently but have to be adjusted in synchrony to accomplish the respiratory requirements of the organism. The continuous adjustment of the systems requires nervous control, and the neuronal structures involved in that control must be linked closely or even combined to form a single entity.

In this chapter we have concentrated on the organization of the neuronal networks within the brain stem and the spinal cord that are involved in the control of cardiorespiratory function. We have described the tonic and rhythmic activities of the respiratory and cardiovascular systems and then have endeavored to relate these peripheral discharges to the activity of central neurons within the appropriate control networks of the brain stem and the spinal cord. The possible structure and pattern of synaptic interaction between these neuronal networks were then discussed on the basis of the results of intracellular analysis in individual elements of the networks. The close similarity of the neural mechanisms controlling these different activities has led us to propose a model for a cardiorespiratory network that describes the interactions of cardiovascular and respiratory neurons. It includes a "cardiorespiratory oscillator" that is common to the systems but that depends on the activity of two antagonistic reticular inputs. Many of the proposed interconnections are based on indirect arguments, and further experiments are necessary to confirm their occurrence. Yet they can explain many physiological properties of cardiovascular and respiratory control.

REFERENCES

Reviews

Camerer, H., Richter, D. W., Röhrig, N., and Meesmann, M. (1979). Lung stretch receptor inputs to Rβ-neurons, a model for "respiratory gating." In: *Central Nervous Control Mechanisms in Breathing*, C. von Euler and H. Lagercrantz (eds.), Pergamon, Oxford, pp. 261–266.

Daly, M. de B. (1972). Interaction of cardiovascular reflexes. In: *Scientific Basis of Medicine Annual Review*, University of London, Atholone Press, London, pp. 307–332.

Euler, C. von (1977). The functional organization of the respiratory phase-switching mechanisms. *Federation Proceedings* 36, 2375–2380.

Euler, C. von (1986). Brain stem mechanisms for generation and control of breathing pattern. In: *Handbook of Physiology*, Section III: *The Respiratory System*, A. P. Fishman, N. S. Cherniack, J. G. Widdicombe, and S. R. Geiger (eds.), American Physiological Society, Bethesda, MD, pp. 1–67.

Feldman, J. L. (1987). Neurophysiology of breathing in mammals. In: *Handbook of Physiology: The Nervous System*, Vol. IV, F. E. Bloom (ed.), American Physiological Society, Bethesda, MD, pp. 463–524.

Gebber, G. L. (1980). Bulbospinal control of sympathetic nerve discharge. In: *Neural Control of Circulation*, M. J. Hughes and C. D. Barnes (eds.), Academic Press, New York, pp. 51–80.

Harding, R. (1984). Function of the larynx in the fetus and newborn. *Annual Review of Physiology* 46, 645–659.

Hilton, S. M., and Spyer, K. M. (1980). Central nervous regulation of vascular resistance. *Annual Review of Physiology* 42, 399–411.

Hopkins, D. A. (1987). The dorsal motor nucleus of the vagus nerve and the nucleus ambiguus; structure and connections. In: *Cardiogenic Reflexes*, R. Hainsworth, P. N. McWilliam, and D. A. G. G. Many (eds.), Oxford University Press, Oxford, pp. 185–203.

Hugelin, A., and Cohen, M. I. (1963). The reticular activating system and respiratory regulation in the cat. *Annals of the New York Academy of Science* 109, 586–603.

Jänig, W. (1985). Organization of the lumbar sympathetic outflow to skeletal muscle and skin of the cat hindlimb and tail. *Review of Physiology, Biochemistry and Pharmacology* 102, 119–213.

Koepchen, H. P. (1962). *Die Blutdruckrhythmik*. D Steinkopff Verlag, Darmstadt.

Koepchen, H. P. (1983). Respiratory and cardiovascular "centres," functional entirety or separate structures? In: *Central Neurone Environment*, M. E. Schläfke, H. P. Koepchen, and W. R. See (eds.), Springer-Verlag, Berlin, Heidelberg, pp. 221–237.

Magoun, H. W. (1950). Caudal and cephalic influences of the brain stem reticular formation. *Physiological Reviews* 30, 459–474.

Merrill, E. G. (1974). Finding a respiratory function for the medullary respiratory neurons. In: R. Bellairs and E. G. Gray (eds.), *Essays on the Nervous System*, Clarendon Press, Oxford, pp. 451–486.

Paintal, A. S. (1973). Vagal sensory receptors and their reflex effects. *Physiological Review* 53, 159–227.

Richter, D. W. (1982). Generation and maintenance of the respiratory rhythm. *Journal of Experimental Biology* 100, 93–107.

Richter, D. W., Ballantyne, D., and Remmers, J. E. (1986a). Respiratory rhythm generation: a model. *News In Physiological Sciences* 1, 109–112.

Schlaefke, M. E. (1981). Central chemosensitivity: A respiratory drive. *Review of Physiology, Biochemistry and Pharmacology* 90, 171–244.

Spyer, K. M. (1981). Neural organization and control of the baroreceptor reflex. *Review of Physiology, Biochemistry and Pharmacology* 88, 23–124.

Spyer, M. K. (1982). Central nervous integration of cardiovascular control. *Journal Experimental Biology* 100, 109–128.

Spyer, K. M. (1984). Central control of the cardiovascular system. In: *Recent Advances in Physiology*, P. F. Porter (ed.), Churchill Livingstone, Edinburgh, pp. 163–200.

Research Papers

Adrian, E. D., Bronk, D. W., and Phillips, G. (1932). Discharges in mammalian sympathetic nerves. *Journal of Physiology (London)* 74, 115–153.

Anders, K., and Richter, D. W. (1987). Morphology of medullary pump-neurones of cats. *Pflugers Archiv* 408, R54.

Anrep, G. V., Pascual, W., and Rössler, R. (1936a). Respiratory variations of the heart rate. I. The reflex mechanism of the sinus arrhythmia. *Proceedings of the Royal Society of London, Series B* 119, 191–217.

Anrep, G. V., Pascual, W., and Rössler, R. (1936b). Respiratory variations of the heart rate. II. The central mechanism of the sinus arrhythmia and the inter-relationships between central and reflex mechanisms. *Proceedings of the Royal Society of London, Series B* 119, 218–230.

Aoki, M., Mori, S., Kawahara, K., Watanabe, H., and Ebata, N. (1980). Generation of spontaneous respiratory rhythm in high spinal cats. *Brain Research* 202, 51–63.

Averill, D. B., Cameron, W. E., and Berger, A. J. (1984). Monosynaptic excitation of dorsal medullary respiratory neurons by slowly adapting pulmonary stretch receptors. *Journal of Neurophysiology* 52, 771–785.

Backman, S. B., Anders, K., Ballantyne, D., Roehrig, N., Camerer, H., Mifflin, S., Jordan, D., Dickhaus, H., Spyer, K. M., and Richter, D. W. (1984). Evidence for a monosynaptic connection between slowly adapting pulmonary stretch receptor afferents and inspiratory beta neurones. *Pflugers Archiv* 402, 129–136.

Bainton, C. R., Richter, D. W., Seller, H., Ballantyne, D., and Klein, J. P. (1985). Respiratory modulation of sympathetic activity. *Journal of the Autonomic Nervous System* 12, 77–90.

Ballantyne, D., and Richter, D. W. (1984). Post-synaptic inhibition of bulbar inspiratory neurones in the cat. *Journal of Physiology (London)* 348, 67–87.

Ballantyne, D., and Richter, D. W. (1986). The non-uniform character of expiratory synaptic activity in expiratory bulbospinal neurones of the cat. *Journal of Physiology (London)* 370, 433–456.

Ballantyne, D., Jordan, D., Spyer, K. M., and Wood, L. M. (1986). Synaptic inhibition of caudal medullary expiratory bulbospinal neurones during hypothalamic stimulation in the cat. *Journal of Physiology (London)* 376, 32P.

Barillot, J. C. (1970). Depolarization presynaptique des fibres sensitives vagales et laryngeales. *Journal of Physiology (Paris)* 62, 273–294.

Barillot, J. C., and Dussardier, M. (1976). Activité des motoneurones larynges expiratoires. *Journal of Physiology (Paris)* 72, 311–343.

Barman, S. M., and Gebber, G. L. (1976). Basis for synchronization of sympathetic and phrenic nerve discharges. *American Journal of Physiology* 231, 1601–1607.

Bartlett, D., Remmers, J. E., and Gauthier, H. (1973). Laryngeal regulation of respiratory airflow. *Respiratory Physiology* 18, 194–204.

Berger, A. J., Cameron, W. E., Averill, D. B., Kramis, R. C., and Binder, M. D. (1984). Spatial distribution of phrenic and medial gastrocnemius motoneurons in the cat. *Experimental Neurology* 86, 559–575.

Bianchi, A. L., and Barillot, J. C. (1982). Respiratory neurons in the region of the retrofacial nucleus: Pontile, medullary, spinal and vagal projections. *Neuroscience Letters* 31, 227–282.

Bradley, D. J., Pascoe, J. P., Paton, J. F. R., and Spyer, K. M. (1987). Cardiovascular and respiratory responses evoked from the posterior cerebellar cortex and fastigial nucleus in the cat. *Journal of Physiology (London)* 393, 107–121.

Champagnat, J., Denavit-Saubie, M., Moyanova, S., and Rondouin, G. (1982). Involvement of amino acids in periodic inhibitions of bulbar respiratory neurones. *Brain Research* 327, 351–365.

Champagnat, J., Denavit-Saubie, M., and Siggins, G. R. (1983). Rhythmic neuronal activities in the nucleus of the tractus solitarius isolated in vitro. *Brain Research* 280, 155–159.

Champagnat, J., Jacquin, T., and Richter, D. W. (1986). Voltage-dependent currents in neurones of the nuclei of the solitary tract of rat brainstem slices. *Pflugers Archiv* 406, 372–379.

Ciriello, J., Caverson, M. M., and Polosa, C. (1986). Function of the ventrolateral medulla in the control of the circulation. *Brain Research Review* 11, 359–391.

Cohen, M. I., and Gootman, P. M. (1969). Spontaneous and evoked oscillations in respiratory and sympathetic discharge. *Brain Research* 16, 265–268.

Cohen, M. I., and Gootman, P. M. (1970). Periodicities in efferent discharge of splanchnic nerve of the cat. *American Journal of Physiology* 218, 1092–1101.

Coleridge, H. M., Coleridge, J. C. G., and Roberts, A. M. (1983). Rapid shallow breathing evoked by selective stimulation of airway C-fibres in dogs. *Journal of Physiology (London)* 340, 415–433.

Connelly, C. A., and Wurster, R. D. (1985a). Spinal pathways mediating respiratory influences on sympathetic nerves. *American Journal of Physiology* 249, R91–99.

Connelly, C. A., and Wurster, R. D. (1985b). Sympathetic rhythms during hyperventilation induced apnea. *American Journal of Physiology* 249, R424–431.

Davidson, N. S., Goldner, S., and McCloskey, D. I. (1976). Respiratory modulation of baroreceptor and chemoreceptor reflexes affecting heart rate and cardiac vagal efferent nerve activity. *Journal of Physiology (London)* 259, 523–530.

Davies, R. O., and Kubin, L. (1986). Projection of pulmonary rapidly adapting receptors to the medulla of the cat: An antidromic mapping study. *Journal of Physiology (London)* 343, 63–86.

Davies, R. O., Kubin, L., and Pack, A. I. (1987). Pulmonary stretch receptor relay neurones of the cat: Location and contralateral medullary projections. *Journal of Physiology (London),* 383, 571–586.

Dembowsky, K., Czachurski, J., and Seller, H. (1985). Morphology of sympathetic preganglionic neurons in the thoracic spinal cord of the cat: An intracellular horseradish peroxidase study. *Journal of Comparative Neurology* 238, 453–465.

Downing, S. E., and Lee, J. C. (1975). Laryngeal chemosensitivity: A possible mechanism of sudden infant death. *Pediatrics* 55, 640–649.

Duron, B., Marlot, D., Larnicol, N., Jung-Caillol, M. C., and Macron, J. M. (1979). Somatotopy in the phrenic motor nucleus of the cat as revealed by retrograde transport of horseradish peroxidase. *Neuroscience Letters* 14, 159–163.

Feldman, J. L., and Grillner, S. (1983). Control of vertebrate respiration and locomotion: A brief account. *The Physiologist* 26, 310–316.

Feldman, J. L., and Speck, D. (1983). Interactions among inspiratory neurons in dorsal and ventral groups in cat medulla. *Journal of Neurophysiology* 49, 472–490.

Fukuda, Y., and Honda, Y. (1983). Effects of hypocapnia on respiratory timing and inspiratory activities of the superiorlaryngeal, hypoglossal, and phrenic nerves in the vagotomized rat. *Japanese Journal of Physiology* 33, 733–742.

Gebber, G. L., and McCall, R. B. (1976). Identification and discharge patterns of spinal sympathetic interneurons. *American Journal of Physiology* 231, 722–733.

Gesell, R., and White, F. (1938). Recruitment of muscular activity and the central neurone after-discharge of hyperpnea. *American Journal of Physiology* 122, 48–56.

Gilbey, M. P., Jordan, D., Richter, D. W., and Spyer, K. M. (1984). Synaptic mechanisms involved in the inspiratory modulation of the vagal cardioinhibitory neurones in the cat. *Journal of Physiology (London)* 356, 65–78.

Gilbey, M. P., Yoshinobu, N., and Spyer, K. M. (1986). Discharge patterns of cervical sympathetic preganglionic neurones related to central respiratory drive in the rat. *Journal of Physiology (London)* 378, 253–266.

Graham, K., and Duffin, J. (1981a). Cross-correlation of medullary expiratory neurons in the cat. *Experimental Neurology* 73, 451–464.

Graham, K., and Duffin, J. (1981b). Cross-correlation of medullary dorsomedial neurones in the cat. *Exp Neurol* 75, 627–643.

Haji, A., Connelly, C., Schultz, S. A., Wallace, J., and Remmers, J. E. (1986). Postsynaptic actions of inhibitory neurotransmitters on bulbar respiratory neurons. In: *Neurobiology of the Control of Breathing,* C. von Euler and H. Lagercrantz (eds.), Raven, New York, pp. 187–194.

Hering, E. (1869). Über den Einfluss der Athmung auf den Kreislauf. I. Über Athembewegungen des Gefässsystems.

Sber Akad Wiss, Wien, Math Nat Kl, II Abtl 60, 829–856.

Hilaire, G., and Monteau, R. (1976). Connexions entre les neurones inspiratoires bulbaires et les motoneurones phreniques et intercosteaux. *Journal of Physiology (Paris)* 72, 987–1000.

Hilaire, G., Monteau, R., and Bianchi, A. L. (1984). A cross-correlation study of interactions among respiratory neurons of dorsal, ventral and retrofacial groups in cat medulla. *Brain Research* 302, 19–31.

Hirst, G. D. S., and McLachlan, E. M. (1986). Development of dendritic calcium currents in ganglionic cells of the rat lower lumbar sympathetic chain. *Journal of Physiology (London)* 377, 349–368.

Hwang, J.-C., Bartlett, D., Jr., and St. John, W. M. (1983). Characterization of respiratory-modulated activities of hypoglossal motoneurons. *Journal of Applied Physiology* 55, 793–798.

Iriuchijima, J., and Kumada, M. (1964). Activity of single vagal fibres efferent to the heart. *Japanese Journal of Physiology* 14, 479–487.

Jordan, D., and Spyer, K. M. (1987). Central neural mechanisms mediating cardiovascular interactions. In: *The Neurobiology of the Cardiorespiratory System.* Taylor, E. W. (ed.), Manchester University Press, Manchester, U.K., pp. 322–341.

Kirkwood, P. A., Munson, J. B., Sears, T. A., and Westgaard, R. H. (1988). Respiratory interneurones in the thoracic spinal cord of the cat. *Journal of Physiology (London)* 395, 161–192.

Koepchen, H. P., Klüssendorf, D., and Sommer, D. (1981). Neurophysiological background of central neural cardiovascular-respiratory coordination. Basic remarks and experimental approach. *Journal of the Autonomic Nervous System* 3, 335–368.

Kunze, D. L. (1972). Reflex discharge patterns of cardiac vagal efferent fibres. *Journal of Physiology (London)* 222, 1–15.

Langhorst, P., Lambertz, M., and Schulz, G. (1981). Central control and interactions affecting sympathetic and parasympathetic activity. *Journal of the Autonomic Nervous System* 4, 149–163.

Lawson, E. E., Richter, D. W., and Bischoff, A. (1988). Intracellular recordings of respiratory neurons in the lateral medulla of the piglet. *Journal of Applied Physiology* (in press).

Lee, J. C., Stoll, B. J., and Downing, S. E. (1977). Properties of the laryngeal chemoreflex in neonatal piglets. *American Journal of Physiology* 233, R30–36.

Lindsay, B. G., Segers, L. S., and Shannon, R. (1987). Functional associations among lateral medullary respiratory neurons in the cat. II. Evidence for inhibitory actions of expiratory neurons. *Journal of Neurophysiology* 57, 1101–1117.

Lipski, J., and Duffin, J. (1986). An electrophysiological investigation of propriospinal inspiratory neurons in the upper cervical cord of the cat. *Experimental Brain Research* 61, 625–637.

Lipski, J., and Merrill, E. G. (1980). Electrophysiological demonstration of the projection from expiratory neurones in rostral medulla to contralateral dorsal respiratory group. *Brain Research* 197, 521–524.

Long, S. E., and Duffin, J. (1984). Cross-correlation of ventrolateral inspiratory neurons in the cat. *Experimental Neurology* 83, 233–253.

Long, S., and Duffin, J. (1986). The neuronal determinants of respiratory rhythm. *Progress in Neurobiology* 27, 101–182.

McAllen, R. M. (1987). Central respiratory modulation of subretrofacial bulbospinal neurones in the cat. *Journal of Physiology (London)* 388, 533–545.

McAllen, R. M., and Spyer, K. M. (1976). The location of cardiac vagal preganglionic motoneurones in the medulla of the cat. *Journal of Physiology (London)* 258, 187–204.

McAllen, R. M., and Spyer, K. M. (1978). Two types of vagal preganglionic motoneurones projecting to the heart and lungs. *Journal of Physiology (London)* 282, 353–364.

McCrimmon, D. R., Speck, D. F., and Feldman, J. L. (1987). Role of the ventrolateral region of the nucleus of the tractus solitarius in processing respiratory afferent input from vagus and superior laryngeal nerves. *Experimental Brain Research* 67, 449–459.

McLachlan, E. M., and Jänig, W. (1983). The cell bodies of origin of sympathetic and sensory axons in some skin and muscle nerves of the cat hindlimb. *Journal of Comparative Neurology* 214, 115–130.

Magoun, H. W., and Rhines, R. (1946). An inhibitory mechanism in the bulbar reticular formation. *Journal of Neurophysiology* 9, 165–171.

Mathew, O. P., Abu-Osba, Y. K., and Thach, B. T. (1982). Genioglossus muscle responses to upper airway pressure changes: Afferent pathways. *Journal of Applied Physiology: Respiratory, Environmental and Exercise Physiology* 52, 445–450.

Merrill, E. G., and Fedorko, L. (1984). Monosynaptic inhibition of phrenic motoneurons: A long descending projection from Bötzinger neurons. *Journal of Neuroscience* 4, 2350–2353.

Merrill, E. G., Lipski, J., Kubin, L., and Fedorko, L. (1983). Origin of the expiratory inhibition of nucleus tractus solitarius inspiratory neurones. *Brain Research* 263, 43–50.

Mifflin, S. W., and Richter, D. W. (1987). Effects of QX-314 on medullary respiratory neurones. *Brain Research* 420, 22–31.

Mifflin, S. M., Spyer, K. M., and Withington-Wray, D. J. (1986a). Hypothalamic inhibition of baroreceptor inputs in the nucleus of the tractus solitarius of the cat. *Journal of Physiology (London)* 373, 58P.

Mifflin, S. M., Spyer, K. M., and Withington-Wray, D. J. (1986b). Respiratory modulation of hypoglossal motoneurones in the cat. *Journal of Physiology (London)* 382, 61P.

Millhorn, D. E., Eldridge, F. L., and Waldrop, T. G. (1980). Prolonged stimulation of respiration by a new central neural mechanism. *Respiratory Physiology* 41, 87–103.

Numao, Y., Koshiya, N., Gilbey, M. P., and Spyer, K. M. (1987). Central respiratory drive-related activity in sympathetic nerves of the rat: The regional differences. *Neuroscience Letters* 81, 279–284.

Pantaleo, T., and Corda, M. (1986). Respiration-related

neurones of the medial nuclear complex of the solitary tract of the cat. *Respiratory Physiology* 64, 135–148.

Polosa, C., Gerber, U., and Schondorf, R. (1980). Central mechanisms of interaction between sympathetic preganglionic neurons and the respiratory oscillator. In: *Central Interaction between Respiratory and Cardiovascular Control Systems*, H. P. Koepchen, S. M. Hilton, and A. Trzebski (eds.), Springer-Verlag, Berlin, Heidelberg, New York, pp. 137–143.

Remmers, J. E., and Bartlett, D., Jr. (1977). Reflex control of expiratory airflow and duration. *Journal of Applied Physiology: Respiratory Environment and Exercise Physiology* 42, 80–87.

Remmers, J. E., Richter, D. W., Ballantyne, D., Bainton, C. R., and Klein, J. P. (1986). Reflex prolongation of the stage I of expiration. *Pflugers Archiv* 407, 190–198.

Richter, D. W., and Seller, H. (1975). Baroreceptor effects on medullary respiratory neurones of the cat. *Brain Research* 86, 168–171.

Richter, D. W., Camerer, H., Meesmann, M., and Röhrig, N. (1979). Studies on the synaptic interconnection between bulbar respiratory neurones of cats. *Pflugers Archiv* 380, 245–257.

Richter, D. W., Champagnat, J., and Mifflin, S. (1986b). Membrane properties involved in respiratory rhythm generation. In: *Neurobiology of the Control of Breathing*, C. von Euler and H. Lagercrantz (eds.), Raven, New York, pp. 141–147.

Richter, D. W., Jordan, G., Ballantyne, D., Meesmann, M., and Spyer, K. M. (1986c). Presynaptic depolarization in myelinated vagal afferent fibres terminating in the nucleus of the tractus solitarius in the cat. *Pflugers Archiv* 406, 12–19.

Richter, D. W., Ballantyne, D., and Remmers, J. E. (1987). The differential organization of medullary post-inspiratory activities. *Pflugers Archiv* 410, 420–427.

St. John, W. M., and Bledsoe, T. A. (1985). Comparison of respiratory-related trigeminal, hypoglossal and phrenic activities. *Respiratory Physiology* 62, 61–78.

Schmidt-Vanderheyden, W., Heinich, L., and Koepchen, H. P. (1970). Investigations into the fluctuations of proprioceptive reflexes in man. I. Fluctuations of the patellar tendon reflex and their relation to the vegetative rhythms during spontaneous respiration. *Pflugers Archiv* 317, 56–71.

Sears, T. A. (1964a). Efferent discharge in alpha and fusimotor fibres of intercostal nerves of the cat. *Journal of Physiology (London)* 174, 295–315.

Sears, T. A. (1964b). Some properties and reflex connexions of respiratory motoneurons of the cat's thoracic spinal cord. *Journal of Physiology (London)* 175, 386–403.

Sears, T. A., Berger, A. J., and Phillipson, E. A. (1982). Reciprocal tonic activation of inspiratory and expiratory motoneurones by chemical drives. *Nature* 299, 728–730.

Segers, L. S., Shannon, R., and Lindsay, B. G. (1985). Interactions between rostral pontine and ventral medullary respiratory neurons. *Journal of Neurophysiology* 54, 318–334.

Segers, L. S., Shannon, R., Saporta, S., and Lindsay, B. G. (1987). Functional associations among lateral medullary respiratory neurons in the cat. I. Evidence for excitatory and inhibitory actions of inspiratory neurons. *Journal of Neurophysiology* 57, 1078–1100.

Seller, H., Langhorst, P., Richter, D., and Koepchen, H. P. (1968). Über die Abhängigkeit der pressoreceptorischen Hemmung des Sympathicus von der Atemphase und ihre Auswirkung in der Vasomotorik. *Pflugers Archiv* 302, 300–314.

Shee, C. D., Ploysongsang, Y., and Milic-Emili, J. (1985). Decay of inspiratory muscle pressure during expiration in conscious humans. *Journal of Applied Physiology* 58, 1859–1865.

Spyer, K. M., and Jordan, D. (1987). Electrophysiology of the nucleus ambiguus. In: *Cardiogenic Reflexes*, R. Hainsworth, P. N. McWilliam, and D. A. G. G. Many (eds.), Oxford University Press, Oxford, pp. 237–249.

Suzue, T. (1984). Respiratory rhythm generation in the in vitro brain stem-spinal cord preparation of the neonatal rat. *Journal of Physiology (London)* 354, 173–183.

Traube, D. (1865). Über periodische Thätigkeits-Äusserungen des vasomotorischen und Hemmungs-Nervencentrums. *Cbl Med Wiss* 56, 881–885.

Viala, D. (1986). Evidence for direct reciprocal interactions between the central rhythm generators for spinal "respiratory" and locomotor activities in the rabbit. *Experimental Brain Research* 63, 225–232.

Younes, M. K., Remmers, J. E., and Baker, J. (1978). Characteristics of inspiratory inhibition by phasic volume feedback in cats. *Journal of Applied Physiology* 45, 80–86.

12

Role of the Cerebral Cortex in Autonomic Function

D. F. CECHETTO AND C. B. SAPER

As early as 1869, the British neurologist John Hughlings Jackson (cited in Hoff et al., 1963), noting the autonomic responses that accompanied motor seizures in epileptic patients, proposed that within the convolutions of the cerebrum were represented not only the voluntary movements of the whole body but also the involuntary movements of the blood vessels and viscera. Jackson's interpretation was prescient in more ways than one: in addition to being the first modern neuroscientist to suggest a cortical visceral representation, his observations underscored the difficulties in distinguishing direct autonomic responses from reflex changes that accompany somatic motor activity, pain, and generalized epileptic discharge. These issues have been inordinately difficult to resolve and remain a problem to this day.

In this chapter, we will first examine the methods that have been used to explore the cerebral cortex for areas involved in autonomic function. Then we will review in detail the anatomical and physiological data on three cortical regions for which such a role has been proposed.

METHODOLOGY

Electrical Stimulation

Historically, experiments using electrical stimulation have played an important part in shaping thought on the role of the cerebral cortex in autonomic function. Shortly after Jackson presented his hypothesis concerning the visceral cortex, a number of investigators began to examine the cardiovascular and other autonomic effects of applying electrical stimulation to different regions of the cerebral cortex. These studies (see historical reviews by Kaada, 1951; Hoff et al., 1963; Delgado, 1960) are difficult to interpret for a variety of reasons. First, the exact sites of stimulation often were not adequately de-

scribed. Second, large voltages were used, so that current spread was difficult to assess. Bard (1929) pointed out that many of the responses could be attributed to activation of subcortical regions, or even to widespread epileptic discharges. Third, due to the above problems as well as to differences in anesthesia, species, and experimental protocol, the results obtained were inconsistent, not only between laboratories but often within a single study.

By the late 1930s a more rigorous approach began to evolve in electrical stimulation studies of cortical autonomic areas. Hoff and Green (1936) and Kaada (1951) systematically mapped the cortical sites from which electrical stimulation elicited autonomic responses. Attempts were made to control for excitation of fibers of passage by demonstrating that adjacent areas were unresponsive, that sectioning fiber tracts below the site of stimulation abolished the responses, that following destruction of the cortex stimulation of subcortical fibers did not reproduce the autonomic responses, and that local cortical anesthesia abolished the responses (see Delgado, 1960 for review).

However, these approaches still did not eliminate the possibility that responses were due to orthodromic excitation of fibers of passage, or antidromic activation of fibers with collaterals that innervate other areas of the brain. These problems are of particular importance in the insular and infralimbic areas, which overlie the main pathways by which many ascending afferents from the brain stem and basal forebrain reach the cortical mantle (see Saper, 1987). Chemical stimulation, for example using excitatory amino acids, can overcome this objection, but has come into common use only in the past few years.

Other problems with stimulation methods remain even in chemical stimulation studies, including the distinction of primary autonomic responses from reflex changes due to the activation of somatic motor or sensory pathways, inconsistency of responses due to variation in depth or type of anesthesia employed (or changes in the behavioral state in awake animals), and differences in the actual stimulation parameters and autonomic variables that are measured (e.g., opposite changes in blood flow in different vascular beds may cause no net change in blood pressure). Consequently, much of the information that has been gathered on the autonomic cortex over the last century using stimulation methods must be viewed with caution. These problems underscore the importance of taking a multidisciplinary approach, and where possible correlating the results of stimulation studies with other modes of neurophysiological and neuroanatomical investigation.

Ablation Studies

These are subject to many of the same problems as stimulation experiments: differentiating the effects of involving local cell bodies versus fibers of passage, distinguishing primary effects on autonomic function from those secondary to involving somatic motor or sensory reflexes, and measuring and interpreting the differences in autonomic function that are seen in terms of behavioral state. An additional problem is that the effects of various unilateral cortical ablations on autonomic function are not striking (see section on Sensorimotor Cortex). On the other hand, bilateral cortical lesions may produce pronounced changes in autonomic reflex control and special visceral afferent (taste) discrimination (see sections on Insular and Medial Prefrontal Cortex). Historically, these studies were among the first to focus attention on areas of the cerebral cortex that are believed to play a role in autonomic function. However, it is difficult to interpret the results except in the context of data gained subsequently from other methods of study.

Electrophysiological Recording

Relatively few studies have attempted to record electrical responses of the cerebral cortex to autonomic stimulation. The best studied visceral sensory modality has been taste. Electrical stimulation studies of the various branches of the oral sensory nerves have been performed while recording evoked potentials in the cerebral cortex (Yamamoto et al., 1980; Norgren, 1984). Recordings of single and multiunit responses to gustatory stimulation have further refined the delineation of taste cortex (see Norgren, 1984, for review; Kosar et al., 1986; Cechetto and Saper, 1987; see section on the Insular Cortex).

Relatively few studies have examined cortical responses to stimulation of general visceral afferents. Studies of the evoked potentials (Bailey and Bremer, 1938; Dell and Olson, 1951) or single unit responses (Radna and MacLean, 1981) elicited by stimulating the proximal end of the cut cervical vagus nerve can be criticized for potentially activating afferents that may produce nonspecific responses associated with pain or arousal (Bonvallet et al., 1954; Bridgers et al., 1985). On the other hand, cortical and thalamic areas identified in these studies agree closely with more recent data from single unit recordings using selective visceral stimuli (Cechetto and Saper, 1987; see discussion on the Insular Cortex).

Neuroanatomical Studies

The early delineation of autonomic cortical regions was impeded by the relative insensitivity of the neuroanatomical methods that were available. The early axonal degeneration methods were not effective for demonstrating small unmyelinated fibers that compose many forebrain autonomic pathways (see Cechetto and Calaresu, 1983). In addition, the anatomical interpretation of degeneration following experimental lesions was hampered by the same fiber-of-passage problem as most physiological approaches.

The introduction of axonal tracer methods, utilizing axonal transport of a variety of markers, in the 1970s largely solved these problems. Not only are the methods extremely sensitive, but they can, if used properly, identify direct cortical connections with the central autonomic control system, without involving fibers of passage. These studies have demonstrated that the medial prefrontal and insular regions have direct projections to areas of the amygdala, hypothalamus, brain stem, and spinal cord that are involved in autonomic control (Saper, 1982a,b; Shipley, 1982; Shipley and Sanders, 1982; Terreberry and Neafsey, 1983; van der Kooy et al., 1984; Yasui et al., 1985; Hurley-Gius et al., 1986). Although it is possible for a cortical area to influence autonomic outflow via polysynaptic routes, the existence of monosynaptic projections into the autonomic outflow system provides important support for the idea that a region of cerebral cortex plays a primary role in autonomic regulation. Nevertheless, it is not possible to be sure that an area that projects into central autonomic pathways, or receives input from them, is primarily autonomic in function. This determination clearly requires correlation of the neuroanatomical substrates with the types of physiological studies outlined above.

Criteria for Identifying Autonomic Cortical Areas

Although each of the methods for defining autonomic cortex has major drawbacks, a multidisciplinary approach tends to minimize the extent to which the investigator may be misled by any one method. Fortunately, the data that have been derived from the different approaches are in fairly good agreement on the cortical areas involved in autonomic control. The results of key investigations (reviewed below) in rats, cats, dogs, and primates indicate that at least three cortical regions can be closely linked with autonomic regulation: the insular cortex, the medial prefrontal cortex, and the sensorimotor cortex.

In the remainder of this chapter, we will examine the evidence relating each of these areas to autonomic control. In each case, the evidence will be evaluated with respect to the following criteria: (1) demonstration of autonomic responses using electrical and/or chemical activation at discrete sites in the cortex, (2) electrophysiological recording of neurons in the cortex that provide evidence of neuronal activity related to autonomic function, and (3) demonstration by neuroanatomical methods that the cortical region has direct connections with subcortical sites involved in autonomic control.

INSULAR CORTEX

Stimulation Studies

Electrical stimulation of the insular cortex in rats, cats, dogs, monkeys, and humans elicits autonomic responses including changes in blood pressure, heart rate, respiration, piloerection, pupillary dilatation, gastric motility, peristaltic activity, salivation, and adrenaline secretion (Kaada, 1951; Wall and Davis, 1951; Hoffman and Rasmussen, 1953; Penfield and Faulk, 1955; von Euler and Folkow, 1958; Delgado, 1960; Hoff et al., 1963; Hall et al., 1977; Ruggiero et al., 1987). The types of responses obtained in these studies are critically dependent on the stimulation parameters, particularly frequency of stimulation, the species, and the type and depth of the anesthesia used in the investigation.

Although each of these studies can be criticized on one or more of the grounds discussed in the beginning of this chapter, the work of Ruggiero and colleagues (1987) was seminal in demonstrating similar responses during both electrical and chemical microstimulation of the insular cortex. Rats, anesthetized with α-chloralose and paralyzed with gallamine, demonstrated a rise in arterial pressure and heart rate during electrical stimulation of the posterior insular cortex with stimulus threshold between 20 and 30 μA and at a most effective frequency of 50–100 Hz. In these experiments increases in arterial blood pressure and heart rate were also obtained by injecting the same site with glutamic or kainic acid. Stimulation of adjacent sites, for example, in the olfactory or somatic sensory cortex, did not produce

these responses. There is, therefore, little doubt that autonomic responses can be obtained with specific stimulation of neuronal cell bodies in the insular cortex. However, elucidation of the role of the insular cortex in normal autonomic function has relied largely on other means of investigation.

Ablation Studies

Cannon and Britton (1925) showed that "sham rage" could be induced in cats following crude decortication (a spatula was inserted into the brain beneath the occiptal lobe, severing the subcortical connections of all cortical regions except for portions of the piriform lobe and amygdala). On innocuous stimulation, such as stroking the fur on the animal's flank, cats would demonstrate all of the somatomotor manifestations of rage (arching the back, extruding the claws, growling, crying, hyperirritability, and hyperactivity), as well as autonomic manifestations of rage (piloerection, dilatation of the pupils, retraction of the nictitating membrane, panting, tachycardia). Kennard (1945) attempted to reproduce this phenomenon with more restricted lesions. In cats, bilateral ablation of the orbitoinsular region of the frontal lobes resulted in a syndrome similar to that of complete decortication or complete removal of the frontal lobes. Although interpretation of these studies is difficult in light of the problems reviewed in the first part of this chapter, these early attempts did suggest a tonic role for the insular region in the regulation of autonomic (particularly sympathetic) response.

The possible nature of this role was illuminated by experiments examining taste responses after cortical ablations. In studies extending back to the turn of the century (for review see Norgren, 1984), lesions involving the anterior insular region in experimental animals and humans have been found to impair gustatory sensory thresholds. The clearest delineation of the cortical area that is critical for gustatory function was the demonstration by Yamamoto and colleagues (1980) that ablation of the insular region that receives lingual sensory afferents (as studied electrophysiologically) in rats can permanently eliminate a conditioned aversive taste discrimination. As taste is a special visceral sensory modality, these studies suggest that the insular area contains a visceral sensory representation.

Electrophysiological Recordings

Additional evidence consistent with a role for the insular cortex in visceral sensation has been provided by electrophysiological recordings. Both single and multiunit studies and evoked potential recordings have demonstrated that taste responses may be obtained from a dysgranular region of anterior insular cortex in the rat and in the monkey (Yamamoto et al., 1980; Pritchard et al., 1986; Cechetto and Saper, 1987) (see Figures 12-1 and 12-2). Yamamoto and colleagues mapped the distribution of evoked potentials obtained from stimulating the different cranial nerves involved in gustatory response. Their data clearly demonstrated an anteroposterior topographic gradient to the representations of the facial, glossopharyngeal, and vagus nerves in the insular cortex. Furthermore, the glossopharyngeal and vagal representations extended considerably further posteriorly than the area specifically devoted to the gustatory cortex.

These studies confirmed earlier investigations using evoked potentials, suggesting the possibility that general visceral sensation may also be represented in the insular cortex. Bailey and Bremer, as early as 1938, had stimulated the proximal end of the cut cervical vagus nerve in the *encephale isolé* cat, demonstrating an increase in the rate and amplitude of cortical electrical activity localized to the orbitoinsular region. Dell and Olson (1951), using

similar methods, showed that the evoked potentials localized to the insular cortex were of short latency (8–10 msec). The rapidity of this response suggests an oligosynaptic pathway. Furthermore, although the sensory modality that is activated cannot be determined in this sort of experiment, the tight localization of the response in the insular region indicates that it is not a nonspecific effect of stimulating nociceptive or arousal systems.

This conclusion is supported by recordings from neurons in the insular cortex of the rat during selective activation of a variety of visceral sensory inputs, including gustatory (saline solution on the tongue), gastric mechanoreceptor (balloon inflation in the stomach), arterial chemoreceptor (10% CO_2 and intravenous low-dose sodium cyanide), and arterial baroreceptor (intravenous phenylephrine) stimuli (Pritchard et al., 1986; Kosar et al., 1986; Cechetto and Saper, 1987) (see Figure 12-3). Neurons responding to gustatory stimulation were localized rostrally in the dysgranular insular area. In contrast, neurons that responded to general visceral stimuli were located more posterodorsally in the granular

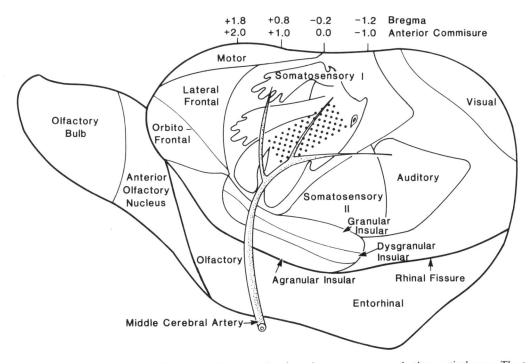

Figure 12-1 Lateral view of the rat forebrain to illustrate the visceral sensory cortex and other cortical areas. The taste cortex is located in the rostral half of the dysgranular insular area, and the general visceral cortex occupies the granular insular region. The rostral granular insular area receives gastric mechanoreceptor afferents, while the more caudal granular insular cortex receives cardiovascular and respiratory information. Note that the taste cortex is adjacent to the gastrointestinal (rostral granular insular) and tongue somatic sensory areas, while the caudal, cardiorespiratory (granular insular) cortex is located in close proximity to the thoracic representation in the second somatosensory area. The distances in millimeters at the top of the drawing are given with respect to the bregma point in the atlas of Paxinos and Watson (1986) and the anterior edge of the crossing of the anterior commissure, and are equivalent to the planes shown in Figure 12-3. (Modified from Finger, 1987.)

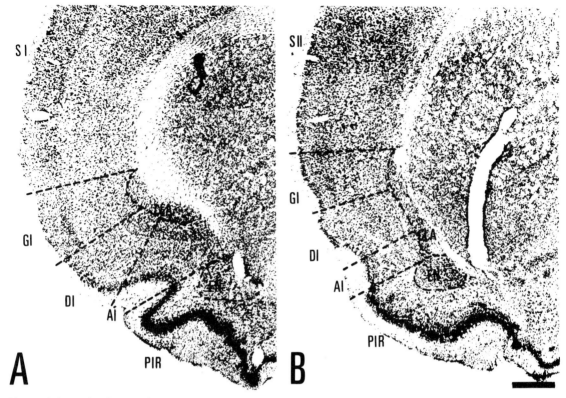

Figure 12-2 A pair of photomicrographs to demonstrate the cytoarchitectonic subdivisions of the rostral (A) and caudal (B) insular cortex in the rat, respectively 2.0 and 0.5 mm anterior to the crossing of the anterior commissure. The granular insular area (GI), containing the general visceral representation, has a well-defined granular layer IV. In the dysgranular insular area (DI), there are only a few clusters of granule cells in layer IV, and layer V is more prominent. In the dorsal part of the agranular insular cortex (AI), layers III and V become denser, resulting in three marked cellular layers, separated by thin bands of white matter. More ventrally, in the fundus of the rhinal fissure, the laminar pattern is lost in the ventral agranular insular area (not separately marked). Note that the dysgranular area becomes less extensive at more caudal levels. CLA, claustrum; EN, endopiriform nucleus; PIR piriform cortex; S I,II, first and second somatic sensory areas. Scale = 500 μm. (Modified from Cechetto and Saper, 1987.)

insular region. Within the general visceral zone, there was a crude viscerotopic organization, with gastrointestinal neurons located most rostrally, cardiovascular neurons most caudally, and arterial chemoreceptor neurons in an intermediate position. Most visceroceptive cortical neurons responded to only one modality, although occasional cases of convergence of cardiovascular and respiratory inputs onto single neurons were observed.

These observations suggest that the insular cortex contains a visceral sensory representation, organized in a manner similar to the somatic sensory cortex (see Figure 12-1). The location of the visceral sensory strip is in close proximity to the somatic sensory areas, with which it is roughly aligned. In fact, the taste area is located just ventral to the tongue somatic sensory region, and the cardiopulmonary region is positioned along the margin of the thoracic representation in the second somatic sensory area. The localization of the cardiovascular region of the insular cortex corresponds closely with the portion of posterior insular cortex from which Ruggerio et al. (1987) obtained blood pressure responses with electrical microstimulation.

Neuroanatomical Studies

Neuroanatomical studies support the view that the insular cortex may serve as a visceral sensory area (Cechetto and Saper, 1987). Using injections of neuroanatomical tracers into the sites of physiologically characterized visceroceptive neurons, we found the taste (dysgranular) insular area to be reciprocally connected with the ventroposteromedial parvocellular nucleus (VPMpc) of the thalamus. The general visceral (granular) area was reciprocally related to a similar, parvocellular area, just lateral to the VPMpc. In congruence with the standard terminology of VPM for the cephalic and VPL for the somatic sensory nuclei of the thalamus, the general visceral parvocellular region was termed the ventroposterolateral parvocellular nucleus (VPLpc). The

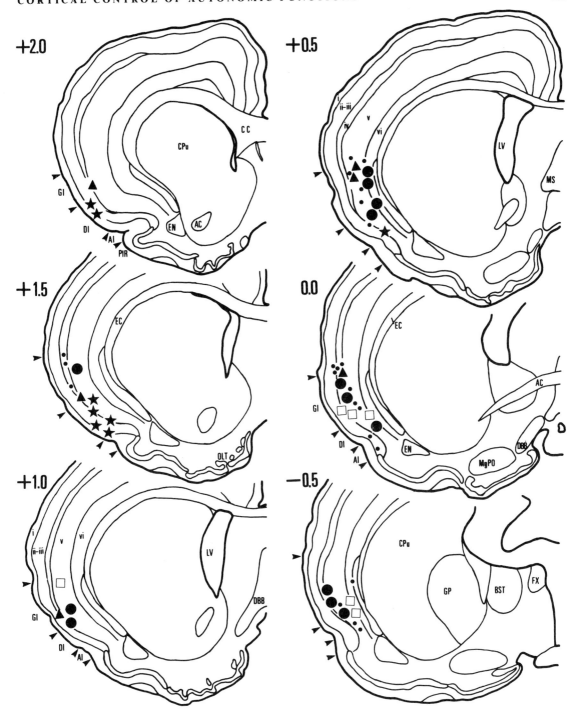

Figure 12-3 A series of drawings of the insular cortex, at six levels arranged from rostral to caudal, demonstrating the distribution of neurons responding to different visceral modalities. Taste units (stars) were located rostrally, within the dysgranular insular cortex. Neurons responding to gastric mechanoreceptors (triangles) were primarily found in the rostral granular insular area, adjacent to the taste cortex. Units responding to respiratory chemoreceptors (circles) or cardiovascular baroreceptors (open squares) were found at progressively more caudal locations in the granular area. Neurons that did not respond to any of these modalities are illustrated by small dots. Numbers at the left of each section indicate distance in millimeters rostral or caudal to the crossing of the anterior commissure. AC, anterior commissure; AI, agranular insular cortex; BST, bed nucleus of the stria terminalis; CC, corpus callosum; CPu, caudate-putamen; DBB, nucleus of the diagonal band of Broca; DI; dysgranular insular cortex; EC, external capsule; EN, endopiriform nucleus; FX, fornix; GI, granular insular cortex; GP, globus pallidus; LV, lateral ventricle; MgPO, magnocellular preoptic nucleus; MS, medial septal nucleus; OLT, olfactory tubercle; PIR, piriform cortex. (Modified from Cechetto and Saper, 1987.)

main source of ascending afferents to the parvocel-lular visceral strip in the thalamus is a topographi-cally organized portion of the contralateral external medial parabrachial nucleus (Cechetto and Saper, 1987). The rostromedial part of the external medial subnucleus projects to the VPMpc, whereas its pos-terolateral part innervates the VPLpc. The topo-graphic organization of afferents from the nucleus of the solitary tract to the parabrachial nucleus has not yet been studied in comparable detail (see Figure 12-4).

The insular cortex also has connections with a large number of subcortical sites involved in auto-nomic control (Figure 12-5). It receives afferents di-rectly from the parabrachial nucleus and from the lateral hypothalamic area (Saper 1982a,b, 1985; Ship-ley and Sanders, 1982). Its efferent fibers innervate the nucleus of the solitary tract, the parabrachial nu-cleus, the lateral hypothalamic area, and the central nucleus of the amygdala (Ross et al., 1981; Saper, 1982a; Shipley, 1982; van der Kooy et al., 1982, 1984; Yasui et al., 1985; Ruggerio et al., 1987). The nucleus of the solitary tract receives a topographi-cally organized projection from the insular cortex. The taste (rostral dysgranular) region of the insular cortex projects to the rostral (gustatory) part of the nucleus of the solitary tract (Saper, 1982b), whereas only the posterior granular (general visceral) insular

area innervates the caudal (general visceral) part of the solitary nucleus (see Chapter 6 for further dis-cussion of the organization of the nucleus of the sol-itary tract).

The insular projections to the parabrachial nu-cleus and lateral hypothalamus primarily innervate those subnuclei that provide reciprocal projections (Saper, 1982a,b; Fulwiler and Saper, 1984). In this regard, they may be considered descending feedback mechanisms, similar to those in other sensory sys-tems for modulating the ascending sensory signal. On the other hand, insular fibers also innervate the parts of the lateral hypothalamus and the parabra-chial nucleus that provide extensive descending pro-jections to the preganglionic cell groups in the me-dulla and spinal cord (Saper et al., 1976; Saper and Loewy, 1980; Berk and Finkelstein, 1982; Hosoya and Matsushita, 1981; Miura et al., 1983; Luiten et al., 1987).

The central nucleus of the amygdala receives an especially intense projection from the insular area (Saper, 1982a; Otterson, 1982; Russchen, 1982a; Cechetto et al., 1983). There are extensive descend-ing projections from the central nucleus of the amygdala to the parabrachial nucleus, the nucleus of the solitary tract, and the parasympathetic pregan-glionic nuclei in the medulla (Mehler, 1980; Price and Amaral, 1981; Schwaber et al., 1980, 1982; Ot-

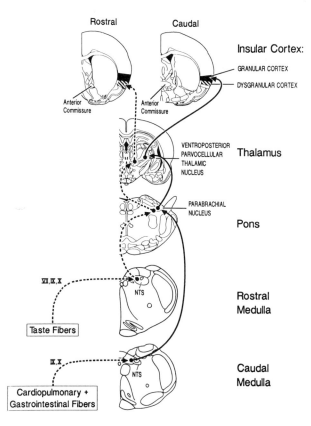

Figure 12-4 A summary drawing, indicating the parallel processing in the special gustatory (dashed lines) and general (solid lines) parasympathetic visceral sensory pathways at several different levels from the brain stem to the cerebral cortex. NTS, nucleus of the solitary tract. (Modified from Cech-etto, 1987.)

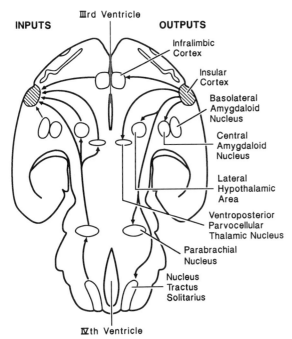

Figure 12-5 A schematic diagram of a horizontal section through a rat brain, illustrating the afferent (left) and efferent (right) connections of the insular cortex).

terson, 1981; Russchen 1982b). In addition, the central nucleus is joined by the nucleus of the solitary tract, parabrachial nucleus, and lateral hypothalamus in innervating the medullary reticular areas involved in coordinating autonomic responses (Loewy and Burton, 1978; Ricardo and Koh, 1978; Saper and Loewy, 1980; Price and Amaral, 1981; Fulwiler and Saper, 1984; Luiten et al., 1987; see Chapter 9). It has been reported that in monkeys, a small number of neurons in the central nucleus may project directly to the spinal cord (Mizuno et al., 1985).

In summary, the insular cortex can be considered on both neurophysiological and neuroanatomical grounds to contain a topographically organized visceral sensory representation. The connections of this region suggest that it may be homologous to the adjacent somatic sensory cortex. Like the somatic sensory cortex, the insular area may provide descending projections into both sensory and motor systems. It therefore may be more accurate to consider the insular region as a visceral sensorimotor area.

MEDIAL PREFRONTAL CORTEX

Electrical Stimulation

It has long been recognized that a variety of autonomic responses can be elicited by electrical stimu-

lation of the medial prefrontal cortex. The responses obtained from this region can be quite dramatic; complete cessation of heart rate may occur in monkeys during stimulation of the cingulate gyrus (Smith, 1945; Ward, 1948). However, as with other cortical areas, variable responses have been obtained in different species and under varying conditions (see Kaada, 1951; Wall and Davis, 1951; Delgado, 1960; Lofving, 1961). In addition, these early studies using large currents may have activated adjacent structures or fiber pathways (see discussion of stimulation studies in the first section of this chapter). Although the responses were sometimes confined to relatively restricted anatomical loci, these are difficult to compare across studies, as few investigators localized their responses to recognized cytoarchitectonic boundaries (see Figure 12-6).

Several recent studies have examined the effects of electrical stimulation with relatively small currents (less than 100 μA) in the medial prefrontal region on heart rate, blood pressure, and gastric motility in the rat (Buchanan et al., 1984, 1985; Hurley-Gius and

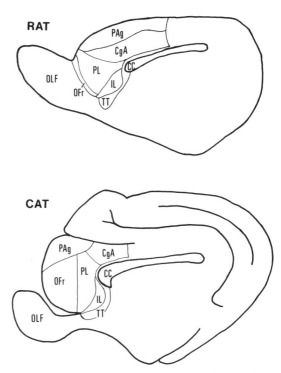

Figure 12-6 A diagram of the medial wall of the cerebral hemisphere of the rat and the cat, to illustrate the relative locations of areas that have been implicated in autonomic regulation. Note that despite the greater development of the cortex in the cat, the infralimbic and prelimbic areas have maintained their relative positions with respect to the genu of the corpus callosum. CC, corpus callosum; CgA, anterior cingulate cortex; IL, infralimbic area; PAg, precentral agranular area; OFr, orbitofrontal area; OLF, olfactory bulb; PL, prelimbic area; TT, taenia tecta.

Neafsey, 1986; Burns and Wyss, 1985). These studies demonstrate in both awake and anesthetized rats and rabbits that the main effects of stimulation are bradycardic, hypotensive, and gastromotor. These responses can be elicited primarily from the prelimbic and infralimbic areas, which constitute the medial bank of the prefrontal cortex just rostral to the genu of the corpus callosum. This localization is consistent with the earlier work of Kaada (1951) in the cat, except that he identified a separate pressor area just ventral to the genu of the corpus callosum (most likely corresponding to the posteroventral infralimbic cortex). However, all of these sites are quite close to the cingulate bundle, which contains a variety of fiber pathways that may have been activated. Further studies employing chemical stimulation will be necessary to determine whether the responses are due to activation of cell bodies.

Ablation Studies

Ablation studies of the medial prefrontal cortex have suggested that the region may play a role in cardiovascular function. Functional ablation with cryoblockade has been reported to reverse renovascular or DOCA-salt hypertension (Szilagyi et al., 1987). Large electrolytic lesions of the medial prefrontal cortex in rats and rabbits also markedly disrupt conditioned heart rate responses (Buchanan and Powell, 1982a,b; Fryzstak and Neafsey, 1987). Verberne and colleagues (1987) used a cytotoxic lesion to study the effects of injury to cell bodies versus fibers of passage in the medial prefrontal cortex. They found that the gain of the baroreceptor reflex (as measured by change in heart rate per change in unit blood pressure) was diminished. However, the lesions in all of these studies were quite large, including both the infralimbic and prelimbic areas, and there has been no attempt to identify the critical locus in the cerebral cortex for blocking these cardiovascular responses.

Electrophysiological Studies

Similarly, there have been relatively few studies on the effects of visceral afferent stimulation on the firing of medial prefrontal neurons, and these have provided little help in identifying a critical locus for autonomic regulation. Stimulation of the cervical vagus nerve has been reported to elicit changes in firing frequencies in about 20% of "cingulate" neurons, but it is not clear exactly which cytoarchitectonic field was being explored nor what modality was being activated (Bachman et al., 1977). Frysinger and Harper (1986) demonstrated neurons in the medial prefrontal cortex that have discharge patterns related either to the respiratory rate or the cardiac

cycle, but did not report the localization of these neurons in detail.

Neuroanatomical Studies

In contrast, neuroanatomical studies indicate that the infralimbic cortex in particular has extensive connections both with the limbic and the autonomic systems. The infralimbic area receives telencephalic afferents from the prelimbic, insular, and entorhinal cortex, and CA1 field of the hippocampus, and parts of the amygdala (Rosene and van Hoesen, 1977; Swanson, 1981; Yasui et al., 1987). In addition, it receives ascending inputs from the VMPpc and VPLpc, the lateral hypothalamus, the parabrachial nucleus, and the nucleus of the solitary tract (Saper, 1982, 1985; van der Kooy et al., 1982, 1984; Fulwiler and Saper, 1984; Yasui et al., 1987). In the rat, a small number of fibers also reach the infralimbic cortex directly from the dorsal horn of the spinal cord (Hurley-Gius et al., 1986).

Infralimbic efferents innervate a number of autonomic sites, including the VPMpc and VPLpc, the lateral hypothalamus, the parabrachial nucleus, and the nucleus of the solitary tract (Terreberry and Neafsey, 1983; Room et al., 1985; Yasui et al., 1986). Other fibers continue through the pyramidal tract into the spinal cord (Hurley-Gius et al., 1986), where they terminate primarily in the marginal zone of the spinal dorsal horn (lamina I) and in the dorsal commissural area (lamina X). A few fibers can be traced from lamina X into the base of the dorsal horn, and at thoracic levels occasional fibers enter the intermediolateral cell column. Electron microscopic evidence will be necessary to determine whether infralimbic fibers terminate on preganglionic neurons. It is interesting to note that a very early study reported fibers from the pyramidal tract to the lateral horn of the spinal cord (Hoff and Hoff, 1934). However, the methods used did not determine the origin of the projection, and even the existence of such a pathway was questioned by later investigators (Wall and Davis, 1951; see section on the Somatic Motor Cortex).

The prelimbic cortex, by comparison, is more closely related to the limbic system, having its main connections with the mediodorsal nucleus of the thalamus and the prefrontal, cingulate, and perirhinal cortical areas (Room et al., 1985). Although it is reciprocally related to the infralimbic cortex (Saper, 1982b; Room et al., 1985; Yasui et al., 1987), it has only sparse descending projections to the hypothalamus and the parabrachial nucleus (Room et al., 1985; Saper, 1982a). Consequently, the anatomical data suggest that the prelimbic cortex may participate in autonomic regulation primarily by serving as a conduit for limbic inputs to the infralimbic cortex.

To summarize, the infralimbic area has a multitude of limbic sensory inputs and a paucity of visceral sensory inputs. The infralimbic cortex receives massive inputs from the hippocampus, the amygdala, and the prelimbic cortex, but only a few fibers from the spinal cord, the nucleus of the solitary tract, the parabrachial nucleus, or the visceral thalamic nuclei. These considerations, as well as the position of the infralimbic cortex at the extreme medial surface of the frontal lobe near the frontal motor areas (in comparison with the insular cortex, at the lateral margin of the hemisphere near the somatic sensory cortex), led Hurley-Gius and Neafsey (1986) to suggest that the infralimbic cortex may act as a visceral motor cortex (see Figure 12-7). The hypothesis is intellectually attractive, but the case would be more compelling if there were stronger electrophysiological evidence. So far, however, key pieces of evidence are lacking, including chemical stimulation and single unit recording studies with accurate localization of the areas that are studied.

SOMATIC MOTOR AND SENSORY CORTEX

Stimulation Studies

As indicated in the introduction, the role of the somatic motor and sensory cortex in central autonomic control has long been a matter of some dispute. It has been known since the experiments of

Dusser de Barenne and Kleinknecht in 1924 that the electrical stimulation of the motor cortex can cause a decrease in blood pressure (cited in Green and Hoff, 1937). Several later studies found similar results (Hsu et al., 1942; Eliasson et al., 1952). Green and Hoff (1937) reported only slight decreases in blood pressure, or none at all, during electrical stimulation of the motor and premotor cortex in cats and monkeys anesthetized with Dial-urethane. On the other hand, stimulation of the motor cortex under ether anesthesia consistently yielded increases in systemic blood pressure in both cats and monkeys. They also measured limb and renal blood volume, reporting that with ether anesthesia stimulation of the motor cortex elicited an increase in limb blood volume and a decrease in renal volume. This study emphasizes the importance of considering responses under different anesthetic conditions, and of measuring autonomic variables more subtle than blood pressure.

As discussed in the first part of this chapter, it is not possible in studies of this sort to be sure whether the response to electrical stimulation is due to the activation of cell bodies as opposed to fibers. Another possibility is that autonomic responses might result from epileptic activity induced by the relatively large voltages used by early experimenters. This issue was examined by Delgado (1960), who recorded the electroencephalogram during electrical stimulation of the motor cortex. He found that cardiovascular responses were not accompanied by changes in spontaneous brain activity, suggesting that generalized seizure activity had not been induced.

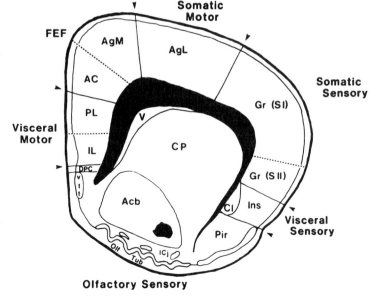

Figure 12-7 A summary figure to show the relationships of the frontal sensory and motor fields, illustrated on a coronal section through the frontal lobe of the rat. Note that the infralimbic (IL) and prelimbic (PL) cortical areas are located at the medial extreme of the hemisphere, adjacent to the frontal eye fields (FEF) and somatic motor cortex. The insular cortex (Ins), in contrast, is located at the lateral extreme of the hemisphere, adjacent to the first (Gr SI) and second (Gr SII) somatic sensory areas. AC, anterior commissure; Acb, nucleus accumbens; AgL, AgM, agranular lateral and medial areas; Cl, claustrum; CP, caudate-putamen; DPC, dorsal peduncular cortex; ICj, islands of Calleja; Olf, Tub olfactory tubercle; Pir, piriform cortex; V, ventricle; vtt, ventral taenia tecta. (Reprinted from Hurley-Gius and Neafsey, 1986, with permission.)

Another problem confounding the interpretation of autonomic responses elicited from the motor cortex is whether stimulation-induced muscle movements are indirectly responsible for changes in blood flow. Green and Hoff (1937) pointed out that electrical stimulation of the motor cortex in cats and monkeys still resulted in changes in limb blood volume even when the voltage used was below the threshold necessary to elicit movements. Furthermore, electrical stimulation of the hindlimb motor cortex of monkeys still elicits an increase in hindlimb blood flow after sectioning the spinal nerves for the limb below the level of the major autonomic outflow, or after paralysis induced by administration of decamethonium bromide (Clarke et al., 1968). These results led to the concept of a central cardiovascular command, generated concomitantly with the motor command, to ready the cardiovascular system for exercise.

Evidence conflicting with a direct cardiovascular response during stimulation of the motor cortex was provided by Hilton and colleagues (1979). In cats under the steroid anesthetic Althesin changes in hind limb blood flow occurred during stimulation of the motor cortex only when there was concomitant muscle contraction. Prevention of muscular contractions by gallamine or spinal cord transection at L4–L5 (which leaves the sympathetic outflow to the hind limb intact) blocked the hind limb vascular response. These experiments can be criticized because gallamine has ganglionic blocking activity. In addition, severing the spinal cord may cause spinal shock not only below the level of the transection, but in the autonomic outflow of the spinal segments immediately rostral to the cut. As the hindlimb blood flow is probably controlled by the upper lumbar sympathetic preganglionic neurons, it is quite possible that their responsiveness was affected by the spinal transection.

An important line of evidence in favor of the central command hypothesis comes from the study of cardiovascular response to muscle exercise (see review by Mitchell and Schmidt, 1984). When the distal end of a cut ventral root is stimulated, the muscles that are innervated can be vigorously exercised without the generation of a central command. Under these conditions, the predominant cardiovascular response is *pressor*. This exercise pressor response is a spinobulbospinal reflex that depends on type III afferent innervation from the exercising muscle. As the stimulation of motor cortex primarily results in *depressor* responses, it is quite unlikely that these could result from muscular activity.

To summarize, the evidence from electrical stimulation studies suggests that the motor cortex may generate a central command for a depressor response. However, further studies are necessary demonstrating a similar response to chemical stimulation.

Ablation studies of the motor cortex have also been cited as supporting a direct role for this cortical area in autonomic regulation. Changes in vasomotor tone have been noted in association with paralysis in humans as a result of damage to the motor cortex (Bucy, 1935; Kennard, 1937; Fulton, 1949). Bucy (1935) reported that a patient suffering right hemiplegia, hemihypesthesia, and motor aphasia also experienced right vasoconstriction, which he interpreted as due to removal of a functional inhibition from the cortex. Other investigators examined this issue by making experimental lesions in animals. In dogs, motor cortex lesions resulted in vasodilatation (see Fulton, 1949), whereas in cats motor and premotor cortex lesions resulted in the paralysis of the mechanism for reflex dilatation in the extremities (Kennard, 1937). In addition, in monkeys both cooling and stimulation of the premotor cortex have been shown to affect gastric motility (Sheehan, 1935). However, none of these studies could distinguish the effects of disrupting fibers of passage versus cell bodies, nor did the experiments control for the possibility that the autonomic changes observed were secondary to somatic motor changes effects of the lesion.

Electrophysiological Studies

There have been few attempts to record autonomic responses from the sensory or motor areas. Dell and Olson (1951), in their wide-ranging evoked potential study, did not report any responses in these areas from stimulation of the vagus nerve. This is not surprising, as there is no evidence for input to the somatic sensory or motor cortex from the vagal *parasympathetic* system (see discussion above on the insular area as a visceral sensory cortex). However, there is evidence that stimulation of *sympathetic* visceral afferent fibers can activate neurons in the somatic sensory cortex.

Stimulation of afferent fibers in the splanchnic nerve in the rabbit, cat, dog, and monkey produces short latency (8–12 msec) responses in the trunk region of the contralateral first and second somatic sensory areas (Amassian 1951a,b; Figure 12-8). This response is eliminated by sectioning the dorsal columns. Short latency (5–6 msec) evoked potentials and single unit responses can also be recorded in the contralateral ventroposterior thalamus of the cat after splanchnic nerve stimulation (Patton and Amassian, 1951; MacLeod, 1958). These units also received cutanous inputs. Evoked potentials can be recorded in the sensorimotor cortex during low

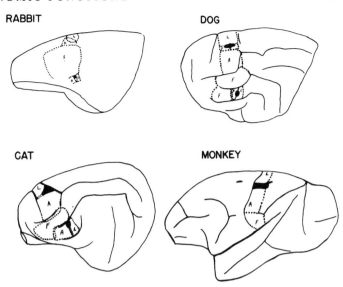

Figure 12-8 A summary diagram showing the locations of areas where evoked potentials could be elicited by electrical stimulation of the splanchnic nerve in four species. In each case, the response was located in the thoracic area of either the first or second somatic sensory areas, or both. The sympathetic afferent system appears to converge with somatic afferents at the first synapse in the spinal cord, and to be carried with the spinothalamic system to the thalamus and cortex (see text). Note that the sympathetic afferent representation in the thoracic area of the second somatic sensory cortex is directly adjacent to the general visceral part of the granular insular cortex (see Figure 12-1). A, arm (forelimb) area; F, face area; L, leg (hindlimb) area; T, thoracic area. (Reprinted from Amassian, 1951a, with permission.)

threshold electrical stimulation of limb venous afferents in the cat (Thompson et al., 1980). Interestingly, the evoked potentials from stimulation of venous afferents from the hindlimb and forelimb mapped to the respective somatic sensory fields for these limbs. Thompson et al. (1980) proposed that this input may provide a feedback for optimal control of limb cardiovascular adjustments to posture and movement.

A mechanism for the convergence of visceral afferent information with somatic sensory inputs has been demonstrated by Foreman and colleagues (Blair et al., 1984; Ammons et al., 1985). In monkeys, spinothalamic neurons (antidromically activated from VPL) that respond to cardiac chemical nociceptors also have somatic sensory peripheral fields. The similarity of the receptive fields of these neurons (left shoulder, arm, and neck) to the sites of referred cardiac pain in humans is striking, leading to the suggestion that this convergence may be the mechanism for referred pain in general. If this were so, one would expect that spinal (sympathetic) visceral afferents would converge with somatic sensory afferents at the level of the dorsal horn, producing a visceral sensory map in the ventrobasal thalamus, and consequently the somatic sensory cortex. To our knowledge this hypothesis has not been formally tested.

Neuroanatomical Studies

It is not clear what pathways might mediate the autonomic responses from the motor cortex. Spiegel and Hunsicker (1936) suggested that both a hypo-thalamic projection and the pyramidal tracts are responsible for mediating autonomic responses from the motor cortex and that damage to the hypothalamic system attenuates pupillary responses more than vasomotor responses. This suggestion has not, to our knowledge, received further study.

The importance of the pyramidal pathway in spinal autonomic control is supported by the demonstration that stimulation of the pyramidal tracts in the decerebrate cat has profound autonomic effects (Landau, 1953). In these experiments, however, it is likely that the autonomic responses were due to the spread of stimulation current to the adjacent ventrolateral medulla. It has been reported that lesions of the pyramidal tracts that reduce somatic motor responses to motor cortex stimulation also reduce the accompanying limb vascular responses (Hilton et al., 1979). Nevertheless, many cortical areas, including the insular and infralimbic regions, send descending fibers through the pyramidal tract. Thus, autonomic responses obtained on stimulating the pyramidal tract cannot necessarily be attributed to the activation of fibers originating in the motor cortex.

To summarize, there is considerable evidence that the sympathetic afferents entering the thoracic spinal cord converge with somatic sensory afferents in the dorsal horn and are thereafter handled as part of the thoracic somatic sensory inflow, including a representation in the somatic sensory cortex. The role of the motor cortex in autonomic response is more controversial. Definitive evidence for the central autonomic command hypothesis, including demonstration of the pathways for this response, would clarify considerably our understanding of the relationship of motor and autonomic control at a cortical level.

SUMMARY

Information from a variety of approaches indicates that at least three cortical areas play a role in autonomic function. The role of the insular area as a visceral sensory cortex, containing an organotopic visceral sensory map, seems the best established. The reciprocal relationship of this region with the infralimbic cortex, and the massive descending projections of the latter into the central autonomic control system, suggests that the infralimbic cortex may serve as an autonomic motor area. The prelimbic cortex, by analogy with the motor system, may be viewed as an autonomic premotor area, mainly receiving limbic afferents, and feeding forward into the infralimbic area, but with little direct autonomic output of its own. The primary sensory and motor areas appear capable, respectively, of receiving visceral afferents and activating autonomic responses, but mainly in coordination with ongoing somatic sensory and motor processes.

This survey of the role of the cerebral cortex in autonomic control reveals a number of questions that remain unanswered: How do these cortical sites integrate autonomic responses with ongoing behaviors? What is the relationship between afferent visceral information and somatic sensations? What is the precise localization of the sites for autonomic responses? What are the specific neural pathways that mediate these responses? In future studies of autonomic cortical areas, it will be important to distinguish sites involved specifically in certain autonomic functions (e.g., cardiovascular or gastrointestinal), and to make more subtle measurements of autonomic variables, such as recording blood flow to various vascular beds rather than blood pressure.

REFERENCES

Reviews

Calaresu, R., Ciriello, J., Caverson, M. M., Cechetto, D. F., and Krukoff, T. L. (1984). Functional neuroanatomy of central pathways controlling the circulation. In: *Hypertension and the Brain,* T. A. Kotchen and C. P. Gurthrie (eds.), Futura, Mount Kisco, NY, pp. 3–21.

Cechetto, D. F. (1987). Central representation of visceral function. *Federation Proceedings* 46, 17–23.

Delgado, J. M. (1960). Circulatory effects of cortical stimulation. *Physiological Reviews* 40; Suppl. 4, 146–178.

Finger, T. E. (1987). Gustatory nuclei and pathways in the central nervous system. In: *Neurobiology of Taste and Smell,* T. E. Finger and W. L. Silver (eds.), Wiley, New York, pp. 331–353.

Fulton, J. F. (1949). Cerebral cortex: Autonomic representation in precentral motor cortex. In: *Physiology of the Nervous System,* J. F. Fulton (ed.), Oxford University Press, New York, pp. 468–484.

Hoff, E. C., Kell, J. F. Jr., and Carroll, M. N., Jr. (1963). Effects of cortical stimulation and lesions on cardiovascular function. *Physiological Reviews* 43, 68–114.

Mitchell, J., and Schmidt, R. F. (1984). Cardiovascular reflex control by afferent fibers from skeletal muscle receptors. In: *Handbook of Physiology. The Cardiovascular System* III, Part 2, American Physiological Society, Bethesda, MD, pp. 623–658.

Norgren, R. (1984). Central neural mechanisms of taste. In: *Handbook of Physiology,* Section I: *The Nervous System,* Vol. III, *Sensory Processes,* I. Darien Smith (ed.), American Physiological Society, Bethesda, MD, pp. 1087–1128.

Smith, D. A., and Devito, J. L. (1984). Central neural integration for the control of autonomic responses associated with emotion. *Annual Review of Neuroscience* 7, 43–65.

Research Papers

Amassian, V. E. (1951a). Cortical representation of visceral afferents. *Journal of Neurophysiology* 14, 433–444.

Amassian, V. E. (1951b). Fiber groups and spinal pathways of cortically represented visceral afferents. *Journal of Neurophysiology* 14, 445–560.

Ammons, W. S., Girardot, M.-N., and Foreman, R. D. (1985). T_2–T_5 spinothalamic neurons projecting to medial thalamus with viscerosomatic input. *Journal of Neurophysiology* 54, 73–89.

Bachman, D. S., Hallowitz, R. A., and MacLean, P. D. (1977). Effects of vagal volleys and serotonin on units of cingulate cortex in monkeys. *Brain Research* 130, 253–269.

Bailey, P., and Bremer, F. (1938). A sensory cortical representation of the vagus nerve with a note on the effects of the low blood pressure on the cortical electrogram. *Journal of Neurophysiology* 1, 405–412.

Bard, P. (1929). The central representation of the sympathetic system. *Archives of Neurology and Psychiatry* 22, 230–241.

Berk, M. L., and Finkelstein, J. A. (1982). Efferent connections of the lateral hypothalamic area of the rat: An autoradiographic investigation. *Brain Research Bulletin* 8, 511–526.

Blair, R. W., Ammons, W. S., and Foreman, R. D. (1984). Responses of thoracic spinothalamic and spinoreticular cells to coronary occlusion. *Journal of Neurophysiology* 51, 636–648.

Bonvallet, M., Dell, P., and Hiebel, G. (1954). Tonus sympathétique et activité electrique cortical. *Electroencephalography and Clinical Neurophysiology* 6, 119–144.

Bridgers, S. L., Spencer, S. S., Spencer, D. D., and Sasaki, C. T. (1985). A cerebral effect of carotid sinus stimulation. Observation during intraoperative electroencephalographic monitoring. *Archives of Neurology* 42, 574–577.

Buchanan, S. L., and Powell, D. A. (1982a). Cingulate damage attenuates conditioned bradycardia. *Neuroscience Letters* 29, 261–268.

Buchanan, S. L., and Powell, D. A. (1982b). Cingulate cortex: Its role in Pavlovian conditioning. *Journal of Comparative and Physiological Psychology* 96, 755–774.

Buchanan, S. L., Powell, D. A., and Buggy, J. (1984). ³H-2-deoxyglucose uptake after electrical stimulation of cardioactive sites in anterior medial cortex in rabbits. *Brain Research Bulletin* 13, 371–382.

Buchanan, S. L., Valentine, J., and Powell, D. A. (1985). Autonomic responses are elicited by electrical stimulation of the medial but not lateral frontal cortex in rabbits. *Behavioral Brain Research* 18, 51–62.

Bucy, P. (1935). Vasomotor changes associated with paralysis of cerebral origin. *Archives of Neurology and Psychiatry* 33, 30–52.

Burns, S. M., and Wyss, J. M. (1985). The involvement of the anterior cingulate cortex in blood pressure control. *Brain Research* 340, 71.

Cannon, W. B., and Britton, S. W. (1925). Studies on the conditions of activity in endocrine glands. XV. Pseudoaffective medulliadrenal secretion. *American Journal of Physiology* 72, 283–294.

Cechetto, D. F., and Calaresu, F. R. (1983). Parabrachial units responding to stimulation of buffer nerves and forebrain in the cat. *American Journal of Physiology* 245, R811–R819.

Cechetto, D. F., and Saper, C. B. (1987). Evidence for a viscerotopic sensory representation in the cortex and thalamus in the rat. *Journal of Comparative Neurology* 262, 27–45.

Cechetto, D. F., Ciriello, J., and Calaresu, F. R. (1983). Afferent connections to cardiovascular sites in the amygdala: A horseradish peroxidase study in the cat. *Journal of the Autonomic Nervous System 8*, 97–110.

Clarke, N. P., Smith, O. A., and Shearn, D. W. (1968). Topographical representation of vascular smooth muscle of limbs in primate motor cortex. *American Journal of Physiology* 214, 122–129.

Dell, P., and Olson, R. (1951). Projections thalamiques corticales et cerebelleuses des afferences viscerales vagales. *Comptes Rendus des Societes Biologiques (Paris)* 145, 1084–1088.

Eliasson, S., Lindgren, P., and Uvnas, B. (1952). Representation in the hypothalamus and the motor cortex in the dog of the sympathetic vasodilator outflow to the skeletal muscles. *Acta Physiologica Scandinavica* 27, 18–37.

Frysinger, R. C., and Harper, R. M. (1986). Cardiac and respiratory relationships with neural discharge in the anterior cingulate cortex during sleep-waking states. *Experimental Neurology* 94, 247–263.

Frysztak, R. J, and Neafsey, E. J. (1987). Effects of rat medial frontal cortex lesions on conditioned emotional responses. *Society for Neuroscience Abstracts* 13, 1551.

Fulwiler, C. E., and Saper, C. B. (1984). Subnuclear organization of the efferent connections of the parabrachial nucleus in the rat. *Brain Research Reviews* 7, 229–259.

Green, H. D., and Hoff, E. C. (1937). Effects of faradic stimulation of the cerebral cortex on limb and renal volumes in the cat and monkey. *American Journal of Physiology* 118, 641–658.

Hall, R. E., Livingston, R. B., and Bloor, C. M. (1977). Orbital cortical influences on cardiovascular dynamics and myocardial structure in conscious monkeys. *Journal of Nuerosurgery* 46, 638–647.

Hilton, S. M., Spyer, K. M., and Timms, R. J. (1979). The

origin of the hind limb vasodilatation evoked by stimulation of the motor cortex in the cat. *Journal of Physiology (London)* 287, 545–557.

Hoff, E. C., and Green, H. D. (1936). Cardiovascular reactions induced by electrical stimulation of the cerebral cortex. *American Journal of Physiology* 117, 411–422.

Hoff, E. C., and Hoff, H. E. (1934). Spinal terminations of the projection fibers from the motor cortex of primates. *Brain* 57, 454–474.

Hoffman, B. L., and Rasmussen, T. (1953). Stimulation studies of insular cortex of *Macaca mulatta*. *Journal of Neurophysiology* 16, 343.

Hosoya, Y., and Matsushita, M. (1981). Brainstem projections from the lateral hypothalamic area in the rat, as studied with autoradiography. *Neuroscience Letters* 24, 111–116.

Hsu, S. H., Hwang, K., and Chu, H. N. (1942). A study of the cardiovascular changes induced by stimulation of the motor cortex in dogs. *American Journal of Physiology* 137, 468–472.

Hurley-Gius, K. M., and Neafsey, E. J. (1986). The medial frontal cortex and gastric motility: Microstimulation results and their possible significance for the overall pattern of organization of rat frontal and parietal cortex. *Brain Research* 365, 241–248.

Hurley-Gius, K. M., Cechetto, D. F., and Saper, C. B. (1986). Spinal connections of the infralimbic autonomic cortex. *Society for Neuroscience Abstracts* 12, 538.

Kaada, B. R. (1951). Somato-motor, autonomic and electrocorticographic responses to electrical stimulation of rhinencephalic and other structures in primates, cat and dog. *Acta Physiological Scandinavica* 24, Suppl. 83, 1–285.

Kennard, M. A. (1937). The cortical influence on the autonomic nervous system. *Bumke und Foersters Handbuch fur Neurologie* 2, 476–491.

Kennard, M. A. (1945). Focal autonomic representation in the cortex and its relation to sham rage. *Journal of Neuropathology and Experimental Neurology* 4, 295–304.

Kosar, E., Grill, H. J., and Norgren, R. (1986). Gustatory cortex in the rat. I. Physiological properties and cytoarchitecture. *Brain Research* 379, 329–341.

Landau, W. M. (1953). Autonomic responses mediated via the corticospinal tract. *Journal of Neurophysiology* 16, 299–311.

Loewy, A. D., and Burton, H. (1978). Nuclei of the solitary tract: Efferent projections to the lower brain stem and spinal cord of the cat. *Journal of Comparative Neurology* 181, 421–450.

Lofving, B. (1961). Cardiovascular adjustments induced from the rostral cingulate gyrus. *Acta Physiologica Scandinavica* 53, Suppl. 184, 1–82.

Luiten, P. G. M., terHorst, G. J., and Steffens, A. B. (1987). The hypothalamus, intrinsic connections and outflow pathways to the endocrine system in relation to the control of feeding and metabolism. *Progress in Neurobiology* 28, 1–54.

MacLeod, J. G. (1958). The representation of the splanchnic afferent pathways in the thalamus of the cat. *Journal of Physiology (London)* 140, 462–478.

Mehler, W. R. (1980). Subcortical afferent connections of the amygdala in the monkey. *Journal of Comparative Neurology* 190, 733–762.

Miura, M., Onai, T., and Takayama, K. (1983). Projections of upper structure to the spinal cardioacceleratory center in cats: An HRP study using a new microinjection method. *Journal of the Autonomic Nervous System* 7, 119–139.

Mizuno, N., Takahashi, O., Satoda, T., and Matsushima, R. (1985). Amygdalospinal projections in the macaque monkey. *Neuroscience Letters* 53, 327–330.

Ottersen, O. P. (1981). Afferent connections to the amygdaloid complex of the rat with some observations in the cat. III. Afferents from the lower brain stem. *Journal of Comparative Neurology* 202, 335–356.

Ottersen, O. P. (1982). Connections of the amydgala of the rat. IV. Corticoamygdaloid and intraamygdaloid connections as studied with axonal transport of horseradish peroxidase. *Journal of Comparative Neurology* 205, 30–48.

Patton, H. D., and Amassian, V. E. (1951). Thalamic relay of splanchnic afferent fibers. *American Journal of Physiology* 167, 815–816.

Paxinos, G., and Watson, C. (1986). *The Rat Brain in Stereotaxic Coordinates,* 2nd ed. Academic Press, Sydney.

Penfield, W., and Faulk, M. E., Jr. (1955). The insula. Further observations on its function. *Brain* 78, 445–470.

Price, J. L., and Amaral, D. G. (1981). An autoradiographic study of the projections of the central nucleus of the monkey amygdala. *Journal of Neuroscience* 1, 1242–1259.

Pritchard, T. C., Hamilton, R. B., Morse, J. R., and Norgren, R. (1986). Projections of thalamic gustatory and lingual areas in the monkey, *Macaca fascicularis. Journal of Comparative Neurology* 244, 213–228.

Radna, R. J., and MacLean, P. D. (1981). Vagal elicitation of respiratory-type and other unit responses in basal limbic structures of squirrel monkeys. *Brain Research* 213, 45–61.

Ricardo, J. A., and Koh, E. T. (1978). Anatomical evidence of direct projections from the nucleus of the solitary tract to the hypothalamus, amygdala, and other forebrain structures in the rat. *Brain Research* 153, 1–26.

Room, P., Russchen, F. T., Groenewegen, H. J., and Lohman, A. H. M. (1985). Efferent connections of the prelimbic (area 32) and the infralimbic (area 25) cortices: An anterograde tracing study in the cat. *Journal of Comparative Neurology* 242, 40–55.

Rose, M. (1927). Gyrus limbicus anterior und regio retrosplenialis (Cortex holoprotoptychos quinquestratificatus). Vergleichende architektonik bei tier und mensch. *Journal fur Psychologie und Neurologie* 35, 65–173.

Rosene, D. L., and van Hoesen, G. W. (1977). Hippocampal efferents reach widespread areas of cerebral cortex and amygdala in the rhesus monkey. *Science* 198, 315–317.

Ross, C. A., Ruggiero, D. A., and Reis, D. J. (1981). Afferent projections to cardiovascular portions of the nucleus of the tractus solitarius in the rat. *Brain Research* 223, 402–408.

Ruggiero, D. A., Mraovitch, S., Granata, A. R., Anwar, M., and Reis, D. J. (1987). Role of insular cortex in cardiovascular function. *Journal of Comparative Neurology* 257, 189–207.

Russchen, F. T. (1982a). Amygdalopetal projections in the cat. I. Cortical afferent connections. A study with retrograde and anterograde tracing techniques. *Journal of Comparative Neurology* 206, 159–179.

Russchen, F. T. (1982b). Amygdalopetal projections in the cat. II. Subcortical afferent connections. A study with retrograde tracing techniques. *Journal of Comparative Neurology* 207, 157–176.

Saper, C. B. (1982a). Reciprocal parabrachial-cortical connections in the rat. *Brain Research* 242, 33–40.

Saper, C. B. (1982b). Convergence of autonomic and limbic connections in the insular cortex of the rat. *Journal of Comparative Neurology* 210, 163–173.

Saper, C. B. (1985). Organization of cerebral cortical afferent systems in the rat. II. Hypothalamocortical projections. *Journal of Comparative Neurology* 237, 21–46.

Saper, C. B. (1987). Diffuse cortical projection systems: Anatomical organization and role in cortical function. In: *Handbook of Physiology, The Nervous System,* V. F Plum (ed.), American Physiological Society, Bethesda, MD, pp. 169–210.

Saper, C. B., and Loewy, A. D. (1980). Efferent connections of the parabrachial nucleus in the rat. *Brain Research* 197, 291–317.

Saper, C. B., Loewy, A. D., Swanson, L. W., and Cowan, W. M. (1976). Direct hypothalamo-autonomic connections. *Brain Research* 117, 305–312.

Schwaber, J. S., Kapp, B. S., and Higgins, G. (1980). The origin and extent of direct amygdala projections to the region of the dorsal motor nucleus of the vagus and the nucleus of the solitary tract. *Neuroscience Letters* 20, 15–20.

Schwaber, J. S., Kapp, B. S., Higgins, G. A., and Rapp, P. R. (1982). Amygdaloid and basal forebrain direct connections with the nucleus of the solitary tract and the dorsal motor nucleus. *Journal of Neuroscience* 2, 1424–1438.

Sheehan, D. (1935). The effect of cortical stimulation on gastric movements in the monkey. *Journal of Physiology (London)* 83, 177–184.

Shipley, M. T. (1982). Insular cortex projection to the nucleus of the solitary tract and brainstem visceromotor regions in the mouse. *Brain Research Bulletin* 8, 139–148.

Shipley, M. T., and Sanders, M. S. (1982). Special senses are really special: Evidence for a reciprocal, bilateral pathway between insular cortex and nucleus parabrachialis. *Brain Research Bulletin* 8, 493–501.

Smith, W. K. (1945). The functional significance of the rostral cingular cortex as revealed by its responses to electrical excitation. *Journal of Neurophysiology* 8, 241–255.

Spiegel, E. A., and Hunsicker, W. C., Jr. (1936). The conduction of cortical impulses to the autonomic system. *Journal of Nervous and Mental Disease* 83, 252–274.

Swanson, L. W. (1981). A direct projection from Ammon's horn to prefrontal cortex in the rat. *Brain Research* 217, 150–154.

Swanson, L. W., and Kuypers, H. G. J. M. (1980). A direct projection from the ventromedial nucleus and retrochiasmatic area of the hypothalamus to the medulla and spinal cord of the rat. *Neuroscience Letters* 17, 307–312.

Szilagyi, J. E., Taylor, A. A., and Skinner, J. E. (1987). Cryoblockade of the ventromedial frontal cortex reverses hypertension in the rat. *Hypertension* 9, 576–581.

Terreberry, R. R., and Neafsey, E. J. (1983). Rat medial

frontal cortex: A visceral motor region with a direct projection to the solitary nucleus. *Brain Research* 278, 245–249.

Thompson, F. J., Lerner, D. N., Fields, K., and Blackwelder, A. (1980). Projection of limb venous afferents to the feline motor-sensory cortex. *Journal of the Autonomic Nervous System* 2, 39–45.

van der Kooy, D., McGinty, J. F., Koda, L. Y., Gerfen, C. R., and Bloom, F. E. (1982). Visceral cortex: A direct connection from prefrontal cortex to the solitary nucleus in the rat. *Neuroscience Letters* 33, 123–127.

van der Kooy, D., Koda, L. Y., McGinty, J. F., Gerfen, C. R., and Bloom, F. E. (1984). The organization of projections from the cortex, amygdala, and hypothalamus to the nucleus of the solitary tract in rat. *Journal of Comparative Neurology* 224, 1–24.

Verberne, A. J. M., Lewis, S. J., Worland, P. J., Beart, P. M., Jarrott, B., Christie, M. J., and Louis, W. J. (1987). Medial prefrontal cortical lesions modulate baroreflex sensitivity in the rat. *Brain Research* 426, 243–249.

von Euler, U.S., and Folkow, B. (1958). The effect of stimulation of autonomic areas in the cerebral cortex upon the adrenaline and noradrenaline secretion from the adrenal gland in the cat. *Acta Physiologica Scandinavica* 42, 313–320.

Wall, P. D., and Pribram, K. H. (1950). Trigeminal neurotomy and blood pressure responses from stimulation of lateral cerebral cortex of *Macaca mulatta. Journal of Neurophysiology* 13, 409–412.

Wall, P. D., and Davis, G. D. (1951). Three cerebral cortical systems affecting autonomic function. *Journal of Neurophysiology* 14, 507–517.

Ward, A. A., Jr. (1948). The cingular gyrus: Area 24. *Journal of Neurophysiology* 11, 13–23.

Yamamoto, T., Matsuo, R., and Kawamura, Y. (1980). Localization of cortical gustatory area in rats and its role in taste discrimination. *Journal of Neurophysiology* 44, 440–455.

Yasui, Y., Itoh, K., Sugimoto, T., Kaneko, T., and Mizuno, N. (1987). Thalamocortical and thalamo-amygdaloid projections from the parvicellular division of the posteromedial ventral nucleus in the cat. *Journal of Comparative Neurology* 257, 253–268.

Yasui, Y., Itoh, K., Takada, M., Mitani, A., Kaneko, T., and Mizuno, N. (1985). Direct cortical projections to the parabrachial nucleus in the cat. *Journal of Comparative Neurology* 234, 77–86.

13

Neural Regulation of Vasopressin-Containing Hypothalamic Neurons and the Role of Vasopressin in Cardiovascular Function

M. C. HARRIS AND A. D. LOEWY

Vasopressin is a peptide hormone that is synthesized in the cell bodies of the magnocellular neurons of the supraoptic and paraventricular nuclei of the hypothalamus. This peptide is transported along with its carrier protein, neurophysin I, in axons that project to the neural lobe of the pituitary gland. Here it is stored in axon terminals and, on physiological demand, released into the hypophysial capillaries. A variety of physiological stimuli, usually involving increases in extracellular fluid osmolality or decreases in blood volume or blood pressure, trigger the release of this hormone.

As with all peptide hormones, vasopressin exerts its biological influence by binding to specialized receptors on the cell membrane. By studying the biological properties of a large number of synthetic analogues of vasopressin (see review by Manning et al., 1987), investigators discovered that there are two general classes of vasopressin receptor. One group (V1 receptors) is located on the vascular smooth muscle cell membrane. Binding of vasopressin to V1 receptors leads to activation of the phosphatidylinositol second messenger system and results in contraction of the muscle. The other group of receptors (V2) is located largely on the cell membranes of the renal tubules. Binding of vasopressin to V2 receptors leads to an increase in the permeability of the basement membrane to water, which is brought about by activation of the adenylate cyclase second messenger system. Vasopressin receptors are not confined to vascular and renal cells. For example, V1 receptors are present on hepatocytes and their activation causes increased glycogenolysis (Michell et al., 1979); as will be seen later, V1 receptors are also located within the central nervous system.

Vasopressin helps to regulate arterial blood pressure by two distinct physiological mechanisms: by acting via the blood vessels themselves through vasoconstriction and by acting through the kidney, resulting in water retention, which leads to expansion of extracellular fluid volume. This latter effect produces an increase in venous return, and, in turn, is responsible for an increase in cardiac output that ultimately can cause an increase in arterial pressure (see Share, 1988 for a review of the historical development of these two areas).

Although vasopressin is a vasoconstrictor peptide, it rarely functions in this way except under extreme physiological conditions, such as during severe dehydration or hemorrhage, because normal plasma levels are too low to cause vasoconstriction. Under normal conditions, the plasma concentration of vasopressin in humans is 2–4 pg/ml and in rats is 3–10 pg/ml. After dehydration for 24–48 hours, these values increase to 10 pg/ml in humans and 15–35 pg/ml in rats (see Cowley and Liard, 1987 for review). The latter values are at the lower limit at which vasopressin has been demonstrated to act as a vasoconstrictor peptide (see Altura and Altura, 1984 for review). Following hypotensive hemorrhage or surgery, plasma concentrations of vasopressin may reach levels of 100–500 pg/ml, that is, 10–100 times the basal values. At this latter concentration, vasopressin can produce profound vasoconstriction in most vascular beds except brain, heart, and lung. Since the concentrations of V1 vasopressin receptors vary in different vascular beds, it follows that at varying plasma concentrations, vasopressin may act as a differential regulator of blood flow by shunting blood from certain vascular beds such as the splanchnic and skeletal muscle circulations to critical tissues such as the brain and heart. In addition, vasopressin can increase the sensitivity of certain reflexes involved in circulatory control as well as potentiating the influence of the sympathetic nervous system.

In this chapter, the neural pathways by which cardiovascular reflexes regulate vasopressin release will be discussed and the peripheral influences of vasopressin on the cardiovascular system will be reviewed. Other issues, such as the role of vasopressin in controlling extracellular fluid osmolality, will not be considered here, but are discussed in Chapter 14 and are the subject of several reviews (Johnson, 1985; Lightman and Everitt, 1986; Bisset and Chowdrey, 1988). In addition, the potential function of oxytocin in cardiovascular control is beyond the scope of this chapter; see Petty (1987) for a discussion.

BACKGROUND

Anatomy of the Magnocellular Hypothalamic Nuclei

The magnocellular portions of the supraoptic and paraventricular nuclei are made up of vasopressin and oxytocin cells that project to the posterior pituitary. In the rat, there are approximately 3,500 vasopressin cells in the supraoptic nucleus and 1,000 in the paraventricular nucleus (see Morris et al., 1987 for review). Vasopressin cells are clustered in the ventral part of the supraoptic nucleus and in the

central part of the paraventricular nucleus (Figure 13-1; Hou-Yu et al., 1986). In the supraoptic nucleus, vasopressin magnocellular neurons project exclusively to the posterior pituitary, but Hatton et al. (1983a) have found that in the rat some vasopressin and oxytocin magnocellular cells in the paraventricular nucleus have axons that send collaterals to the perifornical and lateral hypothalamic areas. The dendrites of most of the supraoptic and paraventricular neurons are confined within the nucleus; however, Golgi studies demonstrate that some magnocellular neurons of both nuclei have dendrites extending beyond their borders (van den Pol, 1982; Leng and Dyball, 1983). Most of the cells that give rise to these extranuclear dendrites lie in the regions of the respective nuclei where oxytocin cells are most concentrated. This implies that connectional studies dealing with the afferent projections to the vasopressin neurons must demonstrate axonal projections directly to these magnocellular regions within each nucleus. However, axonal projections terminating just outside the nuclear limits of the

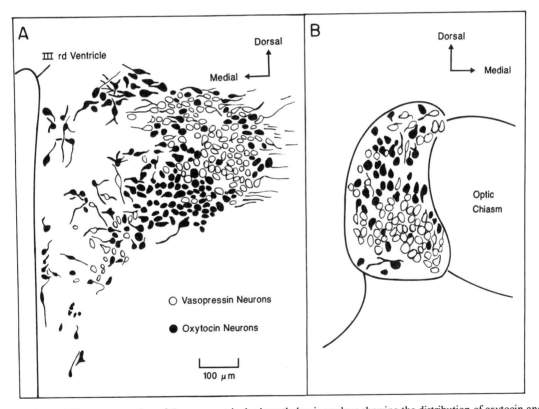

Figure 13-1 (A) Transverse section of the paraventricular hypothalamic nucleus showing the distribution of oxytocin and vasopressin immunoreactive neurons. Note that the oxytocin cells are distributed preferentially around the border of the nucleus, while the vasopressin cells are concentrated in its central part. Dendrites of some of the oxytocin neurons extend beyond the nuclear boundaries. (B) The vasopressin neurons lie in the ventral part by the supraoptic nucleus, while oxytocin cells are concentrated in its dorsal part. (Reproduced with slight modification from Hou-Yu et al., 1986, with permission of the authors and publisher.)

magnocellular cell bodies may affect vasopressin neurons by interneuronal connections or possibly by diffusion of transmitters.

The supraoptic nucelus is relatively homogeneous, but the paraventricular hypothalamic nucleus is a complex structure made up of a series of subnuclei (see reviews by Swanson and Sawchenko, 1983; Swanson et al., 1986; Swanson, 1987). Three main functional regions have been defined (Figure 13-2): First, the magnocellular neurosecretory neurons that synthesize oxytocin and vasopressin form one distinct subnucleus (which has been subdivided into three different groups: anterior, medial, and posterior). These neurons send their axons to the posterior pituitary and release their peptide hormones into the general circulation. Second, the medial and periventricular parvocellular neurosecretory neurons that produce pituitary releasing factors such as corticotropin-releasing factor and thyrotropin-releasing factor form a second functional group. They send their axons to the median eminence,

where they terminate in close proximity to capillaries. Following their release, the hypothalamic-releasing factors are transported by the hypothalamo-hypophyseal portal system to the anterior pituitary where they influence the release of anterior pituitary hormones. Third, a collection of parvocellular neurons that lies dorsal, lateral, and ventral to the magnocellular neurons has widespread connections within the central nervous system. Neurons of this third group project to the autonomic centers of the brain stem and spinal cord. These include mesencephalic central gray matter, parabrachial nucleus, locus coeruleus, caudal raphe nuclei, nucleus of the solitary tract, and intermediolateral cell column (Luiten et al., 1985).

Functional Properties of Vasopressin Neurons

Vasopressin neurons of the magnocellular nuclei are among the few hypothalamic neurons that can be readily identified *in vivo* because of their character-

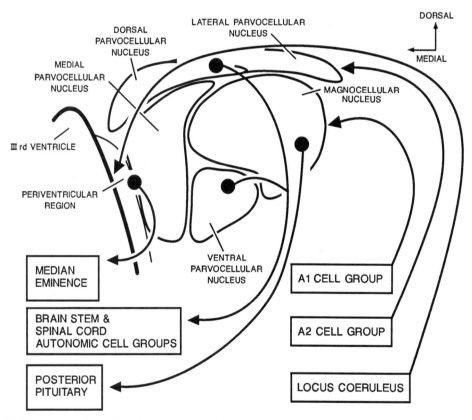

Figure 13-2 The paraventricular hypothalamic nucleus is composed of three functional subdivisions. The magnocellular subdivision contains oxytocin and vasopressin neurons that send axons to the posterior pituitary and release these peptides into the systemic circulation. The medial parvocellular and periventricular subdivisions project to the median eminence and secrete hypothalamic-releasing peptides that are carried to the anterior pituitary via the hypothalamo-hypophyseal portal system. The dorsal, lateral, and ventral parvocellular nuclei project to autonomic centers of the lower brain stem and to the spinal cord. The A1, A2, and locus coeruleus noradrenergic cell groups project to specific regions of the paraventricular hypothalamic nucleus. Only the A1 cell group projects to the magnocellular nucleus. (Adapted from Lightman and Everitt, 1986.)

istic phasic firing pattern (see Wakerley, 1987 for review). Yamashita et al. (1984a) demonstrated by combined intracellular lucifer yellow dye injections and immunohistochemistry that phasically firing neurons in the supraoptic nucleus of rats contain immunoreactive vasopressin. Vasopressin-containing neurons of the paraventricular nucleus also exhibit the same properties (Cobbett et al., 1986). The bursting firing that occurs in the vasopressin neurons may be related to its membrane properties and/or its synaptic inputs. The former factor may be of greater importance since this pacemaker-like activity occurs in both slice preparations (Hatton et al., 1983b) and long-term cultures (Gähwiller and Dreifuss, 1979). The pattern of bursting activity, in all likelihood, is responsible for the basal release of vasopressin, and it has been demonstrated that bursting discharge is the most efficient means of releasing vasopressin (Dutton and Dyball, 1979).

Magnocellular neurons appear to be coupled. When one cell is intracellularly injected with lucifer yellow, there is transfer of the dye from that cell to one or more neurons in the immediate vicinity. This appears not to be a random effect because the labeled pairs or triplets were always the same, viz. either only vasopressin or oxytocin cells (Corbett et al., 1985). The anatomical basis for the dye coupling appears to be mediated by gap junctions between the cells (Andrew et al., 1981). This anatomical specialization could serve to electrotonically couple the vasopressin neurons and promote synchrony of neuronal firing during hormone release (Cobbett et al., 1985).

CARDIOVASCULAR REFLEXES AND VASOPRESSIN RELEASE

Hemorrhage is one of the most potent stimuli for the release of vasopressin. However, the stimulus is complex since hemorrhage can reduce blood pressure as well as blood volume, both of which will release vasopressin (Share, 1962; Beleslin et al., 1967). Changes of blood pressure are sensed by stretch receptors of the carotid sinus and aortic arch on the high-pressure side of the cardiovascular system, and changes of blood volume are sensed by receptors at the junctions of the great veins with the atria of the heart. Which group of receptors is more important in controlling vasopressin liberation is a matter for debate, and may be subject to species variation. It is clear, however, that these receptors impose a tonic inhibitory influence on vasopressin release. Removal of either influence by reducing blood volume or blood pressure will increase circulating vasopressin, the former being more sensitive than the latter. The central neural pathways through which this inhibitory influence is conveyed to the hypothalamus

are incompletely understood. There is general agreement, however, that the ascending catecholamine systems are important, but their precise function is uncertain and is discussed below.

Atrial Receptors

In 1938 Rydin and Verney, using unanesthetized, water-loaded dogs, reported that a slow hemorrhage that did not significantly reduce arterial blood pressure was nevertheless followed by prolonged antidiuresis. Since the kidneys were denervated and the antidiuresis outlasted blood pressure changes by more than an hour, it was concluded that the renal effect followed release of vasopressin. The actual demonstration that hemorrhage causes vasopressin release and the elucidation of the reflexes involved have been the subject of considerable investigation in the 50 years since that first demonstration.

Demonstration of the release of vasopressin during nonhypotensive hemorrhage was achieved by Henry et al. (1968), but in the intervening years it has become evident that a reflex diuresis could be induced by any maneuver, such as negative pressure breathing, that stretches the atrial walls (Gauer et al., 1954). The vagus nerve also showed an increase in discharge during atrial distension and a reduction in nerve activity during small hemorrhage. Moreover, cooling of the vagi abolished the reflex diuresis, which normally followed atrial distension (Henry and Pearce, 1956). From experiments such as these arose the concept that the diuresis that followed atrial distension resulted from the inhibition of vasopressin release. In fact, this is a gross simplification of the complex events linking the cardiovascular and renal responses to expansion of blood volume and atrial distension. The first challenge to the vasopressin hypothesis came from Ledsome and Mason (1972), who attempted to prevent distension-induced diuresis by infusing vasopressin intravenously. The result was that although vasopressin was infused in quantities that would normally produce maximal antidiuresis, it had no influence on the diuresis induced by atrial distension. Unequivocal evidence for a fall in circulating vasopressin was eventually produced by Ledsome et al. (1983) using a sensitive and specifc immunoassay for vasopressin (Figure 13-3). The fall in vasopressin alone was not sufficient, however, to account for the diuresis, nor did it explain the insensitivity to infused vasopressin. This problem has not been totally resolved. As shown by Schultz et al. (1982), atrial distension has profound and complex effects on the circulation by increasing peripheral resistance, arterial blood pressure, and heart rate, all of which may influence renal perfusion.

The interpretation of these data is further complicated by the discovery of atrial natriuretic peptide,

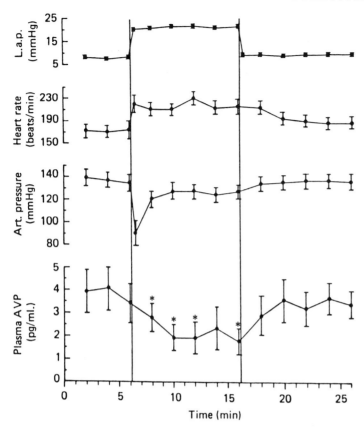

Figure 13-3 A series of graphs showing the changes in the left atrial pressure (L.a.p.), heart rate, mean arterial pressure, and plasma vasopressin (AVP) in response to left atrial distension in the dog during the period between the vertical lines. Each point represents the mean (± standard error of the mean) of measurements (n = 7). Asterisks indicate that the plasma vasopressin value was less than the plasma vasopressin during the control periods ($p <$ 0.05). (Reproduced from Ledsome et al., 1983, with permission of the authors and publisher.)

which is synthesized by the atria of the heart (de Bold, 1982). This peptide, released in response to atrial distension (Ledsome et al., 1985), causes natriuresis and diuresis, which may be accompanied by changes in renal blood flow (see Genest and Cantin, 1988 for review). Nevertheless, the atrial stretch receptors do provide an inhibitory, vagally mediated influence on vasopressin liberation, which is sensitive to quite small changes in blood volume.

Baroreceptors

Atrial receptors are not the only depressor influence on vasopressin release; there is also strong evidence for an inhibitory effect of baroreceptor activation. Share and Levy (1966b) showed in dogs that changing the perfusion pressure of the isolated carotid bifurcation from a pulsatile to nonpulsatile stimulus while maintaining a constant mean pressure resulted in vasopressin release. There is also electrophysiological evidence for an inhibitory influence of baroreceptors on the hypothalamus. In both cats and rats, activation of carotid sinus baroreceptors exerts a powerful inhibitory influence on magnocellular vasopressin neurons of the supraoptic nucleus (Kannan and Yagi, 1978; Harris, 1979; Yamashita and Koizumi, 1979; McAllen and Harris, 1988).

The relative importance of the various high- and low-pressure receptors in controlling vasopressin release is difficult to assess. In dogs, the atrial receptor input seems to be the more important. Thames and Schmid (1979) found that denervation of the high-pressure receptors by sectioning the aortic and carotid sinus nerves, leaving the vagi intact, had little effect on vasopressin levels, but subsequent section of the vagi resulted in a sharp increase in the amount of hormone secreted. In contrast, sectioning the vagal nerves first increased vasopressin output, which was increased again on section of the carotid and sinus nerves. This can be interpreted as showing that both groups of receptors have a tonic depressant effect on vasopressin output, but that normally the vagal influence is the stronger, masking the influence of the arterial baroreceptors. Only on removal of the vagus does the baroreceptor influence become evident.

Whether the same situation occurs in humans is unclear. Much of the early literature suggested that hypotension, which causes an unloading of high-pressure baroreceptors, was a prerequisite for vasopressin release (see Bisset and Jones, 1975 for review), but this may not necessarily be the case. Activation of low-pressure afferents is also involved. There is about a 70% rise in circulating vasopressin following reductions in central blood volume and right atrial pressures (cardiopulmonary low-pressure receptor load), caused by thigh cuff inflation in humans, without changes in mean arterial blood pressure, pulse pressure, or cardiac output (Egan et al., 1984). This suggests that selective unloading of low-pressure receptors will reflexly cause a release of vasopressin in humans.

One further question involves the relative importance of the cardiovascular reflex inputs in the minute-to-minute control of vasopressin output. For example, how important are the cardiovascular influences in comparison with the influence of the changes in plasma osmolality? This is not the place for a detailed discussion of the control of vasopressin by changes in osmolality, a subject involving considerable controversy (see Bie, 1980 and Bisset and Chowdrey, 1988, for reviews). However, it is clear that vasopressin release increases as plasma osmolality is raised above 280 mOsm/kg (Figure 13-4), that is, well within normal physiological variation.

The relative sensitivity of the vasopressin neurons to changes in extracellular fluid osmolality or cardiovascular input is not known and there may be species differences. Electrophysiological experiments by Leng and Dyball (1987) suggest that in rats the influence of blood pressure is not great, but in cats it is possible to record supraoptic neurons whose rate of discharge moves antiphasically with normal small fluctuations in arterial blood pressure (Figure 13-5).

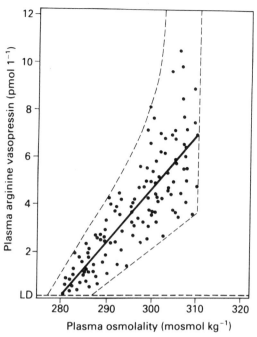

Figure 13-4 This graph shows the direct relationship between plasma osmolality and plasma vasopressin levels. Slight increases in plasma osmolality caused by intravenous infusion of 0.85% NaCl in humans causes rises in plasma vasopressin. (Reproduced from Lightman and Everitt, 1986, with permission of the authors and publisher.)

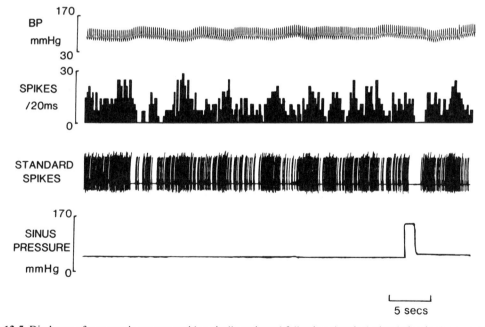

Figure 13-5 Discharge of supraoptic neuron antidromically activated following electrical stimulation in the neural lobe of the cat. The records show that as blood pressure varied naturally, the discharge of the neuron moved in the opposite direction; briefly raising the pressure in a blind sac of the carotid bifurcation on the side ipsilateral to the recording site by about 150 mm Hg completely inhibited the neuronal discharge (McAllen and Harris, unpublished results).

In this connection, Robertson et al. (1976) have put forward an interesting theory concerning the relative interactions of volume and osmotic influences. In both humans and rats, it was found that within normal limits, circulating volume per se had little effect on vasopressin secretion, but it did influence the sensitivity of the magnocellular neurons to osmotic challenge (Robertson and Athar, 1976; Dunn et al., 1973). Thus, isotonic expansion of extracellular volume reduced the release of vasopressin by an osmotic stimulus, whereas reduction of blood volume increased the vasopressin released to an osmotic stimulus of similar magnitude. One can imagine, therefore, that the major role of the cardiovascular inputs is to modulate the magnitude of the response to osmoreceptor challenge, and thus the amount of vasopressin released to the continuously changing osmolality of extracellular fluid.

Chemoreceptors

All the reflex inputs controlling vasopressin release discussed so far have been inhibitory. However, Share and Levy (1966a) noted that perfusion of the isolated carotid bifurcation of the anesthetized dog with deoxygenated blood resulted in pronounced release of vasopressin, suggesting that stimulation of carotid body chemoreceptors may also have a role in influencing hormone output.

Stimulation of carotid body chemoreceptors with an isotonic saline or Ringer's solution saturated with 100% CO_2 activates the phasically firing vasopressinergic neurons in the supraoptic nucleus (Yamashita, 1977; Harris, 1979). However, how important this input is in general control of vasopressin liberation is difficult to assess at the moment.

Muscle Receptors

Vasopressin release may also be influenced by other types of receptors. Electrical or chemical activation of group III (myelinated) and IV (unmyelinated) nociceptive afferents from skeletal muscles and their arteries causes excitation of vasopressinergic supraoptic neurons (Yamashita et al., 1984). This effect can also be produced by intraarterial injections of NaCl, KCl, or bradykinin and is abolished by denervation of the muscle. These muscle nociceptors are probably activated normally by chemical agents released, for example, during extreme exercise (see Chapter 7 for further discussion of the interaction of pain pathways and autonomic function).

The neural pathways that carry group III and IV afferent information to the vasopressin neurons of magnocellular hypothalamic nuclei are only partially understood. Dorsal root fibers convey pain information from free nerve endings in the arteries of

muscles to the spinal cord. Muscle nociceptive afferents synapse on spinal cord neurons located in laminae I and V of the dorsal horn (Craig and Mense, 1983). Although some of these neurons in this region of the spinal cord give rise to the spinothalamic tract, other neurons (or possibly the same cells) also project to the commissural region of the nucleus of the solitary tract and to the parabrachial nucleus (Menetrey and Basbaum, 1987). In addition, some spinal neurons in these areas of the dorsal horn project directly to the hypothalamus, but not to the magnocellular hypothalamic nuclei (Burstein et al., 1987). Just how these ascending pathways affect the vasopressin neurons is unknown.

In summary, vasopressin is under tonic inhibitory influence both from atrial receptors of the heart and from baroreceptors in the aortic arch and carotid sinus. Reduction in the discharge of these receptors by a decrease in blood volume or blood pressure results in the release of vasopressin. The absolute importance of these reflexes in maintaining vasopressin output is uncertain, but they may modulate the sensitivity of the vasopressin-secreting neurons to the continuous osmotic input from the extracellular fluid. An additional excitatory influence on vasopressin release is provided by carotid body chemoreceptors and muscle afferents, but their importance is uncertain.

CENTRAL NEURAL PATHWAYS REGULATING VASOPRESSIN RELEASE

Atrial receptor, baroreceptor, and chemoreceptor afferents terminate in the nucleus tractus solitarius. From this nucleus, multisynaptic pathways pass to the magnocellular hypothalamic nuclei, as well as to other central nervous system sites. These efferent pathways are capable of integrating information necessary for controlling the vasopressin release that occurs with concomitant changes in sympathetic drive to the particular vascular beds and the heart. However, the specific details of how this information is processed remain unexplored. In this section, the anatomy and physiology of these neural circuits will be summarized.

Afferents to the Magnocellular Hypothalamic Nuclei

The central nuclei that provide synaptic inputs to the vasopressin neurons appear to subserve two main functions: regulation of water balance and the cardiovascular system. Although this functional classification is a useful way to categorize the connectional data, it should be stressed that it has not been established that the various inputs relay only one or the other type of information, and it is quite probable that considerable integration occurs at various levels in the brain prior to reaching the final common output—the vasopressin magnocellular neurons.

The inputs to the magnocellular hypothalamic nuclei have been studied in the rat with a variety of neuroanatomical methods. Both nuclei receive direct inputs from the same central nuclei. These include inputs from three forebrain structures: the subfornical organ (a circumventricular organ located in the third ventricle) (Figure 13-6), the median preoptic nucleus (Figure 13-7), and the bed nucleus of the stria terminalis (Figure 13-8) and from three main brain stem nuclei: the pedunculopontine nucleus, the laterodorsal tegmental nucleus (Figure 13-9), and the A1/C1 catecholamine cell group (Figure 13-10) (McKellar and Loewy, 1982; Sawchenko and Swanson, 1983; Tribollet et al., 1985; Tucker et al., 1987; see Swanson and Sawchenko, 1983 and Swanson, 1987 for review). The nucleus tractus solitarius provides another input, but this appears to be relatively minor in terms of the density of its projection (Day and Sibbald, 1988a,b).

Lesion studies have established that both the subfornical organ and the median preoptic nucleus are involved in the neural regulation of water balance (see review by Johnson, 1985, and Chapter 14).

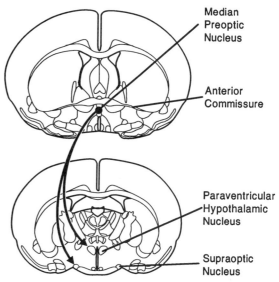

Figure 13-7 Forebrain projections to the magnocellular hypothalamic nuclei arise from the median preoptic nucleus. [Drawings based on figures from Paxinos, G., and Watson, C. (1986). *The Rat Brain in Stereotaxic Coordinates,* 2nd ed., Academic Press, Sydney, with permission of the authors and publisher.]

Other central pathways may be involved as well. For example, changes in plasma osmolality may reach the vasopressin cells via multisynaptic pathways arising from the area postrema. Efferent projections from the area postrema reach the nucleus tractus sol-

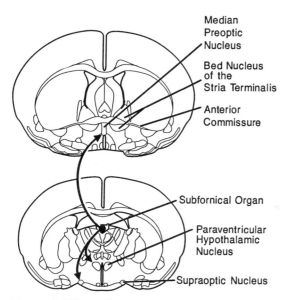

Figure 13-6 Forebrain projections to the magnocellular hypothalamic nuclei arise from the subfornical organ. [Drawings based on figures from Paxinos, G., and Watson, C. (1986). *The Rat Brain in Stereotaxic Coordinates,* 2nd ed., Academic Press, Sydney, with permission of the authors and publisher.]

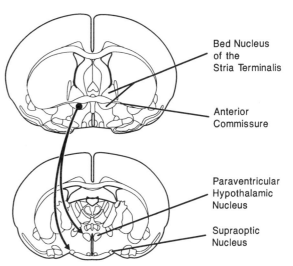

Figure 13-8 Forebrain projections to the magnocellular hypothalamic nuclei arise from the ventral part of the bed nucleus of the stria terminalis. [Drawings based on figures from Paxinos, G., and Watson, C. (1986). *The Rat Brain in Stereotaxic Coordinates,* 2nd ed., Academic Press, Sydney, with permission of the authors and publisher.]

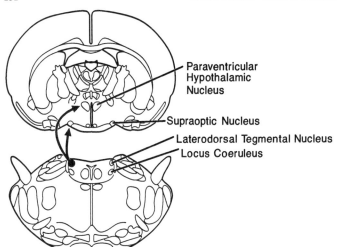

Figure 13-9 Neurons in the laterodorsal tegmental nucleus project to the magnocellular hypothalamic nuclei. [Drawings based on figures from Paxinos, G., and Watson, C. (1986). *The Rat Brain in Stereotaxic Coordinates,* 2nd ed., Academic Press, Sydney, with permission of the authors and publisher.]

itarius and parabrachial nuclei. These, in turn, could affect the release of vasopressin via ascending projections to forebrain sites such as the median preoptic nucleus.

The functions of the other inputs, such as those arising from the bed nucleus of the stria terminalis, are largely unknown. On the basis of connectional data, it can be predicted that this nucleus functions as a site of integration of central cardiovascular and limbic information because this area receives a dense input from the region of the nucleus tractus solitarius known to receive baroreceptor inputs and

chemoreceptor inputs (Ricardo and Koh, 1978) as well as from the amygdala (Weller and Smith, 1982). The functions of the pedunculopontine and laterodorsal tegmental nuclei are unknown. In contrast, the A1 noradrenergic input to the magnocellular hypothalamic nuclei appears to be a critical pathway that relays cardiovascular information to the vasopressin neuron.

Noradrenergic Pathways Involved in Vasopressin Regulation

In this section, the evidence that an ascending noradrenergic pathway is involved in the control of vasopressin will be reviewed. This pathway appears to be involved in the relay of cardiovascular afferent information directly to the vasopressin neurons. Two ideas will be considered: First, noradrenaline acts as an excitatory transmitter of vasopressin neurons. Second, the catecholamine pathway arising from the A1/C1 cell group appears to be the major ascending medullary pathway involved in vasopressin regulation.

Actions of Noradrenaline on Vasopressin Neurons

Noradrenaline acts as a putative excitatory transmitter of vasopressin magnocellular neurons. When noradrenaline is applied by iontophoresis using a very low-current density, it causes neuronal excitation (Arnauld et al., 1983). Randle and co-workers (1986) have repeated these experiments using pressure injection techniques rather than iontophoresis. This has the advantage that various concentrations of noradrenaline can be applied in exact amounts, whereas the exact amount ejected during iontophoresis experiments is impossible to measure accurately. When applied in low concentrations (10 μM),

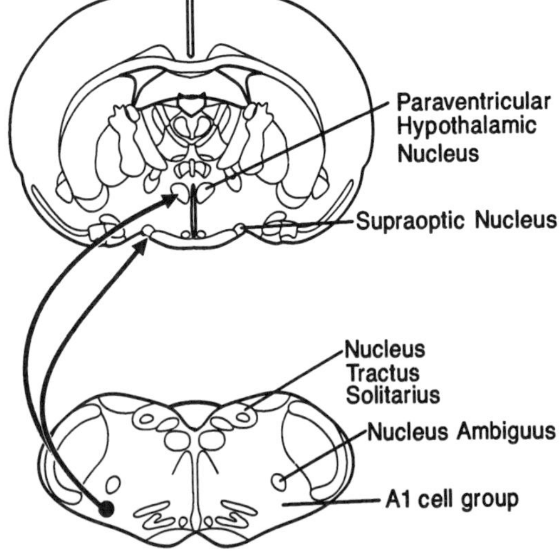

Figure 13-10 A1 noradrenergic and C1 adrenergic neurons of the ventrolateral medulla project to the magnocellular hypothalamic nuclei. [Drawings based on figures from Paxinos, G., and Watson, C. (1986). *The Rat Brain in Stereotaxic Coordinates,* 2nd ed., Academic Press, Sydney, with permission of the authors and publisher.]

noradrenaline was shown to activate neurons, whereas when it was applied at much higher concentrations (millimolar) the effect was inhibitory. The excitatory effects were blocked by the α_1-adrenoreceptor antagonist prazosin, but not by the β-adrenoreceptor antagonist timolol.

Whole animal experiments confirm these observations. Using both anesthetized and unanesthetized rats, Willoughby et al. (1987) demonstrated that microinjection of noradrenaline into supraoptic nucleus causes a release of vasopressin. This is mediated by an α_1-adrenoreceptor because an injection of the α_1-adrenoreceptor agonist phenylephrine increased vasopressin release, whereas neither the α_2-agonist clonidine nor the β-agonist isoproterenol had any effect.

The evidence, therefore, is that when applied directly to vasopressin neurons, noradrenaline is excitatory. However, noradrenaline may not be acting alone. Immunoreactive neuropeptide Y has also been found on both the A1 noradrenaline and C1 adrenergic neurons that project to the magnocellular nuclei (Blessing et al., 1986). However, only sparse to moderate concentrations of neuropeptide Y fibers are present in the regions of the magnocellular nuclei containing vasopressin cell bodies (Sawchenko et al., 1985). Nevertheless, when neuropeptide Y is injected into the supraoptic nucleus, it causes release of vasopressin (Willoughby and Blessing, 1978). Neuropeptide Y causes activation of vasopressin neurons when applied by iontophoresis, but the effect is neither as intense nor as long lasting as that which follows direct application of noradrenaline. Thus, neuropeptide Y may not be a major excitatory transmitter of the A1/C1 cells that project to the neurons, but acts in conjunction with noradrenaline to potentiate the release of vasopressin.

Noradrenergic Pathways

One of the most easily identified projections to the hypothalamus originates from noradrenergic neurons of the lower brain stem. The source of this noradrenergic input is the A1 group of neurons in the ventrolateral medulla, the A2 group in the nucleus tractus solitarius, and the A6 group in the locus coeruleus in the dorsolateral pons. The A1 cell group projects to the supraoptic nucleus and the magnocellular division of the paraventricular nucleus (McKellar and Loewy, 1981, 1982; Sawchenko and Swanson, 1982; Cunningham and Sawchenko, 1988). The A2 cell group projects primarily to the parvocellular region of the paraventricular nucleus, which is the subnucleus involved in autonomic regulation (McKellar and Loewy, 1981; Sawchenko and Swanson, 1982; Cunningham and Sawchenko, 1988). In addition, Day and Sibbald (1988a,b) and Cunningham and Sawchenko (1988) have suggested

that A2 neurons innervate the vasopressin neurons in the supraoptic nucleus—although this projection appears to be sparse. The locus coeruleus projects to the area dorsal to the supraoptic nucleus (but not to the nucleus itself) and to the periventricular division of the paraventricular hypothalamic nucleus (Jones and Yang, 1985; Cunningham and Sawchenko, 1988). These projections are summarized in Figure 13-2. Thus, the A1 cell group appears to be the main noradrenergic cell group that can have a direct effect on the vasopressin neurons.

McNeill and Sladek (1980) noted that within the supraoptic nuclei, the catecholamine fibers tended to be localized within the ventral part of the nucleus where the vasopressin neurons are concentrated, a view that was supported by Swanson et al. (1981). Similarly, catecholamine fibers are concentrated in the dorsal part of the posterior magnocellular subdivision of the paraventricular nucleus where the vasopressin cells are concentrated (see Swanson et al., 1986 for review).

The idea that the A1 noradrenergic cell group is the sole source of the catecholamine-containing fibers projecting to the magnocellular nuclei may be incorrect. For example, Tucker et al. (1987) observed that the majority of the neurons from the ventrolateral medulla that project to the paraventricular hypothalamic nucleus arise not from the A1 noradrenergic neurons, but from the C1 adrenergic neurons at the level of the area postrema and a few millimeters rostral to it. Unfortunately, their analysis did not include a study of the cells that give rise to catecholamine inputs to the supraoptic nucleus. With this reservation aside, it appears that vasopressin neurons of the paraventricular nucleus receive a dual catecholamine innervation from the ventrolateral medulla as well as a sparse input from the A2 neurons. In light of this information, a rethinking of the concepts concerning the ventrolateral medullary regulation of the magnocellular neurons of the hypothalamus will be necessary. In addition, the ventrolateral pathway may be even more complex because some of these catecholamine cells (i.e., both the C1 adrenergic and the A1 noradrenegic neurons) also project to the median preoptic nucleus as well, which is another major source of afferents to the magnocellular nuclei.

The anatomical substrate for a physiological link between baroreceptor and atrial receptor inputs and the release of vasopressin appears to utilize a multisynaptic pathway originating in the nucleus tractus solitarius. This pathway probably projects first to the A1/C1 cell group and then directly to the vasopressin neurons in the magnocellular hypothalamic nuclei. Destruction of this ascending catecholamine system in the mesencephalon by stereotaxic injections of 6-hydroxydopamine, a neurotoxin that is relatively specific for noradrenergic and dopamine-containing fibers, completely abolished the release of vasopressin that normally follows hypotensive hemorrhage (Lightman et al., 1984). However, there is still considerable controversy over whether this is the only central catecholamine pathway that influences vasopressin release.

Destruction of the region of the locus coeruleus with 6-hydroxydopamine abolishes the inhibitory influence of baroreceptor activation on supraoptic vasopressin-secreting neurons in rats (Banks and Harris, 1984). In contrast, 6-hydroxydopamine lesions of the ventrolateral medulla in the region of the A1 cell group block the inhibition that normally follows stimulation of carotid sinus baroreceptors specifically, but not the inhibition that follows a generalized increase in arterial pressure that activates all high-pressure baroreceptors, including those from the aortic arch.

Banks and Harris (1984) have proposed that the major baroreceptor input to supraoptic nuclei was via the locus coeruleus nucleus. Whether this pathway involves the locus coeruleus per se is unresolved. In this context, three anatomical facts have to be considered. First, there is no evidence for a direct anatomical link from the nucleus tractus solitarius to the locus coeruleus in rat (Ricardo and Koh, 1978), unless this pathway terminates on dendrites that extend beyond its nuclear boundaries (Swanson, 1976). Second, neurons in the laterodorsal tegmental nucleus that lie in the central gray matter in close proximity to the locus coeruleus nucleus project directly to the magnocellular hypothalamic nuclei (Figure 13-9; Tribollet et al., 1985); the locus coeruleus does not project directly to the magnocellular nucleus (Jones and Yang, 1985). Since local injections of 6-hydroxydopamine can cause local, nonspecific damage to neurons (Agid et al., 1973), it is possible that the injections used in the experiments by Banks and Harris (1984) destroyed these cells as well. This alternative hypothesis may explain the physiological findings of Banks and Harris (1984). Third, since the A1 noradrenergic cell group projects to the region of the locus coeruleus in the rat (McKellar and Loewy, 1981; Sawchenko and Swanson, 1982), it is quite possible that the local 6-hydroxydopamine injections aimed at the locus coeruleus also disrupted a branch of this ascending A1 pathway. This, too, could account for the findings. A fourth factor has recently emerged, that is, the A2 neurons also project to the supraoptic nucleus (Day and Sibbald, 1988a; Cunningham and Sawchenko, 1988). Just how this system is involved in regulation of vasopressin supraoptic neurons is uncertain.

The observation made by Banks and Harris (1984) that 6-hydroxydopamine lesions of the A1 cell group region only partially abolished the re-

sponse raises two additional questions. First, if C1 adrenergic neurons are involved in this pathway, it is highly probable that they were not destroyed by the 6-hydroxydopamine because adrenergic neurons are refractory to this neurotoxin (Jonsson et al., 1976). Second, if the pathway that arises from the nucleus tractus solitarius possesses a bifurcated (or multibranched) axonal system with one branch projecting to the ventrolateral medulla and the other projecting to the region dorsal to the locus coeruleus nucleus, then destruction of only one branch of this system may be insufficient to eliminate the response. Clearly, further studies will be needed to clarify the circuitry involved in this response.

Central Inhibitory Pathways

Noradrenaline seems to function as an excitatory transmitter of vasopressin magnocellular neuron and one of the major problems in explaining the neural mechanisms causing baroreceptor inhibition of vasopressin release is to localize the site of the inhibition. Two possible physiological mechanisms could account for this inhibition and the two are not necessarily mutually exclusive. First, there could be disfacilitation (i.e., the excitatory inputs could be inhibited at a site outside the magnocellular nuclei) at some point before information is relayed via the ascending catecholamine system. Second, there could be an activation of an inhibitory pathway that, under certain circumstances, could exert a more powerful influence on magnocellular nuclei than the incoming catecholamine afferents.

The pathway and neural transmitters responsible for baroreceptor inhibition of vasopressin neurons are unknown, but a likely site may be in the ventrolateral medulla. Topical application of GABA or glycine on the ventral surface of the medulla in cats prevents the release of vasopressin by bilateral carotid occlusion; application of GABA antagonists to the same region results in vasopressin release (Feldberg and Rocha e Silva, 1978, 1981). Although the concentrations of drugs used in these experiments were very high and probably nonspecific, the results imply that the ventrolateral medulla is a key site in this neural pathway. Additional experiments support this view. For example, microinjection of the GABA antagonist bicuculline into the caudal ventrolateral medulla stimulates vasopressin release (Sved et al., 1985). Blessing and Willoughby (1985) provided further evidence for this idea when they found that microinjection of the long-acting GABA receptor agonist muscimol into the caudal ventrolateral medulla of rabbits abolished the release of vasopressin both after hemorrhage and after constriction of the inferior vena cava. Injection of muscimol into areas close to, but not within the ventrolateral medulla had no effect. In addition, McAllen and Blessing

(1987) recorded from neurons in the A1 region of rabbits that project to the supraoptic nucleus, and demonstrated those neurons to be depressed by baroreceptor activation. On the basis of these data, it is reasonable to hypothesize that the inhibitory influence of baroreceptor stimulation may result from a GABA-mediated depression of A1 neurons. This would serve to inhibit the tonic A1 excitatory drive of the vasopressin neuron. The process of disfacilitation may cause release of vasopressin. This hypothesis has the merit of accounting for the inhibitory influence of baroreceptor stimulation on supraoptic neurons while allowing for the excitatory effects of noradrenaline.

Activation of inhibitory pathways may occur as well. The strongest evidence comes from studies by Jhamandas and Renaud (1986), who reported that baroreceptor-induced inhibition of supraoptic neurons was abolished by direct application of the GABA antagonist bicuculline into this nucleus (Figure 13-11). The source of the GABA input to the magnocellular nuclei is unknown, but GABA terminals have been located in the supraoptic and paraventricular hypothalamic nuclei (Tappaz et al., 1983; van den Pol, 1985). Immunoreactive glutamic

acid decarboxylase cell bodies lie at the periphery of the nucleus (Theodosis et al., 1986), but it has not yet been determined if these cells project to the vasopressin neurons. If they do, it is quite possible that the ascending catecholamine pathways, which terminate in the region dorsal to the supraoptic nucleus, may affect these perinuclear GABA neurons and, in turn, modulate vasopressin release (Jhamandas et al., 1987). An additional possible source may be the GABA neurons of the forebrain, which are thought to project to the regions surrounding the basal forebrain magnocellular nuclei; Jhamandas and Renaud (1986) found that electrical stimulation of this region of the diagonal band of Broca caused an inhibition of vasopressin neurons, which is bicuculline sensitive. However, this cannot be construed as definitive evidence of a pathway because electrical stimulation activates both axons and cell bodies.

There is an additional component of baroreceptor input that is also not explained. Kannan et al. (1981) recorded the activity of neurons ventrolateral to the locus coeruleus that were close to or within the parabrachial nucleus. These neurons were antidromically activated by electrical stimulation of the supraoptic nucleus, inhibited by baroreceptor stim-

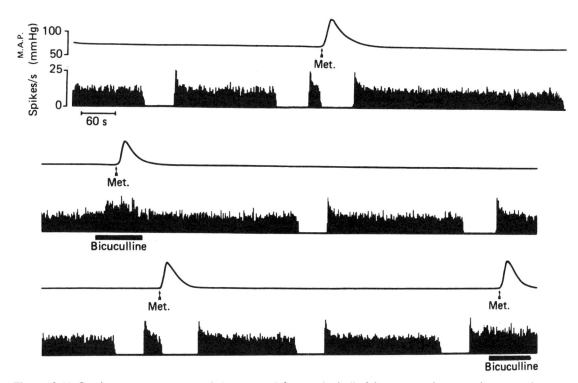

Figure 13-11 Continuous rate-meter records (upper trace) from a phasically firing vasopressin neuron in a rat to demonstrate the reduction in neural firing induced by a rise in mean arterial blood pressure (M.A.P. upper traces) consequent to intravenous administration of metaraminol (Met., arrow). Locally applied bicuculline methiodide (100 μM) by pressure ejection (horizontal line) reversibly abolishes the meteraminol-induced response. (Slight modification from Jahmandas and Renaud, 1986, with permission of the authors and publisher.)

ulation, and excited by carotid occlusion. Their mode of action appears to involve disfacilitation, but they do not fit any of the present theories explaining the action of the baroreceptor system on the vasopressin neurons. Moreover, anatomical studies do not support the idea that there is a direct projection from the parabrachial nucleus to the supraoptic nucleus (Saper and Loewy, 1980). Until detailed studies can be made of this region, its role in vasopressin regulation will remain uncertain.

In summary, the inhibitory influence of baroreceptor and atrial receptor activation on vasopressin liberation is dependent on the ascending catecholamine systems arising from the A1/C1 cell group of the ventrolateral medulla, and possibly from neurons localized in the region near the locus coeruleus. Two hypotheses exist to explain the data. One suggests that inhibition of vasopressin neurons is brought about by disfacilitation following GABA-mediated inhibition of a tonic excitatory influence from the A1/C1 cell group. It is proposed that GABA neurons near the A1/C1 cell group may be involved. The other hypothesis proposes that an excitatory noradrenaline input to GABA neurons localized at some other site, such as near the region of the supraoptic and paraventricular hypothalamic nuclei, causes inhibition of the vasopressin neurons. Other pathways such as projections from the parabrachial and pedunculopontine nuclei may also be involved, but these have not been studied.

Central Chemoreceptor Pathways

Bilateral carotid occlusion releases vasopressin in dogs, cats, and rats (Share and Levy, 1962; Clark and Rocha e Silva, 1967; Harris et al., 1975), and leads to activation of vasopressin neurons in the supraoptic nuclei (Dreifuss et al., 1976). Carotid occlusion can cause activation of carotid body chemoreceptors (Landgren and Neil, 1951), and chemoreceptor stimulation also activates vasopressin neurons in the supraoptic nucleus (Harris, 1979). Therefore, at least part of the release of vasopressin in response to bilateral occlusion of the common carotid arteries may follow activation of carotid body chemoreceptors. It has been found electrophysiologically that carotid body chemoreceptors have no influence on the phasically discharging vasopressin neurons of the paraventricular nucleus (Banks and Harris, 1988), in contrast to their pronounced activation of similar neurons in the supraoptic nucleus (Yamashita, 1977; Harris, 1979). Since the magnocellular region of the paraventricular nucleus receives a pronounced noradrenergic innervation from the A1 cell group, as does the supraoptic nucleus, this mediates against the theory that A1 neurons are responsible for the activation of supraoptic neurons by carotid

body chemoreceptors. In this context, it is interesting to note that in cats, Arita et al. (1988) have localized neurons responsive to carotid body chemoreceptor stimulaton in a region ventrolateral to the retrofacial nucleus, that is considerably rostral to the A1 neurons. Although Arita et al. (1988) made no effort to look at the projection of the chemoreceptor-activated cells, in a study in our own laboratory using rats (Jamieson and Harris, unpublished observations) no evidence was found for carotid body chemoreceptor-induced activation of rostrally projecting neurons in the A1 region. It is possible that these neurons lie rostral to the A1 cell group. Thus, the location of the cell bodies involved and the site of influence of their terminals remain in doubt for the moment.

A final possibility is that an excitatory input to the vasopressin neurons may arise from cholinergic neurons that lie immediately dorsal to the supraoptic nucleus (Meyer and Brownstein, 1980). Pickford (1939, 1947) demonstrated that injection of acetylcholine to the supraoptic nucleus of the dog resulted in vasopressin release. Iontophoretic application of acetylcholine to phasically firing vasopressin supraoptic neurons in rats causes neuronal excitation (Bioulac et al., 1978). Hatton et al. (1983b), using hypothalamic slices, confirmed that acetylcholine excited phasically firing supraoptic neurons and demonstrated that this effect was blocked by nicotinic-blocking agents (turbocurarine and hexamethionium), but not by atropine. By stimulating the areas dorsal and dorsolateral to the supraoptic nucleus where cholinergic neurons are localized, these investigators were able to demonstrate that most of the putative vasopressin neurons were excited and putative oxytocin cells were unaffected. This suggests that the cholinergic cell bodies lying dorsal to the supraoptic nucleus provide an excitatory input to the vasopressin cells. No fully satisfactory physiological explanation for this cholinergic influence has yet been elucidated. Some investigators have suggested that these cells are involved in the osmotic activation of vasopressin release, but the system remains to be fully investigated because a large number of afferents from the lower brain stem project to this region of the hypothalamus.

ACTIONS OF VASOPRESSIN ON THE CARDIOVASCULAR SYSTEM

Vasopressin was originally named because of its pressor property. The discovery that the hormone has antidiuretic effects at doses orders of magnitude lower than those needed to raise blood pressure gave rise to the concept that the pressor effect was an artifact of dosage and did not reflect a physiological function. However, this has been shown not to be true. Vasopressin can affect cardiovascular function either by direct effects on the blood vessels or by effects on the autonomic nervous system at hormone levels well within the range found in plasma under normal physiological conditions. The studies giving rise to this conclusion are summarized below.

In Vitro Studies

Vasopressin has direct effects on vascular smooth muscle at concentrations in the picomolar range (see reviews by Altura and Altura, 1984; Cowley and Liard, 1987), which is well within the physiological plasma concentrations of the hormone. It has a potent vasoconstrictor effect on venules as well as arterioles and arteries in the splanchnic, renal, cutaneous, and skeletal muscle vascular beds, but either has no effect on the cerebral, coronary, and pulmonary arterial beds or causes relaxation (see Altura and Altura, 1984 for review). The threshold for splanchnic and skeletal muscle arteriolar constrictor effects is 10^{-12} to 10^{-13} M.

At threshold of 10^{-11} M, vasopressin causes a relaxation of large cerebral and coronary arteries that is endothelium dependent and appears to be mediated by a V1 receptor (Katusic et al., 1984). Smaller vessels on the surface of the brain are not affected by this peptide (Lassof and Altura, 1980), but when applied to microvessels in the hippocampal slice, vasopressin can cause constriction (Smock et al., 1987).

Until recently, it was thought that vasopressin had no direct effect on the myocardium. Using the isolated perfused rat heart, Boyle and Segel (1986) reported that only at doses of 300–800 pg/ml did vasopressin reduce myocardial oxygen consumption and cardiac output. The authors attributed this to myocardial ischemia following the pronounced coronary artery constriction induced by these large doses of vasopressin. However, Walker et al. (1988), using a more or less identical preparation, found that although doses of vasopressin of 400–500 pg/ml did indeed reduce myocardial function, at doses of 50–100 pg/ml the peptide increased myocardial contractility despite progressive coronary vasoconstriction. All these effects were blocked following administration of a specific V1 receptor antagonist.

Whole Animal Experiments: Systemic Administration of Vasopressin and Vasopressin Antagonists

The detailed examination of a potential role for vasopressin in cardiovascular control is fraught with problems. Recent improvements in techniques for the assessment of regional blood flow and resistance in individual vascular beds in conjunction with the traditional measurement of arterial blood pressure and cardiac output have led to a reevaluation of the cardiovascular function of vasopressin.

Despite these improvements, however, it is important to realize that such data need to be interpreted with caution, taking into account that there are gross differences between species (see Bennett and Gardiner, 1986 for review) and even between strains within species (see Bennett and Gardiner, 1988). Furthermore, it is evident that vasopressin is not the only peptide that influences the cardiovascular system. Nevertheless, in those species submitted to the most detailed study (dog and rat), there is little doubt that vasopressin can exert often quite subtle influences on cardiovascular function. These effects are probably mediated by three factors: (1) direct effects on blood vessels, (2) modulatory effects on baroreflex sensitivity, and (3) modulatory effects on the sympathetic system.

It has been known for some time that animals lacking vasopressin have a rather labile blood pressure that is particularly sensitive to hemorrhage. Errington and Rocha e Silva (1972) and Schwartz and Reid (1981) noted that in dogs, if either the release or the action of vasopressin is prevented, the fall of blood pressure induced by hemorrhage is greater than normal. The same applies to Brattleboro rats which are genetically incapable of synthesizing vasopressin (Laycock et al., 1979; Gardiner and Bennett, 1982). Moreover, this vasopressor influence is probably confined not only to hemorrhage, since even in dehydrated normal rats, the injection of a specific V1 receptor antagonist leads to a fall in arterial blood pressure (Aisenburg et al., 1981; Andrews and Brenner, 1981) and in Brattleboro rats, maintenance of water balance and, therefore, extracellular fluid volume by a nonpressor analogue of vasopressin still results in a lower arterial blood pressure (Woods and Johnson, 1984). The vasoconstrictor influence of the peptide may not always be manifest in changed arterial blood pressure, for Rascher et al. (1985) found that in unanesthetized, water-deprived rats infusion of a V1 antagonist resulted in a reduced total peripheral resistance, but this was compensated for by an increased cardiac output and, consequently, there was no change in arterial blood pressure.

Such subtle influences are also well illustrated by the experiments of Cowley and Liard and their colleagues using dogs. Montani et al. (1980) demonstrated that during intravenous infusion of vasopressin in conscious dogs at doses of 40 fmol/kg/minute (1 fmol = 1.084 pg), there was no change in mean arterial blood pressure, but a 15% increase in total peripheral resistance. This was compensated for by a fall in cardiac output and heart rate. At this dose, plasma vasopressin increased by only about 5 pg/ml above basal levels. This concentration is well above the basal levels observed in normal dogs (2–4 pg/ml) but not beyond the range seen after 36 hours of dehydration (10–40 pg/ml, see Cowley and Liard, 1987). Only when the vasopressin concentration in the infusate was raised to 1,000 fmol/kg/minute or above, so the plasma levels reached approximately 50 pg/ml or more above normal, was there a rise in mean arterial blood pressure.

The mechanisms responsible for these changes in peripheral resistance are complex. Liard (1986a) dehydrated dogs for 48 hours, which resulted in an increase in vasopressin from ~5 to ~11 pg/ml. He measured blood pressure, cardiac output, and regional blood flow in a number of tissues and organs. During the dehydration, there was no change in mean arterial blood pressure, but cardiac output was reduced. Many tissues showed a slight reduction in blood flow, but only in skeletal muscle did this reach statistical significance. However, Liard then investigated the effects on these variables of injecting an antagonist of the V1 (vasoconstrictor) vasopressin receptors and compared it with the influence of an antagonist of both V1 and V2 (antidiuretic) receptors. The effects were dramatic. Injection of the V1 antagonist alone resulted in a ~50% increase in cardiac output and a 25% decrease in peripheral resistance without any change in arterial blood pressure. The fall in peripheral resistance was largely due to increases in blood flow of 60–80% in tissues such as skeletal muscle, skin, fat, bone, and liver. Interestingly, blocking both V1 and V2 receptors resulted in smaller changes in the cardiovascular variables than blocking V1 receptors alone. This implies that the V1 receptor blockade had unmasked a vasodilator component of the V2 receptors in those tissues.

In addition, however, it became evident that even the V1-induced vasoconstriction may have an indirect mechanism. Montani et al. (1980) had earlier shown that when intravenous infusion of vasopressin was given in sufficient quantity to raise plasma levels to 20 pg/ml or greater, changes in peripheral resistance occurred similar to those seen during dehydration. Subsequent experiments by Liard (1986b) demonstrated that *intraarterial* infusions of similar concentrations of vasopressin to the same tissues in conscious dogs did not cause vasoconstriction in skeletal muscle, skin, and gastrointestinal tract. This observation is important because it indicates that at this elevated plasma concentration, circulating vasopressin does not cause a direct vasoconstriction. There are three possible explanations for this phenomenon. First, this vasoconstriction is an indirect effect that is elicited by reflexes (or possibly hormones) originating from the vascular system. Second, vasopressin is directly affecting the sympathetic nervous system peripherally. Third, the response is the result of an effect of vasopressin on the central nervous system. There is evidence to support all three mechanisms, and it is discussed below.

Prior to addressing these mechanisms, the problem that remains to be fully answered is whether vasopressin plays an important vasoconstrictor role in the minute-to-minute control of blood pressure in the normal, healthy mammal, or is it evident only in pathological states such as hemorrhage? From the available evidence, it seems unlikely that the hormone has a dramatic influence on maintenance of blood pressure in the normal hydrated states, particularly in humans. For example, Bussein et al. (1984) examined the influence of a V1 vasopressin antagonist on blood pressure of normally hydrated healthy human subjects and found that it caused no effect on arterial blood pressure. However, studies of this nature are limited because of the difficulty of making accurate measurements of redistribution of regional blood flow in humans. For this reason, a glance at the literature will reveal an almost unparalleled state of confusion (see Bennett and Gardiner, 1986 for review), so at the moment the lack of effect remains to be proved.

Vasopressin and the Reflex Control of the Circulation

The above discussion has concentrated on the direct influence of vasopressin on blood pressure, regional vascular resistance, and blood flow. These data support the idea that under normal conditions vasopressin is not a potent vasoconstrictor hormone. However, this does not negate the importance of this peptide in normal cardiovascular control, for there is evidence favoring the idea that it acts as a "gain enhancer" of cardiovascular function. It appears to augment smooth muscle constriction, sympathetic transmission, and central neural regulation of the cardiovascular system. This idea is based on three lines of evidence. First, vasopressin potentiates the vasoconstrictor action of noradrenaline on vascular smooth muscle (Bartelstone and Nasmyth, 1965). Second, vasopressin may enhance the sensitivity of the baroreceptor reflex by both a peripheral mechanism (Cowley et al., 1974) and through a central mechanism (Undesser et al., 1985). Third, vasopressin can affect the autonomic nervous system directly. In all probability, all three mechanisms work together (Figure 13-12).

The observation that vasopressin potentiates noradrenaline-induced contraction may not be a pharmacological oddity. Hanley et al. (1984) reported the presence of vasopressin-like immunoreactive neurons in the superior cervical, celiac, and thoracic paravertebral sympathetic ganglia. This immunore-

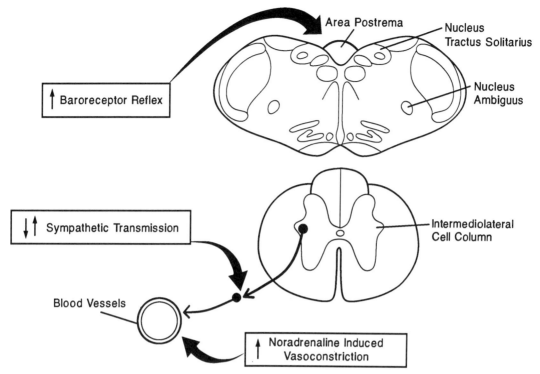

Figure 13-12 Vasopressin can act at three different sites in the body to modify cardiovascular function. It can potentiate the vasoconstrictor action of noradrenaline at blood vessels, modulate sympathetic transmission, and affect the baroreceptor reflex by a central effect mediated by the area postrema.

activity was colocalized with dopamine-β-hydroxy-lase, which suggests that it may function in sympathetic postganglionic neurons as a cotransmitter with noradrenaline. Some of these neurons innervate arteries and may be the anatomical substrate subserving vasopressin potentiation of noradrenaline constriction of vascular smooth muscle.

The theory that vasopressin can enhance the sensitivity of the baroreceptor reflex is based largely on evidence from experiments on dogs. Cowley et al. (1974) demonstrated that the action of vasopressin as a vasoconstrictor hormone is enhanced 8,000-fold when the central nervous system is destroyed. In unanesthetized dogs, the pressor action of vasopressin is also augmented after denervation of the sinoaortic baroreceptors. Cowley et al. (1984) used neurohypophysectomized dogs to examine the aortic pressor response to changes in carotid sinus pressure at three different levels of circulating vasopressin. In the presence of higher levels of vasopressin, the change in aortic pressure was found to be two times, and the increase in peripheral resistance three times that seen for the same change in sinus pressure at normal vasopressin levels. Reduction of sinus pressure below 105 mm Hg increased the open-loop gain of the reflex by a 2-fold factor. Thus, these investigators proposed that the influence of vasopressin on blood

pressure control is a combined effect of its action on the gain of the baroreceptor reflex and the vasoconstriction (see Cowley and Liard, 1987, for review and references).

In rats, the evidence for an influence of vasopressin on baroreflex sensitivity is less certain. Webb et al. (1986) were unable to find any influence in unanesthetized normal rats and in Brattleboro rats. Gardiner and Bennett (1982) found that infusion of vasopressin had no effect on the baroreflex response to an increase in blood pressure, although it did increase the baroreflex sensitivity to depressor stimuli.

In humans, the situation is not clear. There have been reports that humans suffering from idiopathic orthostatic hypotension (a disease that destroys sympathetic preganglionic neurons) show increased sensitivity to vasopressin (Wagner and Braunwald, 1956). O'Callaghan and Sheehan (1986) found that vasopressin infusion in normal subjects had no effect on the cardiac response to carotid sinus suction. However, the interpretation of data from humans is extremely difficult and further assessment is clearly needed (see Bennett and Gardiner, 1986 for discussion of this problem).

The mechanism through which circulating vasopressin influences baroreceptor function is open to debate, but one possibility is that it does so via a direct action on the central nervous system. The hormone may gain access to the brain via the circumventricular organs that lack a blood–brain barrier. One likely site of action may be the area postrema, a circimventricular organ lying in the dorsal medulla oblongata. This structure lies adjacent to the nucleus tractus solitarius and has connections with it (Chapter 14). High-affinity [³H]vasopressin binding sites that are linked exclusively with V1 receptors have been identified in both of these regions (Tribollet et al., 1988).

Whole animal studies support the idea that vasopressin has a central action. Liard et al. (1981) found that infusion of vasopressin into the left vertebral artery of the dog resulted in smaller increases in arterial blood pressure but a larger fall in heart rate than the same infusion into the inferior vena cava. Undesser et al. (1985), using anesthetized rabbits, found that the rise in blood pressure induced by vasopressin infusion was much greater in animals that had area postrema lesions than in controls. This implies that in control animals vasopressin was acting on the area postrema or the tissue close by to enhance the baroreflex response to the rise in blood pressure. The lesions will have inevitably damaged the nucleus tractus solitarius, but they will also have prevented the entry of vasopressin to the central nervous system at this site. Further evidence has been obtained in anesthetized sheep that the sensitivity of the vagal component of the baroreceptor reflex is enhanced by intravenous infusion of vasopressin (Courtice et al., 1984). The same procedure also increases neural activity in cardiac afferent vagal fibers (Lumbers and Potter, 1982; Courtice et al., 1984), an effect that is independent of peripheral vasoconstriction.

Vasopressin can also influence the sympathetic nervous system directly. Kiraly et al. (1986) found high-affinity [³H]vasopressin binding in rat superior cervical ganglion that was displaced by V1 agonists. When vasopressin is applied in low concentrations (nanomolar range) to superior cervical ganglion cells, it causes a reduction in amplitude of fast excitatory postsynaptic potentials generated by electrical stimulation of sympathetic preganglionic nerve fibers. At high concentrations, it causes membrane depolarization (Kiraly et al., 1985; Peters and Kreulen, 1985). Thus, it is quite possible that variable sympathetic responses can be modulated by release of varying amounts of vasopressin. Under emergency conditions, the peptide could act directly on vascular smooth muscle to cause vasoconstriction as well as excitation of sympathetic postganglionic neurons. Under normal conditions, the effects may be a subtle modulation of both of these target organs.

In summary, under emergency conditions, vasopressin causes vasoconstriction in skeletal muscle, skin, gastrointestinal tract, and kidney. It serves to shunt blood from these tissues to the brain, heart, and lungs. Under normal conditions, it acts as a modulator and works in concert with the autonomic nervous system to cause reflex control of cardiovascular function. It can potentiate catecholamine contraction of vascular smooth muscle, modulate synaptic transmission of sympathetic ganglia, and augment the sensitivity of the baroreceptor reflex.

SUMMARY

The vasopressin neurons of the supraoptic and paraventricular nuclei are involved in autonomic regulation. Vasopressin liberation is controlled by cardiovascular reflexes and plasma osmolality. In turn, vasopressin is involved in both the control of blood pressure and water reabsorption in the kidney. The cardiovascular effects of vasopressin occur both by a direct action on vascular smooth muscle and by modulation of some of the neural elements that control cardiovascular reflexes.

Cardiovascular reflex control of vasopressin liberation is controlled mainly through a tonic inhibitory influence of low-pressure receptors located in the atria and high-pressure receptors (baroreceptors) from the carotid sinus and aortic arch. Evidence from dogs suggests that the atrial receptors, responding to changes in blood volume, may be the more important, but baroreceptors are also effective and there may be cross-species and even within-species differences in sensitivity to each input.

The ascending pathways within the central nervous system carrying the input from the nucleus tractus solitarius via multisynaptic pathways to the vasopressin hypothalamic neurons are incompletely understood. The ascending catecholamine systems originating in the A1 noradrenergic and C1 adrenergic cell group of the ventrolateral medulla are probably the main site of integration for many of these systems before they are relayed to the hypothalamus. Since noradrenaline is thought to activate hypothalamic vasopressinergic neurons when acting directly, there is disagreement on the mechanism by which the inhibition of vasopressin output is effected. There are two main theories: (1) Noradrenergic inputs exert a tonic excitatory influence that is blocked at the level of the ventrolateral medulla during baroreceptor/atrial receptor activation, thereby leading to a loss of activation of the vasopressin neurons, that is, disfacilitation. (2) The noradrenergic afferents synapse on GABAergic neurons that lie in close proximity to the magnocellular hypothalamic nuclei, and these second-order cells depress the activity of vasopressin neurons. At present, both theories have their merits, although neither totally accounts for the experimental data.

The physiological role of the cardiovascular reflexes in vasopressin output is not clear, but one attractive hypothesis is that they modulate the sensitivity of the vasopressin neurons to the normal changes in extracellular fluid osmolality that may be the main controlling influence on vasopressin secretion.

Once released into the circulation, vasopressin influences blood volume and blood pressure in at least two ways. First, the well-known influence on water retention by the kidney, and second, via a direct action on peripheral vasculature. The latter effect is complex and not identical across all vascular beds; indeed there may well be vasodilation in some vascular beds such as the cerebral circulation. Although it seems unlikely that the peptide is important for maintaining blood pressure in the normotensive, normally hydrated individual, the amounts of hormone released during a normal dehydration are quite sufficient to help maintain a normal blood pressure. It seems probable, therefore, that the hormone plays a supporting role in the maintenance of blood pressure, a role probably shared with other peptides such as the atrial natriuretic peptide and neuropeptide Y.

The actions of vasopressin on the cardiovascular system may occur indirectly, through the ability of the hormone to increase the sensitivity of the baroreceptor reflex. At the moment, it seems probable that this is a central effect of the peptide that can influence vagal outflow of this central autonomic pathway via its action on the area postrema. This causes an increase in cardiac vagal activity that is independent of peripheral vasoconstriction. Vasopressin can also modulate synaptic transmission in sympathetic ganglia and can act on vascular smooth muscle to potentiate the actions of noradrenaline. Thus, the idea has emerged that vasopressin can act as a "gain enhancer" at multiple sites that affect cardiovascular function.

ACKNOWLEDGMENTS

Sincere thanks go to the authors who kindly allowed us to use illustrations from their work and to Sharon Roberts and Sue Eads who so patiently typed the manuscript.

REFERENCES

Reviews

Altura, B. M., and Altura, B. T. (1984). Actions of vasopressin, oxytocin, and synthetic analogs on vascular smooth muscle. *Federation Proceedings* 43, 80–86.

Bennett, T., and Gardiner, S. M. (1986). Influence of exogenous vasopressin on baroreflex mechanisms. *Clinical Science* 70, 307–315.

Bennett, T., and Gardiner, S. M. (1988). Influence of endogenous vasopressin on cardiovascular regulation: Studies in Long Evans and Brattleboro rats. In: *Vasopressin, Cellular and Integrative Aspects,* A. W. Cowley, et al. (eds.), Raven, New York, pp. 439–446.

Bie, P. (1980). Osmoreceptors, vasopressin and control of renal water excretion. *Physiological Reviews* 60, 961–1048.

Bisset, G. W., and Chowdrey, H. S. (1988). Control of release of vasopressin by neuro-endocrine reflexes. *Quarterly Journal of Experimental Physiology,* 73, 811–872.

Bisset, G. W., and Jones, N. F. (1975). Antidiuretic hormone. In: *Recent Advances in Renal Disease,* N. F. Jones (ed.), Churchill Livingstone, Edinburgh, pp. 350–416.

Cowley, A. W., and Liard, J. F. (1987). Cardiovascular actions of vasopressin. In: *Vasopressin: Principles and Properties,* D. M. Gash and G. J. Boer (eds.), Plenum, New York, pp. 389–433.

Genest, J., and Cantin, M. (1988). The atrial natiuretic factor: Its physiology and biochemistry. *Reviews of Physiology, Biochemistry and Pharmacology* 110, 1–145.

Johnson, A. K. (1985). Role of the periventricular tissue surrounding the anteroventral third ventricle (AV3V) in the regulation of body fluid homeostasis. In: *Vasopressin,* R. S. Schrier (ed.), Raven, New York, pp. 291–298.

Lightman, S. L., and Everitt, B. J. (1986). Water excretion. In: *Neuroendocrinology,* S. L. Lightman and B. J. Everitt (eds.), Blackwell Scientific Publications, Oxford, pp. 197–206.

Manning, M., Bankowski, K., and Sawyer, W. H. (1987). Selective agonists and antagonists of vasopressin. In: *Vasopressin: Principles and Properties,* D. M. Gash and G. J. Boer (eds.), Plenum, New York, pp. 335–368.

Morris, J. F., Chapman, D. B., and Sokol, H. W. (1987). Anatomy and function of the classic vasopressin-secreting hypothalamus neurohypophysial system. In: *Vasopressin: Principles and Properties,* D. M. Gash and G. J. Boer (eds.), Plenum, New York, pp. 1–89.

Petty, M. A. (1987). The cardiovascular effects of the neurohypophysial hormone oxytocin. *Journal of Autonomic Pharmacology* 7, 97–104.

Share, L. (1988). Vasopressin in regulation of water homeostasis and cardiovascular function. In: *Endocrinology: People and Ideas,* S. M. McCann (ed.), American Physiology Society, Bethesda, MD, pp. 1–21.

Swanson, L. W. (1987). The hypothalamus. In: *Handbook of Chemical Neuroanatomy,* Vol. 5. *Integrated Systems of the CNS,* Part I, A. Bjorklund, T. Hokfelt, and L. W. Swanson (eds.), Elsevier, Amsterdam, pp. 1–124.

Swanson, L. W., and Sawchenko, P. E. (1983). Hypothalamic integration: organization of the paraventricular and supraoptic nuclei. *Annual Review of Neuroscience* 6, 269–324.

Swanson, L. W., Sawchenko, P. E., and Lind, R. W. (1986). Regulation of multiple peptides in CRF parvocellular neurosecretory neurons: Implications for the stress response. *Progress in Brain Research* 68, 169–190.

Wakerley, J. B. (1987). Electrophysiology of the central vasopressin system. In: *Vasopressin: Principles and Properties*, D. M. Gash and G. J. Boer (eds.), Plenum, New York, pp. 211–256.

Research Papers

Agid, Y., Javoy, F., Glowinski, J., Bouvet, D., and Sotello, C. (1973). Injections of 6-hydroxydopamine into the substantia nigra of the rat. II. Diffusion and specificity. *Brain Research* 58, 291–301.

Aisenbery, G. A., Handelman, W. A., Arnold, P., Manning, M., and Schrier, R. W. (1981). Vascular effects of arginine vasopressin during fluid deprivation in the rat. *Journal of Clinical Investigation* 67, 961–968.

Andrew, R. D., Mac Vicar, B. A., Dubek, F. E., and Hatton, G. I. (1981). Dye transfer through gap junctions between neuroendocrine cells of rat hypothalamus. *Science* 211, 1187–1189.

Andrews, C. E., Jr., and Brenner, B. M. (1981). Relative contributions of arginine vasopressin and angiotensin II to maintenance of systemic arterial blood pressure in the anesthetised water-deprived rat. *Circulation Research* 48, 254–258.

Arita, H., Kogo, N., and Ichikawa, K. (1988). Locations of medullary neurons with non-phasic discharges excited by stimulation of central and/or peripheral chemoreceptors and by activation of nociceptors in cat. *Brain Research* 442, 1–10.

Arnauld, E., Cirino, M., Layton, B. S., and Renaud, L. P. (1983). Contrasting actions of amino acids, acetylcholine, noradrenaline and leucine enkephalin on the excitability of supraoptic vasopressin-secreting neurons. *Neuroendocrinology* 36, 187–196.

Banks, D., and Harris, M. C. (1984). Lesions of the locus coeruleus abolish baroreceptor-induced depression of supraoptic neurones in the rat. *Journal of Physiology (London)* 355, 383–398.

Banks, D., and Harris, M. C. (1988). Activation of hypothalamic arcuate but not paraventricular neurones following carotid body chemoreceptor stimulation in the rat. *Neuroscience* 24, 967–976.

Bartelstone, H. J., and Nasmyth, P. A. (1965). Vasopressin potentiation of catecholamine action in dog, rat, and cat aortic strip. *American Journal of Physiology* 208, 754–762.

Beleslin, D., Bisset, G. W., Hadlar, J., and Polak, R. L. (1967). The release of vasopressin without oxytocin in response to haemorrhage. *Proceedings of the Royal Society of London Series B* 166, 443–458.

Bioulac, B., Gaffori, O., Harris, M. C., and Vincent, J. D. (1978). Effects of acetylcholine, sodium glutamate and GABA on the discharge of supraoptic neurones in the rat. *Brain Research* 154, 159–162.

Blessing, W. W., and Willoughby, J. O. (1985). Inhibiting the rabbit caudal ventrolateral medulla prevents barore-ceptor-initiated secretion of vasopressin. *Journal of Physiology (London)* 367, 253–265.

Blessing, W. W., Howe, P. R. C., Joh, T. H., Oliver, J. R., and Willoughby, J. O. (1986). Distribution of tyrosine hydroxylase and neuropeptide Y-like immunoreactive neurons in rabbit medulla oblongata, with attention to co-localization studies, presumptive adrenaline-synthesizing perikarya and vagal preganglionic cells. *Journal of Comparative Neurology* 248, 285–300.

Boyle, W. A., III, and Segel, L. D. (1986). Direct cardiac effects of vasopressin and their reversal by a vascular antagonist. *American Journal of Physiology* 251, H734–H741.

Burstein, R., Cliffer, K. D., and Giesler, G. J., Jr. (1987). Direct somatosensory projections from spinal cord to the hypothalamus and telencephalon. *Journal of Neuroscience* 7, 4159–4167.

Bussein, J. P., Walker, B., Nussberger, J., Schaller, M. D., Gavras, H., Hofbaur, K., and Branner, H. R. (1984). Does vasopressin sustain blood pressure of normally hydrated healthy volunteers? *American Journal of Physiology* 246, H143–H147.

Clark, B. J., and Rocha e Silva, M. (1967). An afferent pathway for the selective release of vasopressin in response to carotid occlusion and haemorrhage in the cat. *Journal of Physiology (London)* 191, 529–542.

Cobbett, P., Smithson, K. G., and Hatton, G. I. (1985). Dye-coupled magnocellular peptidergic neurons of the rat paraventricular neuclus show homotypic immunoreactivity. *Neuroscience* 16, 885–895.

Cobbett, P., Smithson, K. G., and Hatton, G. I. (1986). Immunoreactivity to vasopressin- but not oxytocin-associated neurophysin antiserum in phasic neurons of rat hypothalamic paraventricular nucleus. *Brain Research* 362, 7–16.

Courtice, G. P., Kwang, T. E., Lumbers, E. R., and Potter, E. K. (1984). Excitation of the cardiac vagus by vasopressin in mammals. *Journal of Physiology (London)* 354, 547–556.

Cowley, A. W., Jr., Merrill, D., Osborn, J., and Barber, B. J. (1984). Influence of vasopressin and angiotensin on baroreflexes in the dog. *Circulation Research* 54, 163–172.

Cowley, A. W., Jr., Monos, E., Jr., and Guyton, A. C. (1974). Interaction of vasopressin and the baroreceptor reflex system in the regulation of arterial blood pressure in the dog. *Circulation Research* 34, 505–514.

Craig, A. D., and Mense, S. (1983). The distribution of afferent fibers from the gastrocnemius-soleus muscle in the dorsal horn of the cat, as revealed by the transport of HRP. *Neuroscience Letters* 41, 233–238.

Cunningham, E. T., and Sawchenko, P. E. (1988). Anatomical specificity of noradrenegic inputs to the paraventricular and supraoptic nuclei of the rat hypothalamus. *Journal of Comparative Neurology* 274, 60–76.

Day, T. A., and Sibbald, J. R. (1988a). Direct catecholaminergic projections from nucleus tractus solitarius to supraoptic nucleus. *Brain Research* 454, 387–392.

Day, T. A., and Sibbald, J. R. (1988b). Solitary nucleus excitation of supraoptic vasopressin cells via adrenergic afferents. *American Journal of Physiology* 254, R711–R716.

de Bold, A. J. (1982). Tissue fractionation studies on the relationship between an atrial natriuretic factor and specific atrial granules. *Canadian Journal of Physiology and Pharmacology* 60, 324–330.

Dreifuss, J. J., Harris, M. C., and Tribollet, E. (1976). Excitation of phasically firing hypothalamic supraoptic neurones by carotid occlusion in rats. *Journal of Physiology (London)* 257, 337–354.

Dunn, F. L., Brennann, T. J., Nelson, A. E., and Robertson, G. L. (1973). The role of blood osmolality and volume in regulating vasopressin secretion in the rat. *Journal of Clinical Investigation* 52, 3212–3219.

Dutton, A., and Dyball, R. E. J. (1979). Phasic firing enhances vasopressin release from the rat neurohypophysis. *Journal of Physiology (London)* 290, 433–440.

Egan, B., Grekin, R., Ibsen, H., Osterzeil, K., and Stevo, J. (1984). Role of cardiopulmonary mechanoreceptors in ADH release in normal humans. *Hypertension* 6, 832–836.

Errington, M. L., and Roche e Silva, M., Jr. (1972). Vasopressin clearance and secretion during haemorrhage in normal dogs and in dogs with experimental diabetes insipidus. *Journal of Physiology (London)* 227, 395–418.

Feldberg, W. S., and Rocha e Silva, M., Jr. (1978). Vasopressin release produced in anaesthetised cats by antagonists of gamma-aminobutyric acid and glycine. *British Journal of Pharmacology* 62, 99–106.

Feldberg, W. S., and Rocha e Silva, M., Jr. (1981). Inhibition of vasopressin release to carotid occlusion by gamma-aminobutyric acid and glycine. *British Journal of Pharmacology* 72, 17–24.

Gähwiler, B., and Dreifuss, J. J. (1979). Phasically firing neurons in long-term cultures of the rat hypothalamic supraoptic area: Pacemaker and follower cells. *Brain Research* 177, 95–103.

Gardiner, S. M., and Bennett, T. (1982). The control of heart rate in rats with hereditary hypothalamic diabetes insipidus (Brattleboro strain). *Annals of the New York Academy of Science* 394, 363–374.

Gauer, O. H., Henry, J. P., Sieker, O. H., and Wendt, W. E. (1954). The effect of negative pressure breathing on urine flow. *Journal of Clinical Investigation* 33, 287–296.

Hanley, M. R., Benton, H. P., Lightman, S. L., Todd, K., Bone, E., Fretten, P., Palmer, S., Kirk, C. J., and Michell, R. H. (1984). A vasopressin-like peptide in the mammalian sympathetic nervous system. *Nature* 309, 258–261.

Harris, M. C. (1979). Effects of chemoreceptor and baroreceptor stimulation on the discharge of hypothalamic supraoptic neurones in rats. *Journal of Endocrinology* 82, 115–125.

Harris, M. C., Dreifuss, J. J., and Legros, J. J. (1975). Excitation of phasically-firing supraoptic neurons during vasopressin release. *Nature* 258, 80–82.

Hatton, G. I., Cobbett, P., and Salm, A. K. (1983a). Extranuclear axon collaterals of paraventricular neurons in the rat hypothalamus: Intracellular staining, immunocytochemistry and electrophysiology. *Brain Research* 14, 123–132.

Hatton, G. I., Ho, Y. W., and Mason, W. T. (1983b). Synaptic activation of phasic bursting in rat supraoptic nucleus neurones recorded in hypothalamic slices. *Journal of Physiology (London)* 345, 297–317.

Henry, J. P., and Pearce, J. W. (1956). The possible role of cardiac atrial receptors in the induction of changes in urine flow. *Journal of Physiology (London)* 131, 572–585.

Henry, J. P. Gupta, P. D., Meehan, J. P., Sinclair, R., and Share, L. (1968). The role of afferents from the low-pressure system in the release of antidiuretic hormone during non-hypertensive haemorrhage. *Canadian Journal of Physiology and Pharmacology* 46, 287–295.

Hou-Yu, A., Lamme, A. T., Zimmerman, E. A., and Silverman, A. J. (1986). Comparative distribution of vasopressin and oxytocin neurons in the rat brain using a double-label procedure. *Neuroendocrinology* 44, 235–246.

Jhamandas, J. H., and Renaud, L. P. (1986). A gamma-aminobutyric acid-mediated baroreceptor input to supraoptic vasopressin neurones in the rat. *Journal of Physiology (London)* 381, 595–606.

Jhamandas, J. H., Rogers, J., Buijs, R. M., and Renaud, L. P. (1987). Ultrastructural characterization of a GABA-mediated input to rat supraoptic nucleus (SON) from the diagonal band of Broca (DB). *Society for Neuroscience Abstracts* 13, part 2, 1130.

Jones, B. E., and Yang, T. Z. (1985). The efferent projections from the reticular formation and the locus coeruleus studied by anterograde and retrograde axonal transport in the rat. *Journal of Comparative Neurology* 242, 56–92.

Jonsson, G., Fuxe, K., Hökfelt, T., and Goldstein, M. (1976). Resistance of central phenylethanolamine-N-methyl transferase containing neurons to 6-hydroxydopamine. *Medical Biology* 54, 421–426.

Kannan, H., and Yagi, Y. (1978). Supraoptic neurosecretory neurons: Evidence for the existence of converging inputs both from carotid baroreceptors and osmoreceptors. *Brain Research* 14, 385–390.

Kannan, H., Yagi, K., and Sawaki, Y. (1981). Pontine neurones: Electrophysiological evidence of mediating carotid baroreceptor inputs to supraoptic neurones in rats. *Experimental Brain Research* 42, 362–370.

Katusic, Z. S., Shepherd, J. T., and Vanhoutte, P. M. (1984). Vasopressin causes endothelium-dependent relaxations of the canine basilar artery. *Circulation Research* 55, 575–579.

Kiraly, M., Maillard, M., Dreifuss, J. J., and Dolivo, M. (1985). Neurohypophyseal peptides depress cholinergic transmission in a mammalian sympathetic ganglion. *Neuroscience Letters* 62, 89–95.

Kiraly, M., Audigier, S., Tribollet, E., Barberis, C., Dolivo, M., and Dreifuss, J. J. (1986). Biochemical and electrophysiological evidence of functional vasopressin receptors in the rat superior cervical ganglion. *Proceedings of the National Academy of Sciences USA* 83, 5335–5339.

Landgren, S., and Neil, E. (1951). Chemoreceptor impulse activity following haemorrhage. *Acta Physiologica Scandinavica* 23, 158–167.

Lassoff, S., and Altura, B. M. (1980). Do pial terminal arterioles respond to local perivesicular application of the neurophyopophyseal peptide hormones, vasopressin and oxytocin? *Brain Research* 136, 266–269.

Laycock, J. F., Penn, W., Shirley, D. G., and Walter, S. J. (1979). The role of vasopressin in blood pressure regulation immediately following acute haemorrhage in the rat. *Journal of Physiology (London)* 338, 413–421.

Ledsome, J. R., and Mason, J. M. (1972). The effects of vasopressin on the diuretic response to left atrial distension. *Journal of Physiology (London)* 221, 427–440.

Ledsome, J. R., Ngsee, J., and Wilson, N. (1983). Plasma vasopressin concentration in the anaesthetised dog before, during and after atrial distension. *Journal of Physiology (London)* 338, 413–421.

Ledsome, J. R., Wilson, N., Courneya, C. A., and Rankin, A. J. (1985). Release of atrial peptide by atrial distension. *Canadian Journal of Physiology and Pharmacology* 63, 739–742.

Leng, G., and Dyball, R.E.J. (1983). Intercommunication in the rat supraoptic nucleus. *Quarterly Journal of Experimental Physiology* 68, 493–504.

Leng, G., and Dyball, R. E. J. (1987). The role of supraoptic neurones in blood pressure regulation. In: *Organization of the Autonomic Nervous System, Central and Peripheral Mechanisms*, J. Ciriello, F. R. Calaresu, L. P. Renaud, and C. Polosa (eds.), Liss, New York, pp. 447–456.

Liard, J. F. (1986a). Cardiovascular effects associated with antidiuretic activity after blockade of its vasoconstrictor action in dehydrated dogs. *Circulation Research* 58, 631–640.

Liard, J. F. (1986b). Effects of intra-arterial arginine-vasopressin infusions on peripheral blood flows in conscious dogs. *Clinical Science* 71, 713–721.

Liard, J. F., Deriaz, I., Tschopp, M., and Schoun, J. (1981). Cardiovascular effects of vasopressin infused into the vertebral circulation of conscious dogs. *Clinical Science* 61, 345–347.

Liard, J. F., Deraiz, O., Shelling, P., and Thibonnier, M. (1982). Cardiac output distribution during vasopressin infusion or dehydration in conscious dogs. *American Journal of Physiology* 243, H663–H669.

Lightman, S. L., Todd, K., and Everitt, B. J. (1984). Ascending noradrenergic projections from the brainstem: Evidence for a major role in the regulation of blood pressure and vasopressin secretion. *Experimental Brain Research* 55, 145–151.

Luiten, P. G. M., ter Horst, G. J., Karst, H., and Steffens, A. B. (1985). The course of paraventricular hypothalamic efferents to autonomic structures in medulla and spinal cord. *Brain Research* 329, 374–378.

Lumbers, E. R., and Potter, E. K. (1982). The effects of vasoactive peptides on the carotid baroreflex. *Clinical and Experimental Pharmacology and Physiology* Suppl. 7, 45–49.

McAllen, R. M., and Blessing, W. W. (1987). Neurones (presumably A1 cells) projecting from the caudal ventrolateral medulla to the region of the supraoptic nucleus respond to baroreceptor inputs in the rabbit. *Neuroscience Letters* 73, 247–252.

McAllen, R. M., and Harris, M. C. (1988). Long-latency baroreceptor inhibition of supraoptic neurones in the cat. *Neuroscience Letters,* 84, 287–290.

McKellar, S., and Loewy, A. D. (1981). Organization of some brainstem afferents to the paraventricular nucleus of the hypothalamus in the rat. *Brain Research* 217, 351–357.

McKellar, S., and Loewy, A. D. (1982). Efferent projections of the A1 catecholamine cell group in the rat: An autoradiographic study. *Brain Research* 241, 11–29.

McNeill, T. H., and Sladek, J. R., Jr. (1980). Simultaneous monoamine histofluorescence and neuropeptide immunocytochemistry. II. Correlative distribution of catecholamine varicosities and magnocellular neurosecretory neurons in the rat supraoptic and paraventricular nuclei. *Journal of Comparative Neurology* 193, 1023–1033.

Menetrey, D., and Basbaum, A. I. (1987). Spinal and trigeminal projections to the nucleus of the solitary tract: A possible substrate for somatovisceral and viscerovisceral reflex activation. *Journal of Comparative Neurology* 255, 439–450.

Meyer, D. K., and Brownstein, M. J. (1980). Effect of surgical deafferentation of the supraoptic nucleus on its choline acetyltransferase content. *Brain Research* 193, 566–569.

Michell, R. H., Kirk, C. J., and Billah, M. M. (1979). Hormonal stimulation of phosphatidylinositol breakdown, with particular reference to the hepatic effects of vasopressin. *Biochemical Society Transactions* 7, 861–865.

Montani, J. P., Laird, J. F., Schoun, J., and Mohring, J. (1980). Haemodynamic effects of exogenous and endogenous vasopressin at low plasma concentrations in conscious dogs. *Circulation Research* 47, 346–355.

O'Callaghan, P. A., and Sheehan, J. D. (1986). Vasopressin and baroreflex sensitivity in man. *Journal of Physiology (London)* 371, 89P.

Peters, S., and Kreulen, D. L. (1985). Vasopressin-mediated slow EPSPs in a mammalian sympathetic ganglion. *Brain Research* 339, 126–129.

Pickford, M. (1939). The inhibitory effect of acetylcholine on water diuresis in the dog, and its pituitary transmission. *Journal of Physiology (London)* 95, 226–238.

Pickford, M. (1947). The action of acetylcholine in the supraoptic nucleus of the chloralosed dog. *Journal of Physiology (London)* 106, 264–270.

Randle, J. C. R., Day, T. A., Jhamandas, J. H., Bourque, C. W., and Renaud, L. P. (1986). Neuropharmacology of supraoptic nucleus neurones: Norepinephrine and gamma-aminobutyric acid receptors. *Federation Proceedings* 45, 2312–2317.

Rascher, W., Meffle, H., and Gross, F. (1985). Hemodynamic effects of arginine vasopressin in conscious water-deprived rats. *American Journal of Physiology* 249, H29–H33.

Ricardo, J. A., and Koh, E. T. (1978). Anatomical evidence of direct projections from the nucleus of the solitary tract to the hypothalamus, amygdala and other forebrain structures in the rat. *Brain Research* 153, 1–26.

Robertson, G. L., and Athar, S. (1976). The interaction of blood osmolality and blood volume in regulating plasma vasopressin in man. *Journal of Clinical Endocrinology and Metabolism* 42, 613–620.

Robertson, G. L., Shelton, R. L., and Athar, S. (1976). The osmoregulation of vasopressin. *Kidney International* 10, 25–37.

Rydin, H., and Verney, E. B. (1938). The inhibition of water diuresis by emotional stress and by muscular exercise. *Quarterly Journal of Experimental Physiology* 27, 343–373.

Saper, C. B., and Loewy, A. D. (1980). Efferent connections of the parabrachial nucleus in the rat. *Brain Research* 197, 291–317.

Sawchenko, P. E., and Swanson, L. W. (1982). Organization of noradrenergic pathways from the brain stem to the paraventricular and supraoptic nuclei in the rat. *Brain Research Reviews* 4, 275–325.

Sawchenko, P. E., and Swanson, L. W. (1983). The organization of forebrain afferents to the paraventricular and supraoptic nuclei of the rat. *Journal of Comparative Neurology* 218, 121–144.

Sawchenko, P. E., Swanson, L. W., Grzanna, R., Howe, P. R. C., Bloom, S. R., and Polak, J. M. (1985). Co-localization of neuropeptide Y immunoreactivity in brainstem catecholaminergic neurons that project to the paraventricular nucleus of the hypothalamus. *Journal of Comparative Neurology* 241, 138–153.

Schultz, H. D., Fater, D. C., Geer, P. G., and Goetz, K. L. (1982). Reflexes elicited by acute stretch of atrial vs. pulmonary receptors in conscious dogs. *American Journal of Physiology* 242, H1065–H1076.

Schwartz, J., and Reid, I. (1981). Effect of vasopressin blockade on blood pressure regulation during haemorrhage in conscious dogs. *Endocrinology* 109, 1778–1780.

Share, L. (1962). Vascular volume and blood level of antidiuretic hormone. *American Journal of Physiology* 202, 791–794.

Share, L., and Levy, M. N. (1962). Cardiovascular receptors and blood titre of antidiuretic hormone. *American Journal of Physiology* 203, 425–428.

Share, L., and Levy, M. N. (1966a). Effect of carotid chemoreceptor stimulation of plasma antidiuretic hormone titer. *American Journal of Physiology* 210, 157–161.

Share, L., and Levy, M. N. (1966b). Carotid sinus pulse pressure, a determinant of plasma antidiuretic hormone concentration. *American Journal of Physiology* 211, 721–724.

Smock, T., Cach, R., and Topple, A. (1987). Action of vasopressin on neurones and microvessels in the rat hippocampal slice. *Experimental Brain Research* 66, 401–408.

Sved, A. F., Blessing, W. W., and Reis, D. J. (1985). Caudal ventrolateral medulla can alter vasopressin and arterial pressure. *Brain Research Bulletin* 14, 227–232.

Swanson, L. W. (1976). The locus coeruleus: A cytoarchitectonic, Golgi, and immunohistochemical study in the albino rat. *Brain Research* 110, 39–56.

Swanson, L. W., Sawchenko, P. E., Béred, A., Hartman, B. K., Helle, K. B., and Vanorden, D. E. (1981). An immunohistochemical study of the organization of catecholaminergic cells and terminal fields in the paraventricular and supraoptic nuclei of the hypothalamus. *Journal of Comparative Neurology* 196, 271–285.

Tappaz, M. L., Wassef, M., Oertel, W. H., Paut, L., and Pujol, J. F. (1983). Light- and electron-microscopic immunocytochemistry of glutamic acid decarboxylase (GAD) in the basal hypothalamus: Morphological evidence for neuroendocrine gamma-aminobutyrate (GABA). *Neuroscience* 9, 271–287.

Thames, M. D., and Schmid, P. G. (1979). Cardiopulmonary receptors with vagal afferents tonically inhibit ADH release in the dog. *American Journal of Physiology* 237, H299–H304.

Theodosis, D. T., Paut, L., and Tappaz, M. L. (1986). Immunocytochemical analysis of the GABAergic innervation of oxytocin- and vasopressin-secreting neurons in the rat supraoptic nucleus. *Neuroscience* 19, 207–222.

Tribollet, E., Armstrong, W. E., Dubois-Dauphin, M., and Dreifuss, J. J. (1985). Extrahypothalamic afferent inputs to the supraoptic nucleus area of the rat as determined by retrograde and anterograde tracing techniques. *Neuroscience* 15, 135–148.

Tribollet, E., Barberis, C., Jard, S., Dubois-Dauphin, N., and Dreifuss, J. J. (1988). Localization and pharmacological characterization of high affinity binding sites for vasopressin and oxytocin in the rat brain by light microscopic autoradiography. *Brain Research* 442, 105–118.

Tucker, D. C., Saper, C. B., Ruggiero, D. A., and Reis, D. J. (1987). Organization of central adrenergic pathways: I. Relationships of ventrolateral medullary projections to the hypothalamus and spinal cord. *Journal of Comparative Neurology* 259, 591–603.

Undesser, K. P., Hasser, E. M., Haywood, J. R., Johnson, A. K., and Bishop, V. S. (1985). Interactions of vasopressin with the area postrema in arterial baroreflex functions in conscious rabbits. *Circulation Research* 56, 410–417.

van den Pol, A. (1982). The magnocellular and parvocellular paraventricular nucleus of rat: Intrinsic organization. *Journal of Comparative Neurology* 206, 317–345.

van den Pol, A. (1985). Dual ultrastructural localization of two neurotransmitter-related antigens: Colloidal gold-labelled neurophysin-immunoreactive supraoptic neurons receive peroxidase-labelled glutamate decarboxylase or gold-labelled GABA-immunoreactive synapses. *Journal of Neuroscience* 5, 2940–2954.

Wagner, H. N., and Braunwald, E. (1956). The pressor effect of the antidiuretic principle of the posterior pituitary in orthostatic hypertension. *Journal of Clinical Investigation* 35, 1412–1418.

Walker, B. R., Childs, M. E., and Adams, E. M. (1988). Direct cardiac effects of vasopressin: Role of V1- and V2-vasopressinergic receptors. *American Journal of Physiology* 255, H261–H265.

Webb, R. L., Osborn, J. W., and Cowley, A. W. (1986). Cardiovascular actions of vasopressin: Baroreflex modulation in the conscious rat. *American Journal of Physiology* 251, H1244–H1251.

Weller, K. L., and Smith, D. A. (1982). Afferent connections to the bed nucleus of the stria terminalis. *Brain Research* 232, 255–270.

Willoughby, J. O., and Blessing, W. W. (1987). Neuropeptide Y injected into the supraoptic nucleus causes secretion of vasopressin in the unanaesthetised rat. *Neuroscience Letters* 75, 17–22.

Willoughby, J. O., Jervois, P. M., Menadue, M. F., and Blessing, W. W. (1987). Noradrenaline, by activation of alpha-1-adrenoreceptors in the region of the supraoptic nucleus, causes secretion of vasopressin in the unanesthetised rat. *Neuroendocrinology* 45, 219–226.

Woods, R. L., and Johnson, C. I. (1984). Contribution of vasopressin to the maintenance of blood pressure during dehydration. *American Journal of Physiology* 24, F615–F621.

Yamashita, H. (1977). Effect of baro- and chemoreceptor activation on supraoptic nuclei neurons in the hypothalamus. *Brain Research* 126, 551–556.

Yamashita, H., and Koizumi, K. (1979). Influence of carotid and aortic baroreceptors on neurosecretory neurones in supraoptic nuclei. *Brain Research* 170, 259–277.

Yamashita, H., Inenaga, K., Kawata, M., Sano, Y., and Kannan, H. (1984a). Lucifer yellow-filled neurosecretory cells in the supraoptic and paraventricular nuclei. *Biomedical Research* 5, Suppl. 105–114.

Yamashita, H., Kannan, H., Inenaga, K., and Koizumi, K. (1984b). The role of cardiovascular and muscle afferent systems in control of body water balance. *Journal of the Autonomic Nervous System* 10, 305–316.

14

Circumventricular Organs and Their Role in Visceral Functions

A. K. JOHNSON AND A. D. LOEWY

The capillaries of the brain form a unique barrier that permits certain molecules and ions to be transferred from the plasma to the brain by selective regulatory processes that are controlled by the endothelial cells. These cells are connected by an elaborate system of tight junctions and form the blood–brain barrier. This barrier does not exclude all molecules. For example, certain substances such as oxygen, carbon dioxide, and anesthetics that are highly lipid soluble readily pass through this barrier. Other molecules such as amino acids, sugars, and certain ions are also transported across the endothelial cell via various carrier transport systems. However, high-molecular-weight substances such as proteins usually do not gain access to the CNS unless some type of pathological condition has occurred to destroy or to modify the physiology of the endothelial cells.

This barrier is present throughout the CNS, except for a few midline sites along the third and fourth ventricles of the brain. These regions lack a blood–brain barrier and are called *circumventricular organs* (Figure 14-1). At these sites, the capillaries are fenestrated, and this property allows large-molecular-weight substances to pass readily from the plasma to the underlying neural tissue. These sites are first described in a systematic manner by Wislocki and Leduc (1952) after intravenous injections of the vital dye trypan blue. These areas include the organum vasculosum of the lamina terminalis (OVLT), subfornical organ, median eminence, posterior pituitary, intermediate lobe of the pituitary, subcommissural organ, pineal gland, and area postrema. Apart from fenestrated capillaries, all of these regions contain specialized ependymal cells called tanycytes, which traverse the circumventricular organ, having one process that reaches the ventricular surface and another that connects with the surrounding neural tissue. These cells may subserve specialized functions related to transmitting information about the chemical nature of the cerebrospinal fluid of the ventricles to nearby structures (see Gross, 1987, for review).

Three of the circumventricular organs, the area postrema, subfornical organ, and OVLT, have neurons that project to CNS regions involved in regulation of neuroendocrine and autonomic functions. These three circumventricular organs are thought to provide an index of the physiological status of the animal by sampling its internal chemical environment (i.e., plasma and cerebrospinal fluid) and, then, transmitting this information to the CNS. In accordance with this idea, each of these areas has been shown to possess high concentrations of binding sites for peptide hormones such as angiotensin II (van Houten et al., 1980; Mendelsohn et al., 1984), atrial natriuretic peptide (Saavedra, 1987), cholecystokinin (Moran et al., 1986; Zarbin et al., 1983), insulin (van Houten et al., 1979), vasopressin (Tribollet et al., 1988), and probably other peptide hormones as well. In addition, electrophysiological studies have shown that these neurons are responsive to exogenously applied neuropeptides as well as glucose and sodium. Thus, it is quite likely that these neurons act as chemical sensors, and the objective of this chapter will be to review the anatomy and physiology of these three major circumventricular organs (the area postrema, subfornical organ, and organum vasculosum of the lamina terminalis), with particular emphasis on how they regulate body fluid and electrolyte homeostasis and their role in cardiovascular function.

AREA POSTREMA

The area postrema lies at the caudal end of the fourth ventricle of the brain (Figure 14-2). In some mammals, such as rats and rabbits, it is a midline structure lying dorsal to the site where the fourth ventricle communicates with the central canal. In other mammals, such as cats, monkeys, and humans, it is a bilateral structure.

The area postrema, like the other circumventricular organs, lies at an interface between the cere-

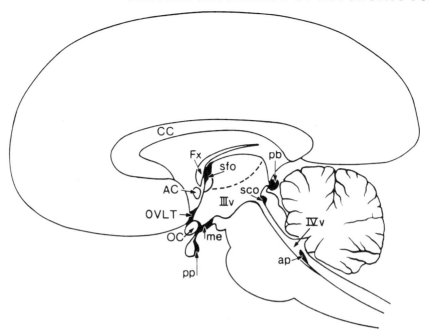

Figure 14-1 Midsagittal section of the human brain showing the location of the circumventricular organs (black shaded areas). These specialized regions surround the third and fourth ventricles, lack a blood–brain barrier, and are highly vascularized. AC, anterior commissure; ap, area postrema; CC, corpus callosum; Fx, fornix; me, mesencephalon; OC, optic chiasm; OVLT, organum vasculosum of the lamina terminalis; pb, pineal body; pp, posterior pituitary; sco, subcommissural organ; sfo, subfornical organ. (Reproduced from Landas et al., 1985, *Neuroscience Letters* 57, 251–256, with permission of the authors and publisher.)

brospinal fluid compartment and the vascular system. Its ventricular surface is covered by a modified, single layer of ependymal cells that has modified microvilli and specialized, narrow intercellular junctions at its apical surface that are permeable to large macromolecules (Leslie, 1986).

The area postrema receives its arterial supply solely from the posterior inferior cerebellar arteries. In rats, these arteries enter from the dorsal surface, but in other species, such as cats, dogs, and humans, the vessels penetrate from the lateral border of the area postrema (Roth and Yamamoto, 1968). These arteries break up and form a network of sinusoids or enlarged capillaries that course throughout the area postrema. At the ventral and ventrolateral border of the area postrema, the sinusoids coalesce to form short connecting vessels that then break up into a second capillary network that transverses through the ventral lying nucleus tractus solitarius (Roth and Yamamoto, 1968). Since the two sets of capillaries are serially connected with one arterial input and one venous outflow, they may constitute a portal system. This vascular relationship may serve as a functional link between the area postrema and the nucleus tractus solitarius (NTS) by providing a potential neurohemal route similar to that seen in the hypothalamo–hypophyseal system. However, direct

physiological evidence supporting this idea is lacking.

Anatomical Connections

The area postrema has specific neural connections. It receives afferent inputs from the carotid sinus nerve (Panneton and Loewy, 1980), vagus nerve (Ciriello et al., 1981), and dorsomedial and paraventricular hypothalamic nuclei (Hosoya and Matsushita, 1981; Luiten et al., 1985) and projects to the commissural-medial region of the NTS and to the lateral parabrachial nucleus (Figure 14-3). These CNS nuclei are part of a central autonomic circuit involved with general visceral functions (see Chapter 6).

Functional Studies

The area postrema is not critical for life. Ablation studies have demonstrated that only subtle abnormalities occur after removal of this structure. Nevertheless, this neural element has been implicated in a wide range of functions such as arousal, control of food and water intake, cardiovascular functions, and chemoreceptive trigger zone for the vomiting response. However, it must be stressed that most of the

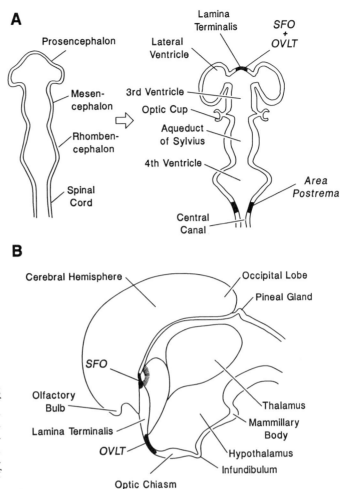

Figure 14-2 (A) Schematic diagram showing the development of the ventricular system of the brain. (B) Midsagittal section of the forebrain indicating the regions of the lamina terminalis that differentiate into circumventricular organs. (Adapted and modified from J. Langman, 1975, *Medical Embryology*, Williams & Wilkins, Baltimore with permission of the publisher.)

functional studies have been based either on surgical lesions or on electrical stimulation methods, and both of these methods have significant limitations. Since the vascular supply of the NTS and area postrema comes from the same source, it is distinctly possible that any surgical lesion of the area postrema that affects the blood supply will also affect the underlying neurons of the NTS as well. To date, this issue has not been considered. It is a potential complicating factor since gastrointestinal afferents project to an NTS area just below the area postrema (see Chapter 6). With the development of excitotoxic agents such as ibotenic acid, which selectively lesion cells and not fibers of passage, it should now be possible to circumvent this problem by making selective lesions of neurons in the area postrema. With the electrical stimulation studies, it is quite likely that both the area postrema neurons as well as nearby NTS neurons were activated with the currents used. In addition, the incoming axons projecting to both these sites may have been antidromically activated

as well. In the latter situation, it is possible that effects ascribed to the area postrema were due to antidromic excitation of the axons and their collaterals of the hypothalamic neurons that project to this structure. This means that the electrical current may have caused excitation or inhibition of other cell groups that receive inputs from these hypothalamic neurons. Since neither of these two potential problems has been controlled in a rigorous way in any of the studies published to date, the functional data regarding the area postrema must be regarded as less than definitive but still worth summarizing to provide an overview of the investigative work already performed.

The area postrema has been implicated as the chemoreceptive emetic trigger zone (see Borison, 1984, for review). Destruction of this structure attenuates or abolishes vomiting that can be induced by chemical emetics (e.g., Borison and Wang, 1951; Wang and Chinn, 1954), by ionizing radiation (e.g., Harding et al., 1985) or by motion sickness (e.g., Brizzee

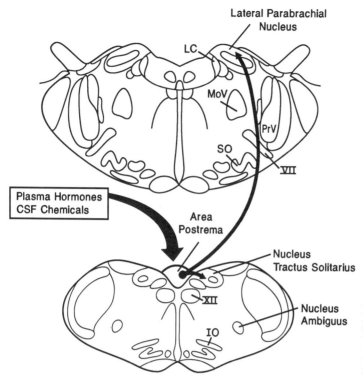

Figure 14-3 Efferent pathways of the area postrema. IO, inferior olivary nucleus; LC, locus coeruleus; MoV, motor trigeminal nucleus; PrV, principal sensory trigeminal nucleus; SO, superior olivary nucleus; VII, facial nerve, XII, hypoglossal nucleus.

et al., 1980). In addition, surgical destruction of the area postrema in humans with intractable vomiting abolishes idiopathic vomiting and alters the emetic threshold to apomorphine (Lindstrom and Brizzee, 1962).

A number of behavioral studies have been directed at evaluating the role of the area postrema in caloric and fluid homeostasis (see reviews by Contreras et al., 1984 and Miselis et al., 1984). Lesions of the area postrema cause changes which include maintenance of lower body weight, permanent polydipsia, elevated salt appetite, and alterations in food preference. The neural basis of how these functions are regulated is unclear, but lesion data presented by Edwards and Ritter (1986) and Edwards et al. (1986) suggest that some aspects of food intake satiety may be controlled by the area postrema. Further support that this area transmits signals related to food and sodium intake comes from Adachi and Kobashi (1985), who have provided electrophysiological evidence that neurons in the area postrema alter their neural activity to glucose and sodium application (see Figure 14-4).

The area postrema has also been implicated in cardiovascular regulation (see review by Ferrario et al., 1987). Lesions of the area postrema in rats produce mild hypotension, bradycardia, and an enhancement of baroreceptor reflex control of heart rate (Skoog and Mangiapane, 1988) and in dogs cause small decreases in cardiac output (Ferrario et al., 1979). Circulating peptide hormones such as angiotensin II and vasopressin exert an indirect effect on the cardiovascular system via an action that is mediated in the area postrema (Otsuka et al., 1986; Undesser et al., 1985). These data are consistent with observations that angiotensin II and vasopressin (as well as other neuroactive agents) cause excitation of neurons in the area postrema (Carpenter et al., 1983). This site of action may also be an important determinant in certain forms of hypertension (Fink et al., 1987).

SUBFORNICAL ORGAN

Anatomical Connections

The subfornical organ (SFO) is a circumventricular organ that lies in the roof of the third ventricle (Figures 14-2 and 14-5). Like the other circumventricular organs, it lacks a blood–brain barrier, possesses a high concentration of peptide hormone-binding sites, and contains neurons that have widespread efferent and afferent connections (see review by Lind, 1987).

The SFO projects heavily to the hypothalamus. Three major areas of termination have been described: (1) the magnocellular paraventricular and

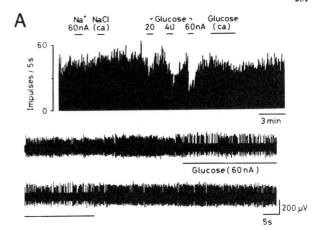

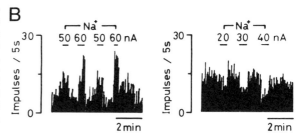

Figure 14-4 (A) Glucose-sensitive neurons of the area postrema. Extracellular electrophysiological recording of a neuron in the area postrema of a rat that is responsive to topical application of glucose. Note that intracarotid application of glucose, which is indicated at the time labeled "ca," produces a weak inhibitory effect. In contrast, when sodium was applied to the same neuron by either direct application or by intravenous infusion, no change in neuronal activity was detected. (B) Sodium-sensitive neurons of the area postrema. Some neurons in the area postrema are excited by exogenous application of Na$^+$ (left) and others are inhibited (right). (Reproduced from Adachi and Kobashi, 1985, with permission of the authors and publisher.)

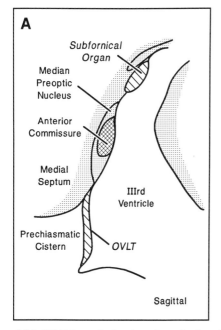

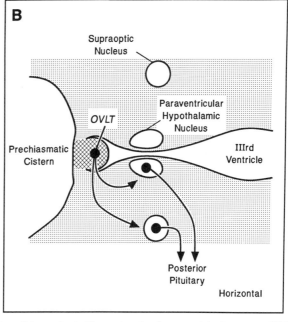

Figure 14-5 (A) Schematic drawing of a sagittal section of the rat brain illustrating the circumventricular organs. (B) Structure of the organ vasculosum of the lamina terminalis and its major efferent pathways.

supraoptic nuclei, (2) the anterior periventricular region surrounding the third ventricle (AV3V region), which includes the median preoptic nucleus, the organum vasculosum of the lamina terminalis (OVLT), and anterior periventricular region, and (3) the perifornical zone of the lateral hypothalamic area (Figure 14-6). The pathway to the paraventricular hypothalamic nucleus terminates in three distinct areas: the magnocellular region, which includes both oxytocin and vasopressin neurons; the medial and lateral parvocellular areas, which project to autonomic centers of the brain stem and spinal cord; and the periventricular zone, which sends fibers to the median eminence (Miselis, 1981 and see Miselis et al., 1987 for review). Since the magnocellular nuclei contain oxytocin and vasopressin neurons that project to the posterior pituitary, this implies that the SFO may regulate the release of these hormones. Electrical stimulation of the SFO excites vasopressin and oxytocin neurons and causes a release of both of these hormones (see review by Renaud et al., 1985; Ferguson et al., 1984b). The SFO projection to the medial parvocellular and periventricular divisions of the paraventricular hypothalamic nucleus affects hypothalamic neurons that project to the median eminence and, thus, modulates anterior pituitary function (Ferguson et al., 1984b). The SFO projection to the lateral parvocellular subnucleus of the paraventricular hypothalamic nucleus (PVH) affects the

sympathetic outflow because this region of the PVH pro-jects throughout the entire intermediolateral cell column. This implies that a variety of sympathetically mediated effects may be modulated by the SFO. This influence on autonomic functions may also be mediated by other SFO → PVH pathways that influence the NTS and the dorsal vagal nucleus (Ferguson and Renaud, 1984; Ferguson et al., 1984a).

The SFO also projects to the AV3V region, which consists of the median preoptic nucleus, OVLT, anterior periventricular nucleus, and medial preoptic region (see Lind, 1987 for review and Figure 14-7). The AV3V region has been implicated as a key area in regulating thirst and the evidence is summarized below. Other forebrain projections are directed to the ventromedial part of the bed nucleus of the stria terminalis—another forebrain region known to receive inputs from other autonomic centers such as the NTS and the parabrachial area and several regions of the hypothalamus (viz., arcuate nucleus, lateral hypothalamic area, dorsomedial hypothalamic nucleus, and zona incerta). In addition, the SFO projects to the substantia innominata in the basal forebrain, to the infralimbic cerebral cortex, to restricted areas in the thalamus, which include the paraventricular thalamic nucleus, central medial nucleus, and nucleus reuniens, and to the dorsal and medial raphe nuclei of the brain stem.

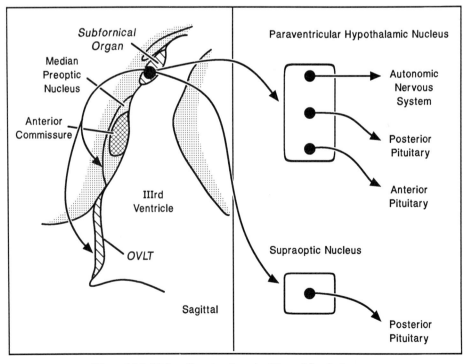

Figure 14-6 Major efferent pathways of the subfornical organ.

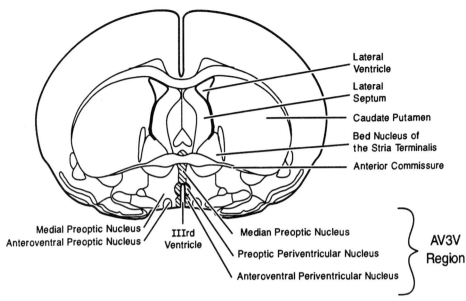

Figure 14-7 Diagram illustration of cell groups that form the AV3V region. Note that the OVLT lies immediately rostral to the anteroventral periventricular nucleus and is considered as part of the AV3V region.

Functional Studies

The SFO appears to be one of the main sites in the CNS involved in the neural regulation of salt and water balance. The key experiments that led to this concept may be traced to a series of microinjection studies performed by Simpson and Routtenberg (1972, 1973) implicating the SFO as an extremely sensitive forebrain region regulating drinking. Prior to these studies, various dipsogenic agents such as the cholinergic agonist, carbachol, and the peptide, angiotensin II, were shown to induce drinking; their effectiveness was very great when given directly in the brain.

Simpson and Routtenberg (1973) examined the role of the SFO in angiotensin II-induced thirst. In comparison to injections made into other brain tissue sites or into the ventricles, application of angiotensin II to the SFO produces drinking at exquisitely low doses. In addition, drinking elicited by systemic administration of angiotensin II was abolished either by SFO lesions or by local application of the angiotensin II receptor antagonist, saralasin, into the SFO (Simpson et al., 1978). Taken together, these results provided a strong case that the SFO is the major target tissue for the dipsogenic action of blood-borne angiotensin II.

Although early studies reported that SFO lesions also abolished the drinking response elicited by centrally applied angiotensin II (Simpson and Routtenberg, 1973), it was later recognized that this effect was not permanent and that it was due to a temporary disruption in the flow of angiotensin II in the

cerebrospinal fluid, so it was prevented from acting at other sites located near the ventricular system (Buggy et al., 1975; Buggy and Fisher, 1976). One of the most sensitive regions for the action of angiotensin II injected into the cerebroventricular system is the periventricular tissue of the anteroventral third ventricle (AV3V region) (Buggy et al., 1975; Buggy and Fisher, 1976; Hoffman and Phillips, 1976; Buggy and Johnson, 1977, 1978). The generation of drinking by angiotensin II gaining access to the AV3V region is in all likelihood due to the mimicking action of an angiotensin II-like substance synthesized within the brain that acts as a neurotransmitter/neuromodulator. This concept will be developed in more detail in a subsequent section, but considerable evidence is now available to support the idea that components of the renin–angiotensin system are synthesized *de novo* in the brain (see Ganten et al., 1972; Printz et al., 1982; Moffett et al., 1987 for reviews) and angiotensin II is likely to function as a neuroactive agent in the CNS.

In addition to the role of the SFO as a target for blood-borne angiotensin II in the generation of thirst, this structure has been implicated in other functions related to the sympathetic nervous system and vasopressin release. Lesions of the SFO attenuate the pressor response produced by systemic infusions of angiotensin II (Mangiapane and Simpson, 1980a and b) and angiotensin II injections into the SFO induce short latency pressor responses (Mangiapane and Simpson, 1980a). In addition, SFO lesions (Mangipane et al., 1984; Iovino and Steardo, 1984) or transections of the ventral stalk (Knepel et al., 1982), which is the major route of efferent outflow of the structure, attenuate the release of vasopressin.

Electrophysiological techniques have been used to characterize the chemical sensitivity of SFO neurons. SFO neurons are responsive to angiotensin II administered intravenously (Tanaka et al., 1985; Ishibashi et al., 1985) and iontophoretically (Felix and Akert, 1974; Nicolaidis et al., 1983; Ishibasdhi et al., 1985). In addition, *in vitro* recordings show SFO neurons to be sensitive to atrial natriuretic peptide, carbachol, serotonin, and glutamate (Buranarugsa and Hubbard, 1979, 1988; Okuya et al., 1987).

In addition to the SFO's role as a target for angiotensin II that is released from the periphery as a chemical signal of hypovolemia and of hypotension, additional evidence suggests that it may also be sensitive to changes in extracellular osmolality and/or sodium concentration. First, *in vitro* recording studies indicate that the SFO is osmosensitive (Sibbald et al., 1988). Second, lesions of the SFO have been reported to attenuate the drinking response to systemic hypertonic saline in the rat (Hosutt et al., 1981; Lind et al., 1984b). Natriuretic responses to intracarotid infusions of hypertonic solutions are blocked by lesions of the SFO of cat (Thornborough et al., 1973).

To summarize, the SFO appears to be a receptor for the hormonal signals related to water and electrolyte status. In addition, it is sensitive to osmolality changes as well. The SFO projects to the AV3V region, the magnocellular hypothalamic nuclei affecting posterior pituitary function, components of the paraventricular hypothalamic nucleus that affect anterior pituitary function, and the autonomic nervous system and other areas of the brain as well. Thus, the SFO projects to several CNS areas involved in the control of body fluid homeostasis, autonomic regulation, and neuroendocrine function.

ORGANUM VASCULOSUM OF THE LAMINA TERMINALIS

The organum vasculosum of the lamina terminalis (OVLT) lies in the ventral portion of the rostral wall of the third cerebral ventricle. During development the SFO arises from the dorsal aspect of the lamina terminalis, and the OVLT arises from the ventral part (Figures 14-2 and 14-5). Both the SFO and the OVLT are highly vascularized, midline structures with unique ependymal faces toward the third ventricle. However, unlike the SFO, the OVLT is bounded by fluid on two sides. The subarachnoid space called the *prechiasmatic cistern* lies immediately rostral to the OVLT so that this circumventricular organ is an isthmus bordered on two sides by cerebrospinal fluid. One part of the OVLT is "inside" the brain and the other is on the "outside" (see reviews by McKinley et al., 1987 and Landas and Phillips, 1987; Figure 14-6). In a dorsoventral direction the OVLT joins the rostrodorsal surface of the optic chiasm with the ventral median preoptic nucleus. Landas and Phillips (1987) estimate that the OVLT in rat is 150 μm wide and 300 μm high.

The parenchyma of the OVLT is comprised of neuronal perikarya, glia, tanycytes, and neuronal processes. Various biogenic amines and neuropeptides have been detected in the OVLT by biochemical and/or histochemical methods. These include dopamine, norepinephrine, serotonin, acetylcholine, luteinizing hormone-releasing hormone (LHRH), somatostatin, vasopressin, oxytocin, neurophysin, angiotensin II, angiotensinogen, and thyrotropin-relasing hormone (see Landas and Phillips, 1987, for review).

Anatomical Connections

Because of its minute dimensions and tenuous dorsal and ventral attachments, it has been very difficult to carry out neuroanatomical tracing studies that require discrete injections of tracer into the OVLT. Phillips and Camacho (1987) have reviewed the anatomical connections of the OVLT. Localized horseradish peroxidase injections into the OVLT result in retrograde cell body labeling in median preoptic nucleus, SFO, perizonal nucleus, which is a region just dorsal to the supraoptic nucleus, medial preoptic area, anterior hypothalamus, posterior hypothalamus, arcuate nucleus, ventromedial hypothalamic nucleus, midbrain central gray matter, and locus coeruleus. Whether these represent projections terminating exclusively in the OVLT or also provide inputs to the tissue around it still has not been resolved. Efferent projections of the OVLT have been identified with either anterograde transport horseradish peroxidase or tritiated amino acids. These are reported to project to the septum, dentate gyrus, cingulate region, an area dorsolateral to the supraoptic nucleus, supraoptic nucleus, stria medullaris, and basal ganglia. The small size of their structure makes them a particularly difficult target to inject without involvement of the periventricular tissue. More discrete injections with the plant lectin PHA-L have been made in the OVLT, and the results indicate that it projects mainly to the supraoptic and paraventricular hypothalamic nuclei (see Figure 14-5). This projection may come from angiotensin II neurons (Wilkin et al., 1989).

Functional Studies

Among the neurochemical constituents of the OVLT, the presence of luteinizing hormone-releasing hormone (LHRH) is quite notable and has given rise to speculation about the role of the OVLT in reproductive functions and behavior. The high concentration of LHRH-like material in the OVLT is due to the presence of dendrites and axons, not cell bodies. The cell bodies that give rise to the LHRH processes appear to reside in the medial septum and medial preoptic region (Kawano and Diakoku, 1981). Lesions of the OVLT (including some surrounding tissue) do not alter basal levels of serum gonadotropins but do markedly attenuate the gonadotropin surge produced by progesterone (Sampson and McCann, 1979). Although such observations provide a suggestion that the OVLT may subserve functions related to sexual function, its relationship to the LHRH system in the brain and its role in sexual function are yet to be defined precisely and await more detailed analysis.

A stronger case has been developed for the OVLT as an important site housing osmoreceptors or sodium receptors. Water intake and vasopressin release occur with dehydration of the cellular fluid compartment (Gilman, 1937; Gilman and Goodman, 1937). Originally, it was proposed that osmosensitive cells located in the brain were responsible for sensing changes in osmolality (Verney, 1947; Andersson, 1953). More recently, Andersson (1971) has suggested that osmoreceptors are in fact sodium receptors. Others have concluded that both osmoreceptors and sodium receptors are likely to exist in the brain (McKinley et al., 1978, 1984). The identification of the precise location and nature of either osmoreceptors or sodium receptors has been a major issue.

In the early 1970s, the site of brain osmoreceptors for thirst was thought to be located in the basal forebrain, specifically the lateral preoptic region (Peck and Novin, 1971; Blass and Epstein, 1971). In subsequent studies, in which the osmosensitivity of the anterior hypothalamic and preoptic regions was mapped in the rat, it was noted that the focus of sensitive sites is actually more medial than the lateral preoptic region (Peck and Blass, 1975). This observation suggested that the major component of CNS osmosensitive tissue may reside close to the third ventricle. Buggy and colleagues (1979) compared the osmosensitivity of injections into the ventral third ventricle with injections into the lateral preoptic region and found the ventricular placements to be more reliable in producing drinking responses. The idea of a focus of osmosensitive elements lying within the periventricular tissue surrounding the anteroventral third ventricle (AV3V region) is supported by the fact that electrolytic lesions that destroy this region produce animals that do not respond by drinking or releasing vasopressin to cellular dehydration (Buggy and Johnson, 1977; see Johnson, 1985a, for review). Similar impairments have been reported with similar lesions in sheep

(McKinley et al., 1984). One of the periventricular structures consistently destroyed by AV3V lesions is the OVLT (see below).

The idea that "the osmoreceptor" is located in a circumventricular organ developed as a result of experiments in which various hyperosmotic solutions were infused centrally or peripherally and both sites of application gave similar responses (sheep: McKinley et al., 1978; dog: Thrasher et al., 1980). In the dog, Thrasher and Keil (1987) have studied the effects of electrolytic lesions that are essentially restricted to the OVLT on the responses to cellular dehydration produced by intravenous infusions of hypertonic saline. The absence of the OVLT markedly elevated the threshold for drinking and vasopressin to this challenge. To totally abolish responses to cellular dehydration, it is necessary to destroy periventricular tissues in addition to the OVLT (see Johnson, 1982 and McKinley et al., 1988 for reviews). Thus, it is reasonable to conclude that the OVLT is involved in osmoreception and/or sodium reception, but it is also likely that the periventricular tissues adjacent to the OVLT are either also osmosensitive or sodium sensitive or that projections from other receptor areas pass into or through this region. At the present time, it is impossible to discriminate between these two possibilities with regard to the locus of osmoreceptors and sodium receptors. However, the periventricular tissue including and adjacent to the OVLT, which has been defined as the AV3V region, does have an important role in the overall regulation of fluid balance and cardiovascular homeostasis.

Understanding the relationship between the area postrema, SFO, OVLT, and the AV3V region is important in understanding the role of the CNS in the regulation of overall body fluid balance and distribution. Such an appreciation might be considered to serve as a conceptual model of the role of the circumventricular organs in other homeostatic processes.

THE CENTRAL CONTROL OF BODY FLUID HOMEOSTASIS

Background

The water of the body resides in both the cellular and extracellular fluid compartments (i.e., plasma and extracellular space). Overall fluid balance depends on the dynamic relationship among water intake, water loss, and the distribution of water between the cellular and extracellular spaces, which is established primarily by the concentration of extracellular sodium. The central nervous system, acting through both hormonal and neural efferent pathways to the kidney, controls the loss of water and sodium from the body and, thereby, can influence the amount of total body salt and water as well as establish the relative volume of each fluid compartment. That is, renal mechanisms can facilitate loss of excess water and/or sodium and, within limits, minimize the rate of dissipation of either substance under conditions of deficit. Although the kidney can optimize available water and sodium resources, behavioral mechanisms associated with water and salt ingestion are necessary to achieve repletion once a deficit in either constituent has accrued.

Because cellular and extracellular fluids have only a loose physical coupling (i.e., through mechanisms establishing extracellular sodium concentration) to one another and because their functions are so markedly different, each compartment is endowed with a different set of receptors and afferent mechanisms for signaling the brain of its momentary status. The cellular compartment is monitored by osmoreceptors or sodium concentration receptors. Such receptors are located both systemically (Baertschi and Vallet, 1981; see review by Haberich, 1968) and centrally (see Andersson, 1971, for review). Peripheral osmoreceptors and sodium receptors are likely to be located in the mesenteric and hepatic vasculature (Baertschi and Vallet, 1981; Haberich, 1968). It is also possible that the humoral factors of osmolality or sodium concentration influence afferent input from high-pressure baroreceptors in the aortic arch and carotid sinus (Kunze and Brown, 1978) and from the kidney (Moss, 1982), as well as in peripheral locations yet to be defined. Central receptors, as previously discussed, are probably associated with one or more of the circumventricular organs and possibly with other central sites that are inside the blood–brain barrier.

Both humoral and neural afferent signals are involved in conveying information about extracellular fluid volume. Angiotensin II, the primary effector peptide of the renin–angiotensin system, conveys humoral information on fluid balance by acting on receptors in the circumventricular organs (see above). In addition, neural afferents reflecting blood volume and blood pressure are located, respectively, in the cardiopulmonary circulation and the aortic arch/carotid sinus regions. Input from pressure/volume receptors reaches the CNS by the IXth and Xth cranial nerves.

The neural inputs from systemic receptors that sense physiological concomitants reflecting the hydrational condition of the cellular and extracellular spaces initially project to the nucleus tractus solitarius (see Chapter 6). The nucleus tractus solitarius receives inputs from the majority of these visceral afferents, but some also terminate in parts of the spinal trigeminal nucleus and in the area postrema. Ascending visceral input is, in turn, relayed to the highest levels of the nervous system involved in the integrative control of fluid balance. The "ascent" from the termination of the first-order afferents to these highest levels may require only a single neuron, although multisynaptic projections via the ventrolateral medulla or parabrachial nucleus are other modes of conduit (see Chapter 6 for a description of ascending pathways).

As discussed in earlier sections, the humoral input that acts directly on the brain appears to target, primarily, the SFO in the case of angiotensin II and the OVLT in the case of osmotic- and sodium-related stimuli. In all probability, the osmotic and sodium information carried as "ascending" input from the brain stem and that derived from the "higher level" input accessing the nervous system through the SFO and OVLT converge within areas of the basal forebrain and hypothalamus. Within these regions of the neuraxis, the multiple sensory inputs arising from widespread and diverse regions of the body are integrated so that, in turn, an optimal pattern of fluid balance-related effector activation is generated. One region in the basal forebrain that is vitally involved in the maintenance of normal fluid balance is the AV3V region. The significance of this region in the global control of fluid homeostasis can best be appreciated from a description of the effects of destruction of this small periventricular area.

The Effects of AV3V Lesions on Body Fluid Balance and Distribution

The AV3V region has been defined on the basis of functional studies mainly involving the characterization of a constellation of physiological changes and deficits produced in animals when this area of the brain is destroyed or isolated from the rest of the nervous system. Although the volume of the typical AV3V lesion in the rat is small, there are several defined anatomical structures destroyed and/or encroached upon by the ablation (see Figure 14-7). An AV3V lesion that produces the changes in body fluid balance control systems described below destroys the periventricular tissue between the anterior commissure and the optic chiasm. It includes the ventral lamina terminalis-associated structures—the OVLT and the ventral portion of the median preoptic nucleus. Within the lesion site is the preoptic periventricular nuclei, which includes the anteroventral periventricular nuclei and extends into the periventricular nuclei of the anterior hypothalamus. The medial preoptic nucleus and anterior hypothalamic region receive little damage (Buggy and Johnson, 1977; Johnson and Buggy, 1978; see Johnson, 1982, 1985a, for reviews). The paraventricular hypothalamic nucleus is not destroyed by the lesion and the supraoptic nucleus is remote from the area of destruction.

The most striking event following ablation of the AV3V region is the abrupt cessation of the ingestion of water. A rat with an AV3V lesion continues to eat and groom and shows normal motor reflexes and locomotor behaviors. The impairment in fluid intake that occurs immediately after removal of the AV3V region is specific for water, for the animals avidly consume palatable liquid diets or sugar- or saccharide-containing solutions. However, water, per se, is responded to as if it were an aversive solution. Even though lesioned adipsic animals are in reality severely dehydrated, they behave toward water as if they were overhydrated.

Associated with the acute AV3V lesion-induced adipsia is a parallel impairment in the release of vasopressin. In spite of severe depletion of fluids in both the cellular and extracellular compartments, vasopressin levels fail to rise (see Johnson, 1985b, for review). Electron microscopic and immunocytochemical examination of the posterior pituitary indicates that massive amounts of vasopressin-like material or related fragments are sequestered in terminals of the posterior pituitary but are not released (see Carithers and Johnson, 1988 for review). Magnocellular neurons themselves do not show the typical morphological changes indicative of increased protein synthesis that are normally associated with dehydration; the cells that are the source of vasopressin appear to be disconnected from the afferent input that would normally promote the release of vasopressin and increase its synthesis.

In the face of adipsia and impaired antidiuretic hormone secretion, most rats with AV3V lesions will die of dehydration within 5 to 10 days postlesion unless they are "therapeutically" hydrated by the investigator. This can be done by gavage, but is most easily accomplished by merely giving the adipsic animal access to a saccharine or sucrose solution. The animal consumes the sweet solution, presumably for its palatable qualities, and adventitiously hydrates itself. Nearly all animals can be "weaned" to water by successively reducing the concentration of the sweetening agent over subsequent days. A group of experimental animals so managed through the postsurgical acute "adipsic" period will have mean daily water intakes comparable to that of a sham lesion group of animals by 10 to 14 days postlesion.

Although *ad libitum* drinking returns to the rat with AV3V lesions in the chronic state, there is still evidence of disordered body fluid regulation that can be revealed by evaluating the functional capacity of the effector systems that maintain hydromineral balance. For example, the "recovered" animals can be evaluated for their capacity to respond to drinking by experimental manipulations that either induce depletions of the fluid compartments of the body (e.g., cellular dehydration produced by systemic hypertonic saline administration or extracellular volume depletion by hemorrhage), simulate hemodynamic changes that accompany severe fluid loss (e.g., ligation of the vena cava), or mimic hormonal changes that accompany fluid depletion (e.g., angiotensin II administration). In all the tests of drinking to all fluid homeostasis-perturbing challenges, rats with chronic AV3V lesions show impaired responses (see Table 14-1). The most severely disrupted responses are those in which the humoral signals, angiotensin II or hyperosmolarity, are the sole stimulus

Table 14-1 Chronic Effects of AV3V Lesions on Experimental Thirst

Stimuli or State Producing Water Intake	Experimental Treatment (Thirst Challenge)	Drinking Response	Reference
Water deprivation (combined cellular and extracellular fluid losses)	Water withheld for 24 hours	Attenuated	Buggy and Johnson (1977)
Cellular dehydration	Systemic injection of hypertonic saline	Abolished	Buggy and Johnson (1977)
Extracellular dehydration Hormonal component	Systemic or central injection of angiotensin II	Abolished	Buggy and Johnson (1977, 1978)
Hormonal and hypotensive components β-Adrenoceptor agonist	Systemic isoproterenol injection	Attenuated	Lind and Johnson (1981)
Reduced cardiac return	Ligation of the inferior vena cava	Attenuated	Shrager and Johnson (197⁹
Hormonal and hypovolemic components without hypotension Sequestration of extracellular fluids	Systemic polyethylene glycol treatment	Attenuated	Buggy and Johnson (1977) Lind and Johnson (1983)

Reproduced from Johnson (1985).

for drinking. Under experimental challenges that involve both humoral and neural afferent input (e.g., drinking to hypovolemia induced by polyethylene glycol treatment) the drinking is significantly impaired (Lind and Johnson, 1983) but not totally abolished. This may be because ascending visceral input can compensate for the loss of sensitivity to the humoral component that mediates the response to the thirst-inducing challenge.

Under *ad libitum* conditions the functional consequence of compromised sensitivity to the humoral signals of dehydration is a degree of loss of fine regulation of fluid homeostasis. Although, as a group, rats with chronic AV3V lesions drink at least a much over a 24-hour period as control animals, any given lesioned animal shows great day-to-day variability in its total response (Lind and Johnson, 1983). In addition, the highly correlated relationship between the amount of food eaten and the volume of water drunk in association with a meal seen in normal animals is abolished in rats with chronic AV3V lesions (Bealer and Johnson, 1980). This observation suggests that the rat with AV3V lesions is not as responsive as a normal animal to internal stimuli (i.e., increased extracellular sodium and/or plasma angiotensin II levels). For example, humoral signals generated as a result of the relative dehydration induced by a dry meal in the stomach may not be detected, and the lesioned rat must rely on larger perturbations in fluid volume to activate systemic pressure or volume receptors.

Paralleling the long-term response deficits in drinking in the "recovered" AV3V lesioned animal are chronic impairments in vasopressin secretion (see Johnson, 1985a for review). As in the case for thirst, the most severe disruptions are in response to the humoral stimuli, that is, hypertonic saline and angiotensin II. Under experimental hypovolemia, which has both neural and humoral afferent signaling components, rats with chronic AV3V lesions do secrete normal amounts of vasopressin (see Johnson, 1985a, for review). Electron microscopic examination of the magnocellular neurons in the paraventricular and supraoptic nuclei of recovered rats with AV3V lesions indicates that the paraventricular hypothalamic nucleus shows evidence of greater recovery in their responsiveness to water deprivation as compared to the supraoptic nucleus. It is possible that either the paraventricular hypothalamic nucleus receives more afferent "ascending" input from pressure/volume receptors than the supraoptic nucleus or that AV3V lesions destroy less "descending" input (see below) to the paraventricular nucleus as compared to the supraoptic nucleus (see review by Carithers and Johnson, 1988, for further discussion).

In addition to impairments in responsiveness to dipsogenic stimuli and capacity to release vasopressin, rats with chronic AV3V lesions also show an in-

teresting impairment in natriuretic responses to volume expansion (Bealer et al., 1983) and water deprivation (Ball et al., 1983). Impairments in natriuretic responses have been suggested to be due to a reduction in the release of a Na^+/K^+-ATPase inhibitor (Bealer et al., 1983).

Taken together, the impairments in capacity to mobilize drinking responses, retain water, and effect an appropriate natriuresis result in an animal with global alterations in fluid balance and distribution. Rats with AV3V lesions have chronic hypernatremia. These animals have the characteristics described in patients with the syndrome of essential (sometimes called neurogenic) hypernatremia (Ross and Christie, 1969; see Table 14-2). The syndrome appears in humans with a wide variety of CNS damage as a result of tumors, stroke, hydrocephalus, or surgery. In the cases where the damage has been assessed in humans, it is described as extending into the region of the optic recess (i.e., the AV3V region). One of the remarkable aspects of some of the case reports in humans is that individuals report not experiencing the sensation of thirst. It should be noted that impairments in both vasopressin and thirst mechanisms release must be manifest for essential hypernatremia to be present. The complete integrity of one of the two systems results in the capacity to maintain normal plasma osmolality.

One of the fascinating aspects of the animal with chronic AV3V lesions is that it is "protected" against most forms of experimental and genetic hypertension (see Table 14-3). In the mid 1970s, it was hypothesized that an action of angiotensin II on the brain may serve as a trigger for the development of renal hypertension (Sweet et al., 1976). This speculation, combined with the fact that rats with AV3V lesions appeared to be "blind" to the effects of systemic angiotensin (at least as far as drinking is concerned), prompted an investigation in which the effects of AV3V lesions on the induction of renal

Table 14-2 Parallels Between Patients with the Syndrome of Essential Hypernatremia and Rats with AV3V Lesions

	Patients with Essential Hypernatremia	Animals with AV3V Lesions
Hypothalamic damage	Yes	Yes
Chronically elevated serum sodium	Yes	Yes
Reduced or absent thirst	Yes	Yes
Elevated plasma renin	Yes	Yes
Elevated aldosterone	No[a]	No
Reduced blood volume	No	No

Reproduced from Johnson (1982).
[a]One patient.

Table 14-3 Effects of AV3V Lesions on Experimental Hypertension

Model	Prevents or Attenuates	Reversed
1 kidney, 1 wrap Grollman hypertension	Yes	Yes (water restricted) No (free access conditions)
2 kidneys, 1 clip Goldblatt hypertension	Yes	Yes
Aortic ligation between the renal arteries	Yes	—
Sinoaortic denervation	Yes	—
Lesions of the nucleus of the solitary tract	Yes	—
DOC-salt hypertension	Yes	—
Conflict stress in borderline hypertensive rats (BHR)	Yes	—
Dahl strain rats	Yes	—
Spontaneously hypertensive rats	No	No
Spontaneously hypertensive, stroke-prone rats	No	—

Based on Johnson (1982).

hypertension were studied (Buggy et al., 1977). Indeed, it was discovered that rats with AV3V lesions do not develop renal hypertension. In addition, subsequent studies indicated that rats with AV3V lesions do not manifest high blood pressure associated with many forms of experimental and genetic hypertension (see Brody and Johnson, 1980, 1981, for reviews). As is apparent from Table 14-3, the hypertensions prevented or attenuated by AV3V lesions include both renin-dependent and -independent forms, as well as neurogenic hypertension, some forms of genetic hypertension, and high blood pressure induced by stress. The only form of experimental/genetic hypertension not interdicted by AV3V lesions is the genetic form present in the spontaneously hypertensive rat (SHR). It is unclear why AV3V lesions prevent hypertension. It may be that the chronic alterations in fluid balance produced by AV3V lesions may be responsible. Rats with AV3V lesions are likely to be impaired in their capacity to expand extracellular fluid volume, a condition that precedes many forms of hypertension (Guyton et al., 1974). In addition, it should be noted that the AV3V region has been demonstrated in functional studies to be involved in the modulation of sympathetic outflow (see Brody and Johnson, 1980, 1981; Brody, 1988 for reviews). At the present time the role of the AV3V region in blood pressure regulation and hypertension is under intensive study.

Neuroanatomical and Functional Relationships of the AV3V Region with Other Central Systems Involved in the Maintenance of Fluid Balance and Cardiovascular Homeostasis

Although many early functional studies clearly indicated a vital role of the AV3V region in the maintenance of body fluid homeostasis, it was quickly recognized that this region of the brain was heterogeneous both in structure and function. Considerable effort has been made recently to learn more about the basic neurobiology of the AV3V region and related functional components of the nervous system. Especially valuable insights have been gained from neuroanatomical studies of the AV3V region and related systems. In many cases it has been possible to generate converging evidence from anatomical and functional studies to give a clearer picture of the role of the AV3V.

Figure 14-8 is a schematic summary of much of what is known about the connections between the AV3V region and other areas of the brain. The demonstration by Miselis and colleagues (1979) that the AV3V region receives efferents (pathway 3) from the SFO conceptually tied together the structures along the lamina terminalis together and suggested that blood-borne information received by the SFO was likely to be passed to nuclei within the AV3V region for further processing. Severing the fibers that emerge from the ventral stalk of the SFO that are en route to the AV3V region renders animals unresponsive to systemically applied angiotensin that produces drinking in normal animals (Eng and Miselis, 1981; Lind and Johnson, 1982a).

Ascending pathways reach the AV3V region from the parabrachial nucleus (pathway 6; Saper and Loewy, 1980) and from several regions containing norepinephrine cell bodies (pathway 5; Saper et al., 1983). Parabrachial lesions produce overdrinking and enhanced vasopressin release. These responses are specific to hypotensive/hypovolemic challenges that are mediated by elevated levels of circulating angiotensin II (Ohman and Johnson, 1986, 1989; Ohman et al., 1988). In contrast, selective depletion of norepinephrine within the AV3V region produces drinking and pressor response deficits to angiotensin II (see below). Together, such observations suggest that the AV3V region may receive and integrate

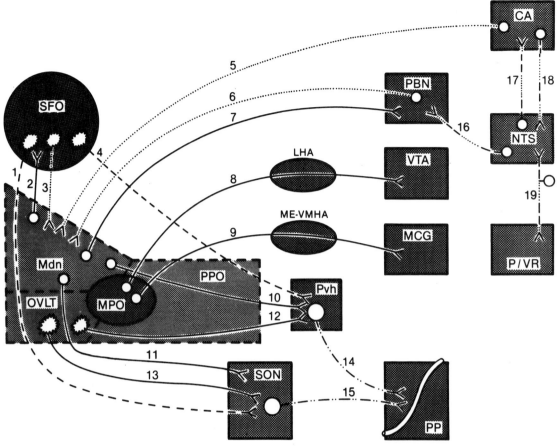

Figure 14-8 Diagram illustrating the cell groups and fiber systems associated with the AV3V region. CA, catecholamine cell groups of the brain stem; LHA, lateral hypothalamic area; MCG, midbrain central gray matter; Mdn, median preoptic nucleus; MPO, medial preoptic area; ME-VMHA, median eminence–ventromedial hypothalamic area; NTS, nucleus of the solitary tract; OVLT, organum vasculosum of the lamina terminalis; PBN, parabrachial nucleus; PP, posterior pituitary; PPO, periventricular preoptic area; Pvh, paraventricular hypothalamic nucleus; SFO, subfornical organ; SON, supraoptic nucleus.

both excitatory and inhibitory ascending inputs from the brain stem that interact to control water intake.

Several efferent pathways from the AV3V region have been found to project to areas implicated in fluid control. Of particular importance are the projections to the paraventricular (pathways 10 and 12) and supraoptic nuclei (pathways 11 and 13) (Miselis, 1981; Silverman et al., 1981; Wilkin et al., 1989), the ventral tegmental area (VTA) via the lateral hypothalamus (pathway 8; Conrad and Pfaff, 1976; Swanson et al., 1978), and the mesencephalic central gray matter via a periventricular route close to the midline (Conrad and Pfaff, 1976; Swanson et al., 1978). The projections to the magnocellular regions have obvious implications for the control of vasopressin and oxytocin release. The pathway coursing through the lateral hypothalamus to the VTA has been suggested to be involved in the control of thirst

(Mogenson and Kucharczyk, 1978; Swanson et al., 1978). The descending periventricular projection (pathway 8) is likely to be involved in conducting information that influences autonomic outflow. Electrical stimulation of the AV3V region or at points along this medial path produces hemodynamic changes that resemble the defense response (Fink et al., 1978) and lesions in the median eminence–ventromedial hypothalamic region, which would interrupt this projection and thereby prevent the development of renal hypertension (Johnson et al., 1981).

In addition to both efferents and afferents associated with the AV3V region there are clearly fibers of passage that course through the region. Some of the most notable of these are the projections from the SFO that descend through the AV3V en route to hypothalamic structures (Miselis, 1981; Lind et al., 1982). Direct projections from the SFO to magnocellular and parvocellular hypothalamic nuclei are likely to function to alter activity in the innervated regions (Ferguson et al., 1984a; Tanaka et al., 1987a,b).

Over recent years the application of modern techniques of neurobiology has been especially effective in providing some understanding of the function of the AV3V region and why AV3V lesions are so disruptive in terms of body fluid homeostasis. Examination of Figure 14-8 indicates that virtually every efferent mechanism that functions in the control of fluid balance and dynamics is impinged upon by the lesion. The emerging picture is that the AV3V contains (1) tissues sensitive to humoral changes (e.g., the OVLT), (2) fibers of passage, and (3) elements involved in the integration of information important for the control of fluid balance. An appreciation of the manner in which the AV3V may function in the latter role can be gained by discussing a current model that has been proposed to account for the role of lamina terminalis-associated structures in the control of extracellular fluid depletion-induced drinking.

A Model for the Role of the AV3V Region in the Control of Extracellular Thirst

The AV3V contains components of systems involved in nearly every aspect of the control of fluid homeostasis. By employing various neurobiological approaches it appears that it will be possible to tease out many of the different components that subserve such functions. For example, one integrative role of the AV3V is hypothesized to involve the control of drinking in response to extracellular volume depletion (i.e., so-called extracellular thirst). Results from several experimental approaches have led to the generation of a model to describe the mode of interaction between two defined neural systems associated with the AV3V region and that appear to have a role in the mediation of drinking to extracellular fluid depletion.

Figure 14-9 presents a current model to account for the role of the SFO, AV3V region, and ascending noradrenergic pathways terminating within the AV3V region in extracellular thirst. The first component of the model involves the SFO and a descending angiotensinergic projection into the AV3V (Lind and Johnson, 1982b). This aspect of the model in effect states that in cases of hypotension/hypovolemia circulating angiotensin II levels rise to act on the SFO (Simpson and Routtenberg, 1973; Simpson et al., 1978). In turn, efferent output from the SFO is carried over a descending pathway that employs angiotensin II (or a related substance) as a neurotransmitter. Components of this pathway, which terminate within the AV3V region, particularly the median preoptic nucleus, release angiotensin II when they are activated. The experimental data that support this component of the model are briefly the demonstration (1) of a major efferent bundle (Miselis et al., 1979; Miselis, 1981; Lind et al., 1984a,b 1985) containing angiotensin II-like material (Lind et al., 1985) that terminates in the median preoptic area, (2) that cutting this bundle abolishes the drinking response to blood-borne an-

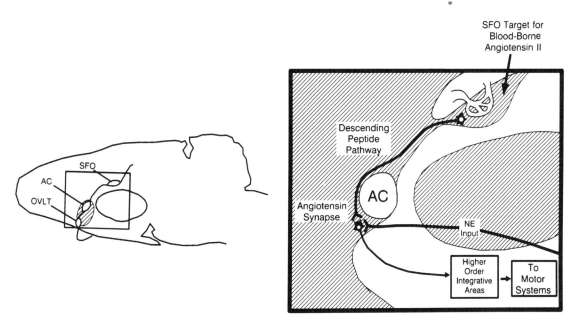

Figure 14-9 Model of the AV3V region in control of thirst.

giotensin II but not CSF-borne angiotensin II (Lind and Johnson, 1982a,b), (3) that SFO ablation abolishes the drinking reponse to blood-borne angiotensin II but not CSF-borne angiotensin II, (4) that drinking induced by blood-borne angiotensin II is blocked by the presence of a CSF-borne angiotensin II receptor antagonist (Johnson and Schwob, 1975) but that CSF-borne angiotensin II does not act on the SFO for its dipsogenic effect (Buggy et al., 1975; Buggy and Fisher, 1976), (5) that cold cream plugs placed in the AV3V region abolish drinking in response to CSF-borne angiotensin II but do not impair the drinking response to systemic angiotensin II, (6) that, in addition to the SFO, the AV3V region contains a high density of angiotensin II receptors (Mendelson et al., 1983; Plunkett et al., 1987), and (7) that the *in situ* hybridization derived signal for angiotensinogen mRNA is high throughout the AV3V (Lynch et al., 1987).

The second neurochemical aspect of this model is an ascending noradrenergic input from brain stem noradrenergic cell groups (Johnson, 1985b; Johnson and Cunningham, 1987; Johnson and Wilkin, 1987). This component is proposed to be activated by hypovolemia/hypotension. The afferent signal from the periphery is carried from arterial baroreceptors and/or cardiopulmonary receptors into the CNS and, in turn, to noradrenergic cell groups in the NTS and ventrolateral medulla, which then project to the median preoptic nucleus (Saper et al., 1983). Functional evidence that supports a role for this ascending noradrenergic input into the AV3V region in extracellular thirst includes the demonstration that (1) central 6-hydroxydopamine (6-OHDA)-induced depletions of forebrain catecholamine produces drinking deficits to angiotensin II (Gordon et al., 1979, 1985), (2) periventricular norepinephrine is a critical catecholamine for the drinking response to angiotensin II (Bellin et al., 1987a), (3) localized depletion of norepinephrine in the median preoptic nucleus/OVLT region results in specific impairments in the drinking response to systemic and centrally applied angiotensin II (Bellin et al., 1987b, 1988; Cunningham and Johnson, 1989), and (4) replacement of norepinephrine in 6-OHDA-depleted animals restores impaired drinking responses to angiotensin II (MacRae-Degeuruce et al., 1986, 1987).

Overall, the model describes the interaction between two converging inputs into the AV3V region. One of the inputs derived from circulating angiotensin II enters the CNS at a high level of the "visceral neuraxis" (Miselis et al., 1987) via the SFO and the second enters the brain stem. Synaptically released angiotensin II and norepinephrine are proposed to interact within the AV3V region to "reinforce" each other's actions. Functional evidence indicating increased turnover of norepinephrine in the median preoptic nucleus in hypovolemic animals (Wilkin et al., 1987) is consistent with this proposal.

SUMMARY

Specialized areas of the brain called *circumventricular organs* lack a blood–brain barrier and function as part of a humoral feedback system involved in a variety of functions, including cardiovascular control, food intake, and water and electrolyte homeostasis. Three of these regions [the area postrema, subfornical organ (SFO), and organum vasculosum of the lamina terminalis (OVLT)] are discussed in this chapter with particular attention to their anatomical connections and potential function(s).

Two of these structures, SFO and OVLT, have been implicated in the neural control of water and electrolyte balance, and the experimental evidence supporting this idea is discussed in detail. In addition, evidence for the presence of central osmoreceptors is reviewed. The experimental findings suggest that the OVLT or nearby periventricular region (which together have been termed the AV3V region) plays a critical role in its function. Lesions of the AV3V region produce alterations in water intake after various peripheral changes such as dehydration and hypovolemia. These changes parallel dysfunctions seen in humans with the syndrome of essential hypernatremia. Lesions of the AV3V region prevent various forms of experimental hypertension. The neural circuitry arising from the AV3V region is reviewed and a comprehensive overview is presented of how this region may regulate vasopressin release, the autonomic nervous system, and behavioral responses.

REFERENCES

Reviews

Andersson, B. (1971). Thirst and brain control of water balance. *American Scientist* 59, 408–415.

Borison, H. L. (1984). History and status of the area postrema. *Federation Proceedings* 43, 2937–2940.

Brody, M. J. (1988). Central nervous system and mechanisms of hypertension. *Clinical Physiology and Biochemistry* 6, 230–239.

Brody, M. J., and Johnson, A. K. (1980). Role of the anteroventral third ventricle region in fluid and electrolyte balance, arterial pressure regulation and hypertension. In: *Frontiers in Neuroendocrinology*, Vol. 6, L. Martini and W. F. Ganong (eds.), Raven, New York, pp. 249–292.

Brody, M. J., and Johnson, A. K. (1981). Role of forebrain structures in models of experimental hypertension. In: *Disturbances in the Neurogenic Control of the Circulation*, Clinical Physiology Series, American Physiological Society, Williams & Wilkins, Baltimore, pp. 105–117.

Carithers, J. R., and Johnson, A. K. (1988). Fine structural studies of the effects of AV3V lesions on the hypothalamo-neurohypophyseal neurosecretory system. In: *Vasopressin*, A. W. Cowley (ed.), Raven, New York, pp. 301–319.

Contreras, R. J., Kosten, T., and Bird, E. (1984). Area postrema: Part of the autonomic circuitry of caloric homeostasis. *Federation Proceedings* 43, 2966–2968.

Ferrario, C. M., Barnes, K. L., Diz, D. I., Block, C. H., and Averill, D. B. (1987). Role of area postrema pressor mechanisms in the regulation of arterial pressure. *Canadian Journal of Physiology and Pharmacology* 65, 1591–1597.

Ganten, D., Granger, P., Ganten, U., Boucher, R., and Genest, J. (1972). An intrinsic renin-angiotensin system in the brain. In: *Hypertension*, J. Genest and E. Koiw (eds.), Springer-Verlag, Heidelberg-Berlin-New York, pp. 423–432.

Gross, P. M. (1987). *Circumventricular Organs and Body Fluids*, Vols. I–III, CRC Press, Boca Raton, FL.

Haberich, F. J. (1968). Osmoreception in the portal circulation. *Federation Proceedings* 27, 1137–1141.

Johnson, A. K. (1982). Neurobiology of the periventricular tissue surrounding the anteroventral third ventricle (AV3V) and its role in behavior, fluid balance, and cardiovascular control. In: *Circulation, Neurobiology and Behavior*, O. A. Smith, R. A. Galosy, and S. M. Weiss (eds.), Elsevier, New York, pp. 277–295.

Johnson, A. K. (1985a). Role of the periventricular tissue surrounding the anteroventral third ventricle (AV3V) in the regulation of body fluid homeostasis. In: *Vasopressin*, R. W. Schrier (ed.), Raven, New York, pp. 319–331.

Johnson, A. K. (1985b). The periventricular anteroventral third ventricle (AV3V): Its relationship with the subfornical organ and neural systems involved in maintaining body fluid homeostasis. *Brain Research Bulletin*, 15, 595–601.

Johnson, A. K., and Cunningham, J. T. (1987). Brain mechanisms and drinking: The role of lamina terminalis-associated systems and extracellular thirst. *Kidney International* 32, S35–S42.

Johnson, A. K., and Wilkin, L. D. (1987). The integrative role of neural systems of the lamina terminalis in the regulation of body fluid homeostasis. In: *Circumventricular Organs and Body Fluids*, Vol. 3, P. M. Gross (ed.), CRC Press, Boca Raton, FL, pp 125–141.

Knepel, W., Nutto, D., and Meyer, D. K. (1982). Effect of transection of subfornical organ efferent projections on vasopressin release induced by angiotensin or isoprenaline in the rat. *Brain Research* 248, 180–184.

Landas, S., and Phillips, M. I. (1987). Comparative anatomy of the organum vasculosum of the lamina terminalis. In: *Circumventricular Organs and Body Fluids*, Vol. 1, P. M. Gross (ed.), CRC Press, Boca Raton, pp. 131–156.

Lind, R. W. (1987). Neural connections of the subfornical organ. In: *Circumventricular Organs and Body Fluids*, Vol. 1, P. M. Gross (ed.), CRC Press, Boca Raton, FL, pp. 27–42.

Lind, R. W., and Johnson, A. K. (1982a). Central and peripheral mechanisms mediating angiotensin-induced thirst. In: *The Renin Angiotensin System in the Brain*, D. Ganten, M. Printz, M. I. Phillips, and B. A. Scholkens

(eds.), Experimental Brain Research (Suppl. 4), pp. 353–364.

McKinley, M. J., Clever, J., Denton, D. A., Oldfield, B. J., Penschow, J., and Rundgren, M. (1987). Fine structure of the organum vasculosum of the lamina terminalis. In: *Circumventricular Organs and Body Fluids*, Vol. 1, P. M. Gross (ed.), CRC Press, Boca Raton, FL, pp. 111–130.

McKinley, M. J., Congiu, M., Miselis, R. R., Oldfield, B. J., and Pennington, G. (1988). The lamina terminalis and osmotically stimulated vasopressin secretion. In: *Recent Progress in Posterior Pituitary Hormones 1988*, S. Yoshida and L. Share (eds.), Elsevier Science Publishers B. V. (Biomedical Division), Amsterdam, pp. 117–124.

Miselis, R. R., Hyde, T. M., and Shapiro, R. E. (1984). Area postrema and adjacent solitary nucleus in water and energy balance. *Federation Proceedings* 43, 2969–2971.

Miselis, R. R., Weiss, M. L., and Shapiro, R. E. (1987). Modulation of the visceral neuraxis. In: *Circumventricular Organs and Body Fluids*, Vol. III, P. M. Gross (ed.), CRC Press, Boca Raton, FL, pp. 144–160.

Moffett, B. R., Bumpus, F. M., and Husain, A. (1987). Minireview: Cellular organization of the brain renin-angiotensin system. *Life Sciences* 41, 1867–1879.

Mogenson, G. J., and Kucharczyk, J. (1978). Central neural pathways for angiotensin-induced thirst. *Federation Proceedings* 37, 2683–2688.

Phillips, M. I., and Camacho, A. (1987). Neural connections of the organum vasculosum of the lamina terminalis. In: *Circumventricular Organs and Body Fluids*, Vol. 1, P. M. Gross (ed.), CRC Press, Boca Raton, FL, pp. 157–169.

Printz, M. P., Ganten, D., Unger, T., and Philips, M. I. (1982). Minireview: The brain angiotensin system. In: *The Brain Renin Angiotensin System*, D. Ganten, M. Printz, M. I. Phillips, and B. A. Scholken (eds.), Springer-Verlag, Heidelberg, pp. 3–52.

Renaud, L. P., Ferguson, A. V., Day, T. A., Bourque, C. W., and Sgro, S. (1985). Electrophysiology of the subfornical organ and its hypothalamic connections—an *in vivo* study in the rat. *Brain Research Bulletin* 15, 83–86.

van Houten, M., and Posner, B. I. (1984). Circumventricular organs: Receptors and mediators of direct peptide hormone action on brain. *Advances in Metabolic Diseases* 10, 269–289.

Research Papers

Adachi, A., and Kobashi, M. (1985). Chemosensitive neurons within the area postrema of the rat. *Neuroscience Letters* 55, 137–140.

Andersson, B. (1953). The effect of injections of hypertonic NaCl-solutions into different parts of the hypothalamus of goats. *Acta Physiologica Scandinavica* 28, 188–201.

Baertschi, A. J., and Vallet, P. G. (1981). Osmosensitivity of the hepatic portal vein area and vasopressin release in rats. *Journal of Physiology (London)* 314, 217–230.

Ball, N. W., Johnson, A. K., and Haywood, J. R. (1983). Factors contributing to arterial pressure and fluid and electrolyte balance during water deprivation in rats with lesions of the AV3V. *Federation Proceedings* 42, 989.

Bealer, S. L., and Johnson, A. K. (1980). Preoptic-hypothalamic periventricular lesions alter food-associated drinking and circadian rhythms. *Journal of Comparative and Physiological Psychology* 94, 547–555.

Bealer, S. L., Haywood, J. R., Gruber, K. A., Buckalew, V. M., Fink, G. D., Brody M. L., and Johnson, A. K. (1983). Preoptic-hypothalamic periventricular lesions reduce natriuresis to volume expansion. *American Journal of Physiology* 244, R51–R57.

Bellin, S. I., Bhatnagar, R. K., and Johnson, A. K. (1987a). Periventricular noradrenergic systems are critical for angiotensin-induced drinking and blood pressure responses. *Brain Reseach* 403, 105–112.

Bellin, S. I., Landas, S. K., and Johnson, A. K. (1987b). Localized injections of 6-hydroxydopamine into lamina terminalis-associated structures: Effects on experimentally-induced drinking and pressor responses. *Brain Research* 416, 75–83.

Bellin, S. I., Landas, S. K., and Johnson, A. K. (1988). Selective catecholamine depletion of structures along the ventral lamina terminalis: Effects on experimentally-induced drinking and pressor responses. *Brain Research* 456, 9–16.

Blass, E. M., and Epstein, A. N. (1971). A lateral preoptic osmosensitive zone for thirst in the rat. *Journal of Comparative and Physiological Psychology* 76, 378–394.

Borison, H. L., and Wang, S. C. (1951). Locus of the central emetic action of cardiac glycosides. *Proceedings of the Society for Experimental Biology and Medicine* 76, 335–338.

Brizzee, K. R., Ordy, J. M., and Mehler, W. R. (1980). Effect of ablation of area postrema on frequency and latency of motion sickness-induced emesis in the squirrel monkey. *Physiology and Behavior* 24, 849–853.

Buggy, J., and Fisher, A. E. (1976). Anteroventral third ventricle site of action for angiotensin induced thirst. *Pharmacology, Biochemistry, and Behavior* 4, 651–660.

Buggy, J., and Johnson, A. K. (1977). Preoptic-hypothalamic periventricular lesions: Thirst deficits and hypernatremia. *American Journal of Physiology* 233, R44–R52.

Buggy, J., and Johnson, A. K. (1978). Angiotensin-induced thirst: Effects of third ventricular obstruction and periventricular ablation. *Brain Research* 149, 117–128.

Buggy, J., Fisher, A. E., Hoffman, W., Johnson, A. K., and Phillips, M. I. (1975). Ventricular obstruction: Effect on drinking induced by intracranial injection of angiotensin. *Science* 190, 72–74.

Buggy, J., Fink, G. D., Johnson, A. K., and Brody, M. J. (1977). Prevention of the development of renal hypertension by anteroventral third ventricular tissue lesions. *Circulation Research* 40, I110–I117.

Buggy, J., Hoffman, W. E., Phillips, M. I., Fisher, A. E., and Johnson, A. K. (1979). Osmosensitivity of rat third ventricle and interactions with angiotensin. *American Journal of Physiology* 236, R75–R82.

Buranarugsa, P., and Hubbard, J. I. (1979). The neuronal organization of the rat subfornical organ *in vitro* and a test of the osmo- and morphine-receptor hypothesis. *Journal of Physiology (London)* 291, 101–116.

Buranarugsa, P., and Hubbard, J. I. (1988). Excitatory effects of atrial natriuretic peptide on rat subfornical organ neurons *in vitro*. *Brain Research Bulletin* 20, 627–631.

Carpenter, D. O., Briggs, D. B., and Strominger, N. (1983).

Responses of neurons of canine area postrema to neurotransmitters and peptides. *Cellular and Molecular Neurobiology* 3, 113–126.

Ciriello, J., Hrycyshyn, A. W., and Calaresu, F. R. (1981). Glossopharyngeal and vagal afferent projection to the brain stem of the cat: A horseradish peroxidase study. *Journal of the Autonomic Nervous System* 4, 63–79.

Conrad, L. C. A., and Pfaff, D. W. (1976). Efferents from medial basal forebrain and hypothalamus in the rat: An autoradiograhic study of the medial preoptic area. *Journal of Comparative Neurology* 169, 185–220.

Cunningham, J. T., and Johnson, A. K. (1989). Decreased norepinephrine in the ventral terminalis region is associated with angiotensin II drinking response deficits following local 6-hydroxydopamine injections. *Brain Research* 480, 65–71.

Edwards, G. L., and Ritter, R. C. (1986). Area postrema lesions: Cause of overingestion is not altered visceral nerve function. *American Journal of Physiology* 251, R575–R581.

Edwards, G. L., Ladenheim, E. E., and Ritter, R. C. (1986). Dorsomedial hindbrain participation in cholecystokinin-induced satiety. *American Journal of Physiology* 251, R971–R977.

Eng, R., and Miselis, R. R. (1981). Polydipsia and abolition of angiotensin-induced drinking after transections of subfornical organ efferent projections in the rat. *Brain Research* 225, 200–206.

Felix, D., and Akert, A. (1974). The effect of angiotensin II on neurones of the cat subfornical organ. *Brain Research* 76, 350–353.

Ferguson, A. V., and Renaud, L. P. (1984). Hypothalamic paraventricular nucleus lesions decrease pressor response to subfornical organ stimulation. *Brain Research* 305, 361–364.

Ferguson, A. V., Day, T. A., and Renaud, L. P. (1984a). Subfornical organ stimulation excites paraventricular neurons projecting to dorsal medulla. *American Journal of Physiology* 247, R1088–R1092.

Ferguson, A. V., Day, T. A., and Renaud, L. P. (1984b). Subfornical organ efferents influence the excitability of neurohypophyseal and tuberoinfundibular paraventricular nucleus neurons in the rat. *Neuroendocrinology* 39, 423–428.

Ferrario, C. M., Barnes, K. L., Szilagyi, J. E., and Brosnihan, K. B. (1979). Physiological and pharmacological characterization of the area postrema pressor pathways in the normal dog. *Hypertension* 1, 235–245.

Fink, G. D., Buggy, J., Haywood, J. R. Johnson, A. K., and Brody, M. J. (1978). Hemodynamic responses to electrical stimulation of areas of rat forebrain containing angiotensin and osmosensitive sites. *American Journal of Physiology* 235, H445–H451.

Fink, G. D., Brunner, C. A., and Mangiapane, M. L. (1987). Area postrema is critical for angiotensin-induced hypertension in rats. *Hypertension* 9, 355–361.

Gilman, A. (1937). The relation between blood osmotic pressure, fluid distribution and voluntary water intake. *American Journal of Physiology* 120, 323–328.

Gilman, A., and Goodman, L. (1937). The secretory response of the posterior pituitary to the need for water conservation. *Journal of Physiology (London)* 90, 113–124.

Gordon, F. J., Brody, M. J., Fink, G. D., Buggy, J., and Johnson, A. K. (1979). Role of central catecholamines in the control of blood pressure and drinking behavior. *Brain Research* 178, 161–173.

Gordon, F. J., Brody, M. J., and Johnson, A. K. (1985). Regional depletion of central nervous system catecholamines: Effects on blood pressure and drinking behavior. *Brain Research* 345, 285–297.

Guyton, A. C., Coleman, T. G., Cowley, A. W., Jr., Manning, R. D., Norman, R. A., Jr., and Ferguson, J. D. (1974). A systems analysis approach to understanding long-range arterial blood pressure control and hypertension. *Circulation Research* 35, 159–176.

Harding, R. K., Hugenholtz, H., Keaney, M., and Kucharczyk, J. (1985). Discrete lesions of the area postrema abolish radiation-induced emesis in the dog. *Neuroscience Letters* 53, 95–100.

Hoffman, W. E., and Phillips, M. I. (1976). Regional study of cerebral ventricle sensitive sites to angiotensin II. *Brain Research* 110, 313–330.

Hosoya, Y., and Matsushita, M. (1981). A direct projection from the hypothalamus to the area postrema in the rat, as demonstrated by the HRP and autoradiographic methods. *Brain Research* 214, 144–149.

Hosutt, J. A., Rowland, N., and Stricker, E. M. (1981). Impaired drinking responses of rats with lesions of the subfornical organ. *Journal of Comparative and Physiological Psychology* 95, 104–113.

Iovino, M., and Steardo, I. (1984). Vasopressin release to central and peripheral angiotensin II in rats with lesion of the subfornical organ. *Brain Research* 322, 365–368.

Ishibashi, S., Oomura, Y, Gueguen, B., and Nicolaidis, S. (1985). Neuronal response in subfornical organ and other regions to angiotensin II applied by various routes. *Brain Research Bulletin* 14, 307–313.

Johnson, A. K., and Buggy, J. (1978). Periventricular preoptic-hypothalamus is vital for thirst and normal water economy. *American Journal of Physiology* 234, R122–R129.

Johnson, A. K., and Schwob, J. E. (1975). Cephalic angiotensin receptors mediating drinking to systemic angiotensin II. *Pharmacology, Biochemistry and Behavior* 3, 1077–1084.

Johnson, A. K., Buggy, J., Fink, G. D., and Brody, M. J. (1981). Prevention of renal hypertension and of the central pressor effect of angiotensin by ventromedial hypothalamic ablation. *Brain Research* 205, 255–264.

Kawano, H., and Daikoku, S. (1981). Immunohistochemical demonstration of LHRH neurons and their pathways in the rat hypothalamus. *Neuroendocrinology* 32, 179–186.

Kunze, D. L., and Brown, A. M. (1978). Sodium sensitivity of baroreceptors: Reflex effects on blood pressure and fluid volume in the cat. *Circulation Research* 42, 714–720.

Leslie, R. A. (1986). Comparative aspects of the area postrema: Fine-structural considerations help to determine its function. *Cellular and Molecular Neurobiology* 6, 95–120.

Lind, R. W., and Johnson, A. K. (1981). Periventricular preoptic-hypothalamic lesions: Effects on isoproterenol induced thirst. *Pharmacology, Biochemistry and Behavior* 15, 563–565.

Lind, R. W., and Johnson, A. K. (1982b). Subfornical organ-median preoptic connections and drinking and pressor responses to angiotensin II. *Journal of Neuroscience* 2, 1043–1051.

Lind, R. W., and Johnson, A. K. (1983). A further characterization of the effects of AV3V lesions on ingestive behavior. *American Journal of Physiology* 245, R83–R90.

Lind, R. W., Van Hoesen, G. W., and Johnson, A. K. (1982). An HRP study of the connections of the subfornical organ of the rat. *Journal of Comparative Neurology* 210, 265–277.

Lind, R. W., Swanson, L. W., and Ganten, D. (1984a). Angiotensin II immunoreactivity in the neural afferents and efferents of the subfornical organ of the rat. *Brain Research* 321, 209–215.

Lind, R. W., Thunhorst, R. L., and Johnson, A. K. (1984b). The subfornical organ and the integration of multiple factors in thirst. *Physiology and Behavior* 32, 69–74.

Lind, R. W., Swanson, L. W., and Ganten, D. (1985). Organization of angiotensin II immunoreactive cells and fibers in the rat central nervous system. *Neuroendocrinology* 40, 2–24.

Lynch, K. R., Hawelu-Johnson, C. L., and Guyenet, P. G. (1987). Localization of brain angiotensinogen mRNA by hybridization histochemistry. *Molecular Brain Research* 2, 149–158.

Lindstrom, P. A., and Brizzee, K. R. (1962). Relief of intractable vomiting from surgical lesions in the area postrema. *Journal of Neurosurgery* 19, 228–236.

Luiten, P. G. M., ter Horst, G. J., Karst, H., and Steffens, A. B. (1985). The course of paraventricular hypothalamic efferents to autonomic structures in medulla and spinal cord. *Brain Research* 329, 374–378.

Mangiapane, M. L., and Simpson, J. B. (1980a). Subfornical organ: Forebrain site of pressor and dipsogenic action of angiotensin II. *American Journal of Physiology* 239, R382–R389.

Mangiapane, M. L., and Simpson, J. B. (1980b). Subfornical organ lesions reduce the pressor effect of systemic angiotensin II. *Neuroendocrinology* 31, 380–384.

Mangiapane, M. L., Thrasher, T. N., Keil, L. C., Simpson, J. B., and Ganong, W. F. (1984). Role of the subfornical organ in vasopressin release. *Brain Research Bulletin* 13, 43–47.

McKinley, M. J., Denton, D. A., and Weisinger, R. S. (1978). Sensors for antidiuresis and thirst—osmoreceptors or CSF sodium detectors? *Brain Research* 141, 89–103.

McKinley, M. J., Congiu, M., Denton, D. A., Park, R. G., Penschow, J., Simpson, J. B., Tarjan, E., Weisinger, R. S., and Wright, R. D. (1984). The anterior wall of the third cerebral ventricle and homeostatic responses to dehydration. *Journal of Physiology (Paris)* 79, 421–427.

McRae-Degueurce, A., Bellin, S. I., Landas, S. K., and Johnson, A. K. (1986). Fetal noradrenergic transplants into amine-depleted basal forebrain nuclei restore drinking to angiotensin. *Brain Research* 374, 162–166.

McRae-Degueurce, A., Cunningham, J. T., Bellin, S., Landas, S., Wilkin, L., and Johnson, A. K. (1987). Fetal noradrenergic cell suspensions transplanted into amine-depleted nuclei of adult rats. *Annals of the New York Academy of Sciences* 495, 757–759.

Mendelsohn, F. A. O., Quirion, R., Saavedra, J. M., Aguilera, G., and Catt, K. J. (1984). Autoradiographic localization of angiotensin II receptors in rat brain. *Proceedings of the National Academy of Sciences USA* 81, 1575–1579.

Miselis, R. R. (1981). The efferent projections of the subfornical organ of the rat: A circumventricular organ within a neural network subserving water balance. *Brain Research* 230, 1–23.

Miselis, R. R., Shapiro, R. E., and Hand, P. J. (1979). Subfornical organ efferents to neural systems for control of body water. *Science* 205, 1022–1025.

Moran, T. H., Robinson, P. H., Goldrich, M. S., and McHugh, P. R. (1986). Two brain cholecystokinin receptors: Implications for behavioral actions. *Brain Research* 362:175–179.

Moss, N. G. (1982). Renal function and renal afferent and efferent nerve activity. *American Journal of Physiology* 243, F425–F433.

Nicolaidis, S., Ishibashi, S., Gueguen, B., Thornton, S. W., and Beaurepaire, R. (1983). Iontophoretic investigation of identified SFO angiotensin and responsive neurons firing in relation to blood pressure changes. *Brain Research Bulletin* 10, 357–363.

Ohman, L. E., and Johnson, A. K. (1986). Lesions in lateral parabrachial nucleus enhance drinking to angiotensin II and isoproterenol. *American Journal of Physiology* 251, R504–R509.

Ohman, L. E., and Johnson, A. K. (1989). Brain stem mechanisms and the inhibition of angiotensin-induced drinking. *American Journal of Physiology* 256, R264–R269.

Ohman, L. E., Shade, R. E., and Haywood, J. R. (1988). Parabrachial nucleus involvement in hypotension-induced vasopressin release. *The FASEB Journal* 2, p. A 1482).

Okuya, S., Inenaga, K., Kaneko, T., and Yamashita, H. (1987). Angiotensin II sensitive neurons in the supraoptic nucleus, subfornical organ and anteroventral third ventricle of rats *in vitro*. *Brain Research* 402, 58–67.

Otsuka, A., Barnes, K. L., and Ferrario, C. M. (1986). Contribution of area postrema to pressor actions of angiotensin II in dog. *American Journal of Physiology* 251, H538–H546.

Panneton, W. M., and Loewy, A. D. (1980). Projections of the carotid sinus nerve to the nucleus of the solitary tract in the cat. *Brain Research* 191, 239–244.

Peck, J. W., and Blass, E. M. (1975). Localization of thirst and antidiuretic osmoreceptors by intracranial injections in rats. *American Journal of Physiology* 228, 1501–1509.

Peck, J. W., and Novin, D. (1971). Evidence that osmoreceptors mediating drinking in rabbits are in the lateral preoptic area. *Journal of Comparative and Physiological Psychology* 74, 134–147.

Plunkett, L. M., Shigematsu, K., Kurihara, M., and Saavedra, J. M. (1987). Localization of angiotensin II receptors along the anteroventral third ventricle area of the rat brain. *Brain Research* 405, 205–212.

Ross, E. J., and Christie, S. B. M. (1969). Hypernatremia. *Medicine* 48, 441–473.

Roth, G. I., and Yamamoto, W. S. (1968). The microcirculation of the area postrema in the rat. *Journal of Comparative Neurology* 133, 329–340.

Saavedra, J. M. (1987). Regulation of atrial natriuretic peptide receptors in the rat brain. *Cellular and Molecular Neurology* 7, 151–173.

Samson, W. K., and McCann, S. M. (1979). Effects of lesions in the organum vasculosum lamina terminalis on the hypothalamic distribution of luteinizing hormone-releasing hormone and gonadotropin secretion in the ovariectomized rat. *Endocrinology* 105, 939–946.

Sanders, B. J., Knardahl, S., and Johnson, A. K. (1989). The effects of lesions of the anteroventral third ventricle (AV3V) on the development of stress-induced hypertension in the borderline hypertensive rat (BHR). *Hypertension* 13, 817–821.

Saper, C. B., and Loewy, A. D. (1980). Efferent connections of the parabrachial nucleus in the rat. *Brain Research* 197, 291–317.

Saper, C. B., Reis, D. J., and Joh, T. (1983). Medullary catecholamine inputs to the anteroventral third ventricular cardiovascular regulatory region in the rat. *Neuroscience Letters* 42, 285–291.

Shapiro, R. E., and Miselis, R. R. (1985). The central neural connections of the area postrema of the rat. *Journal of Comparative Neurology* 234, 344–364.

Shrager, E., and Johnson, A. K. (1979). Drinking to caval ligation following ablation of periventricular tissue surrounding the anteroventral third ventricle (AV3V) is specifically correlated with the postlesion response to angiotensin II. *Society for Neuroscience Abstracts* 5, 224.

Sibbald, J. R. Hubbard, J. H., and Sirett, N. E. (1988). Responses from osmosensitive neurons of the rat subfornical organ *in vitro*. *Brain Research* 461, 205–214.

Silverman, A. J., Hoffman, D. L., and Zimmerman, E. A. (1981). The descending afferent connections of the paraventricular nucleus of the hypothalamus (PVN). *Brain Research Bulletin* 6, 47–61.

Simpson, J. B., and Routtenberg, A. (1972). The subfornical organ and carbachol-induced drinking. *Brain Research* 45, 135–152.

Simpson, J. B., and Routtenberg, A. (1973). Subfornical organ: Site of drinking elicited by angiotensin II. *Science* 181, 1172–1175.

Simpson, J. B., Epstein, A. N., and Camardo, J. S., Jr. (1978). Localization of receptors for the dipsogenic action of angiotensin II in the subfornical organ of rat. *Journal of Comparative and Physiological Psychology* 92, 581–608.

Skoog, K. M., and Mangiapane, M. L. (1988). Area postrema and cardiovascular regulation in rats. *American Journal of Physiology* 254, H963–H969.

Swanson, L. W., Kucharczyk, J., and Mogenson, G. J. (1978). Autoradiographic evidence for pathways from the medial preoptic area to the midbrain involved in the drinking response to angiotensin II. *Journal of Comparative Neurology* 178, 645–660.

Sweet, C. S., Columbo, J. M., and Gaul, S. L. (1976). Central antihypertensive effects of inhibitors of the renin-angiotensin system in rats. *American Journal of Physiology* 231, 1794–1799.

Tanaka, J., Kaba, H., Saito, H., and Seto, K. (1985). Electrophysiological evidence that circulating angiotensin II sensitive neurons in the subfornical organ alter the activity of hypothalamic paraventricular neurohypophyseal neurons in the rat. *Brain Research* 342, 361–365.

Tanaka, J. Saito, H., and Kaba, H. (1987a). Subfornical organ and hypothalamic paraventricular nucleus connections with median preoptic nucleus neurons: An electrophysiological study in the rat. *Experimental Brain Research* 68, 579–585.

Tanaka, J., Saito, H., Kaba, H., and Seto, K. (1987b). Subfornical organ neurons act to enhance the activity of paraventricular vasopressin neurons in response to intravenous angiotensin II. *Neuroscience Research* 4, 424–427.

Thornborough, J. R. (1973). Receptors in cerebral circulation affecting sodium excretion in the cat. *American Journal of Physiology* 225, 138–141.

Thrasher, T. N., and Keil, L. C. (1987). Regulation of drinking and vasopressin secretion: Role of organum vasculosum laminae terminalis. *American Journal of Physiology* 253, R108–R120.

Thrasher, T. N., Brown, C. J., Keil, L. C., and Ramsay, D. J. (1980). Thirst and vasopressin release in the dog: An osmoreceptor or sodium receptor mechanism? *American Journal of Physiology* 238, R333–R339.

Tribollet, E., Barberris, C., Jard, S., Dubois-Dauphin, M., and Dreifuss, J. J. (1988). Localization and pharmacological characterization of high affinity binding sites for vasopressin and oxytocin in the rat brain by light microscopic autoradiography. *Brain Research* 442, 105–118.

Undesser, K. P., Hasser, E. M., Haywood, J. R., Johnson, A. K., and Bishop, V. S. (1985). Interactions of vasopressin with the area postrema in arterial baroreflex function in conscious rabbits. *Circulation Research* 56, 410–417.

van Houton, M., Posner, B. I., Kopriwa, B. M., and Brawer, J. R. (1979). Insulin-binding sites in the rat brain: *In vivo* localization to the circumventricular organs by quantitative radioautography. *Endocrinology* 105, 666–673.

van Houton, M., Schiffrin, E. L., Mann, J. F. E., Posner, B. I., and Boucher, R. (1980). Radioautographic localization of specific binding sites for blood borne angiotensin II in rat brain. *Brain Research* 186, 480–485.

Verney, E. B. (1947). The antidiuretic hormone and the factors which determine its release. *Proceedings of the Royal Society of London, Series B* 135, 25–106.

Wang, S. C., and Chinn, H. I. (1954). Experimental motion sickness in dogs: Functional importance of chemoreceptive emetic trigger zone. *American Journal of Physiology* 178, 111–116.

Wilkin, L. D., Mitchell, L. D., Ganten, D., and Johnson, A. K. (1989). The supraoptic nucleus: Afferents from areas involved in control of body fluid homeostasis. *Neuroscience* 28, 573–584.

Wislocki, G. B., and Leduc, E. H. (1952). Vital staining of the hematoencephalic barrier by silver nitrate and trypan blue, and cytological comparisons of the neurohypophysis, pineal body, area postrema, intercolumnar tubercle, and supraoptic crest. *Journal of Comparative Neurology* 96, 371–413.

Zarbin, M. A., Innis, R. B., Wamsley, J. K., Snyder, S. H., and Kuhar, M. J. (1983). Autoradiographic localization of cholecystokinin receptors in rodent brain. *Journal of Neuroscience* 3, 877–906.

15

Autonomic Control of the Eye

A. D. LOEWY

For the eye to function normally, a variety of functions that are under control of the autonomic nervous system need to be maintained. These functions include autonomic adjustments of smooth muscles controlling the iris and the lens so that a focused image is projected onto the fovea, as well as sympathetic regulation of the uveal blood vessels to provide nutrients to the ocular tissues. This chapter reviews the neural pathways involved in (1) the pupillary light reflex, (2) the accommodation response, (3) the regulation of blood flow to the eye, and (4) the control of intraocular pressure.

PUPILLARY LIGHT REFLEX

The pupillary light reflex serves as an image quality optimizer. As light intensity increases under normal conditions, the pupil constricts, regulating the amount of light reaching the retina. By changing the light aperture, just as in a camera, the pupil serves to improve the visual image reaching the retina. The neural pathways involved in this reflex are summarized in this section. This pathway appears to involve a six neuron arc. After activation of retinal photoreceptors (rods) and a sequential relay through the bipolar cells, the third-order neurons, the retinal ganglion cells, project to the pretectum. The pretectum projects to the Edinger–Westphal nucleus (or its nonprimate mammalian homologue in the ventral tegmental area), which gives rise to the preganglionic parasympathetic fibers. These exit the midbrain in the oculomotor nerve and synapse in the ciliary ganglion. From there, the postganglionic fibers innervate the sphincter muscle of the iris.

The pupillary light reflex is used as an important clinical test to assess the neurological status of patients. Under normal conditions, when a bright light is shined into the patient's eye, the pupils of both eyes constrict. The reaction in the ipsilateral eye is termed the direct light reflex and the response in the contralateral eye is referred to as the indirect or consensual light reflex. The lesions that potentially affect these responses have been reviewed by Patten (1977), Miller (1985), and Thompson (1987) and will not be described here. This section deals with the neural circuitry involved in this reflex.

Innervation of the Iris

The iris is composed of two smooth muscles: the sphincter and the dilator. These muscles change the diameter of the pupil in response to the amount of light entering the eye (pupillary light reflex), in response to a change in gaze from far to near vision (near response), or after other stimuli, including pain or vestibular changes. Each muscle is innervated by a different component of the autonomic nervous system.

The dilator muscle is under sympathetic control. Preganglionic cholinergic sympathetic fibers originate mainly from the neurons in T1 and T2 spinal segments of the intermediolateral cell column. The axons leave the spinal cord in the ventral roots and project to the superior cervical ganglion (Figure 15-1). From here, postganglionic noradrenergic sympathetic fibers travel along with the internal carotid artery and then form a plexus of fibers that travels through the cavernous sinus by joining the ophthalmic branch of the trigeminal nerve to enter the orbit through the superior orbital fissure. Some of the nerve fibers in the plexus form the long ciliary nerves that innervate the blood vessels of the anterior aspect of the eye, and others enter the eye as the short ciliary nerves on their way to the dilator muscle and the choroidal blood vessels.

The dilator muscle is traditionally considered to receive only a noradrenergic innervation from the superior cervical ganglion. Studies by Ehinger (1967) in the cat, however, indicate that this muscle also receives input from acetylcholinesterase-containing fibers that degenerate after removal of the ciliary gan-

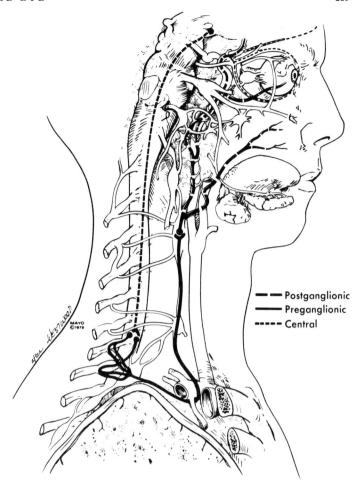

Figure 15-1 Diagram illustrating the sympathetic pathways involved in pupillary dilation in the human. A descending central pathway that originates in the brain at an undetermined site provides an excitatory input to the sympathetic preganglionic neurons that lie within the intermediolateral cell column at the T1 and T2 spinal levels. Preganglionic fibers leave the spinal cord in the ventral roots, form the white rami, and ascend to the superior cervical ganglion. These axons synapse in this ganglion. Postganglionic sympathetic fibers originating from the superior cervical ganglion travel with the internal carotid and its branches to the eye. These fibers innervate the dilator muscle of the iris. [Reprinted from Maloney et al. (1980). *American Journal of Ophthalmology* 90, 394–402, with permission of the authors and publisher. Copyright by the Ophthalmic Publishing Company, Chicago.]

- - Postganglionic
—— Preganglionic
----- Central

glion. The function of this dual innervation is unknown, but it may explain how pupillodilation can occur by stimulating the oculomotor nerve in sympathectomized animals (Paulson and Kapp, 1967).

The sphincter muscle is innervated by acetylcholine-containing postganglionic parasympathetic fibers that originate from the ciliary ganglion. These enter the posterior aspect of the eye as the short ciliary nerves and then course in the superficial aspect of the choroid to innervate the ciliary muscle and the sphincter muscle. The acetylcholine-containing preganglionic fibers that innervate the ciliary ganglion have been assumed to originate from neurons localized in the Edinger–Westphal nucleus in the midbrain. These parasympathetic fibers join the exiting oculomotor nerve and leave the brain from the interpeduncular fossa on the ventral surface of the midbrain. The nerve enters the superior part of the lateral wall of the cavernous sinus and travels rostrally to enter the orbit through the superior orbital fissure. The preganglionic parasympathetic fibers join the inferior branch of the oculomotor nerve, which gives off a branch to the ciliary ganglion.

The iris receives sensory innervation from cell bodies in the trigeminal ganglion. Calcitonin gene-related peptide and substance P trigeminal fibers distribute to both the dilator and constrictor muscles (Terenghi et al., 1985). These two neuropeptides have a parallel distribution in the anterior uvea and coexist in some of the same trigeminal primary sensory neurons. The function of this innervation is unknown.

The site of origin of the oculomotor parasympathetic preganglionic neurons has been studied in a variety of mammals with the retrograde neuronal tracing technique. In the monkey, injections of horseradish peroxidase into the ciliary ganglion result in retrograde cell labeling in the Edinger–Westphal nucleus, the anteromedian nucleus, and the nucleus of Perlia (Burde and Loewy, 1980; see Figure 15-2). In contrast, studies in the cat (Figure 15-3), rat, and rabbit indicate that the major source of the oculomotor parasympathetic preganglionic neurons

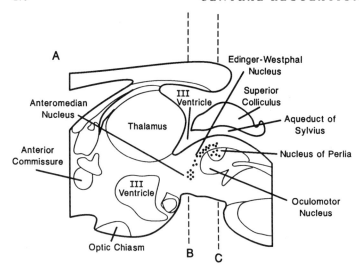

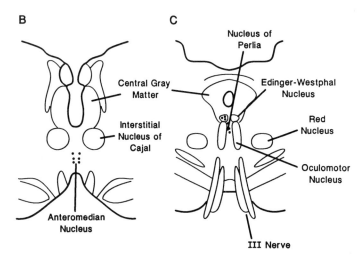

Figure 15-2 (A) Parasagittal section through the mesencephalon of a monkey showing the distribution of retrogradely labeled neurons after a horseradish peroxidase injection into the ciliary ganglion. Three areas contain labeled cells: anteromedian nucleus, Edinger–Westphal nucleus, and the nucleus of Perlia. (B and C) Frontal sections through the mesencephalon of a monkey showing the distribution of retrogradely labeled neurons after a horseradish peroxidase injection into the ciliary ganglion. Three areas contain labeled cells: antermedian nucleus, Edinger–Westphal nucleus, and nucleus of Perlia lying between the oculomotor nuclei. [Adapted and modified from Burde and Loewy (1980). *Brain Research* 198, 434–439, with permission of the authors and publisher.]

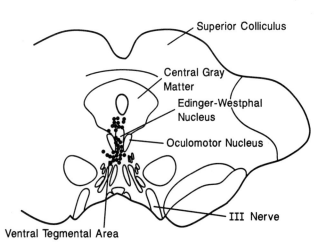

Figure 15-3 Transverse section through the mesencephalon of a cat after a horseradish peroxidase injection into the ciliary ganglion. Retrogradely labeled cells are concentrated in the areas ventral and dorsal to the oculomotor nucleus. In contrast to monkeys (Figure 15-2), very few cells are found in the Edinger–Westphal nucleus. [Modified from Loewy et al. (1978). *Brain Research* 141, 153–159, with permission of the authors and publisher.]

comes from the area immediately ventral to the oc-ulomotor nucleus in the ventral tegmental area. La-beled cells were also found in the central gray mat-ter; only a few were found in the Edinger–Westphal nucleus (cat: Loewy et al., 1978; rat: Martin and Do-livo, 1983; rabbit: Johnson and Purves, 1981). Sim-ilarly, the largest pupilloconstrictor responses elic-ited from electrical stimulation of the midbrain of the cat are from the area ventral to the Edinger–Westphal nucleus, rather than from the nucleus it-self (Sillito and Zbrozyna, 1970). Stimulation of the Edinger–Westphal nucleus or the anteromedian nu-cleus produced only weak pupilloconstrictor responses.

The Edinger–Westphal nucleus provides the main input to the ciliary ganglion in the pigeon. This nu-cleus has been shown to be organized into three regions, each with a distinct function. The medial subnucleus is involved in pupilloconstrictor func-tion, the middle subdivision controls accommoda-tion, and the lateral region regulates choroidal blood flow (see Reiner et al., 1983 for review). The neurons of the medial and middle regions of the Edinger–Westphal nucleus provide distinctive cap-like end-ings that synapse on the large-sized ciliary ganglion cells. The neurons of the lateral subdivision project to a class of small-sized ciliary ganglion cells called the choroidal cells, which are the postganglionic parasympathetic neurons innervating the choroidal blood vessels. These form boutonal endings.

Acetylcholine is thought to be the main transmit-ter of the parasympathetic preganglionic neurons. However, 50% of the synaptic endings of the oculo-motor parasympathetic preganglionic axon termi-nals in the pigeon also contain substance P-like and enkephalin-like immunoreactivity (Reiner et al., 1983). Whether these peptides coexist within acetyl-choline preganglionic fibers has not yet been estab-lished and is an important issue. The demonstration of multiple transmitter-like substances in a single axon terminal in other sites in the nervous system has changed our thinking about neurotransmission. Evidence has been obtained that the parasympa-thetic postganglionic neurons that innervate the sal-ivary glands probably transmit frequency-dependent chemically coded signals (see Lundberg and Hokfelt, 1986 for review). Whether a similar process occurs in the central nervous system is not known. How-ever, on the basis of other studies in the central ner-vous system, substance P has been shown to cause excitatory postsynaptic effects while enkephalin has inhibitory postsynaptic effects. Using this informa-tion, Reiner and co-workers (1983), in their review, hypothesized that acetylcholine may be the primary excitatory transmitter of the preganglionic endings and that neuropeptides modulate this excitation. This model suggests that substance P would increase

on-going excitability induced by acetylcholine, and enkephalin would decrease it.

Although neither enkephalin nor substance P has yet been localized in the oculomotor preganglionic neurons, Katayama and Nishi (1984) have studied the effects of enkephalin on cat parasympathetic cil-iary ganglion cells. Both met- and leu-enkephalin caused hyperpolarization of ciliary ganglion cells. The amplitude of excitatory postsynaptic potentials elicited by preganglionic nerve stimulation in these neurons was reduced by applying enkephalin to these cells and the effect was antagonized by nalox-one. Furthermore, enkephalin had no effect on the depolarization elicited by iontophoresis of acetyl-choline onto the ciliary ganglion cells. This suggests that enkephalin inhibits the postganglionic neuron by reducing the amount of acetylcholine released from the preganglionic fibers.

Somatostatin may also function as a neuromod-ulator in the cat ciliary ganglion (Kondo et al., 1982). When applied to ciliary ganglion neurons, this peptide causes hyperpolarization. The somato-statin input originates from either the trigeminal ganglion or the oculomotor preganglionic neurons, although definitive proof of either projection is lack-ing. Histochemical maps of immunoreactive so-matostatin cell bodies indicate their presence in the ventral tegmental area (Finley et al., 1981)—a po-tential site of origin for the cell bodies that give rise to oculomotor preganglionic neurons.

Neural Pathways Subserving the Pupillary Light Reflex

The pathway subserving the light reflex is generally thought to involve the following central neural com-ponents: (1) a three-neuron relay occurs in the retina [photoreceptors (rods) → bipolar cells → ganglion cells] and then the retinal ganglion cells relay lumi-nance or brightness information via optic tract fibers to the pretectum; (2) neurons from the pretectum project to the pupilloconstrictor neurons of the Edinger–Westphal nucleus; (3) the preganglionic parasympathetic neurons send their axons via the oculomotor nerve to synapse in the ciliary ganglion; and (4) the ciliary ganglion neurons give rise to post-ganglionic parasympathetic axons that travel in the short ciliary nerves to innervate the sphincter muscle of the iris (Figure 15-4).

Retinal Ganglion Cells

The retina has several specialized functions that in-clude detection and central transmission of contrast, pattern, movement, color, and luminance informa-tion. The retina contains three specific classes of ganglion cells that encode this information and pro-ject to distinct central sites (Fukuda and Stone,

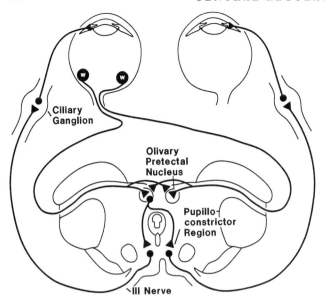

Figure 15-4 Diagram illustrating the neural pathways involved in the pupillary light reflex in the cat. Luminance information is conveyed by W-type retinal ganglion cells to the olivary pretectal nucleus. This projection is bilateral. Second-order neurons originating from the olivary pretectal nucleus project bilaterally to the region of the preganglionic parasympathetic pupilloconstrictor neurons. In monkeys, the preganglionic neurons lie in the Edinger–Westphal nucleus, whereas in the cat these cells lie in the area ventral to the oculomotor nucleus (see Figures 15-2 and 15-3). The preganglionic fibers leave the brain in the oculomotor (III) nerve and synapse in the ciliary ganglion. Postganglionic neurons arising from the ciliary ganglion innervate the sphincter muscle of the iris.

1974; see Stone, 1983 for review). These have been classified as W, X, and Y ganglion cells. Each type has its own distinct receptive field properties, conduction velocities, and specific sites of termination in the brain. The W cells are the smallest type of ganglion cell. Their axons have the slowest conduction velocities and lowest rate of discharge. They project to the pretectum, superior colliculus, pulvinar, ventral lateral geniculate nucleus, and also to lower layers of the dorsal lateral geniculate nucleus. The X cells are medium in size and convey information regarding detail, form, and color mainly to the parvocellular layers of the dorsal lateral geniculate nucleus. Most of these ganglion cells are found in the region of the fovea and they subserve high-resolution vision. The Y cells are the largest ganglion cells and they project to both the superior colliculus and the magnocellular layers of the dorsal lateral geniculate nucleus. The Y cells are concerned primarily with movement, visual attention, and gross features of the visual stimulus.

A subset of retinal W ganglion cells relays luminance information to the pretectum. Barlow and Levick (1969) noted a subclass of retinal ganglion cells whose ongoing firing rate was directly related to luminance levels; they called these cells "luminance detectors." Their firing rate was unaffected by any pattern stimulus. These cells fire tonically and have on-center receptive fields (Fukuda and Stone, 1974). The receptive field centers of these cells are relatively small, varying from 0.5° to 2.0° in diameter. Thus, each of these cells appears to monitor only a small part of the visual field in the cat.

Pretectum

Magoun and Ranson (1935) demonstrated that lesions of the pretectum in the cat impaired the light reflex. Large bilateral lesions eliminated the response, whereas unilateral pretectal lesions severely impaired the light reactions in the contralateral eye. Hare et al. (1935) showed that pupillary constriction in the cat could be elicited by electrical stimulation of the pretectum several weeks after transection of both optic nerves. This work drew attention to the fact that the pretectum contained one of the nuclei involved in the pupillary light reflex and that the response was not due to electrical stimulation of retinal afferent fibers of passage.

Subsequent neuroanatomical studies established that retinal afferents terminate in the pretectum, mainly in the nucleus of the optic tract and the olivary pretectal nucleus (rat: Scalia, 1972; cat: Berman, 1977; monkey: Hutchins and Weber, 1985; see Figure 15-5) and, to a lesser extent, in the posterior and medial pretectal nuclei. These projections are bilateral, with the contralateral side receiving a greater number of afferent fibers.

Electrophysiological studies have established that there are two types of neurons in the pretectum of the rat that are sensitive to changes in light intensity: luminance-sensitive and darkness-sensitive cells (Clarke and Ikeda, 1981, 1985). Luminance-sensitive cells show a graded increased in neuronal firing with increases in brightness (Figure 15-6). Darkness-sensitive cells show a graded increase in firing following decreases in light intensity (Figure 15-7). These

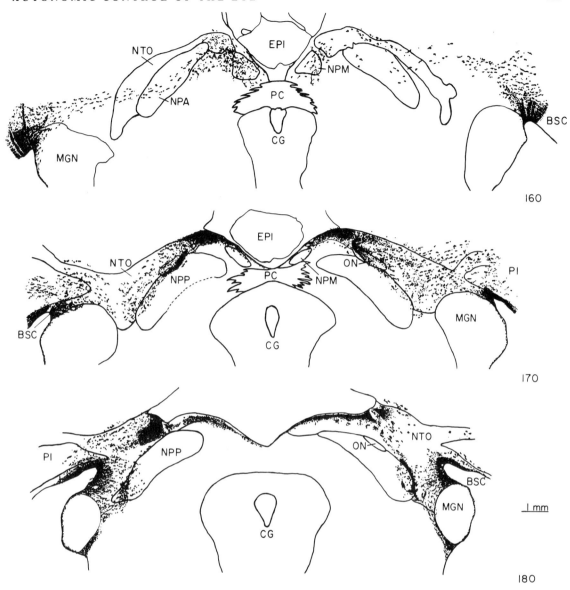

Figure 15-5 Drawings of an autoradiographic preparation through the pretectum of a squirrel monkey after an intraocular injection of [³H]proline in the left eye (on reader's left side). Note the dense concentration of labeling in olivary pretectal nucleus (ON) and nucleus of the optic tract (NTO). The posterior pretectal nucleus (NPP) and the medial pretectal nucleus (NPM) also receive retinal inputs. BSC, brachium of the superior colliculus; CG, central gray matter; EPI, epithalamus; MGN, medial geniculate nucleus; NPA, anterior pretectal nucleus; PC, posterior commissure; PI, inferior pulvinar nucleus. [Reproduced from Hutchins and Weber (1985). *Journal of Comparative Neurology* 232, 425–442, with permission of the authors and publisher. Copyright 1985, Alan R. Liss, Inc., New York.]

two classes of cells are anatomically segregated in separate subnuclei of the pretectum. The luminance detector neurons are found only in the olivary pretectal nucleus, and the darkness detector neurons are clustered in the posterior pretectal nucleus. Clarke and Ikeda (1985) suggested that the olivary pretectal nucleus is involved in control of pupilloconstriction while the posterior pretectal nucleus may be respon-

sible for the oculomotor-controlled pupillary dilatation that can occur during darkness.

Further evidence for the role of the olivary pretectal nucleus in control of pupilloconstriction comes from experiments performed by Trejo and Cicerone (1984); they found that electrical stimulation of the olivary pretectal nucleus in the rat caused pupilloconstriction. This response could be elicited only

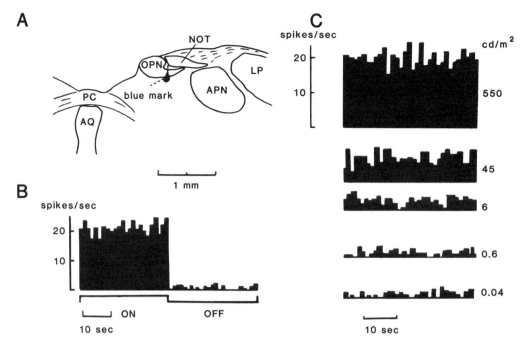

Figure 15-6 (A) Transverse section through the pretectum of a rat illustrating the recording site labeled blue mark where a luminance-sensitive cell was localized. This recording site lies in the ventral portion of the olivary pretectal nucleus (OPN). AQ, aqueduct of Sylvius; APN, anterior pretectal nucleus; LP, lateral posterior thalamic nucleus; NOT, nucleus of the optic tract. PC; PC, posterior commissure. (B) A poststimulus histogram obtained from the cell marked in A. (C) A series of poststimulus histograms of an on-sustained luminance-sensitive neuron in the olivary pretectal nucleus at different levels of brightness. [Reproduced from Clarke and Ikeda (1981). *Documenta Ophthalmologia,* The Hague, Series 30, 53–61, with permission of the authors and publisher. Copyright 1981, W. Junk Publishers, The Netherlands.]

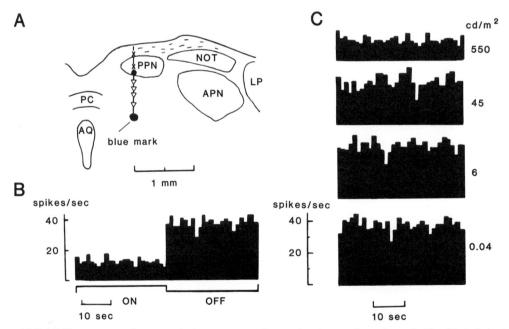

Figure 15-7 (A) Transverse section through the pretectum of a rat showing an electrode track. The filled circle that lies within the posterior pretectal nucleus (PPN) indicates the site where a darkness detector neuron was found. Abbreviations are same as in Figure 15-6. (B) Poststimulus histogram obtained from the darkness detector neuron illustrated in A. (C) Series of poststimulus histograms of an off-sustained darkness detector neuron in the posterior pretectal nucleus to different levels of luminance. Each histogram is a pen-recorder trace of 40-second periods, sampling the rate of firing every 1.25 second. [Reproduced from Clarke and Ikeda (1981). *Documenta Ophthalmologia,* The Hague, Series 30, 53–61, with permission of the authors and publisher. Copyright 1981, W. Junk Publishers, The Netherlands.]

from the region containing the luminance-sensitive cells. Thus, the olivary pretectal nucleus appears to function as the main pretectal nucleus involved in the light reflex, and this reflex, at least in the rat, is almost totally dependent on the oculomotor parasympathetic outflow because superior cervical sympathectomy causes only a minor change in the characteristics of this reflex (Clarke and Ikeda, 1981, 1985). This suggests that during the pupillary light reflex, the parasympathetic system dominates the control of the pupil, although it has been demonstrated that the sympathetic pupillodilator system is inhibited during light reflex (Passatore and Pettorossi, 1976).

There have been several controversies regarding the role of other pretectal nuclei in the pupillary light reflex. First, earlier electrophysiological studies in the cat suggested that the nucleus of the optic tract was involved in pupillomotor control (see Clarke and Ikeda, 1985 for discussion). Subsequent studies have failed to confirm this. The nucleus of the optic tract is more likely to be involved in reflexes related to optokinetic nystagmus because the cells in this region responded preferentially to moving stimuli in the contralateral visual field and not to changes in brightness or darkness. Moreover, this nucleus projects mainly to the inferior olivary nucleus (Mizuno et al., 1974) and not to the region of the oculomotor parasympathetic preganglionic neurons (Berman, 1977; Breen et al., 1983; Steiger and Buttner-Ennever, 1979). Thus, on the basis of the physiological properties and anatomical connections of the nucleus of the optic tract it seems unlikely that this nucleus is involved with pupillary control.

A second unresolved issue is to determine if the nucleus of the posterior commissure plays a role in pupillary regulation. Carpenter and Pierson (1973) suggested that in the monkey this nucleus receives afferent visual information from the pretectum and relays it to the Edinger–Westphal nucleus. Benevento et al. (1977) failed to confirm this finding. Although the nucleus of the posterior commissure projects to the region containing the oculomotor preganglionic neurons (Berman, 1977; Breen et al., 1983), none of these studies established that this pathway provides a synaptic input onto the preganglionic neurons.

Carpenter and Pierson (1973) reported that various unilateral lesions of the pretectum had no effect on the pupillary light reflex, except when they made large lesions that destroyed the region of the nucleus of the posterior commissure. However, these lesions also included the posterior commissure, the dorsal part of the central gray matter, and portions of the pretectum. Since more than the nucleus of the posterior commissure was destroyed in these experiments, these findings must be viewed as equivocal.

It is quite likely that these lesions destroyed the axons emanating from the olivary pretectal neurons that project to the region of the oculomotor preganglionic neurons. Some of the olivary pretectal fibers project to the contralateral preganglionic neurons by first crossing the midline (or sending a collateral branch across the midline) in the posterior commissure and, then, projecting ventrally to the preganglionic neurons (Figure 15-8A). This means that large lesions of the nucleus of the posterior commissure (which lies lateral in the posterior commissure) could theoretically eliminate 75% of the olivary pretectal inputs to the oculomotor preganglionic neurons. In other words, all the inputs from the ipsilateral pretectal olivary nucleus and the crossed inputs from the contralateral pretectal olivary nucleus would be destroyed by these unilateral lesions. Such lesions would be more profound than midline lesions of the posterior commissure because the latter would affect only the crossed projections (see Figure 15-8A). Resolution of whether the nucleus of the posterior commissure is involved in the pupillary light reflex will require restricted lesions of the cell bodies of this area with excitotoxic agents, such as kainic or ibotenic acid, which destroy cell bodies but

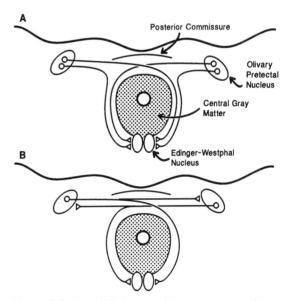

Figure 15-8 (A and B) Two possible arrangements of the central course of axons originating from the olivary pretectal nucleus. (A) The generally held view of the central course of the pupillary light reflex in which olivary pretectal neurons give rise to a bilateral projection to the preganglionic neurons in the Edinger–Westphal nucleus. (B) An interpretation that suggests that the olivary pretectal neurons project to the contralateral olivary pretectal nucleus and the contralateral Edinger–Westphal nucleus. [Modified from a drawing published by Gamlin et al. (1984). *Journal of Comparative Neurology* 226, 523–543.]

do not damage fibers of passage, and subsequent physiological testing.

A third unresolved issue relates to the question: What percentage of fibers from the olivary pretectal nucleus crosses the midline in the posterior commissure? Gamlin et al. (1984) presented two alternate schemes to explain how the olivary pretectal fibers reach the pupilloconstrictor neurons. The first (Figure 15-8A) follows the traditional view that some of the fibers cross the midline in the posterior commissure and the others project to the ipsilateral preganglionic neurons along the lateral border of the central gray matter. In the second scheme (Figure 15-8B), all the fibers cross the midline and innervate the contralateral olivary pretectal nucleus. Gamlin et al. (1984) argue that the second pathway is the more likely one for humans and monkeys because lesions of the posterior commissure totally eliminate the pupillary light response. However, the experimental and clinical studies cited by Gamlin et al. (1984) to support this view are extremely weak. In contrast, Magoun et al. (1935) found that posterior commissure lesions in the cat reduced the response by about 50%, suggesting that the projection from the pretectum to the oculomotor pupillomotor neurons involves a bilateral pathway, as presented in Figure 15-8A. Whether the same holds true in humans and monkeys has not been adequately tested.

A fourth unresolved issue concerns the integration of parasympathetic and sympathetic activity that occurs during light reflex. When the oculomotor parasympathetic fibers are excited, there is a concomitant inhibition of the sympathetic fibers that innervate the dilator muscle (Passatore and Pettorossi, 1976). The level of activity of these sympathetic fibers follows an almost linear, inverse relationship to the intensity of light illuminating the retina. The anatomical basis of this integration of parasympathetic and sympathetic neural activity is unknown. On the basis of lesion experiments Okada et al. (1960) concluded that there was a bilateral, descending pathway originating from the pretectum, with partial decussations at both the midbrain and the T1 level of the spinal cord.

NEURAL PATHWAYS CONTROLLING ACCOMMODATION

The near response involves a series of internal and external eye movements, which brings a nearby visual image into focus onto the fovea. Three changes must occur to allow an object to be focused onto the retina: (1) an increase in the curvature of the lens caused by contraction of the ciliary muscle and a subsequent release of tension on the zonule fibers that connect to the lens (accommodation), (2) pupillary constriction caused by contraction of the sphincter muscle of the iris, and (3) convergence of the eyes brought about by contraction of the medial recti muscles that are under the control of the oculomotor somatic motor neurons. The first two responses are controlled by the oculomotor parasympathetic neurons.

Accommodation Motor Neurons

The organization of the parasympathetic pre- and postganglionic neurons involved in accommodation is generally thought to be very similar to that of the pupilloconstrictor system. However, several studies indicate that the accommodation system may be more complicated.

Preganglionic accommodation neurons may project directly to the eye and bypass the ciliary ganglion. Westheimer and Blair (1973) reported that electrical stimulation of the oculomotor preganglionic nerve in monkeys caused accommodation, but not pupillary constriction, after nicotine was applied to the ciliary ganglion. This result was surprising because it had been assumed that both pupillomotor and accommodation preganglionic neurons synapse in the ciliary ganglion, both use acetylcholine as a transmitter, and both activate nicotinic cholinergic receptors on their respective postganglionic ciliary neurons. Since nicotine impairs ganglionic transmission between pre- and postganglionic neurons, one interpretation may be that the pathway for accommodation does not synapse in the ciliary ganglion. A second interpretation is that the response is not dependent on activation of nicotinic receptors. A third possibility is that the preganglionic neurons may not use acetylcholine as a neurotransmitter. None of these points has yet been resolved.

Retrogradely labeled cells are found in the Edinger–Westphal nucleus after horseradish peroxidase is injected into the eye of monkeys (Jaeger and Benevento, 1980). It is difficult to interpret these findings. On the one hand, they suggest that some oculomotor parasympathetic neurons project directly to the eye. However, on the other hand, this result may be due to transneuronal transfer of the enzyme (Burde, 1988).

The question of a direct oculomotor parasympathetic pathway was addressed by Ruskell and Griffiths (1979). After sectioning the oculomotor nerve in monkeys and waiting for 8–10 days, they found no electron microscopic evidence of nerve fiber degeneration distal to the ciliary ganglion, but the preganglionic fibers and the synaptic terminals in the ciliary ganglion did degenerate. Since a timed sequence of experiments with a broader range of postlesion survival periods was not studied, it is premature to use their data in support of either a direct or indirect parasympathetic pathway to the eye.

The exact localization of the accommodation preganglionic neurons has never been determined. Accommodation neurons have been localized dorsal to the oculomotor nucleus by single unit recordings in awake monkeys (Judge and Cumming, 1986). This region corresponds to the Edinger–Westphal nucleus. Clarke et al. (1985), using electrical stimulation currents of less than 1 μA in marmosets, found that accommodation responses could be elicted throughout the rostrocaudal extent of the Edinger–Westphal nucleus, whereas pupilloconstriction was elicted from the ventral portion of the Edinger–Westphal nucleus. When the anteromedian nucleus was stimulated, no oculomotor responses were elicted. Bando et al. (1981b) recorded from single oculomotor accommodation units in the cat and found them localized in the area of the Edinger–Westphal nucleus and the central gray matter. They did not find such neurons in the anteromedian nucleus. All of the cells were antidromically activated from the oculomotor nerve and orthodromically excited by electrical stimulation of cerebellar or pretectal sites that produced accommodation.

Cerebral Cortex

The major afferent stimulus for accommodation is thought to be an unfocused foveal image and binocular disparity (Cumming and Judge, 1986) as analyzed by the visual cortex. The exact cortical pathways involved in accommodation are unknown. There is evidence of two hierarchical sets of corticocortical projection systems that originate from the primary visual cortex (Brodmann's area 17) and are involved in visual processing (see Maunsell and Newsome, 1987 for review). One pathway is concerned with perception of form and color and is thought to be a continuation of the X-retinal ganglion cell pathway. This system involves a series of connections from visual area 1 (Brodmann's area 17) to visual area 2, then to visual area 3, visual area 3A, visual area 4, and finally to the inferotemporal cortex. The other projection system, involved in processing information related to visual movement and attention, may be a continuation of the Y-retinal ganglion cell pathway. It utilizes a series of corticocortical connections from visual area 1 (Brodmann's area 17) to visual area 2, from this region to visual area 3, then from the middle temporal cortex (an area referred to as MT or visual area 5), and finally to the posterior parietal cortex (Brodmann's area 7) and the frontal eye fields (Brodmann's area 8).

Evidence that this second system (or part of it) may be involved in accommodation is suggested by the work of Jampel (1960). By stimulating the transition zone between the temporal and occipital cortices (the region along the superior temporal sulcus between Brodmann's area 19 and 22), he produced all three components of the near response (Figure 15-9). No other area of the cerebral cortex gave such a response, except that stimulation of the frontal eye fields caused convergence and pupillary constriction but no changes in lens curvature. Recent neuroanatomical studies of the temporal lobe indicate that Jampel's accommodation area probably corresponds with the middle temporal region that lies in the superior temporal sulcus at the rostral border of the occipital lobe (Ungerleider and Desimone, 1986b).

The middle temporal region is visuotopically organized and receives a direct input from the primary visual cortex—Brodmann's area 17. The central part of the visual field projects to the posterior part of the superior temporal sulcus and the peripheral visual field projects to the sulcal floor and a short distance into the anterior bank of the sulcus (Ungerleider and Desimone, 1986b). On the basis of this map, one would predict that the foveal part of the middle temporal region in the posterior bank of the superior

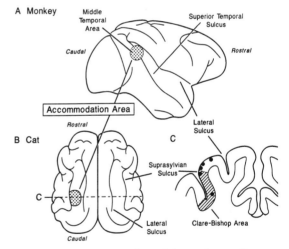

Figure 15-9 (A) Lateral view of the cerebrum of a macaque monkey illustrating the location of the accommodation area as defined by Jampel (1960). This area appears to coincide with the middle temporal area as discussed in the text. (B) Dorsal view of the cerebrum of a cat illustrating the accommodation area as defined by Bando et al. (1981a). (C) Traverse section of the cerebrum of a cat at the A5.0 stereotaxic level showing the sites where accommodation units were recorded. In addition, electrical stimulation of these loci caused pupillary constriction. Some of the units were found within the Clare–Bishop area of the cerebral cortex as defined by Hubel and Wiesel (1969) and others lay medial to this region along the medial bank of the suprasylvian sulcus. [Drawings B and C were modified from Bando et al. (1981a). *Brain Research* 225, 195–199.]

temporal sulcus would be the main cortical region responsible for ocular changes during accommodation. However, Jampel (1960) also elicited accommodation from the area rostral to the superior temporal sulcus, which lies beyond the middle temporal area. It is possible that these responses were due to current spread from this rostral area to the middle temporal region. This issue needs to be reexplored using smaller currents and careful cytoarchitectonic mapping of active sites.

The middle temporal area does not appear to have direct connections with the oculomotor complex, based on the autoradiographic studies of Maunsell and van Essen (1983) and Ungerleider et al. (1984). Presumably, if the middle temporal area functions as an accommodation center it must do so by polysynaptic pathways that have yet to be determined. It is also not known whether lesions of the middle temporal area disrupt accommodation, although Ungerleider et al. (1984) described preliminary studies indicating that animals with middle temporal lesions are impaired in their ability to detect and to grasp small, nearby objects.

Electrophysiological recordings in the middle temporal area show that a large proportion of the cells in this area are specialized for analysis of movement of visual stimuli (Zeki, 1974; see Ungerleider and Desimone, 1986a for additional references; Maunsell and Newsome, 1987, for review). Zeki (1974) pointed out that the neurons found in the middle temporal region of the monkey are similar to those in the Clare–Bishop area in the cat. Cells in both of these regions have large receptive fields, are directionally selective, are insensitive to form, and both receive a direct, visuotopic projection from area 17. Bando et al. (1981a) have recorded from the Clare–Bishop area and found that there were cells along the medial bank of the suprasylvian sulcus whose discharge correlates with the accommodation response (see Bando et al., 1988, for review). Stimulation of this area produced accommodation (Figure 15-9B and C). Thus, it is possible that these cells and the homologous ones in the middle temporal region may be responsible for making the necessary adjustments for near vision.

Cerebellum

The cerebellum is known to be involved in a variety of autonomic functions, including control of the light reflex and accommodation in the cat (Hosoba et al., 1978). Electrical stimulation of the fastigial or interpositus nuclei of the cerebellum, as well as of the cerebellar cortex, causes accommodation (Hosoba and Tsukahara, 1976; Hultborn et al., 1978). Reactive sites were found in lobule VII of the vermis (folium vermis and tuber vermis), lobule simplex,

and lobule paramedianus—all of which correspond to known visual areas in the posterior cerebellar cortex. The response elicited from these cortical areas had a considerably longer latency than those evoked on stimulation of the deep cerebellar nuclei (17 versus 5.5 msec).

The anatomical basis of this response is unknown. Horseradish peroxidase injections into the oculomotor complex of the monkey results in retrograde cell body labeling in the deep cerebellar nuclei and the underlying cell group Y (Gonzalo-Ruiz et al., 1988). However, since anterograde labeling experiments were not performed, it is unknown whether any of these cell groups project directly to the Edinger–Westphal nucleus. Batton et al. (1977) failed to find a direct connection from the fastigial nucleus to the Edinger–Westphal nucleus in the monkey, but did not systematically explore the efferent connections of the other deep cerebellar nuclei. In the cat, Sugimoto et al. (1982) studied the efferent projections of the deep cerebellar nuclei and found no evidence for a pathway to the Edinger–Westphal or anteromedian nuclei. The fastigial nucleus, as well as the other two cerebellar nuclei, project to the ventral portions of the midbrain central gray matter—areas known to give rise to oculomotor preganglionic neurons. The circuitry controlling the cerebellar-accommodation response needs considerable clarification.

REGULATION OF BLOOD FLOW TO THE EYE

A considerable amount of information on ocular blood flow has been gathered by Bill and co-workers (see Bill, 1984, 1985; Alm and Bill, 1987, for reviews).

The blood supply to the eye of primates is derived from two sources: the central artery of the retina, which supplies the inner two-thirds of the retina, and the choroidal arteries, which form a dense vascular plexus surrounding the retina. The choroidal arteries originate from the ophthalmic artery and can be subdivided into three main groups: long posterior ciliary arteries, short posterior ciliary arteries, and anterior ciliary arteries (Figure 15-10). The ciliary arteries provide nutrients to the pigment epithelium and to the layer of rods and cones (outer 100 μm of the retina) as well as to the central part of the retina (fovea) by diffusion. They supply branches to the ciliary body and the iris. The retinal capillaries have tight junctions equivalent to the blood–brain barrier, whereas the choroidal capillaries are fenestrated; however, the pigment epithelium, like choroid plexus epithelium, has tight junctions and intervenes between the fenestrated choroid capillaries and the photoreceptor surface of the retina. The

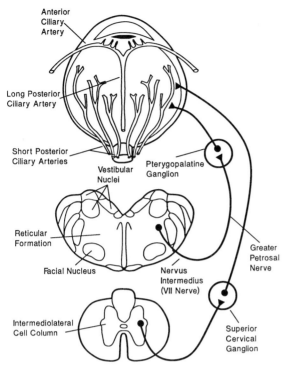

Figure 15-10 Diagram showing the innervation of the arteries of the choroid layer of the eye. The preganglionic sympathetic fibers originate in the intermediolateral cell column at T1 and T2 spinal levels. The postganglionic fibers arise from the superior cervical ganglion. Stimulation of these fibers causes vasoconstriction. The preganglionic parasympathetic fibers originate in the reticular formation of the medulla oblongata. They leave the brain in the nervus intermedius, which travels through the temporal bone and emerges as the greater petrosal nerve before synapsing in the pterygopalatine ganglion. The postganglionic fibers arising from this ganglion innervate the choroidal blood vessels.

fenestrated vessels allow for efficient diffusion of nutrients and waste removal from the posterior or outer retina. The retinal veins and arteries fulfill the same role in the inner retina in primates and other species with vascular retinas. The venous outflow from the eye drains into the vortex veins, which collect to flow into the ophthalmic veins.

The retinal arterioles have an efficient mechanism for autoregulation of blood flow over a wide range of different pressures, a high oxygen extraction rate, and a relatively low blood flow rate (~ 150 ml/min/100g). In contrast, the choroidal vessels are under sympathetic control and have an extremely high flow rate (~ 1200 ml/min/100 g) and a low oxygen extraction rate. The latter blood flow rate is 10 times that for gray matter of the brain (see review by Alm and Bill, 1987). Since the choroidal blood vessels supply nutrients and oxygen to the retina by diffusion (as well as to the overlying sclera, the ciliary

body, and the iris), this extremely high vascular flow ensures metabolic support of the outer retina.

The blood vessels of the eye are regulated by the sympathetic fibers that originate from the superior cervical ganglion and by the parasympathetic fibers of the facial nerve, which originate from the pterygopalatine ganglion (Figure 15-10). The sympathetic fibers that innervate the arteries of the choroid arise from the superior cervical ganglion. Most of these noradrenergic fibers may also contain the putative neurotransmitter neuropeptide Y (Bruun et al., 1984). The sympathetic fibers innervate the choroidal blood vessels but do not affect the retinal blood vessels. Stimulation of the sympathetic nerves or the superior cervical ganglion causes vasoconstriction of the choroidal arterioles and, as would be expected, an increase in choroidal vascular resistance and a decrease in blood flow (Bill, 1985). Similarly, local application of sympathomimetic drugs produces vasoconstriction of the choroidal blood vessels (Ruskell, 1971). The effects of neuropeptide Y on this vascular bed are unknown, but it is likely that neuropeptide Y inhibits the release of noradrenaline by a prejunctional receptor mechanism, as has been shown in other vascular beds (e.g., see Pernow, 1988).

The main function of the sympathetic innervation of the ocular blood vessels is to maintain a carefully regulated blood flow to the eye. The sympathetic fibers control the vasomotor tone of the choroidal arterioles, and these vessels, in turn, alter the metabolic supply of the rods and cones by regulating the amount of nutrients that diffuses to the outer plexiform layer of the retina. In contrast, the retinal blood vessels lack vasomotor nerves and are capable of autoregulation. In humans, however, there are nerve endings with dense core vesicles near the retinal artery just before it enters the retina, which may provide vasomotor control. In these vessels, any severe alteration in arterial pressure can be adjusted locally by the vascular smooth muscle itself to ensure that the retina has a constant blood flow. However, the central artery is under sympathetic control. Microsphere experiments indicate that the ocular sympathetic fibers serve to protect the eye from overperfusion in hypertension (Bill, 1985). When cats are made hypertensive, as long as the cervical sympathetic nerves remain intact, blood flow to the retina, the optic nerve, and the uvea is maintained within the normal range. However, if the cervical sympathetic nerves are cut unilaterally, there is an overperfusion of the uvea and retina on the damaged side. This implies that the sympathetic fibers are activated to protect the ocular tissues during acute episodes of hypertension as normally experienced during exercise or stress.

The parasympathetic innervation of choroidal blood vessels in monkeys originates from the facial nerve (Ruskell, 1971). The facial parasympathetic fibers leave the brain in the intermediate nerve, travel through the temporal bone, and exit the skull as the greater petrosal nerve, which synapses in the pterygopalatine ganglion (Figure 15-10). When the pterygopalatine ganglion is destroyed, there are degenerative changes in the unmyelinated nerves of the choroid and in many nerve terminals on the choroidal arterioles (Ruskell, 1971). Intracranial stimulation of the facial nerve in the rabbit, cat, and monkey results in profound vasodilation of the uveal blood vessels (Stjernschantz and Bill, 1980). Blood flow in the choroid increased by about 150% and in the ciliary body and iris by 30% and 70%, respectively (Stjernschantz and Bill, 1980). This effect could not be abolished by either nicotinic or muscarinic ganglionic blockade, implying that acetylcholine is not the transmitter mediating vasodilation at the pre- or postganglionic sites. Similarly, local application of cholinergic drugs does not produce vasodilation (Ruskell, 1971).

Bill (1985) suggested that the transmitter of the postganglionic neurons of the facial parasympathetic system may be vasoactive intestinal polypeptide. This hypothesis is based on the fact that vasoactive intestinal polypeptide immunoreactive nerve fibers are found in the choroid and in the ciliary body and vasoactive intestinal polypeptide immunoreactive cell bodies are found in the pterygopalatine ganglion (Uddman et al., 1980). In addition, injections of vasoactive intestinal polypeptide into the anterior chamber or intravenously caused dilation of the choroid vasculature (Nilsson and Bill, 1984). However, the magnitude of the vasodilation after intracameral or intravenous injections of vasoactive intestinal polypeptide was considerably smaller than the vascular changes following facial nerve stimulation. The reason for this discrepancy is unknown. It must be emphasized that the additional criteria necessary to establish that vasoactive intestinal polypeptide is the neurotransmitter of the postganglionic neurons have not been established. Thus, it is critical to establish that vasoactive intestinal polypeptide is released during facial nerve stimulation, that facial nerve-induced increases in choroid blood flow can be blocked by a specific vasoactive intestinal polypeptide antagonist, and that vasoactive intestinal polypeptide receptors are present on the choroidal arterioles.

Intracranial stimulation of the oculomotor nerve does not change blood flow in the retina or choroid but produces a marked atropine-sensitive decrease in the iris (Stjernschantz and Bill, 1979). Whether the change is due to a direct neural effect on the blood vessels or is the result of a secondary change induced by contraction of the iris is unknown. In contrast, oculomotor nerve stimulation produces an increase in blood flow in the ciliary body of cats and monkeys, but not in rabbits, where a decrease occurs (Stjernschantz and Bill, 1979). In monkeys, the response is atropine sensitive but in cats, it is atropine insensitive. As mentioned above, it is not certain if this response is due to a direct neural effect or a secondary effect that occurs as a result of ciliary body contraction. To date, there is no anatomical evidence in support of the idea that the oculomotor parasympathetic fibers innervate the blood vessels of either the iris or ciliary body. Thus, it is likely that these effects on blood flow are secondary events following muscle contraction.

CONTROL OF INTRAOCULAR PRESSURE

Aqueous humor is formed continuously by the ciliary epithelium and provides nutrients to the lens and cornea. It flows from the posterior chamber through the pupillary aperture into the anterior chamber where it drains mainly into the venous system through Schlemm's canal (Figure 15-11). The aqueous humor flows through this canal into the aqueous veins that join the intrascleral venous plexus where aqueous humour and venous blood mix together. From here, the intrascleral vessels pierce the sclera to join the episcleral plexus of veins, which lead to the ophthalmic veins. Another route of drainage is the interstitial spaces between the ciliary muscle fibers. This allows some of the aqueous humor to escape through the sclera and ultimately return to the venous circulation through the choroidal vessels (Bill, 1984). The importance of this second system—the uveoscleral or unconventional pathway—varies from one species to another; in monkeys it accounts for 30% of the total outflow, in humans about 5-15%, and in cats about 3% (see reviews by Bill, 1984; Shields, 1987). Thus, Schlemm's canal is the major or conventional outflow pathway.

Intraocular pressure is determined by the amount of aqueous humor that is produced and by its rate of outflow. In humans, the mean intraocular pressure is approximately 15 mm Hg with fluctuations of 1 mm Hg correlating with pulsations in venous blood pressure. The rate of flow of aqueous humor through the pupillary aperture is approximately 2.5 μl/minute. There is a diurnal variation in intraocular pressure reaching its low in the morning and its high in the afternoon. This variation is exaggerated with patients who have glaucoma (Henkind et al., 1973). A similar diurnal rhythm has been demonstrated in rabbits and the increase in intraocular pressure seen in the afternoon is reduced after cervical sympathectomy, whereas the decrease in pressure seen in the morning is only mildly affected (Braslow and Greg-

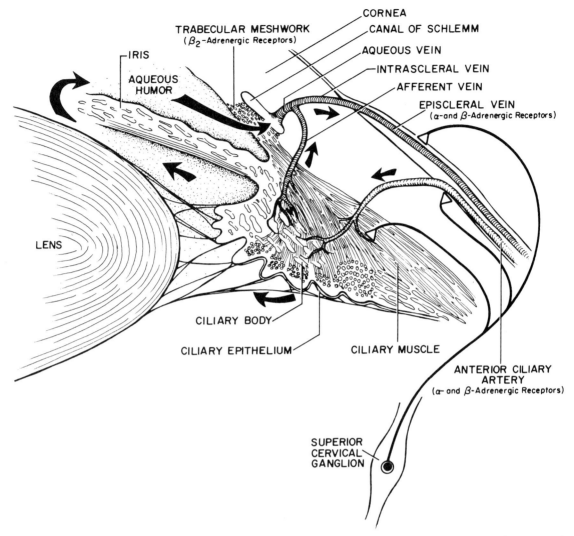

Figure 15-11 Aqueous humor is produced by the ciliary epithelium. It flows into the anterior chamber of the eye and drains into the venous system by first passing through the trabecular meshwork and then into the canal of Schlemm. Aqueous humor and venous blood from the ciliary body and muscle mix together in the aqueous veins. These veins connect with the episcleral veins.

ory, 1987). This implies that some type of central mechanism regulates intraocular pressure (for further discussion see Shields, 1987, p. 423).

Since both the inflow and the outflow of this system are closely related to the vascular system, there have been numerous suggestions that intraocular pressure is regulated by the autonomic nervous system. However, there is no definitive evidence to indicate that the autonomic nervous system directly affects the rate of production of aqueous humor (Bill, 1984). Instead, it is more likely that neurally mediated changes in the vasomotor tone of the intra- and episcleral veins are the main determinants of intraocular pressure.

Electrical stimulation of the superior cervical sym-

pathetic ganglion in the rabbit decreases intraocular pressure (Uusitalo, 1972). The mechanism responsible for this decrease, though not well understood, may be related to the sympathetic innervation of the intra- and episcleral venous system (Figure 15-11). Langham and Palewicz (1977) proposed three potential sites along the venous outflow that can be influenced directly by sympathetic fibers: (1) aqueous veins, (2) afferent veins, and (3) episcleral veins. All three types of veins have been shown to have noradrenergic nerve fibers associated with them (Ehinger, 1966; Laties and Jacobowitz, 1966). Vasoconstriction of the aqueous or episcleral veins would increase intraocular pressure, whereas vasodilatation would decrease it. Vasoconstriction of the afferent veins would decrease vascular filling and increase the channels available for aqueous humor, thereby decreasing intraocular pressure. According to this model, each of these sites possess both α- and β-adrenergic receptors. Although the pharmacological mechanism and site of action are unclear, it is known that α-adrenergic agonists such as epinephrine produce greater decreases in intraocular pressure than β-adrenergic antagonists such as timolol (see Davson, 1980; Potter, 1981; Shields, 1987, for reviews). However, it must be remembered that each of these three types of veins may respond differently to various adrenergic drugs. Thus, it is possible that activation of the α-receptors in one part of this venous system produces vasodilatation, but in another part produces vasoconstriction. In addition, the demonstration of β_2-adrenergic binding sites in the trabecular meshwork (Jampel et al., 1987) lends support to the idea that β-blockers can act directly at this site, possibly to increase the drainage of aqueous humor from the anterior chamber of the eye. However, β-adrenergic inhibitors like timolol appear to lower intraocular pressure mainly by reducing the aqueous humor production, possibly a direct action on the ciliary processes (see Shields, 1987, for discussion).

Electrical stimulation of the oculomotor parasympathetic system increases intraocular pressure by an unknown mechanism (Uusitalo, 1972; Macri and Cevario, 1975). Contraction of the ciliary muscle may increase intraocular pressure by blocking the uveoscleral outflow of aqueous humor. This would occur by elimination of the interstitial spaces between the longitudinal ciliary muscle fibers and, thus, block part of the outflow of the aqueous humor. However, this effect would be of minimal importance because most of the aqueous humor drains through the canal of Schlemm. Contraction of the ciliary muscle increases the rate of aqueous humor outflow by providing posterior traction on the trabecular meshwork. Since this latter structure provides the inner covering leading to Schlemm's canal, traction on it produces greater openings for increased aqueous humor drainage. Although it is still not clear what changes account for the increase in intraocular pressure seen during oculomotor nerve stimulation, there is substantial pharmacological evidence that parasympathomimetic drugs have an opposite effect: they decrease intraocular pressure and increase the outflow of aqueous humor. For example, cholinesterase inhibitors, such as physostigmine and echothiophate, are used routinely in the treatment of glaucoma (see Shields, 1987 for clinical discussion). These drugs potentiate the actions of acetylcholine and cause a prolonged contraction of the ciliary muscle, which allows the pores of the trabecular meshwork to be enlarged for a longer time

so that more aqueous humor drains into the canal of Schlemm. Cholinergic agonists, such as pilocarpine and aceclidine, also decrease intraocular pressure and increase aqueous humor drainage by a direct effect on the ciliary muscle. The mechanism that brings about this drainage is similar to that of the anticholinesterase drugs. It is a direct effect on the ciliary muscle that enlarges the openings of this meshwork leading to Schlemm's canal and thus increases aqueous humor drainage.

SUMMARY

The autonomic nervous system plays an important role in maintaining the normal physiology of the eye. It is involved in optimizing visual acuity by regulating pupil diameter and controlling accommodation. In addition, it maintains the metabolism of the eye by providing a carefully regulated blood supply to the uvea (viz. choroid, ciliary body, and iris). It may also influence intraocular pressure by regulating the outflow of aqueous humor through the episcleral veins.

The diameter of the pupil is regulated by both sympathetic and parasympathetic fibers. When the sympathetic nervous system is activated, it causes pupillary dilation. The neural activity of the cervical sympathetic fibers that innervate the dilator muscle of the iris exhibits a firing pattern that varies inversely with the intensity of the light illuminating the retina. During the light reflex, there is an inhibition of the sympathodilator system. The sympathetic fibers also function under conditions of stress such as occurs in the fight-or-flight situation. The parasympathetic system regulates pupil size directly in response to the level of luminance intensity. It serves to adjust pupillary diameter for maximizing the optics of the eye under various conditions of brightness. The neural circuitry controlling this response is discussed in this chapter.

Accommodation is the mechanism by which the size and shape of the lens are altered to focus visual targets onto the fovea. Under resting conditions, the ciliary body is relaxed and the zonules connecting the ciliary body to the lens are taut, keeping the lens flat and, in a normal individual, focused at a distance. As the visual image comes closer to the individual, the ciliary muscle contracts, allowing the zonules to relax, which in turn allows the lens to become more spherical and stronger in power. A discussion of the cortical mechanism that may be involved is presented in this chapter. In addition, current issues regarding the preganglionic and postganglionic motor neurons controlling accommodation are discussed.

The arterial supply of the eye can be subdivided

into two main groups: retinal and choroidal. The former system of vessels supplies the optic nerve and the retina; they are autoregulated. The latter system provides nutrients to most of the eye, including the optic nerve head, and is under control of the autonomic nervous system and is not autoregulated. When the sympathetic fibers are activated they cause vasoconstriction. These fibers arise from the superior cervical ganglion and release noradrenaline as a neurotransmitter. The parasympathetic fibers innervating the choroidal vessels leave the brain stem in the facial nerve and synapse in the pterygopalatine ganglion. Postganglionic neurons from this ganglion innervate the choroidal blood vessels, but the neurotransmitter released is unknown. It is postulated that vasoactive intestinal polypeptide may be the neurotransmitter used in this system.

Intraocular pressure is controlled by two factors: the rate of production and the rate of outflow of aqueous humor. The autonomic nervous system does not directly influence the rate of production of aqueous humor, but it does control the arterial blood flow in the ciliary body and the aqueous-venous outflow. The latter may be modulated by the sympathetic control of the system of veins that connect the canal of Schlemm to the episcleral venous plexus. Stimulation of the parasympathetic nervous system causes an increase in intraocular pressure. Stimulation of the cervical sympathetic nerve causes a decrease in intraocular pressure. This may be mediated primarily by the episcleral venous system.

REFERENCES

Reviews

Alm, A., and Bill, A. (1987). Ocular circulation. In: *Adler's Physiology of the Eye*, 8th ed., R. A. Moses and W. M. Hart (eds.), Mosby, St. Louis, pp. 183–203.

Bando, T., Toda, H., and Awaji, T. (1988). Lens accommodation-related and pupil-related units in the lateral suprasylvian area in cats. *Progress in Brain Research* 75, 231–236.

Bill, A. (1984). The circulation of the eye. In: *The Microcirculation*, Part 2, *Handbook of Physiology, Section 2*, E. M. Renkin, and C. C. Michel (eds.), American Physiological Society, Bethesda, MD, pp. 1001–1035.

Bill, A. (1985). Some aspects of ocular circulation. *Investigative Ophthalmology and Visual Science* 26, 410–424.

Davson, H. (1980). Aqueous humour and the intraocular pressure. In: *Physiology of the Eye*, Academic Press, New York, pp. 9–81.

Lundberg, J. M., and Hökfelt, T. (1986). Multiple co-existence of peptides and classical transmitters in peripheral autonomic and sensory neurons—functional and pharmacological implications. *Progress in Brain Research* 68, 241–262.

Maunsell, J. H. R., and Newsome, W. T. (1987). Visual processing in monkey extrastriate cortex. *Annual Review of Neuroscience* 10, 363–401.

Miller, N. R. (1985). *Walsh and Hoyt's Clinical Neuro-ophthalmology*, Vol. 2, Williams & Wilkins, Baltimore, pp. 400–457, 469–558.

Patten, J. (1977). *Neurological Differential Diagnosis*. Springer, New York.

Potter, D. E. (1981). Adrenergic pharmacology of aqueous humor dynamics. *Pharmacological Reviews* 33, 133–153.

Reiner, A., Karten, H. J., Gamlin, P. D. R., and Erichsen, J. T. (1983). Parasympathetic ocular control. Functional subdivisions and circuitry of the avian nucleus of Edinger-Westphal. *Trends in Neuroscience* 5, 140–145.

Shields, M. B. (1987). *Textbook of Glaucoma*, 2nd ed. Williams & Wilkins, Baltimore.

Stone, J. (1983). *Parallel Processing in the Visual System*. Plenum, New York.

Thompson, H. S. (1987). The pupil. In: *Adler's Physiology of the Eye. Clinical Application*. R. A. Moses and W. M. Hart (eds.), Mosby, St. Louis, pp. 311–338.

Research Papers

Bando, T., Tsukuda, K., Yamamoto, N., Maeda, J., and Tsukahara, N. (1981a). Cortical neurons in and around the Clare-Bishop area related with lens accommodation in the cat. *Brain Research* 225, 195–199.

Bando, T., Tsukuda, K., Yamamoto, N., Maeda, J., and Tsukahara, N. (1981b). Mesencephalic neurons controlling lens accommodation in the cat. *Brain Research* 213, 201–204.

Barlow, H. B., and Levick, W. R. (1969). Changes in the maintained discharge with adaption level in the cat retina. *Journal of Physiology (London)* 202, 699–718.

Batton, R. R., Jayaraman, A., Ruggiero, D., and Carpenter, M. B. (1977). Fastigial efferent projections in the monkey: An autoradiographic study. *Journal of Comparative Neurology* 174, 281–306.

Benevento, L. A., Rezak, M., and Santos-Anderson, R. (1977). An autoradiographic study of the projections of the pretectum in the rhesus monkey (Macaca mulatta): Evidence for sensorimotor links to the thalamus and oculomotor nuclei. *Brain Research* 127, 197–218.

Berman, N. (1977). The connections of the pretectum in the cat. *Journal of Comparative Neurology* 174, 227–254.

Braslow, R. A., and Gregory, D. S. (1987). Adrenergic decentralization modifies the circadian rhythm of interocular pressure. *Investigative Ophthalmology and Visual Science* 28, 1730–1732.

Breen, L. A., Burde, R. M., and Loewy, A. D. (1983). Brainstem connections to the Edinger-Westphal nucleus of the cat: A retrograde tracer study. *Brain Research* 261, 303–306.

Bruun, A., Ehinger, B., Sundler, F., Tornqvist, K., and Uddman, R. (1984). Neuropeptide Y immunoreactive neurons in the guinea-pig uvea and retina. *Investigative Ophthalmology and Visual Science* 25, 1113–1123.

Burde, R. M., and Loewy, A. D. (1980). Central origin of oculomotor parasympathetic neurons in the monkey. *Brain Research* 198, 434–439.

Burde, R. M., (1988) Direct parasympathetic pathway to the eye: revisited. *Brain Research* 463, 158–162.

Carpenter, M. B., and Pierson, R. J. (1973). Pretectal region and the pupillary light reflex: An anatomical analysis in the monkey. *Journal of Comparative Neurology* 149, 271–300.

Clarke, R. J., and Ikeda, H. (1981). Pupillary response and luminance and darkness detector neurones in the pretectum of the rat. *Documenta Ophthalmologia,* The Hague, Series 30, 53–61.

Clarke, R. J., and Ikeda, H. (1985). Luminance and darkness detectors in the olivary and posterior pretectal nuclei and their relationship to the pupillary light reflex in the rat. I. Studies with steady luminance levels. *Experimental Brain Research* 57, 224–232.

Clarke, R. J., Coimbra, C. J. P., and Alessio, M. L. (1985). Oculomotor areas involved in the parasympathetic control of accommodation and pupil size in the marmoset *(Callithrix jacchus). Brazilian Journal of Medicine and Biological Research* 18, 373–379.

Cumming, B. G., and Judge, J. S. (1986). Disparity-induced and blur-induced convergence eye movement and accommodation in the monkey. *Journal of Neurophysiology* 55, 896–914.

Ehinger, B. (1966). Adrenergic nerves to the eye and to related structures in man and in the cynomologus monkey *(Maccaca irus). Investigative Ophthalmology and Visual Science* 5, 42–52.

Ehinger, B. (1967). Double innervation of the feline iris dilator, *Archives of Ophthalmology* 77, 541–545.

Finley, J. C. W., Maderdrut, J. L., Roger, L. J., and Petrusz, P. (1981). The immunocytochemical localization of somatostatin-containing neurons in the rat central nervous system. *Neuroscience* 11, 2173–2192.

Fukuda, Y., and Stone, J. (1974). Retinal distribution and central projections of Y-, X-, and W-cells of the cat's retina. *Journal of Neurophysiology* 37, 749–772.

Gamlin, P. D. R., Reiner, A., Erichsen, J. T., Karten, H. J., and Cohen, D. H. (1984). The neural substrate for the pupillary light reflex in the pigeon *(Columba livia). Journal of Comparative Neurology* 226, 523–543.

Gonzalo-Ruiz, A., Leichnitz, G. R., and Smith, D. J. (1988). Origin of cerebellar projections to the region of the oculomotor complex, medial pontine reticular formations, and superior colliculus in New World monkeys: A retrograde horseradish peroxidase study. *Journal of Comparative Neurology* 268, 508–526.

Hare, W. K., Magoun, H. W., and Ranson, S. W. (1935). Pathway for pupillary constriction. *Archives of Neurology and Psychiatry (Chicago)* 34, 1189–1194.

Henkin, P., Leitman, M., and Weitzman, E. (1973). The diurnal curve in man: New observations. *Investigation Ophthalmology and Visual Science* 12, 705–707.

Hosoba, M., and Tsukahara, N. (1976). The cerebellar control of accommodation of the eye in the cat. *Proceedings of the Japan Academy* 52, 244–247.

Hosoba, M., Bando, T., and Tsukahara, N. (1978). The cerebellar control of accommodation of the eye in the cat. *Brain Research* 153, 495–505.

Hubel, D. H., and Wiesel, T. N. (1969). Visual area of the lateral suprasylvian gyrus (Clare-Bishop area) of the cat. *Journal of Physiology (London)* 202, 251–260.

Hultborn, H., Mori, K., and Tsukahara, N. (1978). Cerebellar influence on parasympathetic neurones innervating intra-ocular muscles. *Brain Research* 159, 269–278.

Hutchins, B., and Weber, J. T. (1985). The pretectal complex of the monkey: A reinvestigation of the morphology and retinal terminations. *Journal of Comparative Neurology* 232, 425–442.

Jaeger, R. J., and Benevento, L. A. (1980). A horseradish peroxidase study of the innervation of the interal structures of the eye. *Investigative Ophthalmology and Visual Science* 19, 575–583.

Jampel, R. S. (1960). Convergence, divergence, pupillary reactions and accommodations of the eye from faradic stimulation of the macaque brain. *Journal of Comparative Neurology* 115, 371–399.

Jampel, H. D., Lynch, M. G., Brown, R. H., Kuhar, M. J., and De Souza, E. G. (1987). β-Adrenergic receptors in human trabecular meshwork. *Investigative Ophthalmology and Visual Science* 28, 722–779.

Johnson, D. A., and Purves, D. (1981). Post-natal reduction of neural unit size in the rabbit ciliary ganglion. *Journal of Physiology (London)* 318, 143–159.

Judge, S. J., and Cumming, B. G. (1986). Neurons in the monkey midbrain with activity related to vergence eye movement and accommodation. *Journal of Neurophysiology* 55, 915–930.

Katayama, Y., and Nishi, S. (1984). Sites and mechanisms of actions of enkephalin in the feline parasympathetic ganglion. *Journal of Physiology (London)* 351, 111–121.

Kondo, H., Katayama, Y., and Yui, R. (1982). On the occurrence and physiological effect of somatostatin on the ciliary ganglion of cells. *Brain Research* 247, 141–144.

Laties, A. M., and Jacobowitz, D. (1966). A comparative study of the autonomic innervation of the eye in monkey, cat, and rabbit. *Anatomical Record* 156, 383–396.

Langham, M. E., and Palewicz, K. (1977). The pupillary, the intraocular pressure and the vasomotor responses to noradrenaline in rabbits. *Journal of Physiology (London)* 267, 339–355.

Loewy, A. D., Saper, C. B., and Yamodis, N. D. (1978). Re-evaluation of the efferent projections of the Edinger-Westphal nucleus. *Brain Research* 141, 153–159.

Macri, F. J., and Cevario, S. J. (1975). Ciliary ganglion stimulation. I. Effects on aqueous humor inflow and outflow. *Investigative Ophthalmology and Visual Science* 14, 28–33.

Magoun, H. W., and Ranson, S. W. (1935). The central path of the light reflex. A study of the effect of lesions. *Archives of Ophthalmology* 13, 791–811.

Magoun, H. W., Ranson, S. W., and Mayer, L. L. (1935). The pupillary light reflex after lesions of the posterior commissure. *American Journal of Ophthalmology* 18, 624–630.

Maloney, W. F., Younge, B. R., and Moyer, N. J. (1980). Evaluation of the causes and accuracy of pharmacologic localization in Horner's syndrome. *American Journal of Ophthalmology* 90, 394–402.

Martin, X., and Dolivo, M. (1983). Neuronal and transneuronal tracing in the tregeminal system of the rat using herpes virus suis. *Brain Research* 273, 253–276.

Maunsell, J. H. R., and van Essen, D. C. (1983). The connections of the middle temporal visual area (MT) and their relationship to a cortical hierarchy in the macaque monkey. *Journal of Neuroscience* 3, 2563–2586.

Mizuno, N., Nakamura, Y., and Iwohari, S. (1974). An

electron microscope study of the dorsal cap of the inferior olive in the rabbit, with special reference to the pretecto-olivary fibres. *Brain Research* 77, 385–395.

Nilsson, S. F. E., and Bill, A. (1984). Vasoactive intestinal polypeptide (VIP); effects in the eye and on regional blood flows. *Acta Physiologica Scandinavica* 121, 385–392.

Okada, H., Nakano, O., Okamoto, K., Nakayama, K., and Nisida, I. (1960). The central path of the light reflex via the sympathetic nerve in the cat. *Japanese Journal of Physiology* 10, 646–658.

Passatore, M., and Pettorossi, V. E. (1976). Efferent fibers in the cervical sympathetic nerve influenced by light. *Experimental Neurology* 52, 66–82.

Paulson, G. W., and Kapp, J. P. (1967). Dilatation of the pupil in the cat via the oculomotor nerve. *Archives of Ophthalmology* 77, 536–540.

Pernow, J. (1988). Co-release and functional interactions of neuropeptide Y and noradrenaline in peripheral sympathetic vascular control. *Acta Physiologica Scandinavica* 133, Suppl. 568, 1–56.

Ruskell, G. L. (1970). An ocular parasympathetic nerve pathway of facial nerve origin and its influence on intraocular pressure. *Experimental Eye Research* 10, 319–330.

Ruskell, G. L. (1971). Facial parasympathetic innervation of the choroidal blood vessels in the monkeys. *Experimental Eye Research* 12, 166–172.

Ruskell, G. L., and Griffiths, T. (1979). Peripheral nerve pathway to the ciliary muscle. *Experimental Eye Research* 28, 277–284.

Scalia, F. (1972). The termination of retinal axons in the pretectal region of mammals. *Journal of Comparative Neurology* 145, 223–258.

Sillito, A. M., and Zbrozyna, A. W. (1970). The localization of pupilloconstrictor function within the midbrain of the cat. *Journal of Physiology* (London) 211, 461–477.

Steiger, H.-J., and Buttner-Ennever, J. A. (1979). Oculomotor nucleus afferents in the monkey demonstrated with horseradish peroxidase. *Brain Research* 160, 1–15.

Stjernschantz, J., and Bill, A. (1979). Effect of intracranial stimulation of the oculomotor nerve on ocular blood flow in the monkey, cat, and rabbit. *Investigative Ophthalmology and Visual Science* 18, 99–103.

Stjernschantz, J., and Bill, A. (1980). Vasomotor effects of facial nerve stimulation: Noncholinergic vasodilation in the eye. *Acta Physiologica Scandinavica* 109, 45–50.

Sugimoto, T., Mizuno, N., and Uchida, K. (1982). Distribution of cerebellar fiber terminals in the midbrain visuomotor areas: An autoradiographic study in the cat. *Brain Research* 238, 353–370.

Terenghi, G., Polak, J. M., Ghatei, M. A., Mulderry, P. K., Butler, J. M., Unger, W. G., and Bloom, S. R. (1985). Distribution and origin of calcitonin gene-related peptide (CGRP) immunoreactivity in the sensory innervation of the mammalian eye. *Journal of Comparative Neurology* 233, 506–516.

Trejo, L. J., and Cicerone, C. M. (1984). Cells in the pretectal olivary nucleus are in the pathway for the direct light reflex of the pupil in the rat. *Brain Research* 300, 49–62.

Uddman, R., Alumets, J., Ehinger, B., Hakanson, R., Loren, I., and Sundler, F. (1980). Vasoactive intestinal polypeptide nerves in ocular and orbital structure sof the cat. *Investigative Ophthalmology and Visual Science* 19, 878–885.

Ungerleider, L. G., and Desimone, R. (1986a). Cortical connections of visual area MT in the macaque. *Journal of Comparative Neurology* 248, 190–222.

Ungerleider, L. G., and Desimone, R. (1986b). Projections to the superior temporal sulcus from the central and peripheral field representations of V1 and V2. *Journal of Comparative Neurology* 248, 147–163.

Ungerleider, L. G., Desimone, R., Galkin, T. W., and Mishkin, M. (1984). Subcortical projections of area MT in the macaque. *Journal of Comparative Neurology* 223, 368–386.

Uusitalo, R. (1972). Effect of sympathetic and parasympathetic stimulation on the secretion and outflow of aqueous humour in the rabbit eye. *Acta Physiologica Scandinavica* 86, 315–326.

Westheimer, G., and Blair, S. M. (1973). The parasympathetic pathways to internal eye muscles. *Investigative Ophthalmology and Visual Science* 12, 193–197.

Zeki, S. M. (1974). Functional organization of a visual area in the posterior bank of the superior temporal sulcus of the rhesus monkey. *Journal of Physiology (London)* 236, 549–573.

16

Autonomic Control of Endocrine Pancreatic and Adrenal Function

A. V. EDWARDS

With one or two exceptions, such as the adrenal medulla and posterior pituitary, the release of hormones into the circulating blood by endocrine cells used to be thought of as representing an entirely separate way of controlling the activity of peripheral tissues from that exerted by the nervous system. Over the past two decades, however, an enormous amount of evidence has accumulated to show that virtually all endocrine effects can be influenced by the autonomic innervation in one way or another and that such influences are functionally important under normal physiological conditions. The fact that this is still not widely appreciated, with occasional exceptions (see Ganong, 1974 for review), is probably the result of a tendency to assume that persistent secretory activity in a denervated or transplanted endocrine gland eliminates the possibility that the autonomic nervous system exerts any important function in the normally innervated gland. This misconception may have been reinforced by the finding that many endocrine cells respond to appropriate nonnervous stimuli *in vitro.* Of course, the fact that adrenocortical cells release glucocorticoids in response to ACTH, that thyroid cells release thyroxine and triiodothyronine in response to thyroid stimulating hormone, and that β-cells from the islets of Langerhans release insulin in response to glucose under these conditions does not preclude the possibility that the autonomic innervation modifies these responses *in vivo.* In experiments designed specifically to test for neural influences on endocrine glands, particularly those carried out in conscious animals so as to avoid the depressant effect of anesthetics, the autonomic fibers that supply endocrine tissues are generally found to play an important part in controlling secretion, quite apart from any effects they may have on the vasculature.

There is now abundant evidence supporting this contention with regard to the endocrine pancreas and the adrenal gland, both of which are involved in the control of carbohydrate metabolism. This is monitored neurally by glucose-sensitive elements whose firing rate is directly affected (either stimulated or inhibited) by changes in the concentration of glucose in the circulating plasma. These sensors are situated both centrally in the hypothalamus, the nucleus tractus solitarius, the area postrema, and the dorsal vagal nucleus, and peripherally in the gut and the portal bed (see Niijima and Mei, 1987, for review). This information, which is integrated in the hypothalamus, leads to an increase or decrease in the rate of release of insulin or glucagon from the pancreatic islets, as may be appropriate. A sufficiently intense *fall* in plasma glucose concentration may lead to the release of physiologically effective amounts of catecholamines from the adrenal medulla. But this latter response has a much higher threshold than that which occurs normally and probably represents an emergency mechanism designed to oppose life-threatening hypoglycemia rather than to control fluctuations in plasma glucose concentration under normal conditions. Other efferent sympathetic mechanisms that respond to a fall in plasma glucose concentration include the innervation to the liver, causing increased hepatic glycogenolysis, and the endocrine pancreas, causing increased glucagon and decreased insulin release; these may be more responsive during hypoglycemia. However, the most sensitive neuroendocrine responses to fluctuations in plasma glucose concentration within the physiological range are changes in the release of pancreatic glucagon and insulin mediated via vagal parasympathetic pathways (see Edwards, 1984 for review).

THE ADRENAL GLAND

The adrenal gland is composed of two different types of endocrine tissue: adrenal cortex and adrenal medulla. The adrenal cortex completely encapsulates the adrenal medulla. The cells of these two tissues develop from different embryological origins and secrete different types of hormones in response to activation of different primary efferent pathways. However, their anatomical proximity is reflected functionally in the fact that both respond to a wide variety of "stresses" and the responses of both are integrated in the hypothalamus.

Embryologically, the adrenal cortex develops from coelomic mesoderm, near the anterior pole of the mesonephros, close to the genital ridge, where the cells proliferate for this purpose between the fourth and the tenth week of human embryonic life. These masses are later invaded by cells of ectodermal origin that migrate from the neural crest to form the adrenal medulla. The adrenal gland is characterized by an outer capsule of connective tissue beneath which lies three layers of adrenal cortex and the adrenal medulla in the center. The outermost region of cortex, the zona glomerulosa, is comprised of parenchymatous cells arranged in clusters and arcades closely associated with capillaries and sinusoids. Beneath that lie the cells of the zona fasciculata, which are arranged in more regular columns disposed radially around capillaries running in the same direction. The innermost layer of cortex, the zona reticularis, borders on the medulla and consists of an anastomosing network of cells. Each of these three regions secretes lipid-soluble steroid hormones, the structure of which is based on the cyclopentanoperhydrophenanthrene or steroid nucleus (Figure 16-1a), derived initially from cholesterol, but each region produces a predominantly separate type.

The end-products of adrenal steroid biosynthesis are of two main types: the C_{21} steroids, which have a 2-carbon side chain attached to C_{17}, and those with either an $O=$ or $OH-$ group attached at C_{17}, which are referred to as C_{19} steroids and are potent androgens. Removal of a further carbon atom converts androgens to estrogens (Figure 16-1d), and it is these androgens and estrogens that are produced by the zona reticularis. Their function under normal physiological conditions is unclear, but adrenal tumors may lead to feminization (very rarely) due to overproduction of estrogens or, more commonly, to masculinization or precocious puberty due to overproduction of androgens. The zona fasciculata is responsible for the production of glucocorticoids, principally cortisol in humans (Figure 16-1b), and corticosterone, which have widespread effects on carbohydrate, fat, and protein metabolism, the control of water diuresis, circulating leukocytes, maintenance of the excitability of the central nervous system, and gastrointestinal system, metabolism of bone, and anti-inflammatory and immunological effects. In the zona glomerulosa, corticosterone is successively hydroxylated and then dehydrogenated within the mitochondria to the mineralocorticoid al-

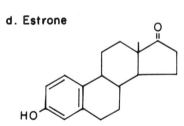

Figure 16-1 The structure and nomenclature of steroids. (a) The numbering system of the steroid nucleus on the 17-carbon cyclic hydrocarbon is illustrated. (b–d) Structural modifications of the steroid nucleus result in steroids with different physiological actions.

dosterone (Figure 16-1c), which is approximately 2,000 times as potent as the glucocorticoids in promoting the reabsorption of Na^+ in the distal convoluted tubule of the kidney and elsewhere. All the steroid hormones act in the cell nucleus to activate DNA and subsequently produce a form of RNA that regulates the synthesis of some specific protein.

In contrast, the adrenal medullae secrete the water-soluble hormones adrenaline and noradrenaline, derived by hydroxylation and decarboxylation, initially from tyrosine. The adrenal medullae represent a specialized part of the sympathetic system and the cells are often referred to as chromaffin cells, because they contain granules in which the catecholamines are synthesized, which stain a deep yellow-brown in the presence of potassium dichromate. They have many features in common with sympathetic postganglionic neurons. Both receive a direct sympathetic preganglionic innervation, and both release catecholamines that produce their characteristic effects peripherally. Adrenal medullary cells differ from sympathetic postganglionic neurons mainly in that some of them contain the enzyme phenylethanolamine *N*-methyltransferase (PNMT), which converts noradrenaline to adrenaline. The neurons are capable of releasing only noradrenaline, which acts as a transmitter within a given tissue close to the site of release, although there is some overspill into the circulation, raising the possibility that it might also produce effects hormonally. The adrenal medullae release a mixture of noradrenaline and adrenaline, in ratios that vary widely among individuals and even more so among species, depending on the proportion of cells in which the gene for PNMT has been expressed (induction of PNMT is dependent on glucocorticoids as is the development of these chromaffin cells; see below) and they are carried as hormones to their sites of action via the blood stream.

Immunohistochemical techniques have revealed that many biologically active peptides are present in the adrenal gland, either in nerve terminals, cells in the medulla or cortex, or in some cases both. The present list includes calcitonin gene-related peptide (Kuramato et al., 1987), vasoactive intestinal peptide (Linnoila et al., 1980; Hökfelt et al., 1981), neuropeptide Y (Allen et al., 1983), enkephalins (Schulzberg et al., 1978), neurotensin (Terenghi et al., 1983), substance P (Kuramato et al., 1985), and corticotropin-releasing factor (Bruhn et al., 1987b). Some of these are said to be colocalized within the same cells or, in the case of neuropeptide Y (Fischer-Colbrie et al., 1986), the same granules as contain the catecholamines. Both arginine vasopressin and oxytocin have been identified in the adrenal cortex and in the adrenal medulla, in which they have been shown to be present within the secretory granules. Furthermore, the presence of their respective neurophysins and of high-affinity receptors for both within the adrenal medulla indicates that they are both synthesized and exert some biological action within this region of the gland (Nussey et al., 1987). However, we know almost nothing about the functions of any of these adrenal neuropeptides.

Adrenal Catecholamines

Adrenaline and noradrenaline (and associated neuropeptides) released from the adrenal medulla are generally supportive of the actions of the rest of the sympathetic nervous system, which depends mainly on the release of noradrenaline, together with co-localized peptides such as neuropeptide Y and gastrin-releasing peptide from noradrenergic postganglionic nerve terminals. In some locations, however, actions of the sympathetic nervous system depend on acetylcholine, together with colocalized peptides such as vasoactive intestinal polypeptide, from cholinergic postganglionic nerve terminals. The fact that the adrenal medullae require more intense stimulation to release biologically effective amounts of catecholamine than does the sympathetic system generally was first recognized by Walter Cannon, who contended that they responded under conditions of "fear, fight and flight" (see Cannon, 1929 for review). This provides a very useful *aide-memoire* for anyone who is unfamiliar with the actions of the catecholamines, because they are generally appropriate to an extreme situation in which an animal is fleeing or fighting for its life. Thus, activation of β-adrenoceptors, which respond preferentially to adrenaline, increases heart rate and the force of myocardial contraction, so increasing cardiac output. Concomitant activation of α-adrenoceptors, which respond preferentially to noradrenaline, leads to vasoconstriction in the skin and gut, whereas activation of β-adrenoceptors, which mediate a vasodilator response in skeletal muscle, leads to diversion of blood from tissues that need it least to muscle that needs it most. At the same time blood will rapidly be enriched with glucose, providing a readily available metabolite for exercising muscle, consequent on β-adrenergic activation of hepatic glycogenolysis and gluconeogenesis. The additional actions of the catecholamines are discussed in Chapter 2.

The actions of the catecholamines released from the adrenal medulla differ from those of noradrenaline released from sympathetic postganglionic nerve terminals in several respects. First, they are much more prolonged, because catecholamines are broken down more slowly in the circulation than they are in the tissues. Second, they are potentially capable of reaching and stimulating every cell in the body, whereas only a small proportion of cells has a direct sympathetic innervation. Circulating catecholamines may well turn out to be of particular significance as a comodulator or mediator affecting the release or action of vasoactive agents from the endothelium such as endothelium-dependent relaxing factor (Furchgott and Zawadzki, 1980) and the novel vasoconstrictor agonist endothelin (Yanagisawa et al., 1988). Third, since adrenaline is usually the predominant amine released from the adrenal medulla and it has a much greater affinity for β-adrenoceptors than noradrenaline, effects mediated via these particular receptors, such as hepatic glycogenolysis, are likely to be promoted most effectively.

No doubt the classical view that adrenal catecholamines fulfill a supportive role in relation to the sympathetic system as a whole is generally correct, but evidence has recently been put forward that indicates that the activities of the two systems can be at least partly dissociated under certain conditions. Thus, during fasting, when hypoglycemia is sufficiently severe, there may be increased adrenal medullary activity associated with relative suppression of sympathetic nervous activity (Young et al., 1984). This combination of changes has also been recorded during acute hypoxia and in association with acute trauma. It leads to a reduction in oxygen consumption, because the sympathetic innervation is much more important than the adrenal medulla in the control of thermogenesis.

Juxtaposition of Adrenal Cortex and Adrenal Medulla

Conventionally, it is thought that the adrenal medulla and cortex are controlled separately, even though they lie in juxtaposition. Adrenaline and noradrenaline are released from the adrenal medulla, together with enkephalins, corticotropin-releasing factor, VIP, and no doubt other biologically active peptides, in response to activation of the sympathetic preganglionic innervation. In contrast, the cortical steroid hormones are released primarily in response to hormonal stimuli: adrenocorticotropic hormone (ACTH) in the case of the glucocorticoids (from the zona fasciculata) and the androgens and estrogens (from the zona reticularis), and angiotensin, in particular, in the case of the mineralocorticoids (from the zona glomerulosa). As we will see in the two sections that follow, there are significant interactions that occur between the two tissues in embryonic and adult life.

Developmental Considerations

The close proximity of these two quite different tissues can be justified teleologically by the fact that the enzyme phenylethanolamine N-methyltransferase, which converts noradrenaline to adrenaline in the adrenal medulla, is induced by glucocorticoids. This is why the ratio of adrenaline to noradrenaline that is secreted gradually rises during fetal and neonatal development as increasing amounts of ACTH, and consequently glucocorticoids, are released. Even more compelling evidence that the anatomical juxtaposition is functionally important comes from the developmental studies of Unsicker and his colleagues. This group has shown that whereas chromaffin cells from adult rat adrenal medullae will grow in culture virtually indefinitely, cells from immature glands (10 days postnatal) die in culture unless they are provided with two distinct growth factors, nerve growth factor and ciliary neurotrophic factor, isolated from the embryonic chick eye. Cells

from even more immature animals (18-day-old embryos) fail to respond to the growth factors and die in culture unless they are exposed to glucocorticoids. Apparently, it is an absolute requirement that embryonic adrenal medullary cells be exposed to glucocorticoids at a concentration of 10^{-10} M, or greater, for a minimum period of 50 minutes to develop into endocrine cells. If they are not so exposed they develop into sympathetic postganglionic neurons instead (Seidel and Unsicker, 1985; see Unsicker, 1986 and Unsicker and Leitze, 1987 for reviews). Therefore, if it were not surrounded by the adrenal cortex, the adrenal medulla would fail to develop.

Neural Control of the Adrenal Cortex

Because the control that is exerted by ACTH can be demonstrated so readily, the possibility that either adrenal medullary agonists (paracrine effect) or a direct neural innervation might influence adrenal cortical function has generally been overlooked. In fact, evidence has accumulated steadily in recent years to show that changes in the concentration of adrenal glucocorticoids cannot always be attributed to changes in plasma ACTH concentration and so must be influenced by some other factor or factors. Diurnal rhythms in adrenocortical sensitivity to ACTH have been demonstrated in rats, dogs, and humans and presumably potentiate the effect of diurnal changes in plasma ACTH concentration that also occur. In dogs, it has been shown that moderate hemorrhage (10–15 ml/kg) produces an increased adrenocortical sensitivity that could not be reproduced by injections of exogenous ACTH (Dempsher and Gann, 1983). Rats maintained on a restricted water schedule exhibit a rapid and pronounced fall in plasma corticosterone concentration immediately after drinking, which cannot be ascribed to a fall in plasma ACTH or to an increase in the rate of steroid catabolism (Wilkinson et al., 1982).

The contention that adrenal cortical function is influenced by the autonomic innervation is strongly supported by morphological evidence of various types of nerve terminal that are present within the zona glomerulosa of the adrenal cortex of a number of different species (reviewed by Holzwarth et al., 1987). In the rat, the adrenal cortical innervation may originate either in the adrenal medulla and respond to activation of the splanchnic nerve or pursue a quite separate pathway or pathways. The fibers may contain classical neurotransmitters or putative peptidergic transmitters, including vasoactive intestinal polypeptide (VIP), neuropeptide Y, leu-enkephalin, somatostatin, and substance P. A catecholaminergic system, thought to be either noradrenergic or dopaminergic (these agonists possibly being colocalized with neuropeptide Y), is apparently independent of the splanchnic nerve supply. On the other hand, VIPergic fibers, which are distributed mainly to the capsule and zona glomerulosa in this species, seem to represent a population of postganglionic sympathetic neurons whose activity depends on a splanchnic preganglionic supply (Holzwarth et al., 1987).

Trophic Considerations

There is also a substantial body of evidence from Dallman and her colleagues that the compensatory growth of the zona fasciculata in the remaining adrenal gland following unilateral adrenalectomy is largely dependent on the innervation and is mediated reflexly (see, for instance, Dallman et al., 1976, 1977). Manipulation of the adrenal gland, and particularly its pedicle, is as effective as removing the gland altogether in this respect, which strongly suggests the involvement of mechanoreceptors (possibly the stretch receptors that have been demonstrated in the adrenal capsule; Kiss, 1951; Niijima and Winter, 1968) and an afferent neural mechanism. The finding that compensatory adrenal growth can be blocked by deafferentation of the ipsilateral posterolateral portion of the mediobasal hypothalamus and ipsilateral lesions of the ventromedial and premammillary hypothalamic nuclei and contralateral hemisection of the spinal cord at T2 (see review by Holzwarth et al., 1987) shows that it is dependent on the nervous system. Clear evidence of the involvement of afferent neural pathways is provided by the finding that the response to manipulation of an adrenal gland can be inhibited by prior administration of local anesthetic. The existence of an efferent component is attested to by the fact that compensatory hypertrophy is abolished in chemically sympathectomized animals. All the available evidence thus suggests that this growth phenomenon, which is manifest in rats within 12 hours, depends on a neural reflex and not on the release of ACTH from the anterior pituitary, although that might fulfill a "permissive" effect. This in no way contradicts the well-established fact that hypophysectomy results in rapid adrenal cortical atrophy and that the administration of exogenous ACTH causes a pronounced increase in adrenal cortical size. The "trophic" effect of ACTH is primarily due to an increase in the size of the cells and adrenal RNA synthesis, whereas the compensatory growth phenomenon is characterized by an increase in the mitotic index and DNA synthesis. Manipulation of one adrenal gland results in compensatory growth of the contralateral adrenal gland 12 hours later, and if that contralateral adrenal gland is then manipulated in the same way the same growth phenomenon is observed in the first gland after another 12 hours has elapsed, illustrating the existence of quite separate neural pathways controlling compensatory growth of the two glands separately. Lowry (1984) has made the suggestion that the adrenal innervation somehow controls the activity of an adrenal proteolytic enzyme that cleaves circulating pro-opiomelanocortin (POMC) to the mitogenic N-POMC$_{1-28}$ and N-POMC$_{2-59}$ forms.

Physiological Evidence for the Neural Control of Glucocorticoid Release

The release of adrenal glucocorticoids can be modifed by neural activity under certain experimental conditions. Stimulation of the peripheral end of the splanchnic nerve in conscious hypophysectomized calves in the absence of exogenous ACTH has no detectable effect on the output of glucocorticoids from the adrenal cortex, although it produces the expected abrupt increase in the rate at which catecholamines and enkephalins are released from the adrenal medulla. In contrast, splanchnic nerve stimulation in calves receiving a continuous intravenous infusion of ACTH results in an abrupt and substantial increase in adrenal cortisol output, which is not associated with any change in mean plasma ACTH concentration, and subsides rapidly when stimulation is discontinued (Figure 16-2). Furthermore, this rise in cortisol output from the adrenal gland is faithfully reflected by an increase in the concentration of cortisol in the peripheral plasma (Edwards and Jones, 1987a). The results of these experiments provide direct evidence that the adrenal cortical response to ACTH is potentiated by splanchnic nerve stimulation.

The normal traffic of efferent impulses in the splanchnic nerves might potentiate adrenocortical responses to ACTH within the usual physiological range. This possibility was investigated by Edwards and Jones (1987b). Noradrenaline was infused intravenously in a group of conscious calves at a dose that produced a moderate increase in the release of endogenous ACTH, and the effects were compared with those of the same dose of noradrenaline administered under precisely similar conditions to another group in which the splanchnic nerves had been cut immediately below the diaphragm a week previously. These infusions raised the concentration of noradrenaline in the circulating plasma about 5-fold, which is within the physiological range, and elicited a similar (3-fold) rise in plasma ACTH concentration in both groups. However, the rise in plasma cortisol in the control group far exceeded that in the group with cut splanchnic nerves, showing that section of these nerves had greatly reduced the sensitivity of the adrenal cortices to ACTH and done so under the most physiological conditions possible (Figure 16-3). In both groups mean cortisol output was linearly related to mean plasma ACTH

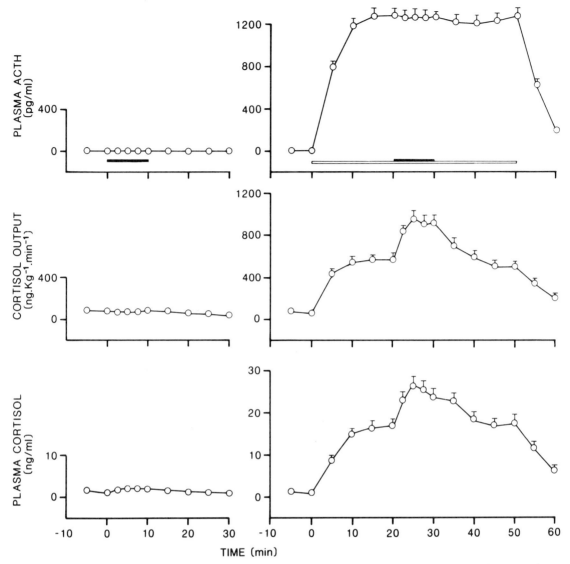

Figure 16-2 Comparison of the changes in mean arterial plasma ACTH and cortisol concentration and right adrenal cortisol output in response to stimulation of the peripheral end of the right splanchnic nerve (4 Hz for 10 minutes) in conscious "functionally hypophysectomized" 2- to 5-week-old calves ($n = 11$) in the presence and absence of exogenous ACTH (5 ng min^{-1} kg^{-1}). Open horizontal bar: duration of ACTH infusion. Closed horizontal bar: duration of electrical stimulation. Vertical bars: SE of each mean value where this exceeds the size of the symbol. (From Edwards and Jones, 1987a, by permission of the *Journal of Physiology*.)

concentration (Figure 16-4) and comparison of the slopes of the two regression lines showed that the effect of splanchnic nerve section had been to reduce adrenal cortical sensitivity to about 30% of normal (Edwards and Jones, 1987b). In a similar study, it was shown in lambs that bilateral section of the splanchnic nerves also substantially reduced the sensitivity of the adrenal cortex to ACTH over the same time period (Edwards et al., 1986). The observation that section of the splanchnic nerve reduces adrenal blood flow in conscious dogs (Engeland et al., 1985)

raises the possibility that this might also be the cause of the reduction in the apparent sensitivity of the adrenal cortex to ACTH, simply by reducing the effective presentation rate. This possiblity has yet to be eliminated.

Possible Mechanisms

Although the underlying mechanism for the sympathetic potentiation of adrenocortical function has still to be elucidated, it needs to be borne in mind

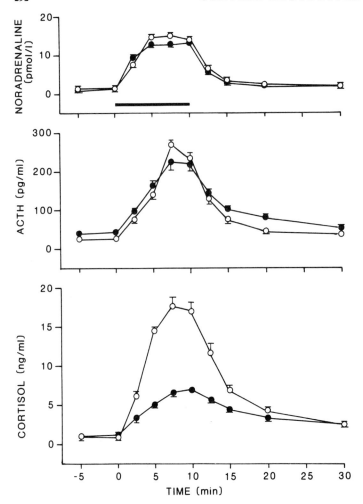

Figure 16-3 Comparison of the changes in mean arterial plasma noradrenaline, ACTH, and cortisol concentration in normal conscious 2- to 6-week-old calves (O, n = 5) and in calves with cut splanchnic nerves (●, n = 6) in response to iv infusions of noradrenaline (333 ng min^{-1} kg^{-1} for 10 minutes). Each animal was atropinized (0.2 mg/kg) to eliminate muscarinic parasympathetic reflex effects. Horizontal bar: duration of infusion. Vertical bars: SE of each mean value where this exceeds the size of the symbol. (From Edwards and Jones, 1987b, by permission of the *Journal of Physiology.)*

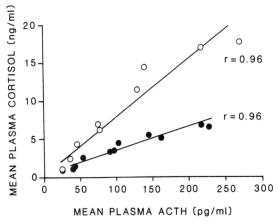

Figure 16-4 Relations between mean plasma ACTH and cortisol concentration in the experiments illustrated in Figure 16-3 and involving the infusion of noradrenaline (333 ng min^{-1} kg^{-1}). O, controls (n = 5); ●, cut splanchnic nerves (n = 6). Regression lines were calculated by the method of least squares. (From Edwards and Jones, 1987b, by permission of the *Journal of Physiology.)*

that bilateral section of the splanchnic nerves involves the severance of both afferent and efferent fibers that innervate the adrenal glands together with other abdominal viscera. However, the original series of experiments yielded direct evidence of the involvement of efferent elements and more recent experiments suggest that efferent vasoactive intestinal polypeptide (VIP) immunoreactive fibers may be responsible for sensitizing the cortex to ACTH under normal conditions. Such fibers have been found to be present in the adrenal cortex in other species, with their axons predominantly in the cortex and nerve cell bodies predominantly in the adrenal medulla, presumably representing a population of sympathetic postganglionic nerve fibers (Hökfelt et al., 1981; Holzwarth, 1984). Furthermore, VIP has been shown to exert a steroidogenic action on adrenal cortical cells *in vitro,* albeit a much less potent effect than ACTH itself (Kowal et al., 1977; Cunningham and Holzwarth, 1988). Stimulation of the peripheral end of the splanchnic nerve in conscious calves results in the release of small but significant amounts of VIP from the adrenal gland, quite sufficient to establish that it is released from intrinsic neurons contained in the adrenal gland under these conditions (Bloom et al., 1988). Finally, the potentiation of cortisol output during ACTH infusions, which occurs in the conscious calf during splanchnic nerve stimulation, can be mimicked by intra-arterial infusions of small doses of VIP into the aorta proximal to the adrenal gland so as to perfuse through it (Figure 16-5; Edwards and Jones, 1987c).

A VIPergic efferent pathway is at least partially responsible for potentiating adrenal cortical secretory responses to ACTH in the calf. Other transmitters could participate in mediating this response both in this and other species. In this connection, it is intriguing to find that large amounts of corticotropin-releasing factor are released in response to splanchnic nerve stimulation both in conscious dogs (Bruhn et al., 1987a) and calves (Edwards and Jones, 1988). Corticotropin-releasing factor is present in the adrenal gland itself (Bruhn et al., 1987b) and is released under these conditions, but the absolute amount is small in comparison with the total amount released, presumably from sympathetic nerve terminals (Edwards and Jones, 1987c). In hypophysectomized calves, intra-aortic infusions of relatively small amounts of corticotropin-releasing factor result in the secretion of significant amounts of cortisol from the adrenal gland, together with detectable amounts of ACTH and pro-opiomelanocortin (A. V. Edwards and C. T. Jones, unpublished observations).

The steroidogenic effect of VIP in the calf could not be accounted for by an increased presentation rate of ACTH to the adrenal gland when this was estimated from the concentration in the arterial plasma together with adrenal plasma flow. However, the possibility that there is a disproportionate increase in blood flow through the adrenal cortex, which could increase the presentation rate of ACTH locally, has yet to be eliminated. In view of the fact that splanchnic nerve stimulation has been found to have no effect on adrenal cortical blood flow in anesthetized dogs while increasing adrenal medullary blood flow 5- to 10-fold (Breslow et al., 1987), it seems unlikely. However, adrenocortical blood flow may already have been maximal, due to endogenous ACTH release, in these acute experiments.

Entirely different mechanisms could be involved in the control of compensatory growth, diurnal rhythms, and the apparent inhibition of glucocorticoid output that occurs with such rapidity after drinking in water-deprived rats. Perhaps there is an inhibitory neural pathway. It could well be so, but the difficulties in devising an experimental protocol to demonstrate this are daunting. One would need to carry out the experiments in hypophysectomized animals with the plasma ACTH concentration held at a constant level and have pharmacological agents with which to block any excitatory transmitter. In view of the fact that no blocking agent is currently available for use in vivo for the only excitatory neurotransmitter that has so far been identified—VIP—it seems unlikely that the question can be resolved at the present time.

VIP in the Adrenal Medulla

VIP has been implicated in the control of catecholamine release from chromaffin cells in the adrenal medulla of the rat (Malhotra and Wakade, 1987a,b). VIPergic transmission is most important in mediating secretion of catecholamines in response to splanchnic nerve stimulation at low frequencies (1 Hz), which is maintained for many hours in the isolated perfused rat adrenal gland preparation, unlike the response to high-frequency stimulation (10 Hz), which fatigues relatively quickly. Pretreatment with atropine and hexamethonium reduced the secretion of catecholamines in response to stimulation at 10 Hz by more than 80%, whereas that which occurred in response to stimulation at 1 Hz was reduced by only about 35% in the presence of these blocking agents (Wakade, 1988). When the catecholamine secretion had declined to very low levels after stimulating at 10 Hz for 100 minutes, reducing the frequency of stimulation caused a sharp increase in secretion, which was reversible and also occurred after the administration of atropine and hexamethonium. A particularly intriguing feature of this mechanism is the fact that it is effectively blocked by naloxone, indicating the involvement of opiate receptors.

VIP is thought to be as potent as acetylcholine in inducing the secretion of catecholamines from the adrenal medulla in the rat (Malhotra et al., 1988). Nicotinic stimulation of chromaffin cells depends on Ca^{2+} entry across the cell membranes, whereas activation of both VIPergic and muscarinic receptors on these same cells results in mobilization of Ca^{2+} from intracellular stores following the generation of inositol 1,4,5-triphosphate (Malhotra et al., 1988). The responses to VIP were effectively blocked both by a growth hormone releasing factor, AC-Tyr^{1}hGRF, which acts as a specific competitive VIP antagonist (Laburthe et al., 1986), and by naloxone.

Release of Aldosterone

The mineralocorticoid hormone aldosterone contributes to the maintenance of constant amounts of sodium and potassium in the body, mainly by increasing the reabsorption of sodium ions in the distal convoluted tubules in the kidney. Any increase in

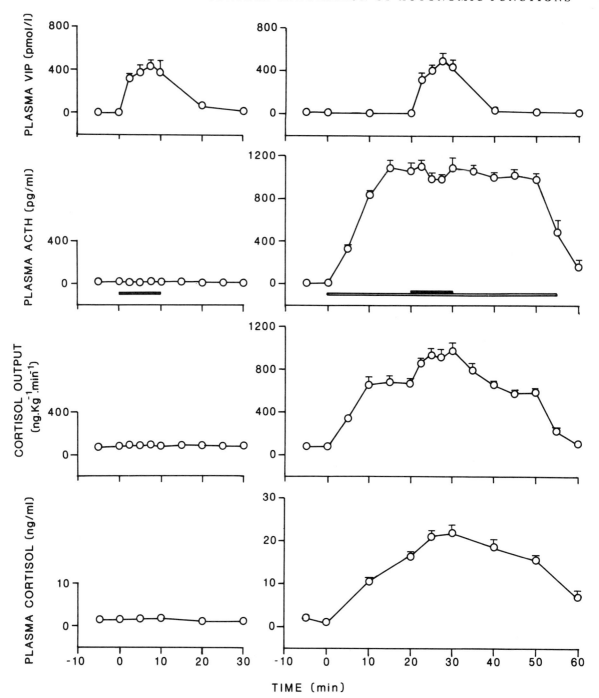

Figure 16-5 Comparisons of the changes in arterial plasma ACTH, adrenal venous affluent plasma VIP, and right adrenal cortisol output in response to intra-aortic VIP (4 μg min^{-1}) in conscious hypophysectomized calves ($n = 6$) in the presence and absence of ACTH (5 ng min^{-1} kg^{-1}). Open bar: duration of ACTH infusion. Closed bar: duration of VIP infusion. Vertical bars: SE of each mean value. (From Edwards and Jones, 1987c, by permission of the *Journal of Physiology.*)

sodium retention promotes the reabsorption of water, together with an increased intake, and so results in expansion of the extracellular fluid. To the extent that this involves expansion of plasma volume, it will tend to increase the blood pressure. An

increased sodium load also acts on the juxtaglomerular apparatus of the kidney, affecting renin release, which is also involved in the regulation of arterial blood pressure. Previously, it was thought that the release of aldosterone is mediated solely by hormonal influences, but this view now needs to be reassessed in terms of evidence considered below.

Anatomical studies demonstrate the presence of fibers containing catecholamines, neuropeptide Y, VIP, substance P, leu-enkephalin, and somatostatin in the zona glomerulosa (Hökfelt et al., 1981; Holzwarth et al., 1984, 1987). The potential sources of these fibers are neurons in the adrenal medulla, sympathetic or dorsal root ganglia and these observations imply that a wide range of neural transmitters can potentially modulate steroidogenesis in this region. Cunningham and Holzwarth (1988) have provided direct evidence of this by demonstrating that VIP promotes the synthesis of aldosterone in a dose-dependent fashion in rat adrenal preparations *in vitro*.

There is, of course, no doubt that the peripheral autonomic system is capable of stimulating aldosterone secretion indirectly via the renal renin–angiotensin system, and possibly by modulating the rate of release of atrial natriuretic factor, as this peptide is capable of inhibiting aldosterone release in response to all known stimuli (Mulrow et al., 1987). Putative mechanisms are represented in the form of a flow diagram in Figure 16.6. No doubt it is a gross oversimplification, but it is consistent with the available evidence at present. ACTH exerts a potent but transient stimulatory effect and potassium also exerts a potent stimulatory effect directly on the glomerulosa cells and indirectly in some way when there is a change in potassium status. Other factors that have been claimed to affect aldosterone release include pro-opiomelanocortin-derived peptides, the so-called aldosterone-stimulating factor (isolated from the pituitary), serotonin, somatostatin, and dopamine. However, further evidence is needed to establish whether any of these fulfills a specific role in relation to the control of aldosterone secretion *in vivo*. In the case of dopamine, there are three possible sites of control. First, it might act directly on the cells of the zona glomerulosa. Second, there is a central dopaminergic pathway in the hypothalamus that appears to be involved in the hormonal control of aldosterone secretion, at least in sheep (Huang et al., 1987). Third, a possible dopaminergic mechanism is via a descending dopaminergic pathway from the paraventricular hypothalamic nucleus to the sympathoadrenal preganglionic neurons (Strack et al., 1989).

Like corticosterone and cortisol, aldosterone is taken up by the brain itself and the steroid receptors, which appear to be quite specific for mineralocorti-

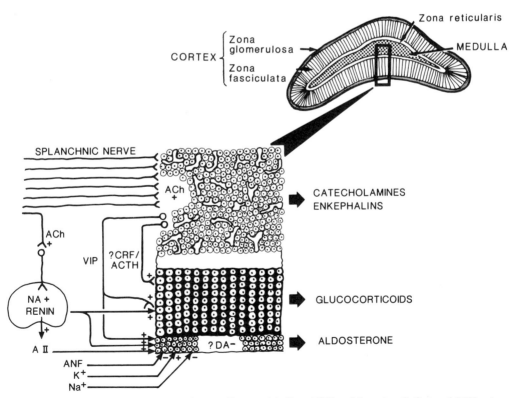

Figure 16-6 Putative adrenal control mechanisms. ACh, acetylcholine; ANF, atrial natriuretic factor; ACTH, adrenocorticotropin; AII, angiotensin II; CRF, corticotropin-releasing factor; DA, dopamine; VIP, vasoactive intestinal polypeptide; +, stimulation; −, inhibition.

coids, are present mainly in the hippocampus, septum, and amygdala (see McEwen et al., 1986 for review). Therefore, it is possible that these sites form part of a feedback loop that monitors and controls the secretion of this hormone. They are also likely to be involved in the behavioral effects it exerts such as suppression of salt appetite in adrenalectomized animals (McEwen et al., 1986). The fact that these steroid receptors are localized to cell nuclei indicates a genomic site of action.

Central Neural Mechanisms Involved in Adrenal Control

Descending Inputs to the Sympathoadrenal Preganglionic Neurons

The inputs to the sympathetic preganglionic neurons innervating the adrenal medulla are incompletely understood. The viral retrograde transneuronal cell body labeling method has been used by Strack et al. (1989) to localize the CNS nuclei that innervate sympathoadrenal preganglionic neurons. Five areas of the brain are involved: the caudal raphe nuclei, ventromedial medulla, rostral ventrolateral medulla, A5 noradrenergic cell group, and paraventricular hypothalamic nucleus (Figure 16-7). The anatomical organization of these different inputs is complicated because some of the axons contain more than one transmitter, such as serotonin, substance P (Appel et al., 1986), neuropeptide Y, and adrenaline (Blessing et al., 1987), and many of these areas project to multiple sites in the brain. In addition, a system of spinal interneurons also seems to be involved in this regulation (Strack et al., 1989). These factors undoubtedly form the neural network affecting control of adrenal catecholamine release.

Receptor autoradiography combined with the retrograde cell body labeling technique has revealed high concentrations of α_2-adrenergic and serotonergic binding sites over the sympathoadrenal preganglionic neurons. Binding sites for mu type opiate and muscarinic cholinergic receptors, which are present in the intermediolateral cell column, are not concentrated in the region over the sympathoadrenal neurons (Seybold and Elde, 1984). Since the A5 noradrenergic cell group and the serotonergic neurons of the raphe pallidus nucleus and related B1 and B3 cell groups of the ventral medulla, which lie lateral to the pyramidal tract, project to the sympathoadrenal preganglionic neurons (Strack et al., 1989), it is clear that these medullary neurons are involved in the control of the adrenal gland.

To date, the only physiological indication that the ventral medulla oblongata regulates the adrenal medulla comes from experiments in which microinjections of an excitatory amino acid (D,L-homocysteic

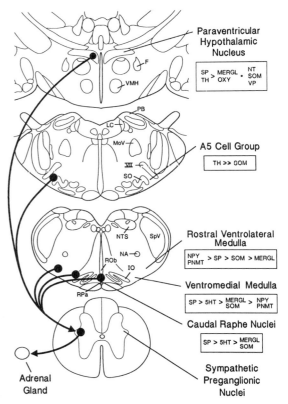

Figure 16-7 Schematic drawing illustrating the major areas in the rat brain that project to the sympathoadrenal preganglionic neurons. The putative neurotransmitters are also summarized. F, fornix; IO, inferior olivary nucleus; LC, locus coeruleus; MERGL, met-enkephalin-Arg-Gly-Leu; MoV, motor trigeminal nucleus; NA, nucleus ambiguus; NPY, neuropeptide Y; NT, neurotensin; NTS, nucleus tractus solitarius; OXY, oxytocin; PB, parabrachial nucleus; PNMT, phenylthanolamine N-methyltransferase; ROb, raphe obscurus nucleus; RPa, raphe pallidus nucleus; SO, superior olivary nucleus; SOM, somatostatin; SP, substance P; SpV, spinal trigeminal nucleus; TH, tyrosine hydroxylase; VII, facial nerve; VP, vasopressin; VMH, ventromedial hypothalamic nucleus. (Reproduced from Strack et al., 1989, with permission of the authors and publisher.)

acid) in this region in cats were found to stimulate release of catecholamines (McAllen, 1986). This response was most probably due to activation of a descending pathway from the ventrolateral medulla to the sympathoadrenal preganglionic neurons.

Another CNS region thought to control adrenal catecholamine release is the paraventricular hypothalamic nucleus. L-Glutamate microinjections in this nucleus cause an increase in adrenal nerve activity (Katafuchi et al., 1988). It is not certain that this effect is due to a direct or indirect excitation of the sympathoadrenal preganglionic neurons, because the paraventricular hypothalamic nucleus has extensive connections in the lower brain stem (see Chapter 6). In addition, the CNS control of adrenal catecholamine release may be quite complex if one considers the data of Darlington et al. (1988), which indicate that in rats there was no change in plasma catecholamines induced by hemorrhage after paraventricular hypothalamic lesions. Since there are multiple inputs to the sympathoadrenal preganglionic neurons, other pathways could compensate for the hypothalamic lesions.

Corticotropin-Releasing Factor

A variety of different stresses are capable of activating both the sympathetic nervous system and the pituitary–adrenal axis. Neurons containing the peptide corticotropin-releasing factor (CRF) play a pivotal role in orchestrating these responses (see reviews by Brown and Fisher, 1985; Gillies and Lowry, 1986). Although the neural pathways that control this dual response are unknown, there is pharmacological evidence that suggests that CRF neurons in the brain may control both responses. This hypothesis is based on the observation that a CRF receptor antagonist, α-helical [Glu^{27}]CRF (9–41), when given into the lateral ventricle of rats, inhibits the release of adrenaline from the adrenal gland after hemorrhage or insulin-induced hypoglycemia (Brown et al., 1986). In addition, this peptide inhibits the hypertension and tachycardia that occur secondary to central administration of CRF. However, since neither the site of action of this peptide nor its biological properties have yet been fully characterized, it is impossible to determine which central neurons have been affected in these experiments. Interpretation of these results is complicated by the fact that this peptide has so far been tested only on ACTH-secreting cells *in vitro*. Furthermore, it is premature to assume that CRF receptors are the same throughout the central nervous system and equally affected by this antagonist peptide.

Intracerebroventricular injections of CRF in conscious rats cause an increase in heart rate and arterial blood pressure that can be blocked by pretreatment with the ganglion blocking agent chlorisondamine (Fisher et al., 1982). Other changes that were attributable to sympathetic stimulation under these same conditions, and were blocked by chlorisondamine, included increases in the concentration of glucose, glucagon, adrenaline, and noradrenaline in the circulating blood. A CNS-selective somatostatin analog effectively blocked the rise in plasma adrenaline without affecting the rise in plasma noradrenaline concentration, yet only partially suppressed the rise in plasma glucose concentration that occurs in response to CRF. It follows that the hyperglycemic effect of CRF was due mainly to the release of noradrenaline from sympathetic postganglionic nerve terminals and only partially, if at all, to the release of adrenaline from the adrenal medulla. It was further established that the effect did not depend on the release of any hormone from the anterior pituitary, the renin–angiotensin system, or circulating vasopressin. This action of CRF can therefore be distinguished from the hyperglycemic effects of other peptides, such as bombesin, thyrotropin-releasing hormone, and β-endorphin, following intraventricular administration, as they are largely dependent on the release of adrenaline from the adrenal medulla (Brown et al., 1982). In dogs, intraventricular administration of CRF also causes a rise in heart rate and aortic blood pressure, both of which depend on activation of the sympathetic system. The fact that the peptide must act directly within the central nervous system is evidenced by the fact that intravenous administration produces a fall in arterial blood pressure, due to a direct vasodilator action in certain vascular beds, which is associated with a reflex tachycardia (Brown and Fisher, 1983).

Immunocytochemical studies in the rat have shown that CRF immunoreactive nerve cell bodies are concentrated in four main sites in the brain: the paraventricular hypothalamic nucleus, the central nucleus of the amygdala, the substantia innominata, and the bed nucleus of the stria terminalis (Olschowka et al., 1982; Swanson et al., 1983; Sakanaka et al., 1987; Figure 16-8). The CRF neurons of the paraventricular hypothalamic nucleus are concentrated in the medial parvocellular and periventricular regions. These areas project to the external lamina of the median eminence and represent the neuroanatomical substrate that is involved in the control of ACTH secretion from the anterior pituitary. Although this accounts for 80% of the CRF neurons in this hypothalamic nucleus, another 15% are localized in the magnocellular division of the paraventricular nucleus, which projects to the posterior pituitary, and the remaining 5% are found in the lateral and dorsal parvocellular subdivision that projects to the medullary and spinal autonomic centers. The CRF neurons in the magnocellular subdivision are concentrated mainly in the part of the nucleus where the neurons that contain oxytocin are found with fewer in the vasopressin area. Some of these cells contain both oxytocin and CRF (Swanson et al., 1983) whereas others contain both vasopressin and CRF (Gillies and Lowry, 1986).

The CRF parvocellular hypothalamic-median eminence pathway appears to be uniquely sensitive to changes in cortisol levels. Adrenalectomy increases the amount of CRF in both the cell bodies and the fibers of this pathway alone without noticeably affecting the other CRF pathways either in the hypothalamus or elsewhere in the brain (Swanson et al., 1983; see Swanson et al., 1986 for review). This is entirely consistent with the presumed function of

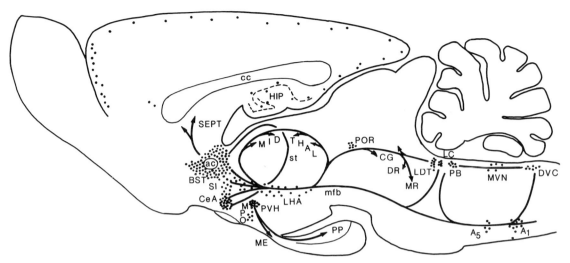

Figure 16-8 Sagittal drawing of the rat brain illustrating the principal CRF-stained cell groups (black dots) (redrawn after Swanson et al., 1982). A_1, A_5, noradrenergic cell groups; BST, bed nucleus of the stria terminalis; CeA, central nucleus of the amygdala; CG, central geniculate; DR, dorsal raphe; DVC, dorsal vagal complex; HIP, hippocampus; LC, locus coeruleus; LDT, laterodorsal tegmental nucleus; LHA, lateral hypothalamic area; ME, median eminence; MPO, medial preoptic area; MR, median raphe; MVN, medial vestibular nucleus; PB, parabrachial nucleus; POR, perioculomotor nucleus; PP, posterior pituitary; PVH, paraventricular hypothalamic nucleus; SEPT, septal region; SI, substantia innominata; ac, anterior commissure; cc, corpus callosum; mfb, medial forebrain bundle; st, stria terminalis.

these cells in the control of the pituitary–adrenal axis.

CRF immunoreactive nerve fibers are found in a number of sites in the central nervous system. They are present in laminae I and II of the spinal cord (Olschowka et al., 1982: Schipper et al., 1983), but there is only one report of CRF immunoreactive fibers in the intermediolateral cell column (Merchenthaler et al., 1983). At this time it is not clear whether this represents a false positive or results from superior histochemical staining. Accordingly, it is not possible to provide a precise description of the route by which centrally administered CRF excites the sympathetic system.

CRF neurons outside the hypothalamus may subserve functions that are complimentary to the CRF hypothalamic neurons. This proposition gains credence from the fact that intraventricular injections of CRF induce a pattern of behavioral changes in rats and monkeys that would be entirely appropriate responses to stress. In rodents, intraventricular injections of CRF induce patterns of behavior reminiscent of anxiety, expression of which is dependent on the environment. In a familiar environment, CRF increases locomotion, rearing, and self-grooming, reproducing the sort of behavior that rats normally exhibit when they are transferred to a strange place (Koob and Bloom, 1985). In a novel environment, CRF decreased locomotion, rearing, and feeding, and increased self-grooming. Both types of behavioral response were reduced by tranquilizing agents.

Injections of minute amounts of CRF into the arcuate nucleus or mesencephalic central gray area of estrogen-treated female rats caused decreased sexual receptivity. CRF produced arousal in monkeys when they were restrained in a chair, but these animals became behaviorally inhibited in response to the peptide when unrestrained in a familiar environment (Kalin, 1985). Thus, the effect of CRF was environment dependent in both species, even though the type of behavior elicited was different: arousal in rodents in a familiar environment and inhibition in the monkeys under the same conditions. It was more recently established that stress-induced fighting in rats is facilitated by quite small doses of CRF administered intraventricularly and, even more significantly, that the CRF antagonist α-helical CRF^{2-41} blocks this behavioral response to high levels of stress (Tazi et al., 1987). This and other evidence strongly suggests that at least under conditions of great arousal, release of CRF within the central nervous system contributes to the behavioral response to stress, in addition to pituitary and sympathetic responses.

Other peptides have also been implicated in the central activation of the sympathetic system. One is bombesin, which, like CRF, causes an increase in the concentration of adrenaline in the circulating plasma following intraventricular administration in the rat. Unlike CRF, it causes a rise in plasma noradrenaline concentration only in relatively high doses. Like CRF, intraventricular injections of bombesin cause hyperglucagonemia and hyperglycemia, but, unlike CRF, both responses depend mainly on the release of adrenaline from the adrenal medulla and are abolished by prior adrenalectomy (Brown and Fisher, 1984). Numerous studies have indicated that the adrenal medulla exhibits a much higher threshold to certain forms of stress (ether anesthesia, exposure to cold, hemorrhage, hypoxia, hypercapnia, and others) than does the rest of the sympathetic system. However, other forms of stress, such as severe hypoglycemia, hypoglycemia combined with cold exposure, acute (but not chronic) hypoxia, and acute ischemic injury, preferentially stimulate the release of adrenal catecholamines while concomitantly suppressing peripheral sympathetic nervous activity (Young et al., 1984). These differences can now be explained by the fact that adrenal activation is probably accomplished via central pathways quite different from those involved in integrating the activity of the rest of the sympathetic system.

The Importance of the Pattern of Nervous Activity

Studies of the effects of stimulation of the peripheral end of the splanchnic nerve have shown that the pattern of the stimulus is an important determinant of adrenal medullary responses (Bloom et al., 1988). This is particularly marked in the case of the release of enkephalins, which is roughly doubled by stimulating intermittently in bursts. In the case of the catecholamines, stimulation in bursts was found to increase the output of both adrenaline and noradrenaline and led to the secretion of proportionately more noradrenaline (Figure 16-9). It has fre-

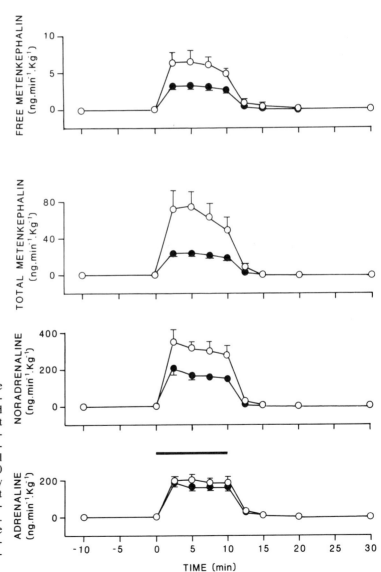

Figure 16-9 Comparison of the changes in mean free and total met[5]-enkephalin-like immunoreactivity and noradrenaline and adrenaline output from the right adrenal gland in conscious 3- to 6-week-old calves in response to stimulation of the peripheral end of the right splanchnic nerve for 10 minutes at either 4 Hz continuously (●, $n = 8$) or at 40 Hz for 1 second at 10-second intervals (○, $n = 7$). Horizontal bar: duration of stimulation. Vertical bars: SE of each mean value where these exceed the size of the stimulus. (After Bloom et al., 1988, by permission of the *Journal of Physiology*.)

quently been reported that the proportions in which these amines are released vary with the particular type of stimulus employed; this observation provides a possible mechanism whereby this might be achieved, without invoking the idea that separate pathways control separate types of chromaffin cells, although the existence of such separate pathways remains an open question. Small amounts of dopamine and a related metabolite, DOPAC, were also released from the adrenal gland in response to splanchnic nerve stimulation, and the average mean output of dopamine during stimulation in bursts was significantly greater than during continuous stimulation (Bloom et al., 1988).

THE ENDOCRINE PANCREAS

The pancreatic islets, or islets of Langerhans, are small ovoid clusters of endocrine cells scattered irregularly between the acini of the exocrine pancreas. Four types of cells are found in a typical islet: α- or A-cells that produce glucagon, β- or B-cells that make insulin, D-cells that synthesize somatostatin, and PP-cells that produce pancreatic polypeptide. The α-cells secrete glucagon, which causes an elevation of blood glucose levels, and so opposes the hypoglycemic effect of insulin, most immediately by stimulating hepatic glycogenolysis, but also by promoting gluconeogenesis and lipolysis. The β-cells secrete insulin, which promotes the uptake of glucose by peripheral cells and so exerts a hypoglycemic effect. Pancreatectomy leads to death from diabetes mellitus, unless insulin therapy is instituted, illustrating the imperative nature of this mechanism. The D-cells produce somatostatin, which is thought to modulate the release of insulin and glucagon via a paracrine type of action. Finally, pancreatic polypeptide-producing cells are widely distributed in the gatrsointestinal tract. They are found in the pancreatic islets, in the exocrine part of the pancreas, and in the gut. This hormone has been shown to exert actions opposite to pancreozymin–cholecystokinin (CCK) and inhibits both gallbladder contractions and exocrine pancreatic secretions. The release of pancreatic polypeptide is controlled by the vagal cholinergic motor system and is regulated by food intake and blood glucose concentrations (see review by Schwartz, 1983). Since relatively little is known about the CNS control mechanisms, it will not be considered in detail here.

The neural control of the islets of Langerhans has been the subject of several reviews (see Miller, 1981; Edwards, 1984; Edwards and Bloom, 1985; Ahrén et al., 1986).

Cholinergic, Adrenergic, and Peptidergic Mechanisms

The importance of the innervation to the pancreatic islets could well be predicted from its density and the intimacy of contact between islet cells and neural elements, which not infrequently results in the formation of "neuroinsular" complexes, as was first recognized by Langerhans (see Table 16-1); for a detailed discussion of the relevant microanatomy see Miller's (1981) review. Physiological studies have established that stimulation of the vagal parasympathetic outflow causes the release of insulin, glucagon, and pancreatic polypeptide, which may be mediated by activation of muscarinic receptors (dog and calf) or by peptidergic transmission implicating VIP and gastrin/CCK (pig, mouse, and probably humans). Stimulation of the sympathetic innervation inhibits release of insulin by an α-adrenergic mechanism and stimulates the release of glucagon and pancreatic polypeptide by α- or β-adrenergic and/or peptidergic mechanisms depending on the species. It is widely

Table 16-1 Pancreatic Neuroendocrine Effector Mechanisms

Neural Pathway	Pancreatic Peptide	Response[a]	Transmitter Mechanisms
Parasympathetic	Insulin	+	Muscarinic[b]
Sympathetic	Insulin	−	α_2-Adrenergic[b]
Sympathetic	Insulin	+	β_2-Adrenergic[b]
Parasympathetic	Glucagon	+	Muscarinic[b]
Sympathetic	Glucagon	+	α_1-Adrenergic[b] ⎫
		+	β_2-Adrenergic ⎬ Species variable
Parasympathetic	Pancreatic polypeptide	+	Muscarinic?[b]
Sympathetic	Pancreatic polypeptide	±	α-Adrenergic,[b] response depends on species
		+	β-Adrenergic
Parasympathetic	Somatostatin	±	Muscarinic?,[b] response depends on species and preparation
Sympathetic	Somatostatin	−	α_1-Adrenergic[b]
Sympathetic	Somatostatin	+	β-Adrenergic

[a] +, stimulation; −, inhibition.

[b] And/or peptidergic in one or more species.

recognized that sympathetic stimulation leads to release of insulin following α-adrenoceptor blockade by a mechanism dependent on β-adrenoceptor activation, but this cannot account for the release of insulin, which occurs in response to splanchnic nerve

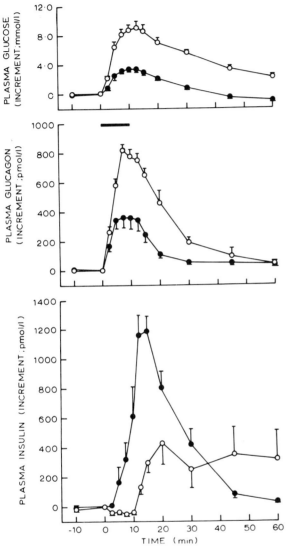

Figure 16-10 Comparison of the changes in mean arterial plasma glucose, pancreatic glucagon, and insulin concentration in conscious adrenalectomized 3- to 6-week-old calves in response to stimulation of the peripheral ends of the splanchnic nerves at 40 Hz for 1 second at 10-second intervals for 10 minutes. O, control calves (n = 6). ●, calves pretreated with propranolol (0.25 mg kg^{-1}) and phentolamine (1.0 mg kg^{-1} and 0.02 mg min^{-1} kg^{-1}, n = 8). Horizontal bar: duration of stimulus. Vertical bars: SE of each mean value. Absolute values at time = 0 in the control group: glucose, 4.3 ± 0.4 mmol/liter; glucagon, 35 ± 8 pmol/liter; insulin, 66 ± 19 pmol/liter. In the group pretreated with propranolol and phentolamine: glucose, 2.7 ± 0.5 mmol/liters; glucagon, 35 ± 8 pmol/liter; insulin, 54 ± 13 pmol/liter. (From Bloom and Edwards, 1984, by permission of the *Journal of Physiology.*)

stimulation in bursts in the calf following the administration of fully effective doses of both propranolol and phentolamine, as illustrated in Figure 16-10. All the evidence suggests that this is mediated by the release of a mammalian bombesin-like peptide from sympathetic postganglionic nerve terminals, either in the pancreas itself or arriving via the blood supply following release elsewhere in the splanchnic region (Bloom and Edwards, 1984). Release of a bombesin-like peptide is unaffected by total adrenergic blockage (Figure 16-11) and the rise in the concentration of the peptide in the plasma during splanchnic nerve stimulation in bursts is sufficient to account for the rise in both plasma insulin and glucagon concentration that occur under these conditions.

Role of the Parasympathetic Innervation

The vagal innervation of the rat pancreas comes solely from the dorsal vagal nucleus (Rineman and Miselis, 1987). Comparable studies have not been done in other species yet. The principal transmitter involved in this system is thought to be acetylcholine. In conscious animals, the release of insulin in response to hyperglycemia is substantially reduced by pretreatment with atropine in species in which transmission is cholinergic. Furthermore, it is well suited to a homeostatic role as the efficacy of increased vagal activity is determined by the existing levels of certain metabolites. Raising the plasma glucose concentration by about 100% completely inhibits the glucagon response to vagal stimulation in the conscious calf and substantially enhances the release of insulin (Figure 16-12), presumably by increasing muscarinic binding sites (Ostenson and Grill, 1987). The glucagon response is restored, without affecting insulin secretion significantly, by intravenous infusions of physiological amounts of a balanced mixture of amino acids, illustrating the specificity of these metabolic modulations. Stimulation via the parasympathetic rather than the sympathetic innervation is also largely responsible for the rise in plasma pancreatic polypeptide concentration that occurs during and after a meal.

Several peptides have been implicated as transmitters in the control of the islets. In the case of the parasympathetic innervation, the evidence is most compelling in respect to VIP. This peptide is co-localized with acetylcholine in certain parasympathetic postganglionic nerve terminals, such as those in the submandibular gland of the cat (Lundberg et al., 1980). In some species, such as the calf, all the pancreatic endocrine responses that are vagally mediated are abolished by atropine in spite of the fact that VIP is released during vagal stimulation, suggesting that transmission is cholinergic. In humans, in which the release of insulin in response to intra-

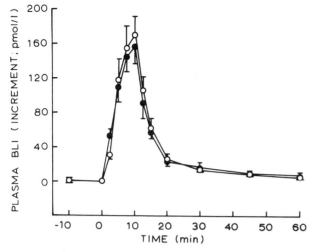

Figure 16-11 Comparison of the changes in mean arterial plasma bombesin-like immunoreactivity (BLI) of 3- to 6-week-old conscious adrenalectomized calves in response to stimulation of the peripheral ends of the splanchnic nerves at 40 Hz for 1 second at 10-second intervals for 10 minutes. O, normal control calves ($n = 6$). ●, calves pretreated with propranolol (0.25 mg kg^{-1}) and phentolamine (1.0 mg kg^{-1} and 0.02 mg min^{-1} kg^{-1}, $n = 8$). The absolute value at time $= 0$ in the control calves was 7 ± 2 pmol/liter and in the other group was 25 ± 3 pmol/liter. (From Bloom and Edwards, 1984, by permission of the *Journal of Physiology*.)

venous glucose is not much affected by atropine, VIP is present in fine nerve terminals throughout the gland and in particularly high concentrations in the islets (Bishop et al., 1980). The peptide stimulates the release of insulin, glucagon, somatostatin, and pancreatic polypeptide (Szecowka et al., 1980; Fahrenkrug et al., 1987). It also strongly potentiates glucagon release in response to carbachol in conscious mice, suggesting that neurally released acetylcholine and VIP might interact in a similar way (Ahrén and Lundquist, 1982), as they are thought to do in the submandibular gland in the cat (Lundberg et al., 1982). This potentiation seems to be quite specific as VIP has no effect on insulin release in response to carbachol in this species (Ahrén and Lundquist, 1981).

In the pig, numerous nerve fibers found in the islet stain with antisera raised against the COOH-terminal tetrapeptide, which is common to cholecystokinin and the gastrins (Larsson, 1979; Rehfeld et al., 1980). These nerve fibers release a low-molecular-weight form of cholecystokinin (presumed to be tetrin) that is a potent stimulant to glucagon and insulin secretion and also exerts important trophic effects on the islets (Rehfeld, 1971; Rehfeld and Lindkaer-Jensen, 1980). The possible roles of other neuropeptides in the control of the endocrine pancreas have been reviewed by Wood et al. (1983) and Ahrén et al. (1986).

Role of the Sympathetic Innervation

No doubt activity of the sympathetic innervation during exercise or in response to stress leads to mobilization of liver glycogen, in part by promoting the release of glucagon and inhibiting the release of insulin, but this is not to say that it does not also contribute a tonic input to the responses to glycemic

stimuli. In both calves and lambs, the release of insulin in response to intravenous glucose is effectively suppressed by pretreatment with propranolol, so long as the splanchnic nerves are intact and phentolamine is not given as well (Bloom and Edwards, 1982, 1985; Figure 16-13). It follows that the release of insulin in response to exogenous glucose is normally modified by both sympathetic α-adrenergic inhibition and β-adrenergic excitation.

Evidence that the central nervous system normally exerts a tonic inhibitory influence on insulin release, presumably via the sympathetic innervation, was obtained by Curry (1983) in an isolated perfused rat pancreas preparation when glucose-induced insulin secretion was compared before and after functional ablation of the central nervous system. The sympathetic innervation may also exert important trophic effects on the pancreatic islets because it has been shown that release of insulin in response to glucose from isolated perfused islets is reduced in tissue taken from rats treated with 6-hydroxydopamine a month previously, which destroys the sympathetic nerve terminals (Burr et al., 1974).

Somatostatin

The secretion of somatostatin from the D cells in the pancreatic islets is also modified by stimulation of the autonomic innervation, being inhibited by vagal or cholinergic and by α-adrenergic stimulation and stimulated by β-adrenergic stimulation (Samols and Wier, 1979; Samols et al., 1981; Holst et al., 1981). This peptide itself exerts a potent inhibitory effect on the release of all three of the pancreatic hormones. This is difficult to reconcile with the effects of adrenergic stimulation because α-adrenergic stimulation, which strongly inhibits insulin release, also inhibits the release of somatostatin, and β-adrenergic stimu-

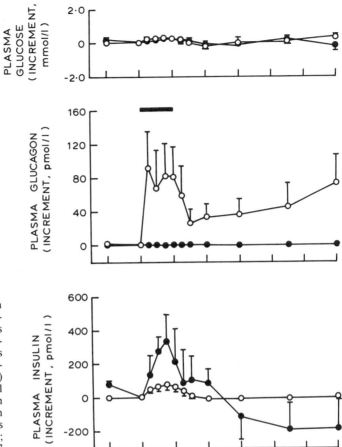

Figure 16-12 Comparison of the changes in mean arterial plasma glucose, pancreatic glucagon, and insulin concentration in conscious 3- to 6-week-old calves in response to stimulation of the peripheral ends of the vagus nerves (40 Hz for 1 second at 10 second intervals for 10 minutes) in the presence (●, $n = 6$) and absence of exogenous glucose (○, 0.5 mmol min^{-1} kg^{-1}, $n = 10$). Horizontal bar: duration of stimulation. Vertical bars: SE of each mean value. Absolute values at time = 0 in calves given glucose: glucose, 5.6 ± 0.8 mmol/liter; glucagon, 1 ± 1 pmol/liter; insulin, 29 ± 7 pmol/liter. (From Bloom and Edwards, 1985, by permission of the *Journal of Physiology*.)

lation, which strongly potentiates the secretion of insulin, also promotes the release of somatostatin. Intravenous infusions of the peptide completely block the release of insulin, glucagon, and pancreatic polypeptide in response to vagal stimulation, whereas release of glucagon in response to stimulation of the sympathetic innervation is unaffected. There is evidence to suggest that the hormonal blockade is achieved by blockage of acetylcholine release from the parasympathetic postganglionic nerve terminals, but this can occur only in restricted regions, as there are numerous other responses that are mediated by muscarinic receptors that are unaffected by somatostatin.

Hormonal Factors

In addition to effects that the autonomic innervation produces directly on the islet cells, release of pancreatic hormones is affected by the release of gastrointestinal hormones during digestion. Hormones such as gastric inhibitory peptide, gastrin, neurotensin,

peptide histidine methionine, and peptide YY, which are released from the gastrointestinal tract in response to oral ingestion of glucose but not intravenous administration of glucose, produce insulinotropic effects (Shuster et al., 1988). This effect—termed the incretin effect—functions as another mechanism that modifies the responses of both α- and β-pancreatic cells. Whether this gut hormonal system is controlled by the intrinsic neurons of the gut is not yet resolved. In any event, it functions as another physiological system that modulates the β-pancreatic and possibly other pancreatic cells.

Central Mechanisms of Islet Control

Afferent Signals

The idea that the pancreatic islets are controlled principally via their autonomic innervation implies the existence of a central control mechanism that is, either directly or reflexly, more sensitive to appropriate signals than the α- and β-pancreatic cells

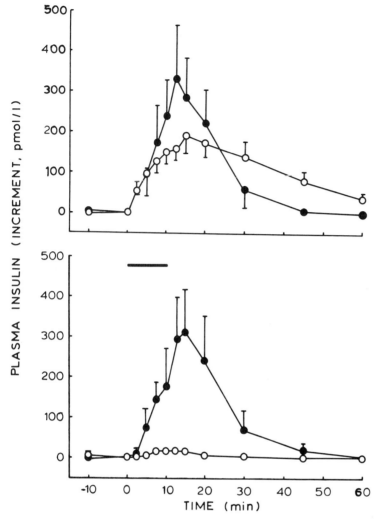

Figure 16-13 Upper panel: comparison of the changes in mean arterial plasma insulin concentration in response to exogenous glucose (0.83 mmol kg^{-1} and 0.05 mmol min^{-1} kg^{-1} iv for 10 minutes) in normal conscious 2- to 6-week-old calves (O, $n = 7$) and calves given phentolamine (0.1 mg kg^{-1} and 0.02 mg min^{-1} kg^{-1}) and propranolol (0.25 mg kg$^-$; ●, n = 7). Lower panel: comparison of the same responses to the same dose of glucose in calves given either propranolol (0.25 mg kg^{-1}, $n = 7$, O) or phentolamine (0.1 mg kg^{-1} and 0.02 mg min^{-1} kg^{-1}, $n = 6$, ●) alone. Horizontal bar: duration of glucose infusion. Vertical bars: SE of each mean value where these exceed the size of the symbol. Absolute values at time = 0: control group, 19 ± 6 pmol/liter; phentolamine + propranolol, 21 ± 1 pmol/liter; propranolol alone, 21 ± pmol/liter; phentolamine alone, 22 ± 1 pmol/liter. (From Bloom and Edwards, 1985; by permission of the *Journal of Physiology.*)

themselves. In the case of both insulin and glucagon release, glucose is obviously one such stimulus, and it is now clear that glucose-sensitive neural elements exist both centrally and peripherally (see reviews by Cryer, 1983; Oomura, 1983; Rohner-Jeanrenaud et al., 1983; Oomura and Yoshimatsu, 1984; Niijima, 1986; Shimazu, 1986).

Central glucoreceptors are located in the lateral hypothalamic area and in the ventromedial hypothalamic nucleus, exhibiting responses opposite to glucose in those two locations. In the lateral hypothalamic area, in which about 25% of the neurons are glucose sensitive, their action is suppressed by direct iontophoretic application of glucose, whereas the activity of those in the ventromedial hypothalamic nucleus is enhanced in a dose-dependent fashion by the same procedure. Other central glucose receptors, of both types, have been identified in the nucleus tractus solitarius.

In the periphery, glucoreceptors have been found

in both the liver and duodenum, with afferent fibers projecting to the nucleus tractus solitarius via the vagi. These respond to glucose with a reduction in firing rate and appear to facilitate the activity of neurons in the lateral hypothalamic area, which are themselves inhibited by glucose, administered either directly or indirectly, via afferents in the portal system. It appears that both central and peripheral "glucoreceptors" are in fact capable of responding not only to other metabolites, such as free fatty acids, but also to insulin and glucagon; those whose discharge is inhibited by gluc se are facilitated by insulin and inhibited by gluca 1. Thus, there is abundant evidence of the existence of a highly sophisticated glycemic sensory system.

Integration

Integration occurs at the level of the hypothalamus, involving the ventromedial hypothalamic nucleus and lateral hypothalamic area in particular, with im-

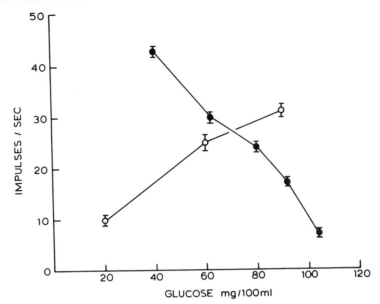

Figure 16-14 The relation between arterial blood glucose concentration and the discharge rate in efferent filaments of the adrenal nerve (●) and the pancreatic branch of the vagus nerve (○) in anesthetized rabbits. Vertical bars: SE of each mean value. (After Niijima, 1975.)

portant inputs from the nucleus tractus solitarius. The relatively crude techniques of stimulation and lesioning have revealed that increased activity of the ventromedial hypothalamic nucleus results in hyperglycemia and hyperglucagonemia, whereas lesions in the lateral hypothalamic area lead to hyperinsulinism, which correlates with the close association that exists between this nucleus and the sympathetic system. Conversely, activity of the lateral hypothalamic area appears to be mediated, at least in part, via the parasympathetic system. An element of reciprocity between the activity in these two nuclei may exist, but it would be naive to suppose that this is of primary importance in such a complex control system. The effect of this integration is illustrated by neural recordings from efferent branches of the vagus and splanchnic nerves, showing how closely, but inversely, the rate of firing in each can be related to plasma glucose concentration (Niijima, 1975; Figure 16-14).

SUMMARY

The autonomic nervous system plays an important part in controlling the activity of both of these endocrine glands. In the adrenal medulla, the control exerted by the sympathetic preganglionic fibers appears to be more subtle than has hitherto been supposed. The pattern of activity seems to be an important determinant of the response. Intermittent high-frequency stimulation of sympathetic fibers innervating the adrenal gland causes the release of noradrenaline and the enkephalins. In particular, it potentiates the release of the large-molecular-weight

forms of enkephalin that have sufficiently long half-lives to enable them to reach peripheral tissues in biologically effective amounts. These responses are regulated by sympathoadrenal preganglionic neurons that are modulated by local spinal interneurons as well as five CNS regions: the caudal raphe nucleus, ventromedial medulla, rostral ventrolateral medulla, A5 cell group, and paraventricular hypothalamic nucleus.

In the adrenal cortex, the steroidogenic response to ACTH is strongly potentiated by some neural mechanism, yet to be identified with certainty, and the sensitivity of the cells to the steroidogenic action of ACTH is substantially reduced by denervating the gland. If the neural pathway has a higher threshold to certain "stresses" than ACTH, it may serve to increase the gain on the pituitary–adrenal cortical axis above a certain level of stress.

In the pancreatic islets, evidence exists that glucose is not the sole controlling mechanism of glucagon and insulin release. Clearly, it is a major factor, but it is the autonomic innervation that provides the direct signals to the α- (glucagon) and β- (insulin) cells together with certain hormonal factors released from the gut. Both divisions of the autonomic nervous system influence the basal rate of glucagon and insulin release by virtue of tonic activity at rest, but they subserve different roles. Responses to glycemic stimuli are mediated primarily via the vagal parasympathetic supply, whereas pancreatic endocrine responses to situations such as exercise or stress are mediated via the sympathetic innervation. Particular areas of the brain, especially the ventromedial and lateral hypothalamic areas that are directly sensitive to glucose plasma levels and also receive afferent information from peripheral glucose receptors, function to integrate both divisions of the autonomic nervous system in such a way as to affect the release of glucagon and insulin from the pancreas and catecholamines from the adrenal gland.

REFERENCES

Reviews

Ahrén, B., Taborsky, G. J., and Porte, D. (1986). Neuropeptide versus cholinergic and adrenergic regulation of islet hormone secretion. *Diabetologia* 29, 827–836.

Brown, M. R., and Fisher, L. A. (1985). Corticotropin releasing factor: Effects on the autonomic nervous system and visceral systems. *Federation Proceedings* 44, 243–248.

Cannon, W. B., (1929). *Bodily Changes in Pain, Hunger, Fear and Rage. An Account of Recent Researches into the Function of Emotional Excitement,* 2nd Ed. New York, Appleton, 404 pp.

Cryer, P. E. (1983). Coordinated responses of glucogenic hormones to central glucopenia: The role of the sympathoadrenal system. *Advances in Metabolic Disorders* 10, 469–483.

Edwards, A. V. (1984). Neural control of the endocrine pancreas. In: *Recent Advances in Physiology 10,* P. F. Baker (ed.), Churchill Livingstone, London, pp. 277–315.

Edwards, A. V., and Bloom, S. R. (1985). Autonomic regulation of insulin secretion. *Trends in Autonomic Physiology* 3, 129–145.

Edwards, A. V., Anderson, P.-O., Järhult, J., and Bloom, S. R. (1984). Studies of the importance of the pattern of autonomic stimulation in relation to alimentary effectors. *Quarterly Journal of Experimental Physiology* 69, 607–614.

Ganong, W. F. (1974). Minireview: The role of catecholamines and acetylcholine in the regulation of endocrine function. *Life Sciences* 15, 1401–1414.

Gillies, G. E., and Lowry, P. J. (1986). Adrenal function. In: *Neuroendocrinology,* S. L. Lightman and B. J. Everitt (eds.), Blackwell Scientific Publications, Oxford, pp. 360–388.

Holzwarth M. A., Cunningham, L. A., and Kleitman, N. (1987). The role of the adrenal nerves in the regulation of adrenal cortical functions. *Annals of the New York Acadmey of Sciences* 512, 449–464.

McEwen, B. S., DeKloet, E. R., and Rostene, W. (1986). Adrenal steroid receptors and actions in the nervous system. *Physiological Reviews* 66, 1121–1188.

Miller, R. E. (1981). Pancreatic neuroendocrinology: Peripheral neural mechanisms in the regulation of the islets of Langerhans. *Endocrine Reviews* 2, 471–494.

Niijima, A. (1986). Neural control of blood glucose level. *Japanese Journal of Physiology* 36, 827–841.

Niijima, A., and Mei, N. (1987). Glucose sensors in viscera and control of blood glucose level. *News in Physiological Sciences* 2, 164–167.

Oomura, Y. (1983). Glucose as a regulator of neuronal activity. *Advances in Metabolic Disorders* 10, 31–65.

Rohner-Jeanrenaud, F., Bobbioni, E., Ionescu, E., Sauter, J.-F., and Jeanrenaud, B. (1983). Central nervous system regulation of insulin secretion. *Advances in Metabolic Disorders* 10, 193–220.

Schwartz, T. W. (1983). Pancreatic polypeptide: A hormone under vagal control. *Gastroenterology* 85, 1411–1425.

Shimazu, T. (1986). Intermediate metabolism. In: *Neuroendocrinology,* S. L. Lightman and B. J. Everitt (eds.), Blackwell Scientific Publications, Oxford, pp. 304–330.

Swanson, L. W., Sawchenko, P. E., and Lind, R. W. (1986). Regulation of multiple peptides in CRF parvocellular neurosecretory neurons: Implications for the stress response. *Progress in Brain Research* 68, 169–190.

Unsicker, K. (1986). Differentiation and phenotypical conversion of adrenal medullary cells: The effects of neuronotrophic, neurite promoting, hormonal and neuronal signals. In: *Neurohistochemistry: Modern Methods and Applications,* Liss, New York, pp. 183–206.

Unsicker, K., and Leitze, R. (1987). Chromaffin cells: Modified neurons that are both targets and storage sites of neuronotrophic and neurite promoting factors. In: *Nato ASI Series H, Vol. 2, Glial-Neuronal Communication in Development and Regeneration,* H. H. Althaus and W. Seifert (eds.), Springer-Verlag, Berlin.

Wood, S. M., Polak, J. M., and Bloom, S. R. (1983). Neuropeptides in the control of the islets of Langerhans. *Advances in Metabolic Disorders* 10, 401–420.

Research Papers

Ahrén, B., and Lundquist, I. (1981). Effects of vasoactive intestinal polypeptide (VIP), secretin and gastrin on insulin secretion in the mouse. *Diabetologia* 20, 54–59.

Ahrén, B. and Lundquist, I. (1982). Interaction of vasoactive intestinal peptide (VIP), with cholinergic stimulation of glucagon secretion. *Experientia* 38, 405–406.

Allen, J. M., Adrian, T. E., Polak, J. M., and Bloom, S. R. (1983). Neuropeptide Y in the adrenal gland. *Journal of the Autonomic Nervous System* 9, 559–563.

Appel, N. M., Wessendorf, M. W., and Elde, R. P. (1986). Co-existence of serotonin- and substance P-like immunoreactivity in nerve fibres apposing identified sympathoadrenal preganglionic neurones in rat intermediolateral column. *Neuroscience Letters* 65, 241–246.

Bishop. A. E., Polak, J. M., Green, I. C., Bryant, M. G., and Bloom, S. R. (1980). The location of VIP in the pancreas of man and rat. *Diabetologia* 18, 73–78.

Blessing, W. W., Oliver, J. R., Hodgson, A. H., Joh, T. H., and Willoughby, J. O. (1987). Neuropeptide Y-like immunoreactive C1 neurons in the rostral ventrolateral medulla of the rabbit project to sympathetic preganglionic neurons in the spinal cord. *Journal of the Autonomic Nervous System* 18, 121–129.

Bloom, S. R., and Edwards, A. V. (1982). Effects of the autonomic nervous system on insulin release in response to exogenous glucose in weaned lambs. *Journal of Physiology (London)* 327, 421–429.

Bloom, S. R., and Edwards, A. V. (1984). Characteristics of the neuroendocrine responses to stimulation of the splanchnic nerves in bursts in the conscious calf. *Journal of Physiology (London)* 346, 533–545.

Bloom, S. R., and Edwards, A. V. (1985). Effects of certain

metabolites on pancreatic endocrine responses to stimulation of the vagus nerves in conscious calves. *Journal of Physiology (London)* 362, 303–310.

Bloom, S. R., Edwards, A. V., and Ghatei, M. A. (1984). Neuroendocrine responses to stimulation of the splanchnic nerves in bursts in the conscious adrenalectomized calf. *Journal of Physiology (London)* 346, 519–531.

Bloom, S. R., Edwards, A. V., and Jones, C. T. (1988). The adrenal contribution to the neuroendocrine responses to splanchnic nerve stimulation in conscious calves. *Journal of Physiology (London)* 397, 513–526.

Breslow, M. J., Jordan, D. A., Thellman, S. T., and Traystman, R. J. (1987). Neural control of adrenal medullary and cortical blood flow during hemorrhage. *American Journal of Physiology* 252, H521–H528.

Brown, M. R., and Fisher, L. A. (1983). Central nervous system effects of corticotropin releasing factor in the dog. *Brain Research* 280, 75–79.

Brown, M. R., and Fisher, L. A. (1984). Brain peptide regulation of adrenal epinephrine secretion. *American Journal of Physiology* 247, E41–46.

Brown, M. R., Fisher, L. A., Spiess, J., Rivier, C., Rivier, J., and Vale, W. (1928). Corticotropin-releasing factor: Actions on the sympathetic nervous system and metabolism. *Endocrinology* 111, 928–931.

Brown, M. R., Gray, T. S., and Fisher, L. A. (1986). Corticotropin releasing factor receptor antagonist: Effects on the autonomic nervous system and cardiovascular function. *Regulatory Peptides* 16, 321–329.

Bruhn, T. O., Engeland, W. C., Anthony, E. L. P., Gann, D. S., and Jackson, I. M. D. (1987a). Corticotropin-releasing factor in the dog adrenal medulla is secreted in response to hemorrhage. *Endocrinology* 120, 25–33.

Bruhn, T. O., Engeland, W. C., Anthony, E. L. P., Gann, D. S., and Jackson, I. M. D. (1987b). Corticotropin releasing factor in the adrenal medulla. *Annals of the New York Academy of Sciences* 512, 115–128.

Burr, I. M., Jackson, A., Culbert, S., Sharp, R., Felts, P., and Olson, W. (1974). Glucose intolerance and impaired insulin release following 6-hydroxydopamine administration to intact rats. *Endocrinology* 94, 1072–1076.

Cunningham, L. A., and Holzwarth, M. A. (1988). Vasoactive intestinal peptide stimulates adrenal aldosterone and corticosterone secretion. *Endocrinology* 122, 2090–2097.

Curry, D. L. (1983). Direct tonic inhibition of insulin secretion by central nervous system. *American Journal of Physiology* 244, E425–429.

Dallman, M. F., Engeland, W. C., and Shinsako, J. (1976). Compensatory adrenal growth: A neurally mediated reflex. *American Journal of Physiology* 231, 408–414.

Dallman, M. F., Engeland, W. C., and McBride, M. H. (1977). The neural regulation of compensatory adrenal growth. *Annals of the New York Academy of Sciences* 297, 373–392.

Darlington, D. N., Shinsako, J., and Dallman, M. F. (1988). Paraventricular lesions: Hormonal and cardiovascular responses to hemorrhage. *Brain Research* 439, 289–301.

Dempsher, D. F., and Gann, D. S. (1983). Increased cortisol secretion after small hemorrhage is not attributable to changes in ACTH. *Endocrinology* 113, 86–93.

Edwards, A. V., and Jones, C. T. (1987a). The effect of splanchnic nerve stimulation on adrenocortical activity in conscious calves. *Journal of Physiology (London)* 382, 385–396.

Edwards, A. V., and Jones, C. T. (1987b). The effect of splanchnic nerve section on the sensitivity of the adrenal cortex to adrenocorticotrophin in the calf. *Journal of Physiology (London)* 390, 23–31.

Edwards, A. V., and Jones, C. T. (1987c). Adrenal cortical responses to vasoactive intestinal peptide in conscious hypophysectomized calves. *Journal of Physiology (London)* 391, 441–450.

Edwards, A. V., and Jones, C. T. (1988). Secretion of corticotrophin releasing factor from the adrenal during splanchnic nerve stimulation in conscious calves. *Journal of Physiology (London)* 400, 89–100.

Edwards, A. V., Hardy, R. N., and Malinowska, K. W. (1974). The effects of infusions of synthetic adrenocorticotrophin in the conscious calf. *Journal of Physiology (London)* 239, 477–498.

Edwards, A. V., Jones, C. T., and Bloom, S. R. (1986). Reduced adrenal cortical sensitivity to ACTH in lambs with cut splanchnic nerves. *Journal of Endocrinology* 110, 81–85.

Engeland, W. C., Lilly, M. P., and Gann, D. S. (1985). Sympathetic adrenal denervation decreases adrenal blood flow without altering the cortisol response to hemorrhage. *Endocrinology* 117, 1000–1010.

Fahrenkrug, J., Holst, J., Pedersen, Y., Yamashita, Y., Ottesen, B., Hökfelt, T., and Lundberg, J. M. (1987). Occurrence of VIP and peptide HM in human pancreas and their influence on pancreatic endocrine secretion in man. *Regulatory Peptides* 18, 51–61.

Fisher-Colbrie, R., Diez-Guerre, J., Emson, P. C., and Winkler, H. (1986). Bovine chromaffin granules: Immunological studies with antisera against neuropeptide Y, met-enkephalin and bombesin. *Neuroscience* 18, 167–174.

Fisher, L. A., Rivier, J., Rivier, C., Spiess, J., Vale, W., and Brown, M. V. (1982). Corticotropin releasing factor (CRF): Central effects on mean arterial pressure and heart rate in rats. *Endocrinology* 110, 2222–2224.

Furchgott, R. F., and Zawadzki, J. V. (1980). The obligatory role of endothelial cells in the relaxation of arterial smooth muscle by acetylcholine. *Nature* 288, 373–376.

Hökfelt, T., Lundberg, J. M., Schultzberg, M., and Fahrenkrug, J. (1981). Immunohistochemical evidence for a local VIP-ergic neuron system in the adrenal gland of the rat. *Acta Physiologica Scandinavica* 113, 575–576.

Holst, J. J., Sottimano, C., Olssen, M., Lindkaer-Jensen, S., and Nielsen, O. V. (1981). Nervous control of gastropancreatic somatostatin secretion in pigs. *Peptides* 2(Suppl. 2), 1–7.

Holzwarth, M. A. (1984). The distribution of vasoactive intestinal peptide in the rat adrenal cortex and medulla. *Journal of the Autonomic Nervous System* 11, 269–283.

Huang, B. S., Malvin, R. L., Lee, J., and Grekin. R. J. (1987). Central dopaminergic regulation of aldosterone secretion in sheep. *Hypertension* 10, 157–163.

Kalin, N. H. (1985). Behavioral effects of ovine corticopin-releasing factor administered to rhesus monkeys. *Federation Proceedings* 44, 249–253.

Katafuchi, T., Oomura, Y., and Kurosawa, M. (1988). Effects of chemical stimulation of paraventricular nucleus on adrenal and renal nerve activity in rats. *Neuroscience Letters* 86, 195–200.

Kiss, T. (1951). Experimental-morphologische analyse der nebennieren-innervation, *Acta Anatomica* 13, 81–89.

Koob, G. F., and Bloom, F. E. (1985). Corticotropin-releasing factor and behavior. *Federation Proceedings* 44, 259–263.

Kowal, J., Horst, I., Pensky, J., and Alfonzo, M. (1977). Vasoactive intestinal peptide (VIP): An ACTH-like activator of adrenal steroidogenesis. *Annals of the New York Academy of Sciences* 297, 314–328.

Kuramoto, H., Kondo, H.,and Fujita, T. (1985). Substance P-like immunoreactivity in adrenal chromaffin cells and intra-adrenal nerve fibres of rats. *Histochemistry* 82, 507–512.

Kuramoto, H., Kondo, H., and Fujita, T. (1987). Calcitonin-gene related peptide (CGRP)-like immunoreactivity in scattered chromaffin cells and nerve fibers in the adrenal gland of rats. *Cell and Tissue Research* 247, 309–315.

Laburthe, M., Couvineau, A., and Rouyer-Fessard, C. (1986). Study of species specificity in growth hormone-releasing factor (GRF) interaction with vasoactive intestinal peptide (VIP) receptors using GRF and intestinal VIP receptors from rat and human: Evidence that Ac-Tyr^{1}nGRF is a competitive VIP antagonist in the rat. *Molecular Pharmacology* 29, 23–27.

Larsson, L.-I. (1979). Innervation of the pancreas by substance P, enkephalin, vasoactive intestinal polypeptide and gastrin/CCK immunoreactive nerves. *Journal of Histochemistry and Cytochemistry* 27, 1283–1284.

Linnoila, R. I., DiAugustine, R. P., Hervonen, A., and Miller, R. J. (1980). Distribution of [met^5]- and [leu^5]-enkephalin-, vasoactive intestinal polypeptide- and substance P-like immunoreactivities in human adrenal glands. *Neuroscience* 5, 2247–2259.

Lowry, P. J. (1984) Pro-opiocortin: The multiple adrenal hormone precursor. *Bioscience Reports* 4, 467–482.

Lundberg, J. M., Anggärd, A., Fahrenkrug, J., Hökfelt, T., and Mutt, V. (1980). Vasoactive intestinal polypeptide in cholinergic neurons of exocrine glands: Functional significance of coexisting transmitters for vasodilation and secretion. *Acta Physiologica Scandinavica* 113, 317–327.

Lundberg, J. M., Hedlund, B., and Bartfai, T. (1982). Vasoactive intestinal polypeptide enhances muscarinic ligand binding in cat submandibular salivary gland. *Nature* 295, 147–149.

Malhotra, R. K., and Wakade, A. R. (1987a). Vasoactive intestinal polypeptide stimulates the secretion of catecholamines from rat adrenal gland. *Journal of Physiology (London)* 388, 285–294.

Malhotra, R. K., and Wakade, A. R. (1987b). Non-cholinergic component of rat splanchnic nerves predominates at low neuronal activity and is eliminated by naloxone. *Journal of Physiology (London)* 383, 639–652.

Malhotra, R. K., Wakade, T. D., and Wakade, A. R. (1988). Vasoactive intestinal polypeptide and muscarine mobilize intracellular Ca^{++} through breakdown of phosphoinositides to induce catecholamine secretion. Role of IP$_3$ in exocytosis. *Journal of Biological Chemistry* 263, 2123–2126.

McAllen, R. M. (1986). Action and specificity of ventral medullary vasopressor neurones in the cat. *Neuroscience* 18, 51–59.

McDougal, J. G. (1987). The physiology of aldosterone secretion. *News in Physiological Sciences* 2, 126–128.

McEwen, B. S., Lambdin, L. T., Rainbow, T. C., and De Nicola, A. F. (1986). Aldosterone effects on salt appetite in adrenalectomized rats. *Neuroendocrinology* 43, 38–43.

Merchenthaler, I., Hynes, M. A., Vigh, A., Schally, A. V., and Petrusz, P. (1983). Immunocytochemical localisation of corticotropin releasing factor (CRF) in the rat spinal cord. *Brain Research* 275, 373–377.

Mulrow, P. J., Takagi, M., and Franco-Saenz, R. (1987). Inhibitors of aldosterone secretion. *Journal of Steroid Biochemistry* 27, 941–946.

Niijima, A. (1975). Studies on the nervous regulatory mechanisms of blood sugar levels. *Pharmacology, Biochemistry and Behavior* 3(Suppl. 1), 139–143.

Niijima, A., and Winter, D. L. (1968). Baroreceptors in the adrenal gland. *Science* 159, 434–435.

Nussey, S. S., Prysor-Jones, R. S., Taylor, A., Ang, V. T. Y., and Jenkins, J. S. (1987). Arginine vasopressin and oxytocin in the bovine adrenal gland. *Journal of Endocrinology* 115, 141–149.

Olschowka, J. A., O'Donohue, T. L., Mueller, G. P., and Jacobwitz, D. M. (1982). The distribution of corticotropin releasing factor-like immunoreactive neurons in the rat brian. *Peptides* 3, 995–1015.

Oomura, Y., and Yoshimatsu, H. (1984). Neural network of glucose monitoring system. *Journal of the Autonomic Nervous System* 10, 359–372.

Ostenson, C.-G., and Grill, V. (1987). Evidence that hyperglycemia increases muscarinic binding in pancreatic islets of the rat. *Endocrinology* 121, 1705–1710.

Rehfeld, J. F. (1971). Effect of gastrin and its C-terminal tetrapeptide on insulin secretion in man. *Acta Endocrinologica (Copenhagen)* 66, 169–176.

Rehfeld, J. P., Larsson, L.-I., Goltermann, N. R., Schwartz, T. W., Holst, J. J., Jensen, S. L., and Morley, J. S. (1980). Neural regulation of pancreatic hormone secretion by the C-terminal tetrapeptide of CCK. *Nature* 284, 33–40.

Rehfeld, J. F., and Lindkaer-Jensen, S. (1980). The effect of gastrin and cholecystokinin on the endocrine pancreas. *Frontiers in Hormone Research* 7, 107–118.

Rinaman, L., and Miselis, R. R. (1987). The organization of vagal innervation of rat pancreas using cholera toxin-horseradish peroxidase conjugate. *Journal of the Autonomic Nervous System* 21, 109–125.

Sakanaka, M., Shibasaki, T., and Lederis, K. (1987). Corticotropin releasing factor-like immunoreactivity in the rat brain as revealed by a modified cobalt-glucose oxidase-diaminobenzidine method. *Journal of Comparative Neurology* 260, 256–298.

Samols, E., and Weir, G. D. (1979). Adrenergic modulation of pancreatic A, B, and D cells α-adrenergic suppression and β-adrenergic stimulation of somatostatin secretion, α-adrenergic stimulation of glucagon secretion in the perfused dog pancreas. *Journal of Clinical Investigation* 63, 230–238.

Samols, E., Stagner, J. I., and Weir, G. C. (1981). Autonomic function and control of pancreatic somatostatin. *Diabetologia* 20, 388–392.

Schipper, J., Steinbusch, H. W. M., Vermes, I., and Tilders, F. J. H. (1983). Mapping of the CRF-immunoreactive nerve fibres in the medulla oblongata and spinal cord of the rat. *Brain Research* 267, 145–150.

Schulzberg, M., Lundberg, J. M., Hökfelt, T., Ternius, L., Brandt, J., Elde, R. P., and Goldstein, M. (1978). Enkephalin-like immunoreactivity in gland cells and nerve terminals of the adrenal medulla. *Neuroscience* 3, 1169–1186.

Seidle, K., and Unsicker, K. (1985). Glucocorticoids trigger initial expression of phenylethanolamine N-methyl transferase (PNMT) and adrenaline (A) in chromaffin cells of embryonic rats. *European Journal of Cell Biology* 39(Suppl. 12), 33.

Seybold, V. S., and Elde, R. P. (1984). Receptor autoradiography in thoracic spinal cord: Correlation of neurotransmitter binding sites with sympathoadrenal neurons. *Journal of Neuroscience* 4, 2533–2542.

Shuster, L. T., Go, V. L. W., Rizza, R. A., O'Brien, P. C., and Service, F. J. (1988). Potential incretins. *Mayo Clinic Proceedings* 63, 794–800.

Strack, A. M., Sawyer, W. B., Platt, K. B., and Loewy, A. D. (1989). CNS cell groups regulating the sympathetic outflow to adrenal gland as revealed by transneuronal cell body labeling with pseudorabies virus. *Brain Research* 491, 274–296.

Swanson, L. W., Sawchenko, P. E., Rivier, J., and Vale, W. W. (1983). Organization of ovine corticotropin-releasing factor immunoreactive cells and fibers in the rat brain: An immunohistochemical study. *Neuroendocrinology* 36, 165–186.

Szecowka, J., Sandberg, E., and Efendic, S. (1980). The interaction of vasoactive intestinal polypeptide (VIP), glucose and arginine on the secretion of insulin, glucagon, and somatostatin in the perfused rat pancreas. *Diabetologia* 19, 137–142.

Tazi, A., Dantzer, R., Le Moal, M., Rivier, J., Vale, W., and Koob, G. F. (1987). Corticotropin-releasing factor antagonist blocks stress-induced fighting in rats. *Regulatory Peptides* 18, 37–42.

Terenghi, G., Polak, J. M., Varndell, I. M., Lee, Y. C., Wharton, J., and Bloom, S. R. (1983). Neurotensin-like immunoreactivity in a subpopulation of noradrenalin-containing cells of the cat adrenal gland. *Endocrinology* 112, 226–233.

Wakade, A. R. (1988). Noncholinergic transmitter(s) maintains secretion of catecholamines from rat adrenal medulla for several hours of continuous stimulation of splanchnic neurons. *Journal of Neurochemistry* 50, 1302–1308.

Wilkinson, C. W., Shinsako, K., and Dallman, M. F. (1982). Rapid decreases in adrenal and plasma corticosterone concentrations after drinking are not mediated by changes in plasma adrenocorticotropin concentration. *Endocrinology* 110, 162–169.

Yanagisawa, M., Kurihara, H., Kimura, S., Tomobe, Y., Kobayashi, M., Mitsoui, Y., Yazaki, Y., Goto, K., and Masaki, T. (1988). A novel potent vasoconstrictor peptide produced by vascular endothelial cells. *Nature* 332, 411–415.

Young, J. B. Rosa, R. M., and Landsberg, L. (1984). dissociation of sympathetic nervous system and adrenal medullary responses. *American Journal of Physiology* 247, E35–E40.

17

Autonomic Regulation of the Urinary Bladder and Sexual Organs

W. C. DE GROAT AND W. D. STEERS

Urogenital functions, such as micturition, penile erection, and seminal emission, are completely dependent on neural mechanisms that involve both the brain and lumbosacral spinal cord. This dependence on central nervous system control distinguishes the urogenital tract from many other visceral structures (e.g., the gastrointestinal tract and cardiovascular system) that maintain a certain level of function even after elimination of extrinsic neural input.

The urogenital organs are also unusual in their pattern of activity and the complexity of their neural regulation. For example, the lower urinary tract and male sex organs exhibit two principal modes of operation: storage and periodic elimination. Thus, many of the neural circuits controlling these organs exhibit switch-like or phasic patterns of activity in contrast to the tonic patterns occurring in the autonomic pathways to the cardiovascular organs. In addition, certain urogenital functions (storage and release of urine) are clearly under voluntary control, whereas others (seminal emission) are involuntary (reflex) but are subject to modulatory influences from the brain and endocrine system. Thus, some urogenital mechanisms depend on learned behavior and exhibit marked changes during postnatal development, whereas others are affected by sexual maturation and hormonal changes that occur at puberty.

Many urogenital functions also depend on the integration of autonomic and somatic efferent mechanisms within the lumbosacral spinal cord. This is necessary during voiding or ejaculation when the activity of pelvic visceral structures must be coordinated with that of the perineal striated muscles.

The dependence of urogenital functions on complex central networks renders these functions very susceptible to a considerable number of neurological disorders. Indeed, changes in the activity of the urogenital organs are often the first signs of systemic diseases such as multiple sclerosis or diabetic neuropathy.

Because of the clinical importance and unusual physiological properties of the neural pathways to the urogenital organs, there has been considerable interest among clinical investigators as well as basic neuroscientists in the central mechanisms regulating these organs. This chapter will review anatomical and physiological studies in animals and humans that have provided insights into the reflex pathways and transmitters involved in the neural control of urogenital function.

LOWER URINARY TRACT

Innervation

The storage and periodic elimination of urine depend on the activity of two functional units in the lower urinary tract: (1) a reservoir (the urinary bladder) and (2) an outlet consisting of bladder neck, urethra, and striated muscles of the urethral sphincter. These structures are in turn controlled by three sets of peripheral nerves: sacral parasympathetic (pelvic nerves), thoracolumbar sympathetic (hypogastric nerves and sympathetic chain), and sacral somatic nerves (pudendal nerves) (Figure 17-1) (see reviews by Kuru, 1965; de Groat and Kawatani, 1985; Torrens and Morrison, 1987; Wein and Barrett, 1988).

Sacral Parasympathetic Pathways

The sacral parasympathetic outflow provides the major excitatory input to the urinary bladder. Cholinergic preganglionic neurons located in the intermediolateral cell column of the S2–S4 levels of the sacral spinal cord send axons via the pelvic nerves to ganglion cells that lie in the pelvic plexus and in the wall of the bladder (Figure 17-2). The ganglion cells,

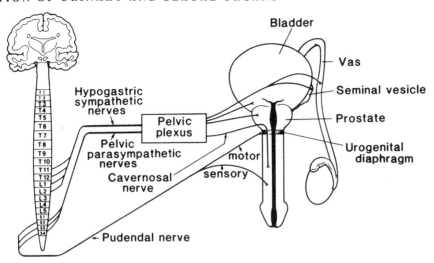

Figure 17-1 Schematic diagram of the innervation of the urinary bladder and male sex organs. [Reproduced from E. A. Klein (1988). In: *Disorders of Male Sexual Function,* Yearbook Medical Publishers, Chicago, with permission of the author and publisher.]

in turn, excite bladder smooth muscle via the release of cholinergic (acetylcholine) and, in some species, noncholinergic-nonadrenergic transmitters. Cholinergic excitatory transmission is mediated by muscarinic receptors, which are blocked by atropine, whereas noncholinergic transmission is thought to be mediated by the purinergic transmitter, adenosine triphosphate (ATP), acting on P_2 purinergic receptors (see Burnstock, 1986 for review) (Table 17-1).

Thoracolumbar Sympathetic Pathways

Anatomical and physiological studies have shown that sympathetic pathways to the lower urinary tract of the cat originate in the lumbosacral sympathetic chain ganglia as well as in the prevertebral ganglia (inferior mesenteric ganglia) (see Figure 17-2; de Groat and Kawatani, 1985). Input from the sacral chain ganglia passes to the bladder via the pelvic nerves, whereas fibers from the upper lumbar and inferior mesenteric ganglia travel in the hypogastric nerves. Sympathetic efferent pathways in the hypogastric and pelvic nerves in the cat elicit similar effects in the bladder consisting of (1) inhibition of detrusor muscle via β-adrenergic receptors, (2) excitation of the bladder base and urethra via α-receptors, and (3) inhibition and facilitation in bladder parasympathetic ganglia via α_2- and α_1-receptors, respectively (Table 17-1) (de Groat and Booth, 1980).

Somatic Efferent Pathways

The efferent innervation of the periurethral and external urethral striated muscles in various species originates from cells in a circumscribed region of the ventral horn, which is termed Onuf's nucleus or the somatic motor nucleus of the external urethral sphincter. These cells send their axons into the pudendal nerve. The sphincter motor nucleus exhibits a number of morphological and histochemical characteristics that distinguishes it from other motor nuclei controlling the limb muscles. For example, the sphincter motor nucleus more closely resembles the sacral autonomic nucleus in terms of its dendritic patterns and spectrum of peptidergic inputs, with which it has a close functional relationship (de Groat et al., 1986).

Afferent Pathways

Afferent axons innervating the lower urinary tract are present in the three sets of nerves (see de Groat, 1986; Jänig and Morrison, 1986 for reviews). The most important afferents for initiating micturition are those passing in the pelvic nerve to the sacral spinal cord (Kuru, 1965). These afferents are small $A\delta$ and C-fibers that convey impulses from tension receptors in the bladder wall to neurons in laminae I, V, VII, and X of the spinal cord (Morgan et al., 1981; de Groat et al., 1981; Roppolo et al., 1985) (Figure 17-3). Electrophysiological studies have shown that bladder afferents in the pelvic nerve of the cat respond in a graded manner to passive distension as well as active contraction of the bladder (see Jänig and Morrison, 1986, for review). The intravesical pressure thresholds for activation of $A\delta$ afferents range from 5 to 15 mm Hg, which is consistent with pressures at which humans report the first sensation of filling during cystometry. Specific high-threshold afferents have not been detected. Therefore, noxious events in the bladder may be encoded by different patterns or high rates of firing in afferent

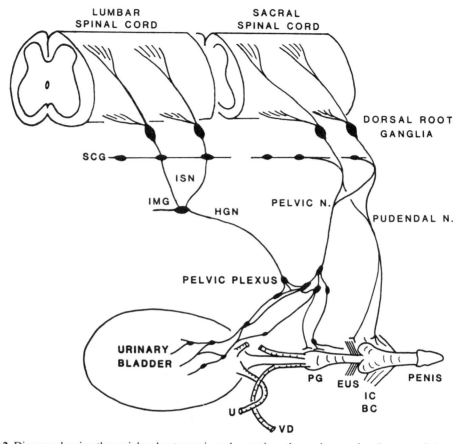

Figure 17-2 Diagram showing the peripheral autonomic and somatic pathways innervating the urogenital tract and urogenital diaphragm of the male cat. Sympathetic preganglionic pathways emerge from the lumbar spinal cord and pass to the sympathetic-chain ganglia (SCG) and then via the inferior splanchnic nerves (ISN) to the inferior mesenteric ganglia (IMG). Preganglionic and postganglionic sympathetic axons then travel in the hypogastric nerve (HGN) to the pelvic plexus and the urogenital organs. Parasympathetic preganglionic axons that originate in the sacral spinal cord pass in the pelvic nerve to ganglion cells in the pelvic plexus and to distal ganglia in the organs. Sacral somatic pathways are contained in the pudendal nerve, which provides an innervation to the penis, the ischiocavernosus (IC), bulbocavernosus (BC), and external urethral sphincter (EUS) muscles. The pudendal and pelvic nerves also receive postganglionic axons from the caudal sympathetic-chain ganglia. These three sets of nerves contain afferent axons from the lumbosacral dorsal-root ganglia. U, ureter; PG, prostate gland, VD, vas deferens. (Reproduced from de Groat and Steers, 1988, with permission of the authors and publisher.)

Table 17-1 Receptors for Putative Transmitters in the Lower Urinary Tract[a]

Tissue	Cholinergic	Adrenergic	Other
Bladder body	$+(M_2)$	$-(\beta_2)$	+ Purinergic (P_2)
			− VIP
			+ Substance P
Bladder base	$+(M_2)$	$+(\alpha_1)$	0 Purinergic
			− VIP
Ganglia	$+(N)$	$-(\alpha_2)$	− Enkephalinergic (δ)
	$+(M_1)$	$+(\alpha_1)$	− Purinergic (P_1)
		$+(\beta)$	+ Substance P
Urethra	$+(M)$	$+(\alpha_1)$	± Purinergic
		$\pm(\alpha_2)$	− VIP
		$-(\beta_2)$	+ NPY
Sphincter striated muscle	$+(N)$		

[a]Letters in parentheses indicate receptor type, e.g., M (muscarinic) and N (nicotinic). +, −, and 0 indicate excitatory, inhibitory, and weak or no effects, respectively.

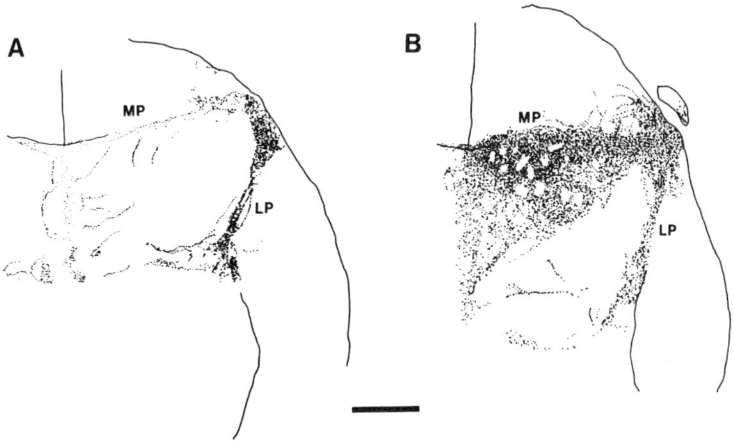

Figure 17-3 The central projection of dorsal root axons and terminals in the sacral spinal cord of visceral afferents in the pelvic nerve (A) and somatic afferents in the pudendal nerve (B) of the monkey as shown by the transganglionic HRP transport method to these nerves. Bar = 400 μm. MP, medial pathway; LP, lateral pathway. (Reproduced from Roppolo et al., 1985, with permission of the authors and publisher.)

pathways, which also transmit nonnoxious information from the bladder.

Mechanoreceptor afferents from the bladder and urethra have also been identified in the sympathetic nerves (hypogastric and inferior splanchnic) passing to the lumbar spinal cord (see Jänig and Morrison, 1986, for review). These afferent pathways consist of myelinated as well as unmyelinated axons and respond in a manner similar to the afferents in the pelvic nerve. The function of sympathetic nerve afferents in the control of micturition is uncertain; however, these afferents can transmit noxious information from the pelvic organs.

Afferent pathways from the striated sphincter muscles and urethral afferents transmit the sensations of temperature, pain, and passage of urine travel in the pudendal nerve to the sacral spinal cord where they terminate in many regions of the dorsal horn receiving visceral afferent input (Figure 17-3). These afferents have a modulatory influence on micturition, as well as other lumbosacral visceral reflexes (see Thor et al., 1986; Torrens and Morrison, 1987 for reviews).

Reflex Mechanisms Controlling the Lower Urinary Tract

The central pathways controlling lower urinary tract function are organized as simple on–off switching circuits that maintain a reciprocal relationship between the urinary bladder and urethral outlet. The principal reflex components of these switching circuits are listed in Table 17-2.

The reflexes involved in urine storage and elimination have been studied with various techniques: (1) measurement of effector organ activity, including intravesical pressure (a cystometrogram, CMG; Figure 17-4), intraurethral pressure, and electrical activity of the striated urethral sphincter muscles (electromyogram, EMG; Figure 17-4) and (2) measurement of neuronal activity in the micturition reflex pathway.

Intravesical pressure measurements during bladder filling in both humans and animals reveal that bladder pressure is maintained at a low and relatively constant level (5–10 cm H_2O) when bladder volume is below the threshold for inducing voiding

Table 17-2 Reflexes to the Lower Urinary Tract

Afferent Pathway	Efferent Pathway	Central Pathway
Urine storage Low level vesical afferent activity (pelvic nerve)	1. External sphincter contraction (somatic nerves) 2. Internal sphincter contraction (sympathetic nerves) 3. Detrusor inhibition (sympathetic nerves) 4. Ganglionic inhibition (sympathetic nerves) 5. Sacral parasympathetic outflow inactive	Spinal reflexes
Micturition High level vesical afferent activity (pelvic nerve)	1. Inhibition of external sphincter activity 2. Inhibition of sympathetic outflow 3. Activation of parasympathetic outflow	Spinobulbospinal reflexes

From de Groat and Booth (1984).

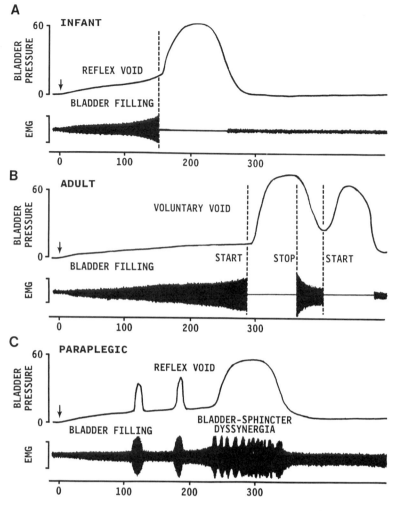

Figure 17-4 Combined cystometrograms and external urethral sphincter electromyograms (EMG) comparing reflex voiding responses in an infant (A) and in a paraplegic patient (C) with a voluntary voiding response in an adult (B). In all the records, the abscissa represents bladder volume in milliliters; the ordinates represent bladder pressure in cm H_2O and electrical activity of the EMG recording. On the left side of each trace, the arrows indicate the start of a slow infusion of fluid into the bladder (bladder filling). Vertical dashed lines indicate the start of sphincter relaxation, which precedes by a few seconds the bladder contraction in A and B. In part B note that a voluntary cessation of voiding (stop) is associated with an initial increase in sphincter EMG followed by a reciprocal relaxation of the bladder. A resumption of voiding is again associated with sphincter relaxation and a delayed increase in bladder pressure. On the other hand, in the paraplegic patient (C), the reciprocal relationship between bladder and sphincter is abolished. During bladder filling transient uninhibited bladder contractions occur in association with sphincter activity. Further filling leads to more prolonged and simultaneous contractions of the bladder and sphincter (bladder sphincter dyssynergia). Loss of the reciprocal relationship between bladder and sphincter in paraplegic patients interferes with bladder emptying.

(Figure 17-4). A low intravesical pressure during urine storage is essential to allow urine flow from the kidney through the ureters at a low pressure head. The accommodation of the bladder to increasing volumes of urine is primarily a passive phenomenon that depends on the intrinsic properties of the vesical smooth muscle and quiescence of the parasympathetic efferent pathway (de Groat et al., 1982; Torrens and Morrison, 1987; Wein and Barrett, 1988). In addition, in some species urine storage is also facilitated by sympathetic reflexes that mediate an active inhibition of the vesical smooth muscle, inhibition of transmission in vesical ganglia, closure of the bladder neck, and contraction of the proximal urethral (Table 17-2, Figure 17-5). Although the importance of these sympathetic reflexes in humans is still uncertain, their contribution to urine storage in animals (cats, dogs) is generally accepted. During bladder filling the activity of the sphincter EMG also increases, reflecting an increase in efferent firing in the pudendal nerve and an increase in outlet resistance,

which contributes to the maintenance of urinary continence. The somatic and sympathetic reflexes that occur during urine storage are initiated by a low level of afferent activity from tension receptors in the bladder, which is conveyed in the pelvic nerve to the sacral spinal cord (Table 17-2, Figure 17-5).

The storage phase of the urinary bladder can be switched to the expulsion phase (voiding) either involuntarily (reflexly) or voluntarily (Figure 17-4). The former is readily demonstrated in the human infant or in the anesthetized animal when the volume of urine exceeds the micturition threshold. At this point, increased afferent firing from tension receptors in the bladder wall reverses the pattern of efferent outflow, producing firing in the sacral parasympathetic pathways and inhibition of sympathetic and somatic pathways. The expulsion phase consists of an initial relaxation of the urethral sphincter (Figure 17-4A) followed in a few seconds by a contraction of the bladder and an increase in bladder pressure and flow of urine. Secondary reflexes elicited by

SPHINCTER REFLEXES

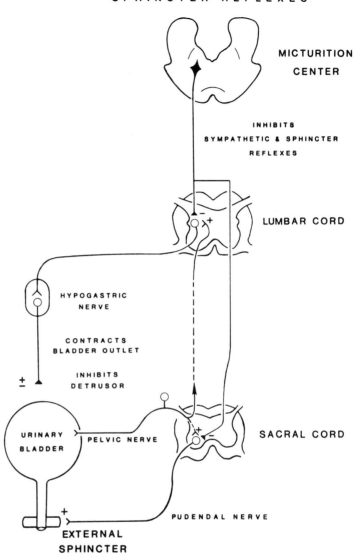

Figure 17-5 Diagram showing detrusor-sphincter reflexes. During the storage of urine, distention of the bladder produces low-level vesical afferent firing, which in turn stimulates (1) the sympathetic outflow to the bladder outlet (base and urethra) and (2) pudendal outflow to the external urethral sphincter. These responses occur by spinal reflex pathways and represent "guarding reflexes," which promote continence. Sympathetic firing also inhibits detrusor muscle and transmission in bladder ganglia. At the initiation of micturition, intense vesical afferent activity activates the brain stem micturition center, which inhibits the spinal guarding reflexes. (Reproduced from de Groat and Booth, 1984, with permission of the authors and publisher.)

the passage of urine through the urethra reinforce the bladder contraction and facilitate bladder emptying (see Kuru, 1965; Wein and Barrett, 1988 for reviews).

During postnatal maturation of the central nervous system, the reflex mechanisms involved in voiding are eventually brought under the control of higher centers in the cerebral cortex and diencephalon, leading to the development of voluntary micturition, which usually occurs in humans between 3 and 5 years of age. The mechanisms involved in the voluntary control of micturition are still uncertain. For example, there may be direct cortical control of the autonomic outflow to the bladder or indirect control exerted via an alteration of the activity of the striated sphincter muscles surrounding the urethra.

Most evidence suggests an indirect mechanism, since the initial event in micturition is a voluntary relaxation of the urethral sphincter (Figure 17-4B) and the pelvic floor and a contraction of the diaphragm and abdominal muscles. The latter produce an increase in intraabdominal pressure and, in turn, an increase in intravesical pressure. These responses coupled with a descent of the pelvic floor and bladder base, which leads to a decrease in urethral closure pressure, are thought to initiate a reflex detrusor contraction and urine flow. Voiding can be terminated voluntarily first by a contraction of the striated urethral sphincter followed by relaxation of the bladder (Figure 17-4B).

The basic reflex mechanisms underlying urine storage and release require the integrative action of

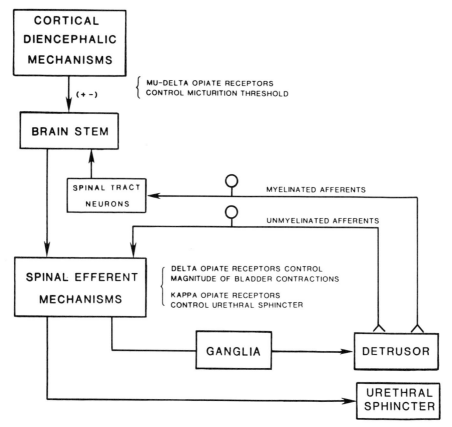

Figure 17-6 Diagram of the central reflex pathways and enkephalinergic mechanisms that regulate micturition in the cat. In animals with intact neuraxis, micturition is initiated by a supraspinal reflex pathway passing through a center in the brainstem. The pathway is triggered by myelinated afferents (Aδ) connected to tension receptors in the bladder wall. In chronic spinal animals, connections between the brain stem and the sacral spinal cord are interrupted and micturition is initially blocked. However, in chronic spinal animals a spinal reflex mechanism emerges that is triggered by unmyelinated (C-fiber) vesical afferents. The C-fiber reflex pathway is usually weak or undetectable in animals with an intact nervous system. Pharmacological studies have shown that in the brain μ or δ opiate receptors control micturition threshold and bladder capacity, whereas in the spinal cord δ opiate receptors control the magnitude of bladder contractions and κ opiate receptors mediate a depression of the pudendal motor outflow to the external urethral sphincter. (Reproduced from de Groat and Kawatani, 1985, with permission of the authors and publisher.)

neuronal populations at various levels of the neuraxis (Figures 17-5–17-8). Certain reflexes, for example, those mediating the excitatory outflow to the sphincters and the sympathetic inhibitory outflow to the bladder, are organized at the spinal level (Figure 17-5), whereas the parasympathetic outflow to the detrusor has a more complicated central organization involving spinal and supraspinal pathways (Figure 17-6).

Storage Reflexes

The sympathetic and pudendal efferent pathways to the lower urinary tract, although not essential for either the storage or release of urine, do, in many species, make a significant contribution to the neural control of bladder capacity and outlet resistance during the storage phase of bladder function.

Studies in animals indicate that sympathetic input

to the lower urinary tract is tonically active during bladder filling. Surgical or pharmacologic blockade of the sympathetic pathway can reduce urethral resistance, reduce bladder capacity, and increase the frequency and amplitude of bladder contractions (Edvardsen, 1968; de Groat and Kawatani, 1985).

Sympathetic firing is initiated at least in part by a sacrolumbar intersegmental spinal reflex pathway that is triggered by vesical afferent activity in the pelvic nerves (de Groat and Lalley, 1972; Figure 17-5). This vesicosympathetic reflex represents a negative feedback mechanism whereby an increase in bladder pressure triggers an increase in inhibitory input to the bladder, thus allowing the bladder to accommodate larger volumes of urine. In the cat the reflex pathway is inhibited during micturition (Edvardsen, 1968; de Groat and Lalley, 1972). This inhibition is abolished by transection of the spinal cord at the

A

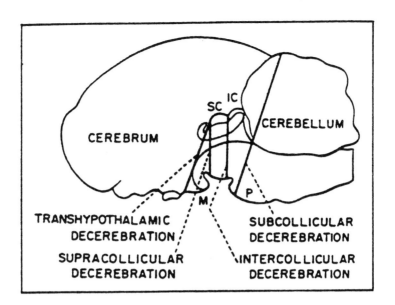

B

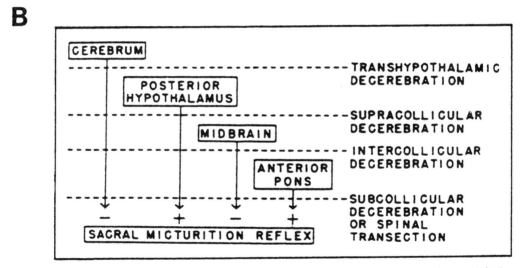

Figure 17-7 (A) Drawing of a sagittal section of the cat brain showing various levels of brain transections made in the study of the supraspinal control of micturition. SC, IC, superior and inferior colliculi; M, midbrain, P, pons. (B) Diagram indicating the net facilitatory and inhibitory actions of the various levels of the brain identified by the transection procedures shown in part A. (Reproduced from Tang, 1955, and from Tang and Ruch, 1956, with permission of the authors and publisher.)

thoracic level, indicating that it originates at a supraspinal site, possibly the pontine micturition center (see discussion below).

Somatic pathways to the striated urethral sphincter exhibit a similar reflex organization. During bladder filling pudendal motoneurons are activated by vesical afferent input, whereas during micturition pudendal motoneurons are reciprocally inhibited. The inhibition is dependent in part on supraspinal mechanisms, since in chronic spinal animals and

paraplegic patients it is weak or absent. Indeed, in these patients the uninhibited spinal vesicosphincter excitatory reflex pathway commonly initiates a striated sphincter contraction in concert with a contraction of the bladder (bladder–sphincter dyssynergia) (Figure 17-4C). This reflex interferes with bladder emptying. In some species (e.g., rat and dog), rhythmic contractions of the sphincter also occur in normal animals during the latter phase of micturition. The function of these contractions is unknown,

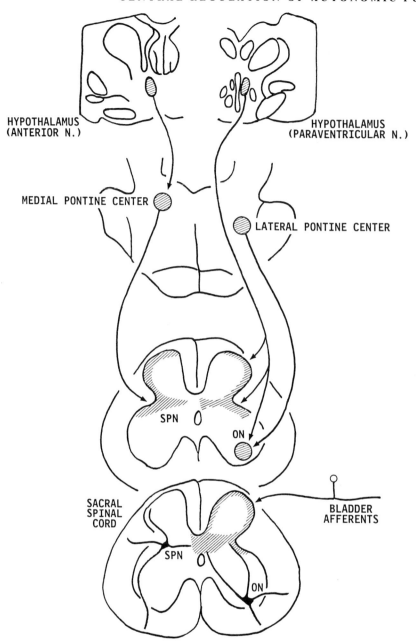

Figure 17-8 Neural connections between the brain and the sacral spinal cord that may be involved in the regulation of the lower urinary tract in the cat. Lower section of spinal cord shows the location and morphology of a preganglionic neuron in the sacral parasympathetic nucleus (SPN), a sphincter motoneuron in Onuf's nucleus (ON), and the sites of central termination of afferent projections from the urinary bladder. (Based on the studies of Nadelhaft et al., 1980; Morgan et al., 1981; Thor et al., 1989.) Upper section of the spinal cord shows the sites of termination of descending pathways arising in the pontine micturition center (medial), the pontine sphincter or urine storage center (lateral), and the paraventricular nuclei of the hypothalamus. Section through the pons shows the projection from the anterior hypothalamic nuclei to the pontine micturition center. (Based on studies of Holstege, 1987; Holstege et al., 1986.)

however, it is clear that they do not interfere with urine flow but rather may enhance bladder emptying, possibly by inducing intermittent isometric contractions of the bladder (Maggi et al., 1986).

Retrograde cell body labeling experiments have revealed that the external urethral sphincter motoneurons in the cat have an unusual dendritic morphology that correlates with the physiological properties of the cells (Figure 17-8) (Thor et al., 1988). These neurons lie in Onuf's nucleus, found in the

S2–S4 ventral horn. One longitudinal and three bundles of transverse dendritic projections have been identified extending (1) dorsolaterally into the region of the sacral parasympathetic nucleus and lateral lamina V, (2) dorsomedially to the dorsal commissure, (3) laterally in the ventrolateral funiculus, and (4) rostrocaudally within Onuf's nucleus. Afferent projections from the urinary bladder terminate in the region of the dorsal dendrites, whereas projections from the lateral pons and the medial hypothalamus descend in the lateral funiculus and terminate in Onuf's nucleus (Figure 17-8). Some investigators have designated the lateral pontine area as the urine storage center since electrical stimulation in this region not only excites the urethral sphincter, but also inhibits activity of the urinary bladder (Holstege et al., 1986). In the dog, this area has been identified in the region of the nucleus subcoeruleus and nucleus reticularis pontis oralis (Nishizawa et al., 1987).

Intracellular recording in pudendal motoneurons revealed that activation of bulbospinal pathways elicited large excitatory and inhibitory postsynaptic potentials (EPSPs and IPSPs) consistent with their mediation by axosomatic synapses. On the other hand, segmental afferent inputs elicited small amplitude EPSPs that reflect weaker synaptic connections on distal dendrites (Mackle, 1979). Thus, it is clear that the activity of sphincter motoneurons is strongly regulated by descending pathways from the brain as well as by spinal reflex mechanism.

Voiding Reflexes

Micturition is dependent primarily on activation of the sacral parasympathetic efferent pathway to the bladder and reciprocal inhibition of the somatic pathway to the urethral sphincter (Table 17-2) (Figure 17-6). Studies in cats using brain lesioning techniques revealed that neurons in the brain stem at the level of the inferior colliculus have an essential role in the control of the parasympathetic component of micturition (Figure 17-7). Removal of areas of the brain above the inferior colliculus by intercollicular decerebration usually facilitated micturition by elimination of inhibitory inputs from more rostral areas of the brain (Tang, 1955; Tang and Ruch, 1956) (Figure 17-7). However, transections at any point below the colliculi abolished micturition. Bilateral lesions in the rostral pons in the region of the locus coeruleus in cats or the lateral dorsal tegmental nucleus in rats abolished micturition, whereas electrical stimulation at these sites triggered bladder contractions and micturition (see reviews by Kuru, 1965; Torrens and Morrison, 1987). These observations led to the concept of a spinobulbospinal micturition reflex pathway that passes through a center in the rostral brain stem (the pontine micturition center). The pathway functions as an "on–off" switch that is activated by a critical level of afferent activity arising from tension receptors in the bladder (de Groat, 1975). This switch is, in turn, modulated by inhibitory and excitatory influences from areas of

Figure 17-9 Diagram showing the reflex pathway for inducing penile erection. Horseradish peroxidase axonal tracing studies in the cat have shown the relationship between sacral parasympathetic preganglionic neurons and afferent projections from the penis. Penile afferents in the pudendal nerve project to the medial side of the dorsal horn (DH) and the dorsal commissure (DCM) in the S2 segment of the spinal cord. Preganglionic neurons send dendrites into regions of afferent termination. DCOL, dorsal column; VH, ventral horn; CC, central canal. In the rat electrical stimulation of the penile afferents in the dorsal nerve of the penis elicits reflex firing in efferent pathways to the penis. Inset is an example of a reflex discharge in parasympathetic postganglionic axons in penile nerves. The reflexes that occur at a long latency (mean 75 msec) are present in normal and chronic spinal rats and are blocked by section of the pelvic nerve. Stimulus marked by arrows. Horizontal calibration 20 msec, vertical calibration 10 μV. (Reproduced from de Groat and Steers, 1988, with permission of the authors and publisher.)

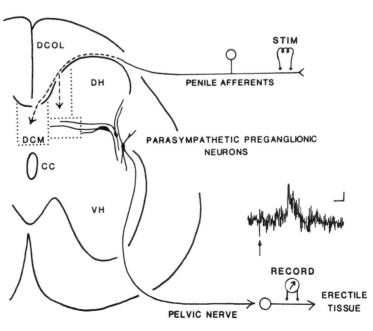

the brain rostral to the pons (e.g., diencephalon and cerebral cortex) (Figures 17-6 and 17-7).

Electrophysiological and neuroanatomical studies in cats and rats provide further support for a spinobulbospinal micturition reflex, but demonstrate a spinal reflex mechanism as well (de Groat et al., 1981, 1986). In cats and rats, the spinobulbospinal reflex pathway is the most prominent when the neuroaxis is intact. Recordings from sacral parasympathetic preganglionic neurons innervating the urinary bladder show that reflex firing occurs with a long latency (65–100 msec) following stimulation of myelinated (Aδ) vesical afferents in the pelvic nerve (de Groat and Ryall, 1969; de Groat, 1975). Afferent stimulation also evokes negative field potentials in the rostral pons at latencies of 30–40 msec, whereas stimulation in the pons evokes firing of preganglionic neurons at latencies of 45–60 msec (de Groat, 1975). The sum of the latencies for the spinobulbar and bulbospinal components of the reflex pathway approximate the latency for the entire reflex. The spinobulbospinal reflex is present in decerebrate animals but is absent in acute or chronic spinal animals.

Single unit recordings in the pontine micturition center of cats and rats have identified several populations of cells exhibiting firing correlated with bladder activity. One group of cells fired just prior to and during reflex contractions of the bladder, whereas another group was inhibited during bladder contractions. The all-or-none-pattern of activity of these units, coupled with pharmacological data (see below), raises the possibility that this region of the pons may contain the neuronal switching circuit responsible for controlling the storage/voiding cycle of the lower urinary tract.

On the other hand, there is also evidence that a switching or gating circuit is present in the spinal cord (Denny-Brown and Robertson, 1933; de Groat and Ryall, 1969; de Groat, 1975; McMahon and Morrison, 1982). For example, in chronic spinal animals, reflex mechanisms controlled within the lumbosacral spinal cord are capable of duplicating many of the functions performed by the reflex pathways in the intact animal. Furthermore, the firing of sacral preganglionic neurons elicited by bladder distension in chronic spinal cats following recovery from spinal shock is similar to that occurring in intact cats (de Groat and Ryall, 1969; de Groat et al., 1982).

Despite these similarities, electrophysiological studies in rats and cats have shown that the reflex pathways in intact and chronic animals are markedly different. In both species, the central delay for the micturition reflex in chronic spinal animals is considerably shorter (< 5 msec in rats; 15–40 msec in cats) than in intact animals (60–75 msec). In addition, in chronic spinal cats the afferent limb of the micturition reflex consists of unmyelinated (C-fiber) afferents, whereas in intact cats it consists of myelinated (Aδ) afferents (Figure 17-6) (see de Groat et al., 1981, 1986, for reviews). Thus, there seems to be a considerable reorganization of reflex connections in the spinal cord following the interruption of descending pathways from the brain. C-fiber afferent-evoked reflexes that are weak and occur in only 60% of cats with an intact neuraxis are facilitated in chronic spinal animals, whereas Aδ afferent reflexes are completely eliminated. Similarly, the short latency spinal micturition reflex that occurs in only 30% of intact rats occurs in 100% of chronic spinal rats. Thus, two distinct central pathways (supraspinal and spinal) utilizing different peripheral afferent limbs (A- and C-fiber) can mediate detrusor-to-detrusor reflexes (Figure 17-6). The supraspinal pathway seems to have the major role in the initiation of bladder contractions in animals with an intact neuraxis. Although the function of the spinal reflex pathway in normal animals is uncertain, this pathway is essential for the development of automatic micturition in paraplegic animals. It is not known whether the spinal switching circuit that mediates automatic micturition is functional in normal animals or whether this circuit becomes functional as a consequence of synaptic reorganization following spinal cord damage (see Thor et al., 1986 for review) or other pathological disorders such as urethral obstruction (see Steers and de Groat, 1988 for review).

Synaptic reorganization in the reflex pathways to the urinary bladder is also known to occur during postnatal development. In many species (e.g., rats and cats), the spinobulbospinal reflex, which is essential for micturition in adult animals, is nonfunctional in neonates, and micturition depends on an exteroceptive somatobladder reflex mechanism triggered when the mother licks the genital or perineal area of the young animal (see reviews by de Groat et al., 1981; Thor et al., 1986). The exteroceptive reflex is organized in the sacral spinal cord and has an afferent limb in the pudendal nerve and an efferent limb in the pelvic nerve. In kittens near the age of weaning (5–7 weeks), this reflex becomes progressively weaker and eventually disappears as the bladder-to-bladder spinobulbospinal reflex emerges as the major regulator of bladder function in older animals. The exteroceptive reflex is essential for survival of the newborn kitten or rat since isolation of the newborn from the mother leads to urinary retention.

Although the spinobulbospinal micturition reflex is nonfunctional in kittens, it is apparently intact and can be unmasked by the administration of general anesthetics such as chloralose or ketamine (Thor et al., 1986). Under general anesthesia, the immature reflex pathway exhibits a very long central delay

(225–325 msec) in comparison to the delay in adult cats (60–75 msec) (de Groat et al., 1981), presumably due to the very slow conduction velocity of the immature central axons in the newborn animal. The latency of the reflex progressively shortens during the first 8 postnatal weeks, reaching the adult latency by 2–3 months of age. The long latency reflex in anesthetized neonatal kittens is eliminated by spinal cord transection and is replaced after a period of a few days by a short latency spinal reflex. This change in reflex patterns in paraplegic kittens is similar to that occurring in adult paraplegic animals.

On the other hand, the somatobladder exteroceptive reflex in young kittens is not eliminated by spinal cord transection. Furthermore, in adult cats and older kittens in which this reflex had disappeared, spinal cord transection causes the reemergence of the reflex. This suggests that the neonatal reflex is suppressed during maturation of the micturition pathways in the brain stem and that removal of these pathways by spinal cord transection leads to unmasking of the reflex. Similar excitatory somatobladder reflexes are present in the human infant, disappear during maturation, and reappear in paraplegic patients (see review by Thor et al., 1986, for references).

The synaptic mechanisms underlying these prominent developmental and injury-induced changes in bladder reflexes are relatively unexplored. There is some evidence that spinal injury reverses developmental changes in afferent projections to the spinal cord, leading to expansion of afferent terminal fields, possibly through the process of axonal sprouting (see Thor et al., 1986, for review). In addition, certain drugs that interact with serotonergic receptors can mimic reversibly the effects of spinal injury on the somatobladder reflex. This raises the possibility that postnatal development of the bulbospinal serotonergic system may be involved in maturation of the spinal micturition reflex pathways.

Anatomical studies have also examined the question of brain–spinal cord integration in regard to the control of lower urinary tract function. Anterograde axonal tracing techniques have revealed direct projections from the pontine micturition center to the sacral spinal cord (Loewy et al., 1979; Holstege et al., 1986) (Figure 17-8). In the cat, neurons in the dorsolateral pons send direct projections to the sacral parasympathetic nucleus and to lamina I on the lateral edge of the sacral dorsal horn, an area that contains dendritic projections from the sacral preganglionic neurons and afferent inputs from the bladder (Nadelhaft et al., 1980; Morgan et al., 1981; de Groat et al., 1986). Thus, the sites of termination of descending projections from the pontine micturition center are optimally located to regulate reflex mechanisms at the spinal level. A second area located

somewhat more laterally in the pons sends projections to the sphincter motor nucleus in the sacral spinal cord (Holstege et al., 1986). Electrical stimulation of this dorsolateral area elicits sphincter contractions and inhibits bladder activity, whereas stimulation of the more medial pontine area produces the opposite effects: inhibition of sphincter activity and excitation of the bladder.

The dorsal pontine tegmentum receives spinal cord afferents that arise from neurons located in lateral laminae I, V, and VII of the sacral spinal cord. The cell bodies of these ascending spinal projection neurons are located at sites in spinal gray matter that receive dense projections from bladder afferent pathways (Figure 17-8) and respond to distension or contraction of the bladder (de Groat et al., 1981). It is assumed that these neurons represent the spinal ascending limb of the micturition reflex pathway. Thus, a considerable body of neuroanatomical and electrophysiological data support the concept of a spinobulbospinal micturition pathway as outlined in Figure 17-6. It is believed that this pathway is, in turn, subject to complex modulatory influences from more rostral sites in the brain (Figures 17-6 and 17-7).

The organization of suprapontine pathways controlling micturition is less well defined, despite the fact that there is a large body of literature dealing with the responses of the lower urinary tract to lesions or electrical stimulation of the brain. This literature is beyond the scope of this chapter and will be summarized only briefly here; however, the topic has been reviewed in detail in a number of monographs (e.g., Torrens and Morrison, 1987; Wein and Barrett, 1988).

Studies in humans indicate that the voluntary control of micturition depends on connections between (1) the frontal cortex (medial frontal gyrus and anterior cingulate lobe) and the septal and the preoptic region of the hypothalamus and (2) the paracentral lobule and the brain stem and spinal cord. Lesions to these areas of cortex resulting from tumors, aneurysms, or cerebrovascular disease appear to remove inhibitory control over the anterior hypothalamic area that normally provides an excitatory input to micturition centers in the brain stem.

Electrical stimulation of anterior and lateral hypothalamic regions induces bladder contractions and voiding, whereas stimulation of posterior and medial hypothalamic areas inhibits bladder activity (Torrens and Morrison, 1987). According to results obtained in cats, the inhibitory and excitatory effects of hypothalamic stimulation are believed to be mediated, respectively, by activation of sympathetic inhibitory pathways and activation of parasympathetic excitatory pathways to the bladder (Gjone, 1965; Torrens and Morrison, 1987).

Axonal tracing studies in cats have shown that the anterior hypothalamic area sends direct projections through the medial forebrain bundle to the pontine micturition center (Figure 17-8) (Holstege, 1987). On the other hand, medial and posterior hypothalamic areas including the paraventricular nucleus send direct projections to the sacral parasympathetic nucleus, the sphincter motor nucleus (Onuf's nucleus), and certain sites of bladder afferent termination (laminae I and X) in the sacral spinal cord (Holstege, 1987). The modulatory effects of hypothalamic centers on the reflex pathways to the lower urinary tract are no doubt mediated at least in part through these direct spinal connections.

Hypothalamic areas also send diverse projections to areas of the brain stem that may have an important role in the control of bladder function. For example, the lateral hypothalamic area projects to the parabrachial nucleus (Holstege, 1987), which reportedly has facilitatory effects on micturition (Torrens and Morrison, 1987). On the other hand, the anterior, medial, and paraventricular areas of the hypothalamus project to the central gray matter and medullary raphe nuclei. Electrical stimulation of these areas and adjacent reticular formation (e.g., nucleus reticularis gigantocellularis) has been shown to exert prominent modulatory effects on bladder and urethral sphincter activity (Torrens and Morrison, 1987). Thus, hypothalamic control may be mediated by direct inputs to pontine and sacral micturition centers or via indirect mechanisms through other brain stem regions.

Neurotransmitters in Micturition Reflex Pathways

The sacral parasympathetic reflex pathway to the urinary bladder is essentially a positive feedback circuit (Figure 17-6). In the absence of inhibitory modulation this circuit would trigger voiding at very low bladder volumes and therefore not allow adequate urine storage, a situation that does occur with injuries or diseases of the central nervous system (Torrens and Morrison, 1987; Wein and Barrett, 1988). Thus, it is clear that the reflex must be under tonic inhibitory control. There has been considerable interest in defining the properties and, in particular, the neurotransmitters involved in the putative inhibitory mechanisms.

Glycine

Recurrent inhibition has been identified in the sacral parasympathetic pathways to the bladder of the cat (de Groat and Ryall, 1968; de Groat, 1976). It was shown that antidromic activation of the sacral ventral roots at frequencies of 10–20 Hz depressed the firing of parasympathetic preganglionic neurons and activity of the urinary bladder. The inhibition exhibited a number of important differences from recurrent inhibition of motoneurons, but like the latter it was antagonized by the intravenous administration of strychnine, a glycine receptor antagonist. Strychnine also blocked the depressant actions of glycine on sacral parasympathetic neurons, raising the possibility that this amino acid may be the transmitter in the inhibitory pathway. Unfortunately, the role of spinal glycinergic mechanisms in the regulation of storage and voiding reflexes has yet to be studied.

Enkephalins

Immunocytochemical and pharmacological experiments have focused attention on the role of central enkephalinergic inhibitory mechanisms in the regulation of micturition. Enkephalinergic varicosities are very prominent in the region of the sacral parasympathetic nucleus and the external urethral sphincter motor nucleus (Onuf's nucleus) in the sacral spinal cord as well as in the region of the pontine micturition center of various species (de Groat et al., 1983, 1986).

Administration of exogenous enkephalins or opiate drugs to the brain by intracerebroventricular injection or to sacral spinal cord by intrathecal injection in the cat and rat depresses micturition and sphincter reflexes (de Groat and Kawatani, 1985; de Groat et al., 1986; Maggi and Meli, 1986). Three types of opiate receptors mediate these depressant effects (μ, δ, and κ). In the cat spinal cord δ opiate receptors are primarily responsible for inhibition of the micturition reflex, whereas both μ and δ opiate receptors mediate inhibition in the cat brain (Figure 17-6). Sphincter reflexes are resistant to the actions of μ and δ opiate agonists administered to the spinal cord, but are inhibited by the intrathecal administration of κ receptor agonists. The situation is somewhat different in the rat where both μ and δ receptors are involved in the brain and spinal cord in the inhibition of bladder reflexes. In humans, intrathecal or epidural administration of various opiate drugs with actions on μ receptors also depresses bladder function, however the epidural administration of pentazocine, which is a κ receptor agonist, produces analgesia but does not elicit urinary retention (de Groat and Kawatani, 1985).

The role of endogenous opioid peptides in the control of micturition in animals has been examined by administering drugs that enhance or antagonize the actions of opioid peptides. Thiorphan, a substance that inhibits the metabolism of enkephalins, depresses bladder reflexes in the cat following intrathecal or intracerebroventricular injection. The inhibitory effect of thiorphan is blocked by naloxone, an opioid antagonist. Naloxone also has direct effects on micturition in the absence of thiorphan, indicating that endogenous opioid peptides have a role in controlling micturition (de Groat et al., 1983, 1986; Maggi and Meli, 1986). The administration of naloxone systemically, intrathecally, intracerebroventricularly, or by microinjection into the pontine micturition center facilitates the micturition reflex. In low doses, naloxone reduces the bladder volume necessary to evoke micturition. Naloxone also increases the frequency and magnitude of low-amplitude pressure waves on the tonus limb of the cystometrogram in chloralose-anesthetizeed cats. These pressure waves are similar to uninhibited contractions seen in patients with hyperactive bladder reflexes. Injections of small doses of naloxone into the pontine micturition center of decerebrate cats also lowers the micturition threshold. In high doses, the drug produces sustained contractions of the bladder and firing on bladder postganglionic nerves. The effect is noted in anesthetized animals with an intact neuraxis or in decerebrate unanesthetized animals, but not in acute spinal animals where the spinobulbospinal micturition reflex pathway is interrupted.

However, in chronic paraplegic cats and rats that exhibit automatic micturition, naloxone administered systemically or injected intrathecally induces rhythmic bladder contractions and spontaneous urination, and facilitates somatobladder reflexes (Thor et al., 1986; de Groat et al., 1986). These data indicate that the spinal pathways mediating micturition in paraplegic cats are also under tonic enkephalinergic inhibitory control. This is in contrast to normal animals where intrathecal naloxone does not change bladder capacity. Thus, bladder capacity in normal animals appears to be controlled by enkephalinergic mechanisms in the brain, whereas in paraplegic animals this function shifts to the spinal cord.

Naloxone also affects bladder function in man (see review by de Groat and Kawatani, 1985). In normal patients, a significant rise in intravesical pressure (i.e., decreased bladder compliance) has been noted during cystometry following naloxone. Naloxone also increases instability during cystometry in patients with incomplete suprasacral spinal cord lesions, reducing by approximately one-third the bladder volume necessary to induce micturition. These data suggest that endogenous enkephalinergic mechanisms in the brain and spinal cord have an important role in regulating the storage and release of urine.

γ-Aminobutyric Acid (GABA)

Injections of GABA agonists intracerebroventricularly, into the pontine micturition center or intrathecally, inhibit the micturition reflex. Bicuculline, a GABA antagonist, administered into the pontine micturition center in decerebrate unanesthetized cats blocks the inhibitory effects of GABA agonists and also decreases the bladder volume threshold for inducing micturition (Roppolo et al., 1986). The latter data indicate that GABAergic inhibitory mechanisms in the pons are involved in regulating bladder capacity.

5-Hydroxytryptamine (Serotonin)

The lumbosacral sympathetic and parasympathetic autonomic centers receive a dense serotonergic input from the raphe nuclei in the caudal brain stem. Systemic administration of the serotonergic precursor, 5-hydroxytryptophan, inhibits the parasympathetic micturition reflex, but facilitates the vesicosympathetic reflex (see de Groat et al., 1979 for review). Since electrical stimulation of the serotonergic neurons in raphe nuclei also inhibits bladder activity (see Torrens and Morrison, 1987 for review), it is possible that bulbospinal serotonergic pathways are involved in modulating the micturition reflex pathway at sites in the spinal cord.

SEXUAL ORGANS

In humans, the physiological responses initiated by erotic stimuli are divided into four phases: excitement, plateau, orgasm, and resolution, which collectively comprise the "sexual response cycle" (Masters and Johnson, 1970; de Groat and Booth, 1984). Although anatomic differences obviously precluded identical responses in the male and female during each phase of the cycle, it is clear that similar vascular (penile and clitoral erection), secretory (stimulation of prostatic, urethral, and vaginal secretions), as well as smooth and striated muscle responses occur in both sexes. The major components of the sexual response cycle are also conserved across a range of mammalian species despite the considerable variation in the pattern of sexual behavior in different animals. This section will focus on the autonomic and somatic neural mechanisms regulating male sexual functions (erection, secretion, emission, and ejaculation).

Innervation

The sex organs, like the lower urinary tract, receive an innervation from three sets of nerves: sacral parasympathetic (pelvic), thoracolumbar sympathetic (hypogastric and lumbar sympathetic chain), and somatic (pudendal) nerves (Figure 17-1).

Sacral Parasympathetic Pathways

Activation of the parasympathetic pathways traveling in the pelvic nerves and subsequent excitation of the postganglionic neurons that give rise to the cav-

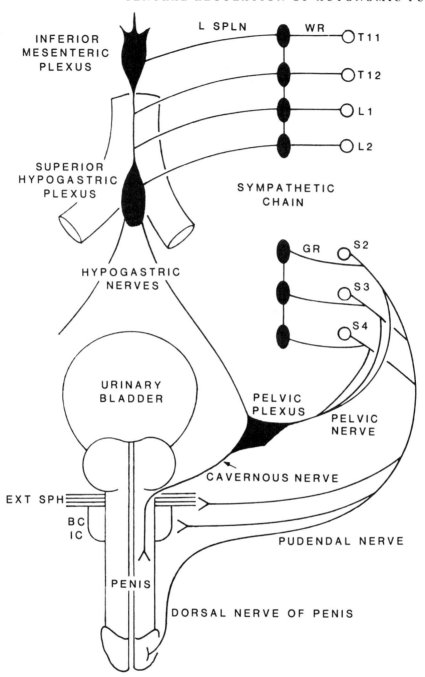

Figure 17-10 Schematic drawing showing the sympathetic, parasympathetic, and somatic efferent pathways to the penis. Thoracolumbar sympathetic pathway emerges from the T11 to L2 segments of the spinal cord and passes via the white rami (WR) to the sympathetic chain ganglia and then via the lumbar splanchnic nerves (L SPLN) to the prevertebral ganglia in the inferior mesenteric and superior hypogastric plexuses, from which fibers travel in the hypogastric nerves to the pelvic plexus. Sympathetic preganglionic fibers also descend in the sympathetic chain to the sacral ganglia from which postganglionic fibers pass in gray rami (GR) to the sacral nerves, at which point they join the pelvic or pudendal nerves. Sacral parasympathetic preganglionic axons arise in the S2 to S4 segments of the spinal cord and pass in the pelvic nerve to the pelvic plexus. Ganglion cells in the pelvic plexus send axons into the cavernous nerve, which passes in close proximity to the prostate gland en route to the penis. Branches of the pudendal nerve innervate the external sphincter (EXT SPH) and the bulbocavernosus (BC) and ischiocavernosus (IC) muscles, as well as providing sensory fibers to the dorsal nerve of the penis. The pudendal nerve arises in the S2 to S4 segments of the spinal cord. (Reproduced from de Groat and Steers, 1988, with permission of the authors and publisher.)

ernous (penile) nerves (Figure 17-10) elicit erection. This causes dilation of the penile arteries and relaxation of the muscles in the walls of the sinusoids and the arterioles supplying the erectile tissue. As a result, blood flow in erectile tissue increases, leading to a rise in intracavernous pressure and expansion of the cavernous spaces to produce extension and rigidity of the penis (see Figure 17-11; Lue and Tanagho, 1988, for review). The veins draining the erectile tissue are surrounded by a dense connective tissue called the tunica albuginea (Figure 17-11). As blood volume in the penis increases, this leads to a partial compression of these emissary veins and, as a result, erection occurs.

By analogy with parasympathetic pathways to other organs, it might be expected that acetylcholine is the neurotransmitter in the vasodilator pathway to the penis. However, in many species, including humans, there is evidence that a noncholinergic transmitter plays a major role (see de Groat and Steers, 1988, for review). For example, in some animals, atropine, a muscarinic cholinergic antagonist, reduces but does not completely block penile erections, whereas in other species, including humans, atro-

pine has little effect. Thus, attention has focused on the possible role of neuropeptides, such as vasoactive intestinal polypeptide (VIP), which has been identified as a cotransmitter with acetylcholine in some parasympathetic postganglionic neurons (Dail, 1987). VIP is present in postganglionic nerves in the penis and is released during penile erection. Exogenous VIP produces vasodilation, relaxes penile smooth muscle, and when administered locally to the penis of humans, monkeys, and dogs increases penile volume (see de Groat and Steers, 1988 for review). Further studies are needed to determine whether the coordinated actions of VIP and acetylcholine initiate penile erection or whether additional transmitter substances are also involved.

Lumbar Sympathetic Pathways

The sympathetic innervation to the reproductive organs arises in prevertebral as well as paravertebral ganglia and follows three routes: (1) the hypogastric nerves, (2) the pelvic nerves, and (3) the pudendal nerves (Figure 17-2). The sympathetic nerves provide an input to penile and clitoral erectile tissue and to vascular and nonvascular smooth muscle as well

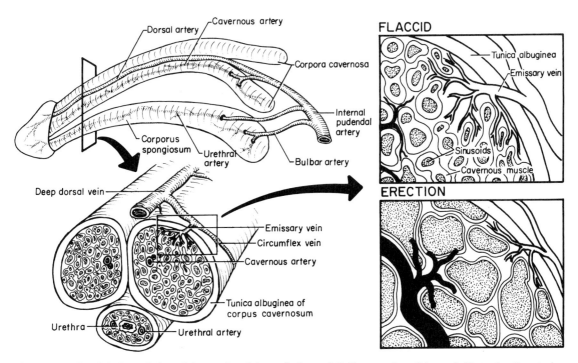

Figure 17-11 Top left: Lateral view of the arteries of the penis. Lower left: Cross section of the penis illustrating the arteries within the erectile tissue. Note the connective tissue sheath (tunica albuginea) surrounding the corpora cavernosa and corpus spongiosum. Each of the corporeal bodies has a main artery (or pair of arteries). When these dilate, blood volume in the erectile tissues increases. Right: Cross section illustrating the relationship of the erectile tissue, its venous drainage, and the tunica albuginea. Vascular changes in the flaccid state are shown on the left while the morphological changes during erection are illustrated on the right. As the penile arteries and sinusoids dilate, blood volume in the erectile tissue increases and the veins become partially compressed against the tunica albuginea; this results in erection. (Adapted and modified from Lue and Tanagho, 1988, with permission of the authors and publisher.)

as glandular tissue throughout the reproductive organs (see reviews by Bell 1972; Elbadawi and Goodman 1980). Sympathetic postganglionic neurons are thought to release primarily noradrenaline; however, other substances such as acetylcholine, adenosine triphosphate (ATP), and neuropeptides have also been identified as transmitters in these neurons (see reviews by Burnstock, 1986; Dail et al., 1985).

Sympathetic inputs to the erectile tissue can initiate tumescence as well as detumescence by release of different transmitters. Inputs from the caudal sympathetic ganglia that contain noradrenaline and neuropeptide Y produce vasoconstriction of penile blood vessels and detumescence via actions on α-adrenergic and peptide receptors (see de Groat and Steers, 1988 for review). On the other hand, inputs from the hypogastric nerve, which passes through ganglionic relay stations in the pelvic plexus, can produce vasodilation and penile erection. Pharmacological experiments indicate acetylcholine and noncholinegic transmitters, such as VIP, mediate the erectile response.

Sympathetic nerves provide excitatory inputs to the ductus deferens, seminal vesicles, and prostate gland (Bell, 1972; Elbadawi and Goodman, 1980). These excitatory responses are mediated primarily by an action of noradrenaline on α-adrenergic receptors. However, in the ductus deferens and seminal vesicles a second excitatory transmitter, ATP, is co-released with noradrenaline and acts on nonadrenergic, purinergic receptors (Burnstock, 1986).

Sacral Somatic Pathways

The pudendal nerves arising from α-motor neurons located in the lumbosacral segments of the spinal cord provide efferent excitatory input to the bulbocavernosus and ischiocavernosus muscles (Figure 17-2) which are responsible for ejaculation in males and contribute to the rhythmic perineal contractions during orgasm in females (Levin, 1980; Hart and Leedy, 1985; Sachs and Meisel, 1988). In many species, including cat, monkey, and humans, the motor neurons innervating these muscles are located in Onuf's nucleus, whereas in the rat they are located in a separate nucleus in the medial part of the ventral horn.

Afferent Pathways

Afferent pathways to the penis, clitoris, and vagina are present in the pudendal nerves (see reviews by Levin, 1980; Hart and Leedy, 1985). Afferent pathways to deeper structures such as the uterine cervix and uterine horns are present in the pelvic and hypogastric nerves, respectively. Electrophysiological studies have shown that afferents from the penis respond to tactile stimuli, whereas the great majority of afferents from the uterus are of the polymodal type that respond to nonnoxious and noxious mechanical and chemical stimuli (see Sachs and Meisel, 1988 for review).

Reflex Mechanisms Controlling Sexual Function

Penile Erection

Penile erection is primarily an involuntary or reflex phenomenon that can be elicited by a variety of stimuli and by at least two distinct central mechanisms: reflexogenic or psychogenic (de Groat and Booth, 1984) (Table 17-3). The central control of clitoral engorgement is likely to be organized in a similar manner, but has not been examined in detail. However, other aspects of female sexual behavior have been studied using various animal models (see review by Levin, 1980).

Reflexogenic penile erections elicited by exteroceptive stimulation of the genital regions are mediated by a sacral spinal reflex mechanism, having an afferent limb in the pudendal nerve and an efferent limb in the sacral parasympathetic outflow. The spinal organization for reflexogenic erections has been investigated in several species. Axonal tracing methods in the cat and rat reveal that pudendal afferent pathways terminate in the dorsal commissure and medial dorsal horn (Figures 17-3 and 17-9) (Nunez et al., 1986; Roppolo et al., 1985; Booth et al., 1986). Interneurons in these regions are activated by tactile stimulation of the penis and are presumably involved in transmitting sensations to the brain in addition to activating the sacral preganglionic neurons that initiate penile erection. The parasympathetic preganglionic neurons are located in the intermediolateral nucleus and send dendritic projections to the same regions that receive penile afferent input (Figure 17-9). These relatively few neural components presumably form the anatomical sustrate for reflexogenic erections.

Electrophysiological experiments in the rat have also provided insight into the pathways and mechanisms involved in reflexogenic erections (Steers et al., 1988). Electrical stimulation of the terminal branch of the pudendal nerve, known as the dorsal nerve of the penis, can elicit long latency reflex discharges (50–150 msec) in postganglionic neurons passing from the major pelvic ganglion into the penile nerves (Figure 17-10). Since stimulation of the dorsal penile nerve evokes reflexes that are unaffected by acute or chronic spinal cord transection but can be abolished by pelvic nerve section, it is apparent that they are mediated by a polysynaptic spinal reflex pathway involving sacral preganglionic neurons. These reflexes presumably follow the same pathway as those mediating penile erection in response to tactile stimulation of the penis.

Table 17-3 Male Sexual Reflexes

Response	Afferent Nerves	Efferent Nerves	Central Pathway	Effector Organ
Penile erection				
Reflexogenic	Pudendal nerve	Sacral parasympathetic	Sacral spinal reflex	Dilation of arterial supply to corpus cavernosum and corpus spongiosum
Psychogenic	Auditory, imaginative, visual, olfactory	Sacral parasympathetic Lumbar sympathetic	Supraspinal origin	
Glandular secretion	Pudendal nerve	Sacral parasympathetic Lumbar sympathetic	Sacral spinal reflex	Seminal vesicles and prostate
Seminal emission	Pudendal nerve	Lumbar sympathetic	Intersegmental spinal reflex (sacrolumbar)	Contraction of vas deferens, ampulla, seminal vesicles, prostate, and closure of bladder neck
Ejaculation	Pudendal nerve	Somatic efferents in pudendal nerve	Sacral spinal reflex	Rhythmic contractions of bulbocavernosus and ischiocavernosus muscles

From de Groat and Booth (1984).

Penile erection in some species such as the horse, dog, and rat is not entirely under autonomic control (see reviews by Hart and Leedy, 1985; Sachs and Meisel, 1988). Contraction of the bulbocavernosus and ischiocavernosus striated muscles, although not essential, appears to facilitate penile erection as well as contribute to other aspects of species-specific copulatory behavior (Hart and Leedy, 1985). The efferent neurons mediating these somatic contractions are contained within a region of the sacral spinal cord known as the bulbocavernosus nucleus or Onuf's nucleus (Arnold and Breedlove, 1985). In the rat, penile afferent neurons project into the ventral horn and appear to make synaptic contacts with the soma and dendrites of motor neurons (Nunez et al., 1986). These connections could be involved in the somatic reflex mechanisms involved in copulation.

Psychogenic erections are initiated by supraspinal centers in response to auditory, visual, olfactory and imaginative stimuli (Table 17–3). The efferent limb of the reflex pathway can be in either the thoracolumbar or the sacral autonomic outflow. Under normal conditions it is likely that psychic and reflexogenic stimuli act synergistically in producing erections. Conversely, it is also known that psychological factors, such as guilt and hostility, can interfere with erectile reflexes. In patients with lower motoneuron lesions involving the sacral spinal cord or cauda equina, reflexogenic erections are abolished but psychogenic erections may still occur via the sympathetic innervation to the penis (Bors and Comarr, 1960; Chapelle, et al., 1980). However, in patients with spinal cord lesions above the T12 level, psychogenic erections are abolished but reflexogenic erections persist.

The supraspinal mechanisms involved in erectile function have been examined in various species using lesioning as well as electrical and chemical stimulation techniques. Studies in primates and rodents indicate that hypothalamic and limbic pathways play a key role in erection and that the medial preoptic-anterior hypothalamic region functions as an integrating center for erection as well as other sexual responses (de Groat and Steers, 1988; Sachs and Meisel, 1988). Electrical stimulation at this site produces full erections in anesthetized and unanesthetized animals, whereas lesions at the same site generally suppress sexual behavior. However, since these two methods affect both cell bodies as well as fibers of passage, it is still uncertain which CNS nuclei are involved.

Electrical brain stimulation in freely moving, socially interacting male rhesus monkeys revealed that stimulation of the lateral hypothalamus and dorsomedial nucleus of the hypothalamus as well as the preoptic area induced penile erection and copulatory responses. Stimulation at the former two sites, but not the latter site, also promoted ejaculation.

In humans, a loss of libido and erectile failure has been noted after the placement of bilateral lesions in the ansa lenticularis for the relief of hyperkinetic behavior. These lesions extended into the dorsomedial nucleus of the hypothalamus, the ventral thalamic peduncle, and the perifornical hypothalamic region, sites corresponding to those in monkeys where electrical stimulation also induced erection.

Efferent pathways from the medial preoptic-anterior hypothalamic region enter the medial forebrain bundle and then pass caudally into the midbrain tegmental region near the lateral part of the substantia nigra. In male rats, lesions of the medial forebrain bundle or the dorsolateral tegmentum eliminate sexual behavior, whereas lesions in the substantia nigra that deplete nigrostriatal dopamine stores impair but do not block mating behavior.

Caudal to the midbrain, the efferent pathway for eliciting erection in monkeys travels in the ventrolateral part of the pons and medulla. The exact details regarding this pathway remain obscure. Several studies have demonstrated that the descending hypothalamic pathways that have connections with the autonomic centers in the spinal cord transverse the ventrolateral pontine region (see Holstege, 1987 for additional references). For example, neuroanatomical studies in cats have demonstrated direct projections from the paraventricular hypothalamic nucleus to both the thoracic and sacral spinal cord, where some of the fibers terminate in the lumbosacral autonomic centers involved in erectile function, as well as in the sacral ventral horn—viz. Onuf's nucleus (Holstege, 1987). It is noteworthy that Onuf's nucleus is the only somatic motor nucleus to receive direct projections from the hypothalamus.

The neurons in the paraventricular hypothalamic nucleus contain the peptidergic neurotransmitter, oxytocin, which has allowed the axons from these cells to be traced with immunocytochemical techniques. It is noteworthy that the descending hypothalamic oxytocinergic pathway follows a route similar to the one for erection described in earlier studies by MacLean and co-workers (1963). Pharmacologic evidence implicating oxytocinergic pathways in penile erection has recently been obtained in rats (see below).

In contrast to the well-established role of the hypothalamus in mediating sexual responses, the function of higher centers in the brain is less clear. Based on the responses to electrical stimulation in animals, it seems likely that diverse areas of the brain may modulate penile erection. This diversity is not unexpected based on the variety of stimuli (i.e., visual, olfactory, etc.) that are known to elicit erectile responses. Thus inputs to the hypothalamus from (1) thalamic nuclei (which are known to process somatosensory and visual sensory information), (2) the rhinencephalon, including the cingulate gyrus, septum, and hippocampus (which receive olfactory information), and (3) limbic structures, such as the temporal and frontal cortical lobes and the hippocampus (which are involved in emotion and memory) provide the anatomical substrates for the very complex cerebral modulation of sexual function. More detailed descriptions of these pathways are contained in reviews by de Groat and Steers (1988) and Sachs and Meisel (1988).

Secretion

The first and second phases of the sexual response cycle are associated with mucus secretion from the bulbourethral and Littre's glands, and secretion from seminal vesicles and the prostate gland in the male. This secretion is thought to be regulated by both sacral and thoracolumbar preganglionic neurons (de Groat and Booth, 1984 (Table 17–3), however, this conclusion is based primarily on the pharmacology of the neuroeffector region rather than neurophysiological methods. For example, acetylcholine has been implicated as the efferent transmitter in postganglionic neurons since cholinomimetic agents mimic neurally evoked secretion following hypogastric stimulation. However, it has not been established that acetylcholine mediates neurally evoked secretion. The central pathways controlling secretion have not been investigated.

Emission/Ejaculation

The third phase of the sexual response in the male begins with sympathetically mediated contractions of the epididymis and vas deferens and is accompanied by the release of seminal and prostate fluid into the posterior urethra. This is called emission. All of these events occur as a result of activaton of the T12–L2 sympathetic preganglionic neurons (Table 17–3) (Chapelle et al., 1988).

The fourth phase of the male sexual response is ejaculation. The expulsion of this fluid is accompanied by closure of the bladder neck (i.e., sympathetically mediated constriction of the internal urinary sphincter), and contractions of the bulbocavernosus and ischiocavernosus muscles mediated by the firing of efferent somatic ventral horn motor neurons located within the bulbocavernosus nucleus. The bulbocavernosus muscle fibers are organized in an oblique fashion so that their contraction produces a massive wrenching action to propel the semen (see Hutch, 1972 for review). This contraction is coordinated with an initial urethral dilation followed by a closure of the proximal part of the membranous urethra to prevent reflux of semen into the prostate gland and seminal vesicles. This ensures anterograde propagation of the semen. Damage or pharmacological blockade of sympathetic pathways interferes with closure of the internal urinary sphincter and causes retrograde ejaculation into the bladder (for further discussion see review by Newman et al., 1982).

The visceral afferent neurons responsible for triggering ejaculation have not been identified, but are thought to convey information from the posterior urethra or the accessory sex organs. The afferent information conveyed from the contraction of the smooth muscles of the vas deferens, prostate gland, and seminal vesicles, the build up and release of pressure in the urethra, and the perineal somatic musculature contractions trigger the sensations associated with orgasm. The relative importance of each afferent component and the central pathways involved in orgasm are unknown. However, for further discussion of the neural basis of orgasm in the male, see Newman et al. (1982) for a review.

Neuroendocrine Mechanisms

Since sexual potency depends on a proper hormonal environment, the reduction of androgen levels after castration or as a consequence of endocrine disorders can lead to a loss of libido and reduced erectile and ejaculatory function. In many instances, these effects can be reversed by the systemic administration of testosterone or by the injection of testosterone into brain sites (medial preoptic–anterior hypothalamic area) that control sexual behavior. Autoradiographic studies showed that these sites also accumulate large quantities of testosterone after systemic administration. Thus, nerve cells as well as peripheral effector organs are targets for hormonal modulation.

Sex hormones can influence synaptic transmission and also induce morphologic changes in the nervous system resulting in differences (sexual dimorphism) in cell number, structure, and synaptic organization (see Arnold and Breedlove, 1985; Sachs and Meisel, 1988 for review). These effects are most obvious in mammalian species during the prenatal or early postnatal periods, when hormones exert an organizing effect on certain aspects of central nervous system function, including the establishment of neural responsivity to subsequent hormonal stimulation throughout adult life. A number of neural structures in the spinal cord (e.g., the sacral bulbocavernous nucleus or Onuf's nucleus) and in the hypothalamic-limbic system (e.g., the medial preoptic area) important for reproductive behavior are sexually dimorphic as a result of the neonatal sex hormone environment.

Androgens also appear to influence the morphology and synaptic connections of certain sexually dimorphic nuclei in adult animals (see Arnold and Breedlove, 1985, for review). For example, castration in rats and dogs produces a dramatic decrease in somal size and dendritic length of spinal motoneurons that innervate the bulbocavernosus muscles. The changes are reversed by the administration of testosterone. These data are consistent with behavioral studies in rats that showed that sexual reflexes in chronic spinal rats were influenced by androgen actions on neural elements in the spinal cord. An excellent review of the hormonal influences on sexual behavior and associated neural mechanisms has been published by Sachs and Meisel (1988).

Neurotransmitters in Sexual Reflex Pathways

Pharmacological studies in animals have implicated many neurotransmitter systems in the central control of sexual function. The literature relevant to this topic is extensive (see review by Bitran and Hull, 1988) and will be summarized very briefly in this section.

Monoamines

The monoaminergic transmitters (5-hydroxytryptamine, dopamine, and noradrenaline) appear to have varied roles in the central mechanisms underlying sexual behavior. For example, pharmacological blockade or destruction of the 5-hydroxytryptamine (5-HT)-containing pathways in the brain facilitates sexual activity in male rats and rabbits, whereas the administration of a 5-HT precursor decreases sexual activity. These data indicate that 5-HT pathways in the brain exert a general depressant effect on sexual motivation. However, other studies imply that at the level of the spinal cord 5-HT mechanisms facilitate seminal emission, but diminish penile erections in the rat.

The effects of 5-HT in the CNS are due to an action on a variety of 5-HT receptors broadly classified as either 5-HT$_1$ or 5-HT$_2$. The 5-HT$_1$ receptors are further subdivided into 5-HT$_{1A}$, 5-HT$_{1B}$, 5-HT$_{1C}$, and 5-HT$_{1D}$. Systemically administered 5-HT$_{1A}$ or 5-HT$_2$ agonists or 5-HT releasing agents inhibit penile erection (see Bitran and Hull, 1988; de Groat and Steers, 1988, Steers and de Groat, 1988 for reviews) but stimulate emission and ejaculation in rats. However, the 5-HT$_{1B}$ agonist m-chlorophenylpiperazine (mCPP) induces penile erections in rats and primates (Berensen and Broekkamp, 1987; Steers and de Groat, 1988) but does not affect emission or ejaculation. Electrophysiological analysis of the effect of mCPP on penile erection in the rat has revealed that this agent elicits efferent discharges on the penile nerve accompanied by a rise in intracavernous pressure (Steers and de Groat, 1988). This firing is abolished by pelvic nerve transection and 5-HT antagonists, but remains after acute and chronic thoracic spinal cord transection indicating an action at the level of the spinal cord.

Dopaminergic pathways have a facilitatory effect on male copulatory behavior in the rat (Bitran and Hull, 1988). Administration of L-DOPA, a precursor of dopamine, or the administration of dopamine receptor agonists, such as apomorphine, increase mounting, intromissions, and ejaculations in male rats. The facilitatory effects of apomorphine on penile erection can also be elicited following injections into the medial preoptic area and paraventricular nucleus of the hypothalamus. The responses can be blocked by either dopamine or oxytocin antagonists, indicating an interaction between dopaminergic and oxytocinergic mechanisms in the control of erectile function. Lesions of the dopamine system depress copulatory behavior.

Noradrenergic pathways exert an inhibitory influence on sexual function. Clonidine, a centrally acting α_2-adrenergic receptor agonist, inhibits erections and copulatory activity in rats. The inhibitory effects of clonidine are reversed by yohimbine, an α_2-adrenergic receptor antagonist. The administration of yohimbine alone increases sexual motivation, suggesting that sexual activity is tonically inhibited by a noradrenergic pathway.

Neuropeptides and GABA

Oxytocin, a neuropeptide present in efferent pathways from the hypothalamus to spinal and brain stem autonomic centers, facilitates penile erectile mechanisms in the rat when administered in nanogram quantitites into the cerebral ventricles or injected into the paraventricular nucleus of the hypothalamus (Argiolas et al., 1987). However, the intrathecal administration of oxytocin does not influence sexual responses. This finding is somewhat unexpected since oxytocin is present in hypothalamospinal projections and might be expected to function as a transmitter in these pathways. Oxytocin levels in blood and cerebrospinal fluid increase during sexual activity and orgasm in animals and humans (Carmichael et al., 1987; Hughes et al., 1987). It has been suggested that circulating oxytocin "primes" the smooth muscle of the genital tract for sexual activity whereas central oxytocin facilitates sexual reflexes.

Endogenous opioid peptides and GABA have also been implicated as inhibitory transmitters in sexual pathways. These agents inhibit copulatory behavior when administered into the brain of male rats, whereas the administration of receptor antagonists for either type of transmitter facilitates copulatory behavior. For example, the opioid antagonist, naloxone, given within the medial preopotic–anterior hypothalamic area (1) facilitates copulation, (2) facilitates oxytocinergic effects, (3) increases peripheral oxytocin levels during sexual activity, and (4) prevents inhibition of sexual activity by other hypothalamic peptides.

Thus, a broad spectrum of neurotransmitters seems to be involved in the control of sexual behavior in the rodent. It is clear, however, that behavioral

pharmacological studies of sexual function must be interpreted with the realization that putative transmitters may be involved in a variety of synaptic mechanisms, some of which even exert opposing effects on the same reflex pathway at different levels of the neuraxis. Thus, determining the physiological significance of a drug effect following systemic or intraventricular administration can be extremely difficult in a neural control system as complicated as the one regulating sexual function. The pharmacological literature concerning neurotransmitter mechanisms and sexual function is replete with variable or contradicting observations (Bitran and Hull, 1988). Some apparently contradictory reports appear to be related to the effects of different doses of drugs on heterogeneous populations of receptors. This problem can be resolved by the use of selective agonists and antagonists. There are also problems in determining whether findings in rodents are generally applicable to humans. However, the susceptibility of human sexual function to a broad range of drugs suggests that sexual behavior in humans, as in rodents, depends on a variety of neurochemical mechanisms.

SUMMARY

Pelvic organs, such as the urinary bladder and sex organs, have two principal modes of operation: storage and periodic elimination. Both functions involve coordinated motor responses controlled by the autonomic and somatic nervous systems.

Micturition is regulated by three sets of nerves: sacral parasympathetic, thoracolumbar, and pudenal somatic. Each of these motor outflows is controlled by higher neural centers. The sacral parasympathetic outflow arises from the S2–S4 levels of the intermediolateral cell column; these fibers synapse on second-order parasympathetic postganglionic neurons located in the pelvic plexus. This outflow provides an excitatory influence on the smooth muscle of the urinary bladder. Activation of this motor system depends on various spinal and brain stem reflex pathways that arise from receptors on the bladder and urethra. The thoracolumbar sympathetic outflow originates mainly from sympathetic preganglionic neurons in the T12–L2 levels of the spinal cord. These fibers synapse on sympathetic postganglionic neurons of the upper lumbar sympathetic and inferior mesenteric ganglia. The second-order neurons innervate the smooth muscle of the internal urinary sphincter. The main function of this pathway is to provide contraction of the internal urinary sphincter. Other functions include a β-adrenergic-mediated inhibition of the detrusor muscle and modulation of neurotransmission of the bladder parasympathetic ganglia. The somatic outflow originates from motor neurons in the ventral horn of the S2–S4 spinal segments. These fibers innervate the external urinary sphincter and related striated skeletal muscles of the urogenital diaphragm. These are under tonic contraction. During voiding, central descending pathways inhibit these motor neurons to allow for relaxation of the external urinary sphincter. Each of these motor pathways is accompanied by sensory fibers that function to provide feedback.

The motor outflow to the bladder and its related sphincters are controlled by several cell groups in the brain, including the paraventricular hypothalamic nucleus and the pontine micturition center. The paraventricular hypothalamic nucleus provides a direct input to the sympathetic and parasympathetic preganglionic neurons, as well as to the α-motor neurons innervating the external urinary sphincter. Since the paraventricular hypothalamic nucleus projects to laminae I and X of the spinal cord, areas that receive bladder afferent fibers, it is thought that this nucleus may modulate sensory afferent reflexes as well.

The sex organs are innervated by three sets of nerves: sacral parasympathetic, thoracolumbar sympathetic, and somatic. The present chapter reviews the innervation of male sex organs. Penile erection is under sacral parasympathetic control. The neurotransmitters involved in this response may involve both acetylcholine and vasoactive intestinal polypeptide. In addition, sympathetic fibers may also alter blood flow to the erectile tissue. Sympathetic fibers provide an excitatory input to the vas deferens, seminal vesicles, prostate gland, and internal urinary sphincter. During emission, the sympathetic nerves innervating each of these organs are activated so that semen is transmitted into the posterior urethra and the internal urinary sphincter is closed to prevent retrograde ejaculation into the bladder. During ejaculation, axons of ventral horn neurons traveling in the pudendal nerve cause contraction of bulbocavernosus and ischiocavernosus muscles.

REFERENCES

Reviews

Arnold, A. P., and Breedlove, S. M. (1985). Organizational and activational effects of sex steroids on brain and behavior: A re-analysis. *Hormones and Behavior* 19,469–498.

Bell, C. (1972). Autonomic nervous control of reproduction: Circulatory and other factors. *Pharmacological Reviews* 24,657–736.

Bitran, D., and Hull, E. M. (1988). Pharmacological analysis of male rat sexual behavior. *Neuroscience and Biochemical Reviews* 11,365–389.

Bors, E., and Comarr, A. E. (1960). Neurological disturbances in sexual function with special reference to 529

patients with spinal cord injury. *Urological Survey* 10,191–222.

Burnstock, G. (1986). The changing face of autonomic neurotransmission. *Acta Physiologica Scandinavica* 126,67–91.

de Groat, W. C. (1986). Spinal cord projections of visceral afferent neurones. In: *Visceral Sensation. Progress in Brain Research,* F. Cervero and J. F. B. Morrison (eds.), Elsevier, Amsterdam, pp. 165–188.

de Groat, W. C., and Booth, A. M. (1984). Autonomic systems to bladder and sex organs. In: *Peripheral Neuropathy,* 2nd ed., P. J. Dyck, P. K. Thomas, E. Lambert, and R. Bunge (eds.), Saunders, Philadelphia, pp. 285–299.

de Groat, W. C., and Kawatani, M. (1985). Neural control of the urinary bladder: Possible relationship between peptidergic inhibitory mechanisms and detrusor instability. *Neurourology and Urodynamics* 4,285–300.

de Groat, W. C., and Steers, W. D. (1988). The neuroanatomy and neurophysiology of penile erection. In: *Contemporary Management of Impotence and Infertility,* E. Tanagho, T. Lue, and T. McClure (eds.), Williams & Wilkins, Baltimore, pp. 3–27.

de Groat, W. C., Booth, A. M., Milne, R. J., and Roppolo, J. R. (1982). Parasympathetic preganglionic neurons in the sacral spinal cord. *Journal of the Autonomic Nervous System* 5,23–43.

de Groat, W. C., Booth, A. M., Krier, J., Milne, R. J., Morgan, C., and Nadelhaft, I. (1979). Neural control of the urinary bladder and large intestine. In: *Integrative Functions of the Autonomic Nervous System,* C. M. Brooks, K. Koizumi, and A. Sato (eds.), University of Tokyo Press, Tokyo, pp. 50–67.

de Groat, W. C., Nadelhaft, I., Milne, R. J., Booth, A. M., Morgan, C., and Thor, K. (1981). Organization of the sacral parasympathetic reflex pathways to the urinary bladder and large intestine. *Journal of the Autonomic Nervous System,* 3,135–160.

de Groat, W. C., Kawatani, M., Hisamitsu, T., Lowe, I., Morgan, C., Roppolo, J. R., Booth, A. M., Nadelhaft, I., Kuo, D., and Thor, K. (1983). The role of neuropeptides in the sacral autonomic reflex pathways of the cat. *Journal of the Autonomic Nervous System* 7,339–350.

de Groat, W. C., Kawatani, M., Hisamitsu, T., Booth, A. M., Roppolo, J. R., Thor, K., Tuttle, P., and Nagel, J. (1986). Neural control of micturition: The role of neuropeptides. *Journal of the Autonomic Nervous System* Suppl. 369–387.

Elbadawi, A., and Goodman, D. C. (1980). Autonomic innervation of accessory male genital organs. In: *Male Accessory Sex Glands,* E. Spring-Mills and E. S. E. Hafey (eds.), Elsevier, Amsterdam, pp. 101–128.

Hart, B. L., and Leedy, M. G. (1985). Neurological basis of male sexual behavior. In: *A Handbook of Behavioral Neurobiology,* N. Adler, D. Pfaff, and R. W. Goy (eds.), Plenum, New York, pp. 373–422.

Hutch, J. A. (1972). *Anatomy and Physiology of the Bladder, Trigone, and Urethra.* Appleton-Century-Crofts, New York.

Jänig, W., and Morrison, J. F. B. (1986). Functional properties of spinal visceral afferents supplying abdominal and pelvic organs, with special emphasis on visceral nociception. In: *Visceral Sensation. Progress in Brain Re-*

search, F. Cervero and J. F. B. Morrisson (eds.), Elsevier, Amsterdam, pp. 87–114.

Kuru, M. (1965). Nervous control of micturition. *Physiological Reviews* 45,425–494.

Levin, R. J. (1980). The physiology of sexual function in women. *Clinics in Obstetrics and Gynaecology* 7,213–251.

Lue, T. F., and Tanagho, E. A. (1988). Functional anatomy and mechanism of penile erection. In: *Contemporary Management of Impotence and Infertility,* E. A. Tanagho, T. F. Lue, and R. D. McClure (eds.), Williams & Wilkins, Baltimore, pp. 39–50.

Maggi, C. A., and Meli, A. (1986). The role of neuropeptides in the regulation of the micturition reflex. *Journal of Autonomic Pharmacology* 6,133–162.

Masters, W. H., and Johnson, V. E. (1970). *Human Sexual Inadequacy.* Little, Brown, Boston.

Newman, H. F., Reiss, H., and Northup, J. C. (1982). Physical basis of emission, ejaculation, and orgasm in the male. *Urology* 19,341–350.

Sachs, B. D., and Meisel, R. L. (1988). The physiology of male sexual behavior. In: *The Physiology of Reproduction,* E. Knobil and J. Neill (eds.), Raven, New York, pp. 1393–1482.

Thor, K., Kawatani, M., and de Groat, W. C. (1986). Plasticity in the reflex pathways to the lower urinary tract of the cat during postnatal development and following spinal cord injury. In: *Development and Plasticity of the Mammalian Spinal Cord,* M. Goldberger, A. Gorio, and M. Murray (eds.), Fidia Research Series, Vol. III. Fidia Press, Padova, Italy, pp. 65–81.

Torrens, M., and Morrison, J. F. B. (1987). *The Physiology of the Lower Urinary Tract.* Springer-Verlag, Berlin.

Wein, A. J., and Barrett, D. M. (1988). *Voiding Function and Dysfunction: A Logical and Practical Approach.* Year Book Medical Publishers, Chicago.

Research Papers

Argiolas, A., Melis, M. R., Mauri, A., and Gessa, G. L. (1987). Paraventricular nucleus lesion prevents yawning and penile erection induced by apomorphine and oxytocin but not by ACTH in rats. *Brain Research* 421,349–352.

Berendsen, H., and Broekkamp, C. L. E. (1987). Drug-induced penile erections in rats: Indications of serotonin 1B receptor mediation. *European Journal of Pharmacology* 135,279–287.

Booth, A. M., Roppolo, J. A., and de Groat, W. C. (1986). Distribution of cells and fibers projecting to the penis of the cat. *Society for Neuroscience Abstracts* 12,1056.

Carmichael, M. S., Humbert, R., Dixen, J., Calmusano, G., Greenleaf, W., and Davidson, J. M (1987). Plasma oxytocin increases in the human sexual response. *Journal of Clinical Endocrinology and Metabolism* 64,27–31.

Chapelle, P. A., Durand, J., and Lacert, P. (1980). Penile erection following complete spinal cord injury in man. *British Journal of Urology* 52,216–219.

Chapelle, P. A., Roby-Brami, A., Yakovleff, A., and Bussel, B. (1988). Neurological correlations of ejaculation and testicular size in men with a complete spinal cord section. *Journal of Neurology, Neurosurgery, and Psychiatry* 51,197–202.

Dail, W. G. (1987). Autonomic control of penile erectile tissue. *Experimental Brain Research* 16,340–344.

Dail, W. G., Manzanares, K., Moll, M. A., and Minorsky, N. (1985). The hypogastric nerve innervates a population of penile neurons in the pelvic plexus. *Neuroscience* 6,1041–1046.

de Groat, W. C. (1975). Nervous control of the urinary bladder of the cat. *Brain Research* 87,201–211.

de Groat, W. C. (1976). Mechanisms underlying recurrent inhibition in the sacral parasympathetic outflow to the urinary bladder. *Journal of Physiology* 257,503–513.

de Groat, W. C., and Booth, A. M. (1980). Inhibition and facilitation in parasympathetic ganglia. *Federation Proceedings* 39,2990–2996.

de Groat, W. C., and Lalley, P. M. (1972). Reflex firing in the lumbar sympathetic outflow to activation of vesical afferent fibers. *Journal of Physiology (London)* 226,289–309.

de Groat, W. C., and Ryall, R. W. (1968). Recurrent inhibition in sacral parasympathetic pathways to the bladder. *Journal of Physiology (London)* 196,579–591.

de Groat, W. C., and Ryall, R. W. (1969). Reflexes to sacral preganglionic parasympathetic neurones concerned with micturition in the cat. *Journal of Physiology (London)* 200,87–108.

Denny-Brown, D., and Robertson, E. G. (1933). On the physiology of micturition. *Brain* 56,149–190.

Edvardsen, P. (1968). Nervous control of the urinary bladder in cats. I. The collecting phase. *Acta Physiologica Scandinavica* 72,157–171.

Gjone, R. (1966). Excitatory and inhibitory bladder responses to stimulation of "limbic", diencephalic and mesencephalic structures in the cat. *Acta Physiologica Scandinavica* 66,91–102.

Holstege, G. (1987). Some anatomical observations on the projections from the hypothalamus to brainstem and spinal cord: An HRP and autoradiographic tracing study in the cat. *Journal of Comparative Neurology* 260,98–126.

Holstege, G., Griffiths, D., De Wall, H., and Dalm, E. (1986). Anatomical and physiological observations on supraspinal control of bladder and urethral sphincter muscles in the cat. *Journal of Comparative Neurology* 250,449–461.

Hughes, A. M., Everitt, B. J., Lightman, S. L., and Todd, K. (1987). Oxytocin in the central nervous system and sexual behaviour in male rats. *Brain Research* 414,133–137.

Loewy, A. D., Saper, C. B., and Baker, R. P. (1979). Descending projections from the pontine micturition center. *Brain Research* 172,533–538.

Mackel, R. (1979). Segmental and descending control of the external urethral and anal sphincters in the cat. *Journal of Physiology (London)* 294,105–122.

MacLean, P. D., Denniston, R. H., and Dua, S. (1963). Further studies on cerebral representation of penile erection: Caudal thalamus, midbrain, and pons. *Journal of Neurophysiology* 26,274–293.

Maggi, C. A., Giuliani, S., and Santicioli, P. (1986). Analysis of factors involved in determining urinary bladder voiding cycle in urethan-anesthetized rats. *American Journal of Physiology* 251,R250–R257.

McMahon, S. B., and Morrison, J. F. B. (1982). Spinal neurones with long projections activated from the abdominal viscera of the cat. *Journal of Physiology (London)* 332,1–20.

Morgan, C., Nadelhaft, I., and de Groat, W. C. (1981). The distribution of visceral primary afferents from the pelvic nerve within Lissauer's tract and the spinal gray matter and its relationship to the sacral parasympathetic nucleus. *Journal of Comparative Neurology* 201,415–440.

Nadelhaft, I., Morgan, C., and de Groat, W. C. (1980). Localization of the sacral autonomic nucleus in the spinal cord of the cat by the horseradish peroxidase technique. *Journal of Comparative Neurology* 193,265–281.

Nadelhaft, I., Roppolo, J. R., Morgan, C., and de Groat, W. C. (1983). Parasympathetic preganglionic neurons and visceral primary afferents in the monkey sacral spinal cord revealed following the application of horseradish peroxidase to the pelvic nerve. *Journal of Comparative Neurology* 216,36–52.

Nishizawa, O., Sugaya, K., Noto, H., Harada, T., and Tsuchida, S. (1987). Pontine urine storage center in the dog. *Tohoku Journal of Experimental Medicine* 153,77–78.

Nunez, R., Ross, G. H., and Sachs, B. D. (1986). Origin and central projections of rat dorsal penile nerve: Possible direct projection to autonomic and somatic neurons by primary afferents of nonmuscle origin. *Journal of Comparative Neurology* 247,417–429.

Roppolo, J. R., Nadelhaft, I., and de Groat, W. C. (1985). The organization of pudendal motoneurons and primary afferent projections in the spinal cord of the rhesus monkey revealed by horseradish peroxidase. *Journal of Comparative Neurology* 234,475–488.

Roppolo, J. R., Mallory, B. S., Ragoowansi, A., and de Groat, W. C. (1986). Modulation of bladder function in the cat by application of pharmacological agents to the pontine micturition center. *Society for Neuroscience Abstracts* 12,644.

Steers, W. D., and de Groat, W. C. (1990). mCPP, a 5-$HT_1\beta$ agonist, facilitates penile and inhibits urinary bladder function. *Americal Journal of Physiology,* (in press).

Steers, W. D., Mallory, B., and de Groat, W. C. (1988). Electrophysiological study of neural activity in penile nerve of the rat. *American Journal of Physiology,* 254,R989–R1000.

Tang, P. C. (1955). Levels of brainstem and diencephalon controlling the micturition reflex. *Journal of Neurophysiology,* 18,583–595.

Tang, P. C., and Ruch, T. C. (1956). Localization of brainstem and diencephalic areas controlling the micturition reflex. *Journal of Comparative Neurology,* 106,213–245.

Thor, K., Morgan, C., Nadelhaft, I., Houston, M., and de Groat, W. C. (1989). Organization of afferent and efferent pathways in the pudendal nerve of the cat. *Journal of Comparative Neurology,* 288,263–279.

18

Functions of the Sympathetic Innervation of the Skin

W. JÄNIG

The skin is the interface between the body and the external environment, acting as a medium for the exchange of information and energy between the two, protecting the body against physical and chemical damage, and assisting in the retention of body fluids. The functions of the skin are of utmost importance for the constancy of the internal milieu and for its adaptation during perturbations in the environment. The central nervous system contains the neuronal mechanisms that regulate these functions. The efferent sympathetic and afferent innervation of the skin are essential for the physiological coordination of these functions. This chapter concentrates mainly on the functions of the sympathetic nervous innervation of the skin.

GENERAL FUNCTIONS OF THE SKIN

Figure 18-1 summarizes the functions of the skin that are regulated by the sympathetic nervous system. These functions are generally concerned with transfer of information and energy:

Function 1 is the encoding of physical stimuli impinging on the body surface, in space and time. The palmar surfaces of the hands and the finger tips are heavily involved in this function. Optimal performance of afferent encoding is linked to the control of blood flow through the skin and of sweating, the former producing tissue turgor and the latter maintaining skin flexibility and increasing friction between the skin and environmental surfaces. Both processes are controlled by the sympathetic nervous system.

Function 2 includes all mechanisms that protect the organism against harmful physical and chemical stimuli. For this purpose the skin has highly efficient mechanical properties: it is nearly waterproof and is impermeable to many other substances. It maintains osmotic gradients and is the body's first immunolog-

ical line of defense (see reviews by Bos and Kapsenberg, 1986; Edelson and Funck, 1985). Harmful or threatening stimuli acting on the skin are encoded by nociceptive unmyelinated and thin myelinated afferent fibers originating from dorsal root and trigeminal ganglion cells, both of which act as local neurogenic defense mechanisms (Chahl et al., 1984) and send warning signals to the central nervous system (CNS). The CNS initiates various alerting responses and protective reflexes in which sympathetic outflow to the skin is also involved (for review see Jänig, 1985b).

Function 3 is closely linked to the development of emotional behavior. In some warm-blooded animals, the skin and its appendages (hairs, quills, feathers) are used to express emotional states. In humans, complex emotional and behavioral signals are displayed by blushing. This function is particularly evident in animals like the porcupine, which uses piloerection as a defense reaction. These signals have social connotations. In humans, the skin of the face is particularly important in signaling. The main component in the expression of emotions is the autonomic effector organs in the skin (sweat glands, blood vessels, erector pili muscles) that are controlled by the sympathetic nervous system.

Function 4 is the expression of the state of the inner organs and of deep somatic structures (e.g., skeletal muscle) on the body surface (in particular body trunk). It is based on a reciprocal segmental efferent (sympathetic) and afferent innervation of skin, viscera, and deep somatic body structures via the spinal cord and may be particularly important under pathophysiological conditions (see Jänig, 1985b, 1989 for reviews).

Function 5 is the maintenance of the constancy of the body core temperature, which is very important in regulating heat loss. This function is effected through the regulation of cutaneous blood flow for convective heat transfer and sweat production by the eccrine sweat glands for evaporative heat loss. Both

INTERIOR OF BODY   SKIN   ENVIRONMENT

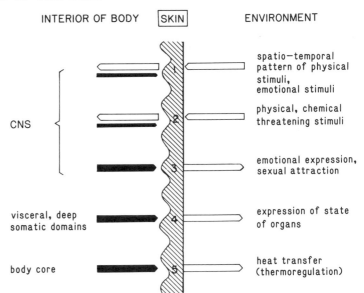

spatio—temporal
pattern of physical
stimuli,
emotional stimuli

physical, chemical
threatening stimuli

emotional expression,
sexual attraction

expression of state
of organs

heat transfer
(thermoregulation)

CNS

visceral, deep
somatic domains

body core

Figure 18-1 General functions of the skin in which the sympathetic supply is directly or indirectly involved.

mechanisms are controlled by the sympathetic nervous system.

Without the reciprocal (afferent and efferent sympathetic) communication between the skin and central nervous system the organism would be threatened. Therefore the skin has a high density of afferent and efferent (sympathetic) innervation. There are considerable regional differences in the functions of the skin (e.g., the skin of the palm, forearm, face, top of the head, and genital region). These differences are probably also reflected in considerable regional differences in the composition and density of afferent and efferent sympathetic innervation.

SYMPATHETIC INNERVATION OF THE SKIN AND ITS TARGET ORGANS

Pathways and Numerical Aspects

The postganglionic neurons supplying the skin are situated in the paravertebral ganglia: those supplying the skin of the head are found in the superior cervical ganglion as well as in the middle cervical ganglion and those supplying the skin of the upper extremities are found in the stellate ganglion. The cell bodies of the sympathetic postganglionic neurons innervating the lower extremities are located in the lower lumbar paravertebral ganglia and those projecting to the trunk are located in the corresponding segmental paravertebral ganglia. The axons of most postganglionic cells in a particular paravertebral ganglion project through the corresponding gray

rami or postganglionic nerves (e.g., the internal carotid nerve to the trigeminal ganglion; see Matthews and Robinson, 1980) and the spinal or trigeminal nerves to the skin. All postganglionic axons reach the skin via the corresponding somatic (or segmental) nerves and not along the blood vessels (see review Jänig, 1985b). The spatial organization of the sympathetic supply of the skin is the basis of sweating, piloerection, and vasomotor reactions, which may occur in the corresponding dermatomes (Head's zones) on the trunk during diseases of internal organs (see Jänig, 1985b, 1989 for reviews).

Very little is known about the number of sympathetic postganglionic neurons that project to the skin. From work in the cat it is known that about 30% of all unmyelinated axons in nerves to hairy skin of the lower hindleg are sympathetic and that this proportion increases in nerves to the plantar surface (McLachlan and Jänig, 1983).

Topographic Organization of Sympathetic Preganglionic Neurons

It is generally assumed that most sympathetic preganglionic neurons are located in the intermediolateral cell column of the thoracic and lumbar spinal cord. However, sympathetic preganglionic neurons are distributed throughout the whole intermediate zone of the thoracolumbar spinal cord, extending from the white matter to the central canal, with the highest concentration of neurons occurring in the intermediolateral cell column. An important question is whether functionally different types of sympathetic preganglionic neurons are situated at different sites of the intermediate zone in the spinal cord.

This question has been addressed in the cat for the lumbar sympathetic supply of pelvic organs and that destined for skin and skeletal muscle. The first projects through the lumbar splanchnic nerves and synapses with postganglionic neurons in the inferior mesenteric ganglion and further distally in the pelvic plexus. The latter projects through the distal lumbar sympathetic trunk and synapses with postganglionic neurons in the distal lumbar and sacral paravertebral ganglia (Figure 18-2A). Retrograde labeling of the sympathetic preganglionic neurons with the enzyme horseradish peroxidase has shown that the sympathetic preganglionic neurons associated with skin and skeletal muscle were located in the lateral funiculus and of the intermediolateral cell column of the spinal cord, whereas most visceral sympathetic preganglionic neurons were situated medial to these latter ones (Figure 18-2B; Jänig and McLachlan, 1986a,b, 1987). Hence, functionally different types of sympathetic preganglionic neurons are located at different sites in the spinal cord; whether differences exist between the location of sympathetic preganglionic neurons projecting to skin and skeletal muscle and whether this differential location applies to other parts of the sympathetic preganglionic cell column await further analysis.

Target Organs of the Sympathetic Supply of the Skin

The target organs of the sympathetic postganglionic neurons in the skin are blood vessels, eccrine sweat glands, erector pili muscles, and possibly apocrine sweat glands. Sebaceous glands are not innervated and we know very little about the innervation of apocrine sweat glands (Millington and Wilkinson, 1983). Other possible target organs of the sympathetic innervation of the skin (such as cutaneous receptors, capillaries, and lipocytes) will not be discussed further since little is known about them (see Jänig, 1985a for review).

The cutaneous vascular bed has a complex organization. Functionally it consists of resistance vessels, exchange vessels (capillaries), capacity vessels (veins), and shunt vessels (arteriovenous anastomoses, Figure 18-3). The latter have been found only in the hands, feet, and ears and are most numerous in the nail beds and palmar and plantar surfaces of the hands and feet. The shunt vessels are coiled muscular vessels that connect arterioles and venules in the dermis, usually deep in the papillary plexus but superficial to the sweat glands (Figure 18-3). Blood flowing through these anastomoses is shunted from high-resistance arterioles and capillaries to the papillary plexus. All sections of the cutaneous vascular bed (with the probable exception of the capillaries) are innervated by sympathetic postganglionic neu-

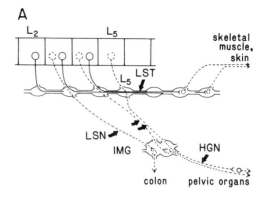

A

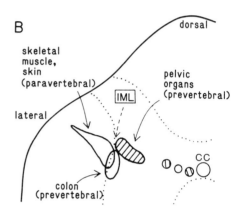

B

Figure 18-2 Location of sympathetic preganglionic neurons in the lumbar spinal cord of the cat. Most preganglionic neurons in the lumbar segments L2–L5 project in the lumbar sympathetic trunk (LST) or lumbar splanchnic nerves (LSN) to the inferior mesenteric ganglion (IMG) or further through the hypogastric nerves (HGN) to the pelvic organs (A). The cut axons of these neurons were labeled with the enzyme horseradish peroxidase at the indicated sites (arrows). The enzyme was taken up by the axons and transported to the cell bodies in the spinal cord. After histochemical processing of serial horizontal sections through the intermediate zone of the spinal segments L2–L5 the labeled preganglionic cell bodies were made visible. The positions of the labeled cells were reconstructed for the three populations of preganglionic neurons (LST, LSN, HGN) using a computer. From these spatial reconstructions the locations of functionally different classes of preganglionic neurons as outlined schematically in B were obtained. IML, intermediolateral cell column. [From Jänig, W. (1987). Functional organization of the lumbar sympathetic outflow to pelvic organs and colon. In: *Organization of the Autonomic Nervous System: Central and Peripheral Mechanism,* J. Ciriello, F. R. Calaresu, L. P. Renaud, and C. Polosa (eds.), Liss, New York, pp. 57–66. Data from Jänig and McLachlan, 1986a,b.]

rons. The cutaneous vascular bed is most important for heat exchange, with the most efficient exchange occurring via the superficial capillary loops because the temperature gradient from blood to tissue is greatest and the surface-to-volume ratio is high.

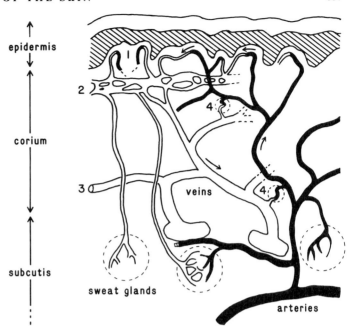

epidermis

corium

subcutis

sweat glands

veins

arteries

Figure 18-3 The vascular bed of the glabrous skin. (1) Papillary capillaries; (2) subpapillary (superficial) plexus; (3) intermediate plexus; (4) arteriovenous anastomoses.

Backup mechanisms include heat exchange first via the venous plexus and second via the shunting blood from the arteriolar side to the venous plexus through the arteriovenous anastomoses (see reviews by Greenfield, 1963; Roddie, 1983).

FUNCTIONAL CHARACTERISTICS OF THE SYMPATHETIC SUPPLY TO THE SKIN

The Final Common Sympathetic Motor Paths to the Skin

Electrical stimulation of the preganglionic axons in the sympathetic trunk initiates impulses in the preganglionic axons that are chemically transmitted to the postganglionic neurons and from here to the target organs. The target organs react in a graded manner to these electrical stimuli at frequencies from less than 1 Hz to about 10 Hz or more with vasoconstriction, sweat production, and piloerection. In the sympathetic neurons the systems normally work at very low frequencies of less than 1 Hz to about 3 Hz (see reviews by Jänig, 1985a, 1988a). Maximal responses occur at frequencies of about 10 Hz or less (Folkow and Neil, 1971). The response of the sweat glands is produced by cholinergic sudomotor neurons and can be blocked by atropine, a muscarinic blocking agent. The vasoconstrictor response is produced by noradrenergic vasoconstrictor neurons and the piloerection by noradrenergic pilomotor neurons. The cutaneous vascular bed is probably also innervated

by sympathetic vasodilator neurons: electrical stimulation of sympathetic axons leads to vasodilation of cutaneous vessels after blockade of the noradrenergic transmission (Bell et al., 1985). The transmitter of these vasodilator neurons is unknown (Figure 18-4).

In the sympathetic ganglia several, or many, preganglionic axons converge onto one postganglionic neuron, and it is generally assumed that a postganglionic neuron is excited when several postsynaptic potentials summate and reach the firing threshold: this is certainly true for most postganglionic sympathetic neurons in the prevertebral ganglia that project to the gastrointestinal tract and associated organs. These neurons integrate preganglionic synaptic input and afferent synaptic input from the periphery (see reviews by Jänig, 1988b; Jänig and McLachlan, 1987; Szurszewski, 1981).

The postganglionic neurons in the paravertebral ganglia including those supplying the skin probably have only a relay function. Thus, they transmit the activity in the preganglionic neurons faithfully to the postganglionic neurons and do not receive afferent synaptic input from the periphery. Despite considerable convergence of preganglionic axons onto any one postganglionic neuron (see review by Gabella, 1976), it is likely that very few preganglionic axons determine the output of the paravertebral neurons. Excitation of these preganglionic inputs generates postsynaptic potentials that are always suprathreshold, whereas excitation of the other preganglionic axons produce postsynaptic potentials that are always far below firing threshold. The first type of syn-

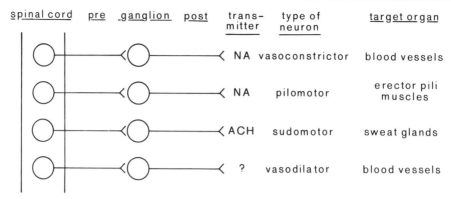

Figure 18-4 Final common sympathetic motor paths. NA, noradrenaline; ACH, acetylcholine. [Modified from Jänig et al., 1983.]

aptic input is produced by "strong" synapses, which function like the neuromuscular endplate; the second type of synaptic input is produced by "weak" synapses (Figure 18-5) (for review see Jänig and McLachlan, 1987). There are no convincing experimental (morphological and neurophysiological) data showing that spinal afferent fibers have modulatory effects on postganglionic neurons in paravertebral ganglia.

The synaptic organization of the paravertebral ganglia (Figure 18-5), the distinct target organs of the paravertebral postganglionic neurons (Figure 18-4), and the distinct functional contexts in which the target organs may be used (thermoregulation, regulation of arterial blood pressure, protective reactions, etc.) indicate that there are separate pre- and postganglionic lines of transmission of impulses to the different target organs, that is, separate final com-

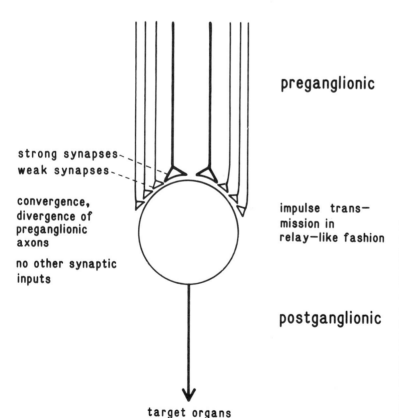

Figure 18-5 A model of impulse transmission in paravertebral ganglia from preganglionic axons to postganglionic neurons. A postganglionic neuron receives a few "strong" synaptic inputs and many "weak" synaptic inputs. A strong synaptic input invariably initiates action potentials in postganglionic neurons by releasing sufficient numbers of quanta of acetylcholine so that the neuron is always depolarized well above the threshold. It resembles the skeletal neuromuscular endplate. A weak synapse evokes subthreshold excitatory potentials by releasing only a few quanta of acetylcholine.

mon sympathetic motor paths (Figure 18-4). That this is indeed the case is supported by analysis of the reflex (reaction) patterns in paravertebral postganglionic neurons and preganglionic neurons in the cat (see reviews by Jänig, 1985a, 1986) and in humans (see Jänig et al., 1983). These discharge patterns will be described in the next sections for the sympathetic postganglionic supply to the skin. They are different from those in neurons projecting to skeletal muscle and pelvic viscera (see reviews by Jänig, 1985a, 1986, 1988a; Jänig and McLachlan, 1987), and these depend on the central sympathetic pathways controlling them.

Vasoconstrictor Neurons

The largest group of sympathetic neurons supplying the skin is probably the noradrenergic vasoconstrictor neurons. These neurons display a typical reflex pattern to natural stimulation of afferents from the body surface and from the interior of the body. Figure 18-6 illustrates a typical reflex pattern in cutaneous vasoconstrictor neurons in an anesthetized and artificially ventilated cat, and, for comparison, the reflex neural activity of a muscle vasoconstrictor neuron that is typical of vasoconstrictor neurons innervating resistance vessels is shown. Most cutane-

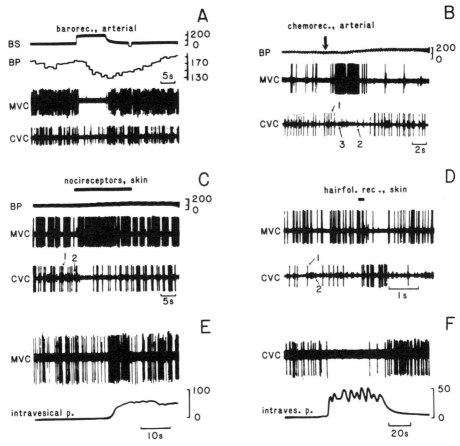

Figure 18-6 Reflex patterns in postganglionic cutaneous vasoconstrictor neurons (CVC) and muscle vasoconstrictor neurons (MVC) supplying the cat hindlimb. Cats were anesthetized with chloralose, artificially ventilated, and immobilized. Activity was recorded from postganglionic axons that were isolated in thin strands from branches of the deep peroneal nerve (skeletal muscle, MVC) and of the superficial peroneal nerve (hairy skin, CVC). (A) Stimulation of arterial baroreceptors by increase of the pressure in the left carotid blind sac (BS), which was vascularly isolated from the arterial system. The left carotid sinus nerve was left intact; the right carotid sinus nerve and both vagoaortic nerves were cut. MVC, multiunit bundle; CVC, two units. (B) Stimulation of arterial chemoreceptors in the left carotid glomus by a bolus injection (0.8 ml) of CO_2–Ringer's solution in the lingual artery close to the glomus. This solution produces a strong excitation of the chemoreceptors. (C) Mechanical noxious stimulation of the skin of a toe of the ipsilateral hindpaw. (D) Stimulation of hair follicle receptors by air jets. Traces superimposed 10 times. This effect is not included in Figure 18-7. (E, F) Isovolumetric contraction of the urinary bladder. The reflexes were elicited by stimulation of visceral (lumbar and sacral) afferents from the bladder. B, C, and D are the same experiment and the same postganglionic units (MVC, one unit; CVC, two units). A, E, and F are different experiments. BP, blood pressure. The ordinate scales are pressure in millimeters of mercury. [Modified from Jänig, 1985b.]

ous vasoconstrictor neurons have a low rate of discharge, which can be modulated only slightly by the
activity of either the arterial baroreceptors or reflexes
associated with the respiratory system, but are
strongly inhibited by noxious stimulation of the skin
area they innervate, or by other afferents arising
from the urinary bladder and colon, arterial chemoreceptors, and central warm sensing structures in

the spinal cord and hypothalamus (Figure 18-7).
This reflex pattern is in striking contrast to that in
all other types of sympathetic neurons, whether they
project to other target organs in the skin, to skeletal
muscle (Figure 18-6), to the viscera, or to the head
(Boczek-Funcke et al., 1988; see Figure 18-7). However, some cutaneous vasoconstrictor neurons are in
their discharge pattern very similar to muscle vaso-

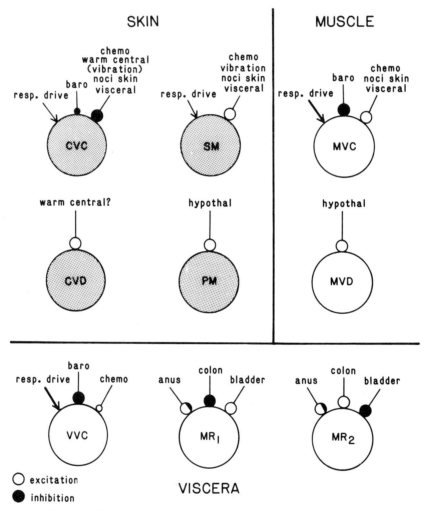

Figure 18-7 Summary diagram of the functional inputs that converge onto sympathetic neurons. This information has
been obtained from anesthetized cats with intact neuraxis. The open and closed circles indicate excitatory and inhibitory
actions, respectively, when the indicated afferents are stimulated. The afferents were stimulated adequately: **anus,** stimulation of the mucosal skin of the anus by mechanical shearing stimuli; **baro,** arterial baroreceptors; **bladder,** distension and
contraction of the urinary bladder; **chemo,** arterial chemoreceptors; **colon,** distension and contraction of the colon; **noci
skin,** cutaneous nociceptors; **vibration,** Pacinian corpuscles in hindpaw; **visceral,** visceral afferents from urinary bladder and
colon; **warm central,** thermosensitive neurons in spinal canal and hypothalamus responding to increase of temperature;
resp. drive, discharges correlated with respiration (phrenic nerve discharges); **hypothal,** the PM and MVD systems are under
hypothalamic control. CVC, cutaneous vasoconstrictor; CVD, cutaneous vasodilator; MR$_1$, MR$_2$, motility regulating neurons projecting to pelvic organs; MR$_1$ neurons may be associated with the hindgut and MR$_2$ neurons with the urinary
bladder (Jänig, 1986; Jänig and McLachlan, 1987); MVC, muscle vasoconstrictor; MVD, muscle vasodilator; PM, pilomotor; SM, sudomotor; VVC, visceral vasoconstrictor. [Modified from Jänig, W. (1988). The function of the autonomic
system as interface between body and environment. Old and new concepts: W. B. Cannon and W. R. Hess revisited. In:
Neurobiological Approaches to Human Disease, D. Helhammer, I. Florin, and H. Weiner (eds.), Hans Huber, Toronto, pp.
143–173, with permission of the publisher.]

constrictor neurons (Figure 18-7); these latter neurons are found to innervate mainly the proximal skin areas of the extremities (Hilbers and Jänig, unpublished observation).

The reflex pattern typical of cutaneous vasoconstrictor neurons is found in the postganglionic supply to the cat hindpaw and hairy skin proximal to the hindpaw and in preganglionic neurons projecting in the distal lumbar sympathetic trunk and in the cervical sympathetic trunk (Boczek-Funcke et al., 1988). Three comments should be made:

1. The neural discharge pattern of cutaneous vasoconstrictor neurons as found in the anesthetized cat is seen only partially and is probably masked in unanesthetized humans (Jänig et al., 1983). This difference is certainly not due to species differences. In the unanesthetized human, the cutaneous vasoconstrictor activity is dominated by the activity of higher brain centers: emotional and arousal stimuli lead to excitation of these neurons in the unanesthetized state; thus, reflexes that depend largely on spinal pathways are not seen in humans (Jänig et al., 1983). The inhibitory reflex elicited in cutaneous vasoconstrictor neurons by noxious stimulation of skin probably also exists in humans (Blumberg and Wallin, 1987).
2. In chronic spinal cats, some reflexes are preserved in cutaneous vasoconstrictor neurons. Stimulation of visceral afferents from the colon and urinary bladder elicits excitation in these neurons as it does in chronic spinal humans (Guttmann, 1976; Jänig, 1985a, 1986; Jänig and Kümmel, 1981; Jänig and Spilok, 1978; Kümmel, 1983).
3. It is unknown whether different sections of the cutaneous vascular bed are innervated by different types of vasoconstrictor neurons (Jänig, 1985a).

Sudomotor Neurons

Sweat glands are innervated by cholinergic postganglionic sympathetic sudomotor neurons. No convincing evidence exists that sweat production is controlled by noradrenergic postganglionic sympathetic neurons in primates, cats, and dogs. However, they are possibly responsive to circulating catecholamines, which may be important for thermoregulation (see review by Robertshaw, 1975).

Neurons supplying sweat glands in the paw of the cat are unlikely to participate in thermoregulation. They are either unaffected or only weakly excited by warming of the hypothalamus and the spinal cord, whereas cutaneous vasoconstrictor neurons decrease their activity during central warming (Gregor et al., 1976; Jänig and Kümmel, 1981). Sudomotor neu-

rons do, however, show distinct excitatory reflexes on stimulation of visceral receptors from colon and urinary bladder, of cutaneous nociceptors, and of vibrational receptors (Pacinian corpuscles). These reflexes have spinal pathways. The latter ("vibrational") reflex is *unique* for the neuronal activation of the sudomotor neurons (Jänig and Kümmel, 1977; Jänig and Räth, 1977). Conceptually, it would be ideal if the sudomotor neurons were automatically activated via a spinal reflex pathway during manipulation (which excites the low-threshold mechanoreceptors) to keep the skin flexible and to increase friction. The same reflex has been observed in young human hyperhydrotic patients who suffer from uninhibited profuse sweating. In these patients, who were otherwise healthy, the sweat glands in the palmar skin can be activated by stimulation of low-threshold mechanoreceptors, probably via a spinal reflex pathway. This reflex may normally be inhibited and may be used only under special functional conditions).

The sudomotor system, although not under the control of the arterial baroreceptors, may be coupled to the neural regulation of respiration (Figure 18-7; Jänig and Kümmel, 1977; Jänig et al., 1980). In humans sudomotor neurons are controlled by the thermoregulatory system, being activated during body heating and silenced during body cooling (see Bini et al., 1980a,b). The sudomotor neurons supplying the palmar and plantar skin surfaces have a higher thermal threshold for neural activation than the neurons supplying sweat glands in more proximal skin areas and are probably homologous to the sudomotor neurons of the cat (Bini et al., 1980a; Jänig et al., 1983). Any mental stimuli lead to an activation of sudomotor neurons, in both unanesthetized humans and cats. The discharge pattern of the sudomotor system in the cat is almost reciprocal to that of the cutaneous vasoconstrictor system (Figure 18-7) and is partially preserved in chronic spinal animals (Jänig 1985a; Jänig and Kümmel, 1981). It means that neural activation of the sweat glands is accompanied by a vasodilation of cutaneous blood vessels and therefore by an enhanced blood supply and heat transport to the body surface.

Pilomotor Neurons

Very little is known about the properties of sympathetic neurons that innervate erector pili muscles (pilomotor neurons). In humans, hair functions mainly as a somatic sensory structure, especially at the openings of the body surface such as the nostrils, the external auditory meatus, the eye, and the anogenital orifices. The vestigial functions of the erector pili muscles in humans are illustrated by "goose skin," which may occur during cold stimuli applied to the body surface and during emotional stress. The first indicates that an important function of the coat of hairs in furred mammals is a protective insulation against a cold (and hot!) environment; the latter indicates that neurally induced piloerection in furred mammals might signal emotional states to other members of the same or other species. Both functions, thermoregulation and expression of emotions, are thought to be primarily controlled by the hypothalamus. Therefore it is not surprising that pilomotor neurons to the tail of the anesthetized cat are silent and cannot be activated by any innocuous and noxious stimuli. In the unanesthetized cat, these neurons may be activated during defense behavior and in cold ambient temperatures. It is therefore likely that the preganglionic pilomotor neurons are predominantly controlled by the hypothalamus and activated in very specific behavioral contexts.

Vasodilator Neurons

In humans, body heating induces an increase of blood flow through the skin, which closely parallels increased sweating. Blocking the nerves to the forearm and hand abolishes the sweating at the peak of the vasodilator response in the innervated skin areas and most of the vasodilation in the forearm skin but *not* the vasodilation in the hand. It is therefore concluded that the increase of blood flow through the forearm (as well as upper arm, thigh, and calf) is elicited largely by active vasodilation and only to a small degree by release of vasoconstrictor activity, and that the increase of blood flow through the hands (and feet) is elicited by release of vasoconstrictor activity (see Roddie, 1983; Rowell, 1981, 1983 for reviews).

From the coincidence of sweating and cutaneous vasodilation it was assumed that both effector responses are coupled in the periphery. This peripheral coupling may occur in the following ways:

1. The activated sweat glands might release a substance (e.g., bradykinin) that induces the vasodilation. This mechanism has largely been refuted for the eccrine sweat glands (see review by Rowell, 1983).
2. The cholinergic postganglionic sudomotor axons release a substance that induces vasodilation. Acetylcholine is certainly not this substance because the vasodilation is atropine resistant. Vasointestinal polypeptide (VIP), which is colocalized in cholinergic sympathetic neurons supplying sweat glands, could be the ideal candidate to elicit the vasodilation in the skin. VIP is released at stimulation frequencies of the sudomotor neurons of 2–3 Hz or more and has vasodilator effects on the blood vessels (Lundberg, 1981).

However, it has not yet been convincingly shown that VIP is released during body heating. Furthermore, it is difficult to understand how VIP could induce a vasodilation of the cutaneous vascular bed (arterioles, veins, shunt vessels) when it is locally released at the deeply situated sweat gland acini (see Figure 18-3).
3. Finally, the vasodilation in hands and feet during body heating could simply be explained by release from vasoconstrictor activity, with no active vasodilation coupled to the activation of the sweat glands required (see Rowell, 1983 for review).

Indirect evidence from experiments on dogs and cats indicates that the skin is supplied by a separate population of vasodilator neurons. Spinal cord heating and electrical stimulation of the preganglionic axons in the lumbar sympathetic trunk produce an atropine-resistant vasodilation in the hindpaw skin, which has been pharmacologically denervated from its noradrenergic vasoconstrictor supply (Bell et al., 1985; Schönung et al., 1972; Jänig, 1985a). Recording from single unmyelinated fibers to the cat hindpaw has shown that some units can be vigorously activated during graded spinal cord warming. Interestingly, it was not proved that these fibers passed through the sympathetic chain and that they were truly postganglionic (Gregor et al., 1976; Jänig and Kümmel, 1981).

The experiments performed on humans and animals indicate that the skin may be innervated by a set of functionally distinct sympathetic vasodilator neurons. However, the strict coincidence between sweating and cutaneous vasodilation could be explained easily by the reciprocal organization of the sudomotor pathway and the cutaneous vasoconstrictor pathway in the neuraxis (probably in the spinal cord; see Figure 18-7) and does not require an active neural vasodilation system (at least to the hands and feet of humans). An active vasodilator system would be favorable for fast and large convective heat transfer to the body surface during dangerous overheating.

Interpretation of the Discharge Patterns in Sympathetic Neurons Supplying Skin

The neural discharge patterns of the sympathetic neurons (viz., its resting activity and its relation to respiration and to reflexes elicited by natural stimulation of afferents from the body surface and from the interior of the body) are functional characteristics of each type of neuron. Figure 18-7 illustrates these patterns for four types of neurons of the lumbar sympathetic outflow to skin, two types to skeletal muscle, and three types to pelvic organs. Each type of neuron has its more or less characteristic discharge pattern. These patterns are the "readouts" of the organization of the systems in the neuraxis as seen under special well-defined experimental test conditions and provide insight into the central neuronal processing. Decoding these "readouts" helps to work out the central structure of the systems ("the hardware") and to understand how the systems work under the conditions of ongoing regulation (e.g., thermoregulatory and nonthermoregulatory control of skin blood flow and sweating).

The experimental work undertaken so far shows that various elements in the reflex patterns depend on different levels of the neuraxis; for example, most somatosympathetic and viscerosympathetic reflexes affecting sudomotor and cutaneous vasoconstrictor neurons utilize pathways contained solely within the spinal cord, whereas the reflexes elicited from arterial baro- and chemoreceptors use pathways to and from the medulla oblongata. The reflex induced by central warm stimuli affecting cutaneous vasoconstrictor neurons uses both a spinal as well a hypothalamic pathway. In contrast, the reflex pattern of the muscle vasoconstrictor neurons (Figures 18-6 and 18-7) is almost entirely determined by the medulla oblongata and the reflex pattern of the "motility regulating" neurons (Figure 18-7) is almost entirely determined by the spinal cord (for details, see Jänig, 1985a, 1986; Jänig and McLachlan, 1987).

The reflex patterns of the different types of sympathetic neurons are outlined schematically in Figure 18-7. These are artificial "snapshots" of the functions of the systems and do not reveal how these systems work during ongoing regulations of the autonomic target organs. However, the cutaneous vasoconstrictor neurons and sudomotor neurons disclose some interesting features in their reflex patterns, which are important in the present context:

1. The cutaneous vasoconstrictor system and the sudomotor system are largely reciprocally organized, indicating that activation of the sudomotor neurons associated with inhibition of cutaneous vasoconstrictor activity is centrally preprogrammed, probably at the level of the spinal cord (see Jänig and Kümmel, 1981; Jänig, 1985a).
2. Cutaneous vasoconstrictor activity is inhibited on stimulation of nociceptors of the skin area that is innervated by the vasoconstrictor neurons concerned. Noxious stimulation of other skin areas elicits either weaker inhibition, excitation, or no reflexes. This spatially organized inhibitory reaction has a spinal pathway and is probably a protective reflex (Jänig, 1985a).
3. Cutaneous vasoconstrictor neurons are inhibited in a graded manner by warming of the spinal cord and hypothalamus, indicating a typical thermoregulatory behavior, even in the cat, which normally does not use the skin very much for convective heat transfer. Many cutaneous vasoconstrictor neurons are also weakly inhibited by stimulation of arterial baroreceptors; some even have a reflex pattern that is very similar to that of the muscle and visceral vasoconstrictor neurons that are primarily involved in regulation of peripheral resistance for blood pressure control (see Figure 18-7). This may indicate that cutaneous vasoconstrictor neurons serve not only thermoregulatory homeostatic functions under the predominant control of the hypothalamus, but probably also nonthermoregulatory homeostatic functions such as control of arterial blood pressure. The latter can be shown in humans during heavy exercise when thermoregulatory and nonthermoregulatory demands compete for the blood volume (see reviews by Brengelmann, 1983; Johnson, 1986; Nadel, 1985; Rowell, 1983). Under these conditions of excessive heat production, the nonthermoregulatory processes may partially take over at the cost of a higher body core temperature.

THERMOREGULATION AND SYMPATHETIC SUPPLY OF THE SKIN

General Concept of Thermoregulation

The body temperature of most warm-blooded animals is maintained within fairly narrow limits (in humans close to 37°C) as a result of an interplay between heat production in the body and heat dissipation from the surface of the body. In response to a decrease in environmental temperature heat is generated, in addition to heat produced by the basic metabolism, by shivering, which involves activity of skeletal muscle. Nonshivering thermogenesis is brought about by consumption of brown fat in newborns and small cold-adapted animals (see reviews by Hensel, 1981; Nicholls and Locke, 1984). This heat production is supplemented by heat-conserving mechanisms such as vasoconstriction in the skin and piloerection (in furred animals). Cutaneous blood vessels dilate and the surface cooling of the blood is increased in response to an increased environmental temperature and an increased heat load through exercise. The most effective mechanism of heat loss is the evaporation of sweat secreted by the eccrine sweat glands (Figure 18-8).

Information about the temperature in the body core is provided by thermosensitive neurons in the anterior hypothalamus, but also in other parts of the central nervous system, notably in the spinal cord

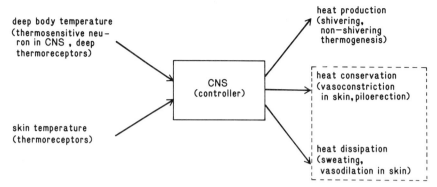

Figure 18-8 Afferent and efferent components of thermoregulation.

and the brain stem (see reviews by Simon, 1974; Thauer, 1970). Information on the temperature of the skin is provided by thermoreceptors, some of which may also be situated deep in the body. Both peripheral thermoreceptors and central thermosensitive neurons are activated either by an increase or decrease in the temperature in their environment; thus they are either warm or cold receptive, the first being more important in the central nervous system and the latter in the periphery. The activity of the different types of thermoreceptors is passed to the control centers in the neuraxis, mainly the hypothalamus. From this control center(s), the thermoregulatory responses are initiated, depending on the impending or real change in the core temperature from a value ("set point") at which heat dissipation and heat conservation are in balance and at a minimum. This "set point" is not rigidly fixed but is variable, depending on the state of the organism. It may change with the state of arousal, the state of sleep, the circadian rhythm, exercise, or other factors (such as plasma osmolality and extracellular fluid volume). Thus, it depends virtually on more or less all regulations that contribute to maintenance and adaption of the internal environment of the organism (Figure 18-8).

The neural organization of the thermoregulatory connections in the neuraxis is poorly understood. This is particularly true for the organization of the control centers and the efferent pathways to the final common sympathetic and somatic motor pathways and their interaction with the neuronal programs of other autonomic controls. (For details see Bligh, 1979; Boulant, 1981; Brück and Hinckel, 1982; Hensel, 1981; Simon et al., 1986.)

Reaction of Sympathetic Target Organs in Skin to Heat and Cold

The main autonomic thermoregulatory effector mechanisms in the skin for heat dissipation and con-

servation are regulation of sweating and blood flow (Figure 18-8). Figure 18-9 illustrates the quantitative change of heat production (A), evaporative heat loss (B), and convective heat transport to the body surface by the blood stream (C) in relation to the core temperature and the skin temperature in humans. These three processes depend on an intact neuronal control with its multiple afferent and efferent links. Their reactions can be quantitatively studied only in unanesthetized humans or animals in which all physiological variables are rigidly controlled. Anesthesia leads to severe distortion and impairment of all three processes. Measurements on single neurons (e.g., cutaneous vasoconstrictor neurons) in anesthetized animals (Jänig, 1985a) and on populations of postganglionic cutaneous vasoconstrictor and sudomotor neurons with microneurography (Bini et al., 1980a,b) illustrate, at least qualitatively, that controlled evaporative heat loss and convective heat transfer from the core to the surface of the body fully depend on efferent sympathetic impulse activity from the central nervous system. The aim of this multiple loop regulation is to maintain the core temperature as far as possible within narrow limits. The activity from thermoreceptors in the skin that monitor the ambient temperature enables the central controller to anticipate changes in body core temperature and to react in advance (Heller et al., 1978).

A decrease of the core temperature leads to a nearly linear increase of the metabolic heat production at constant skin temperature (i.e., at constant afferent inflow from the cutaneous thermoreceptors; Figure 18-9A). A decrease in skin temperature increases the sensitivity of the metabolic heat production induced by a decrease in the core temperature, that is, the effects of the peripheral and central thermosensors are multiplicative (see changes of slope of the curves with changing skin temperature in Figure 18-9A). An alternative strategy of the central controller, used in some mammalian species, is that an increase in the ambient temperature leads to a de-

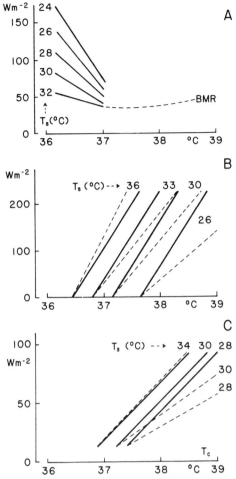

Figure 18-9 Changes of heat production (A), evaporative heat loss (B), and convective heat transfer (C) in relation to core temperature (T_c, abscissa scales; activity of central thermosensors) and skin temperature (T_s, activity of cutaneous thermoreceptors) in humans. The evaporative heat loss and the convective heat transfer are outlined without local temperature effects, that is, only in relation to the sympathetic output to the effector organs (solid lines) and with the effects of local temperature on the sweat glands (B) and blood vessels (C; dashed lines). Ordinate scales, watts/m²; BMR, basic metabolic rate. [Data redrawn, replotted, and schematized from Stolwijk and Hardy, 1977.]

crease in the core temperature threshold for heat production without a change in the slope, that is, that peripheral and central thermosensors interact additively (Figure 18-9A; Benzinger, 1969; Heller et al., 1978; Stolwijk and Hardy, 1977).

A rise in core temperature leads to an increase in evaporative heat loss and convective heat transfer by the blood stream to the body surface at a constant temperature of the skin (Figure 18-9B and C). The first is induced by neural activation of eccrine sweat glands via the sudomotor neurons, although in many mammalian species such as the dog and rabbit

hyperventilation may also play a role. The second component of the response is induced by dilatation of the cutaneous vascular bed as a result of a decrease in the activity of cutaneous vasoconstrictor neurons, particularly to the hands and feet, and perhaps by an increase of discharge of vasodilator neurons (e.g., to forearm skin; see section on Vasodilator Neurons). These neural processes are usually well integrated under normal thermoregulatory conditions. Changing the skin temperature shifts the quantitative relation between core temperature and effector responses in parallel to the right or the left and varies the central threshold for evaporative heat loss and convective heat transfer in the appropriate direction (solid lines in Figure 18-9B and C). The parallel shift means that peripheral and central thermosensory activities are used additively by the control center, if the direct effect of the ambient temperature on the effector organs, namely, sweat glands and blood vessels, is ignored (see below).

Local Effects of Temperature on Effector Organs in the Skin

Local temperature has modifying influences on responses of cutaneous blood vessels and sweat glands to neural impulses. These local effects are of considerable quantitative significance and play an important role in the responses of effector organs (Hensel, 1981). The thermal effects are strictly limited to the area affected by the temperature change. They amplify the thermoregulatory effects exerted by the central controller on the cutaneous effector organs via the sympathetic nervous supply.

A decrease in the local skin temperature attenuates sweat secretion induced by sudomotor impulses. As a result of this local factor, sweat secretion virtually ceases at low temperatures even if the central neuronal drive is high or—conversely—high ambient temperature enhances sweat secretion. The effect of low skin temperatures on evaporative heat loss at high sudomotor drive to the sweat glands is shown by the difference between the solid and the dashed line curves in Figure 18-9B. The changing slope of the dashed line curves indicates that local temperature changes and neural drive multiply each other.

Changes of local skin temperature in the physiological range (20–40°C) also have powerful effects on the responses of cutaneous blood vessels to the vasoconstrictor drive and to circulating catecholamines. Lowering the skin temperature increases the effectiveness of the impulse activity in the postganglionic vasoconstrictor neurons on these blood vessels and leads to a reduction of the convective heat transfer to the body surface (see dashed line curves in Figure 18-9C). Local warming depresses the constrictor response of cutaneous blood vessels to nor-adrenergic sympathetic stimulation. Local temperature changes and vasoconstrictor drive multiply interactively, as expressed by the changing slope of the curves in Figure 18-9C with changing skin temperature (Hensel 1981, Stolwijk and Hardy, 1977).

The mechanisms producing these local temperature effects are not well understood, but local temperature changes in the physiological range have virtually no effect on the autonomic effector organs in the skin after denervation. It is believed that the neuroglandular transmission and the responsiveness of the vascular smooth muscle to noradrenalin and probably other substances are affected (see Vanhoutte, 1980 for review). It has been shown in the smooth muscle cells of the main caudal artery of the rat that neurally induced fast conductance changes that initiate excitatory junction potentials and slow conductance changes resulting from α-adrenergic activation vary differentially with decreasing temperature: the excitatory junction potentials in isolated segments of this artery are reduced in amplitude and prolonged in time course as temperature is lowered. The slow depolarization is considerably slowed in terms of time and not greatly affected in amplitude as temperature is lowered. The interaction of both neurally induced membrane processes shows that the neurovascular transmission is enhanced with decreasing temperature under physiological conditions (Cassell et al., 1988).

At very low temperatures of less than 10°C, the constrictive effects of activity in postganglionic vasoconstrictor neurons or of catecholamines on cutaneous blood vessels may cease, resulting in a dilation of the blood vessels. This phenomenon is the basis of cold vasodilation. This reaction is principally independent, but modified by the efferent innervation of the blood vessels. The arteriovenous anastomoses are particularly involved in this phenomenon. The cold vasodilation of the skin is a local protective reaction of considerable biological importance against freezing (Greenfield, 1963; Hensel, 1981).

SUMMARY

The skin is the interface between the body and environment, serving as a medium for the reciprocal transfer of energy and information, protecting the body against physical and chemical stimuli, and restricting the loss of body fluids. It is densely innervated by somatic primary afferents arising from dorsal root and trigeminal ganglia and by sympathetic postganglionic neurons. This cutaneous innervation is essential for the maintenance of the integrity of the animal.

The sympathetic postganglionic neurons projecting to cutaneous target organs originate in the paravertebral chains and are situated in the intermediolateral cell column and lateral funiculus of the thoracic spinal cord. The target organs within the skin of the sympathetic postganglionic neurons (so far identified) are blood vessels, eccrine sweat glands, and erector pili muscles. Impulses from preganglionic to postganglionic neurons are probably transmitted in separate lines in a relay-like fashion in that a few preganglionic axons may form strong synapses with a postganglionic neuron and determine its output. Integration probably does not occur in these paravertebral ganglion under normal conditions. Thus, the skin is supplied by several final sympathetic motor pathways.

Functionally different types of sympathetic neurons supply the autonomic target organs in the skin: noradrenergic vasoconstrictor neurons innervate blood vessels (arterioles, arteriovenous anastomoses, veins), noradrenergic pilomotor neurons innervate erector pili muscles, cholinergic sudomotor neurons innervate eccrine sweat glands, and possibly vasodilator neurons (transmitter unknown) innervate blood vessels. Vasoconstrictor neurons and sudomotor neurons exhibit distinct reflex patterns on natural stimulation of receptors in the skin and in the interior of the body. Both reflex patterns are reciprocally organized; they differ considerably from the reflex patterns seen in other types of sympathetic neurons that project to skeletal muscle and viscera. Central activation of sudomotor neurons is associated with depression of the activity in cutaneous vasoconstrictor neurons. These reflex patterns appear to be functional labels of the sympathetic neurons and express the organization of the systems in the neuraxis (spinal cord, brain stem, hypothalamus). Pilomotor neurons are normally silent and exhibit no reflex influence and may be activated only in very special behavioral contexts. Little is as yet known of the properties of cutaneous vasodilator neurons. It is assumed that they play an important role in the cutaneous vasodilation of the human skin proximal to hands and feet during heat load.

A major function of the human skin is convective heat transfer from the body core to the body surface by the blood stream and heat dissipation by evaporation of sweat. Both functions are regulated by the sympathetic supply of blood vessels and sweat glands. A rise in core temperature leads to an increase in sweat secretion and vasodilation. The neuronal sudomotor drive and the concomitant release of vasoconstrictor activity (and the possible vasodilator drive) are attenuated by a decrease in skin temperature, that is, by activation of cutaneous cold-receptive afferents. Both peripheral and central thermoreceptive inputs work additively with respect to the changes of the sympathetic outputs to the skin. The ambient temperature has, in addition, powerful direct effects on the thermoregulatory effector organs in the skin. Vasoconstriction is enhanced by low local temperatures and sweat production by high temperatures.

REFERENCES

Reviews

Benzinger, T. H. (1969). Heat regulation: Homeostasis of central temperature in man. *Physiological Reviews* 49, 671–759.

Bligh, J. (1979). The central neurology of mammalian thermoregulation. *Neuroscience* 4, 1213–1236.

Bos, J. D., and Kapsenberg, M. L. (1986). The skin immune system. Its cellular constituents and their interactions. *Immunology Today* 7, 235–240.

Boulant, J. A. (1981). Hypothalamic mechanisms in thermoregulation. *Federation Proceedings* 40, 2843–2850.

Brengelmann, G. L. (1983). Circulatory adjustments to exercise and heat stress. *Annual Review of Physiology* 45, 191–212.

Brück, K., and Hinckel, P. (1982). Thermoafferent systems and their adaptive modifications. *Pharmacological Therapy* 17, 357–381.

Chahl, L. A., Szolcsanyi, J., and Lembeck, F. (ed.) (1984). *Antidromic Vasodilation and Neurogenic Inflammation.* Akademiai Kiado, Budapest.

Edelson, R. F., and Funck, J. M. (1985). The immunologic function of skin. *Scientific American* 252/6, 34–41.

Folkow, B., and Neil, E. (1971). *Circulation.* Oxford University Press, New York.

Gabella, G. (1976). *Structure of the Autonomic Nervous System.* Chapman & Hall, London.

Greenfield, A. D. M. (1963). The circulation through the skin. In: *Circulation. Vol. II, Handbook of Physiology, Section 2,* W. F. Hamilton, (ed.), American Physiological Society, Bethesda, MD, pp. 1325–1351.

Guttmann, L. (1976). *Spinal Cord Injuries,* 2nd ed. Blackwell Scientific Publications, Oxford.

Heller, H. C., Crawshaw, L. I., and Hammel, H. T. (1978). The thermostat of vertebrate animals. *Scientific American* 239(2), 102–113.

Hensel, H. (1981). Thermoreception and temperature regulation. *Monographs of the Physiological Society No. 38.* Academic Press, New York.

Jänig, W. (1985a). Organization of the lumbar sympathetic outflow to skeletal muscle and skin of the cat hindlimb and tail. *Reviews of Physiology, Biochemistry and Pharmacology* 102, 119–213.

Jänig, W. (1985b). Systemic and specific autonomic reactions in pain: Efferent, afferent and endocrine components. *European Journal of Anaesthesiology* 2, 319–346.

Jänig, W. (1986). Spinal cord integration of visceral sensory systems and sympathetic nervous system reflexes. In: *Visceral Sensation,* F. Cervero and J. F. B. Morrison (eds.), *Progress in Brain Research,* New York, Elsevier, Vol. 67, pp. 255–277.

Jänig, W. (1988a). Pre- and postganglionic vasoconstrictor neurons: Differentiation, types and discharge properties. *Annual Review of Physiology* 50, 525–539.

Jänig, W. (1988b). Integration of gut function by sympathetic reflexes through the spinal cord and the prevertebral ganglia. In: *Ballière's Clinical Gastroenterology,* Vol. 2, D. Grundy and N. W. Read (eds.), Balière Tindall, London, pp. 45–62.

Jänig, W. (1989). Autonomic nervous system. In: *Human Physiology,* R. F. Schmidt and G. Thews (eds.), Springer-Verlag, Berlin, pp. 333–370.

Jänig, W., and McLachlan, E. M. (1987). Organization of lumbar spinal outflow to the distal colon and pelvic organs. *Physiological Reviews* 67, 1332–1404.

Johnson, J. M. (1986). Nonthermoregulatory control of human skin blood flow. *Journal of Applied Physiology* 61, 1613–1622.

Millington, P. F., and Wilkinson, R. (1983). *Skin.* Cambridge University Press, Cambridge.

Nadel, E. R. (1985). Recent advances in temperature regulation during exercise in humans. *Federation Proceedings* 44, 2286–2292.

Nicholls, D. G., and Locke, R. M. (1984). Thermogenic mechanisms in brown fat. *Physiological Reviews* 64, 1–64.

Robertshaw, D. (1975). Catecholamines and control of sweat glands. In: *Endocrinology Vol. VI: Adrenal Gland, Handbook of Physiology, Section 7,* H. Blaschko, G. Sayers, and A. D. Smith (eds.), American Physiological Society, Bethesda, MD, pp 591–603.

Roddie, I. C. (1983). Circulation to skin and adipose tissue. In: *The Cardiovascular System. Vol. III, Part 1, Handbook of Physiology, Section 2,* J. T. Shepherd and F. M. Abboud (eds.), American Physiological Society, Bethesda, MD, pp 285–317.

Rowell, L. B. (1981). Active neurogenic vasodilatation in man. In: *Vasodilatation,* P. M. Vanhoutte and I. Leusen (eds.), Raven, New York, pp. 1–17.

Rowell, L. B. (1983). Cardiovascular adjustments to thermal stress. In: *The Cardiovascular System. Vol. III, Part 2, Handbook of Physiology, Section 2,* J. T. Shepherd and F. M. Abboud (eds.), American Physiological Society, Bethesda, MD, pp. 967–1024.

Simon, E. (1974). Temperature regulation: The spinal cord as a site of extrahypothalamic thermoregulatory functions. *Reviews of Physiology, Biochemistry and Pharmacology* 71, 1–76.

Simon, E., Pierau, F.-K., and Taylor, D. C. M. (1986). Central and peripheral thermal control of effectors in homeothermic temperature regulation. *Physiological Reviews* 66, 235–300.

Stolwijk, J. A. J., and Hardy, J. D. (1977). Control of body temperature. In: *Reactions of Environmental Agents, Handbook of Physiology, Section 9,* D. H. L. Lee, H. L. Falk, and S. D. Murphy (eds.), American Physiological Society, Bethesda, MD, pp. 45–68.

Szurszewski, J. H. (1981). Physiology of mammalian prevertebral ganglia. *Annual Review of Physiology* 43, 53–68.

Thauer, R. (1970). Thermosensitivity of the spinal cord. In: *Physiological and Behavioral Temperature Regulation,* J. D. Hardy, A. Ph. Gagge, and J. A. J. Stolwijk (eds.), Charles C Thomas, Springfield, Ill., pp. 472–492.

Vanhoutte, P. M. (1980). Physical factors of regulation. In: *The Cardiovascular System. Vol. II: Vascular Smooth Muscle, Handbook of Physiology, Section 2*, D. F. Bohr, A. P. Somlyo and H. V. Sparks, (eds.), American Physiological Society, Bethesda, MD, pp. 443–474.

Research Papers

Bell, C., Jänig, W., Kümmel, H., and Xu, H. (1985). Differentiation of vasodilator and sudomotor responses in the cat paw pad to preganglionic sympathetic stimulation. *Journal of Physiology (London)* 364, 93–104.

Bini, G., Hagbarth, K.-E., Hynninen, P., and Wallin, B. G. (1980a). Thermoregulatory and rhythm-generating mechanisms governing the sudomotor and vasoconstrictor outflow in human cutaneous nerves. *Journal of Physiology (London)* 306, 537–552.

Bini, G., Hagbarth, K.-E., Hynninen, P., and Wallin, B. G. (1980b). Regional similarities and differences in thermoregulatory vaso- and sudomotor tone. *Journal of Physiology (London)* 306, 553–565.

Blumberg, H., and Wallin, B. G. (1987). Direct evidence of neurally mediated vasodilatation in hairy skin of the human. *Journal of Physiology (London)* 382, 105–121.

Boczek-Funcke, A., Dembowsky, K., Häbler, H.-J., Jänig, W., McAllen, R., and Michaelis, M. (1988). Functional differentiation of sympathetic preganglionic neurones projecting in the cervical sympathetic trunk. *Pflügers Archiv* 411, Suppl. 1, R141.

Cassell, J. F., McLachlan, E. M., and Sittiracha, T. (1988). The effect of temperature on neuromuscular transmission in the main caudal artery of the rat. *Journal of Physiology (London)* 397, 31–44.

Gregor, M., Jänig, W., and Riedel, W. (1976). Response pattern of cutaneous postganglionic neurones to the hindlimb on spinal cord heating and cooling in the cat. *Pflügers Archiv* 363, 135–140.

Jänig, W., and Kümmel, H. (1977). Functional discrimination of postganglionic neurones to the cat's hindpaw with respect to the skin potentials recorded from the hairless skin. *Pflügers Archiv* 371, 217–225.

Jänig, W., and Kümmel, H. (1981). Organization of the sympathetic innervation supplying the hairless skin of the cat's paw. *Journal of the Autonomic Nervous System* 3, 214–230.

Jänig, W., and McLachlan, E. M. (1986a). The sympathetic and sensory components of the caudal lumbar sympathetic trunk in the cat. *Journal of Comparative Neurology* 245, 62–73.

Jänig, W., and McLachlan, E. M. (1986b). Identification of distinct topographical distributions of lumbar sympathetic and sensory neurons projecting to end organs with different functions in the cat. *Journal of Comparative Neurology* 246, 104–112.

Jänig, W., and Räth, B. (1977). Electrodermal reflexes in the cat's paws elicited by natural stimulation of skin. *Pflügers Archiv* 369, 27–32.

Jänig, W., and Spilok, N. (1978). Functional organization of the sympathetic innervation supplying the hairless skin of the hindpaws in chronic spinal cats. *Pflügers Archiv* 377, 25–31.

Jänig, W., Kümmel, H., and Wipprich, L. (1980). Respiratory rhythmicities in vasoconstrictor and sudomotor neurones supplying in the cat's hindlimb. In: *Central Interaction between Respiratory and Cardiovascular Control Systems*, H. P. Koepchen, S. M. Hilton, and A. Trzebski (eds.), Springer-Verlag, Berlin, pp. 128–135.

Jänig, W., Sundlöf, G., and Wallin, B. G. (1983). Discharge patterns of sympathetic neurons supplying skeletal muscle and skin in man and cat. *Journal of the Autonomic Nervous System* 7, 239–256.

Kümmel, H. (1983). Activity of sympathetic neurons supplying skin and skeletal muscle in spinal cats. *Journal of the Autonomic Nervous System* 7, 319–327.

Lundberg, J. (1981). Evidence for coexistence of vasoactive intestinal polypeptide (VIP) and acetylcholine in neurons of cat exocrine glands. Morphological, biochemical and functional studies. *Acta Physiologica Scandinavica* Suppl. 496, 11–57.

Matthews, B., and Robinson, P. P. (1980). The course of post-ganglionic sympathetic fibres distributed with the trigeminal nerve in the cat. *Journal of Physiology (London)* 303, 391–401.

McLachlan, E. M., and Jänig, W. (1983). The cell bodies of origin of sympathetic and sensory axons in some skin and muscle nerves of the cat hindlimb. *Journal of Comparative Neurology* 214, 115–130.

Schönung, W., Wagner, H., and Simon, E. (1972). Neurogenic vasodilatatory component in the thermoregulatory skin blood flow response of the dog. *Naunyn-Schmiedeberg's Archiv für Pharmakologie* 273, 230–241.

19

Autonomic Changes in Affective Behavior

D. JORDAN

The purpose of this chapter is to review what is known about the autonomic responses that accompany affective behavior and to provide a description of the neural mechanisms that integrate autonomic and somatic motor functions. In attempting this task, it is necessary to compare the neural sites responsible for producing patterns of behavior with those responsible for patterns of autonomic response. The discussion focuses on how these behavioral and autonomic sites coincide and interact to provide integrated responses appropriate for particular physiological situations. Much of the experimental work in this area has been done on awake animals in the laboratory. This is an important point since many of the responses evoked under these experimental conditions may not compare equally with those evoked by natural stimuli. The chapter concludes with a discussion of how the integrated response to fear or other emotions can be conditioned to occur on presentation of previously neutral stimuli; the focus here is on the neural pathways mediating such responses. Further discussions of this field can be found in reviews by Kaada (1967), Mancia and Zanchetti (1981), Smith et al. (1980, 1982, 1986), Hilton (1986), and LeDoux (1986, 1987).

DEFINITION OF AFFECTIVE BEHAVIOR

Affective behavior involves integrated somatic and visceral responses elicited by emotions, which are triggered by various stimuli. These responses are generally directed toward a particular object. However, this type of behavior is difficult to define in precise terms. Since much of the experimental work has been carried out on animals, the problem becomes even more difficult when we are asked to define what emotions animals experience. For this reason, research in this field has concentrated on stereotyped behavior patterns, particularly those related to aggression or territorial defense.

At least three different types of behavioral patterns are termed *aggressive behavior:* affective attack, predatory attack, and the flight reaction. On studying the literature, it is often unclear whether the same term is used by different investigators to describe the same behavioral response pattern. This problem of terminology may explain at least some of the inconsistencies in the literature, and it has been discussed at length elsewhere (Glusman, 1974; also see reviews by Kaada, 1967; Siegel and Edinger, 1981).

Affective attack, commonly referred to as the *defense reaction,* is the most commonly described aggressive behavior. For example, cats manifest a stereotypic response by crouching, retracting their ears, vocalizing, and exhibiting pupillary dilation. There is no directed attack at any particular prey or individual. Rather, the attack is directed against any moving object. This contrasts with a predatory attack, in which the behavior pattern is directed against an aggressor or a prey. In this case, autonomic activity is reduced as the animal stalks its prey. Following a period of stalking, the animal will pounce on its prey and bite it.

The type of aggressive behavior elicited in any particular situation depends on the stimulus presented. For example, a defense response can be elicited by a wide range of different environmental stimuli that could be considered a threat to the survival of the individual. It is, therefore, considered a multifactorial process, whereas predatory attack is clearly a response to a specific stimulus (e.g., sight of prey) that has a specific goal. When challenged with the same stimulus, an animal may show a defense reaction if placed in an enclosed environment or if faced with a smaller adversary. However, if an exit is present or if faced with a dominant opponent, the animal will escape. During this flight reaction, autonomic responses such as piloerection and pupillary dilation are still evident.

One question that has yet to be answered is how independent the attack and flight responses are. Under natural circumstances, there are clearly close similarities in the type of stimuli that elicit them. In addition, evidence from electrical stimulation studies suggest that the anatomical substrates in the brain that control the fight and flight areas are closely apposed. Increasing the intensity of stimulation in either the attack or the flight area has been shown to convert an attack response to escape, or vice versa (Hunsperger, 1956), but verification of this result has been controversial (Romaniuk, 1965; Wasman and Flynn, 1962). Two possibilities may account for the differences in results. First, distinct and independent mechanisms for the initiation of flight and fight may exist that when activated would each lead inevitably to such an end result. Alternatively, it is possible to envisage a common system of output, the pattern of which can be switched, depending on the information presented to the integrating system. The second system would allow the individual to both grade the intensity of the responses and provide the flexibility to modify the response if environmental cues change. As yet, no evidence is available to substantiate either possibility.

NEURAL SITES MEDIATING AFFECTIVE BEHAVIOR

A wide range of neural sites have been considered to be important in the initiation and mediation of affective behavior. The three behavior patterns appear to be controlled by separate, but overlapping sites within the brain. Much of this work has been carried out on decerebrate cats, with only the midbrain, lower brain stem, and spinal cord intact. These animals can be induced to produce a pattern of somatic activity regarded as imitating anger and defense when exposed to painful stimulation of the skin; the responses have been termed pseudoaffective reactions (Woodworth and Sherrington, 1904). Higher neural centers such as the limbic system and cerebral cortex are not involved in these reactions and the animal cannot evaluate the significance of the stimulus or the appropriateness of the response. Thus, it is generally thought that the midbrain and lower brain stem provide the minimal neural circuits capable of producing an organized pattern of affective behavior. The behavioral responses elicited in animals with brain stem transections caudal to the midbrain are not well organized (Bard and Macht, 1958 for review).

The central gray matter appears to be a key area integrating the defense response. Electrical or chemical stimulation of this region elicits behavioral and autonomic responses similar to the naturally evoked defense reaction (Hunsperger, 1956; Bandler and Carrive, 1988). This includes pupillary dilation, piloerection, hissing, and cardiovascular changes. Electrolytic lesions of this area abolish defense behavior evoked by electrical stimulation of more rostral CNS sites such as the hypothalamus. In contrast, more rostral lesions do not alter responses evoked by stimulation of the central gray matter. Although the central gray matter appears to be a central site of integration for these behavioral patterns, this region may also subserve other functions including pain perception (see Chapter 7). Since it has not yet been possible to determine if there are spatially separate functional centers within the central gray matter, the possibility remains that the autonomic responses evoked from this region are a reflection of activation of neuronal systems involved in nociceptive functions.

The hypothalamus is another site thought to be involved in the integration of affective behavior. Electrical stimulation of specific hypothalamic loci in free moving animals elicits certain patterns of somatic and autonomic responses that are typical of a range of affective behaviors. The three distinct aggressive behavior patterns can be evoked from the hypothalamus: the defensive reaction can be evoked from the perifornical hypothalamic area and the region just dorsal to the ventromedial hypothalamic nucleus (Hunsperger, 1956). This defense region extends from the anterior to the posterior hypothalamus (Nakao, 1958; Romaniuk, 1965; Wasman and Flynn, 1962). Dorsal to it, there is a hypothalamic region that on electrical stimulation evokes the flight reaction (Romaniuk, 1965). Escape can also be elicited by electrical stimulation of rostral sites in the anterior hypothalamus (Nakao, 1958) as well as lateral hypothalamus (Wasman and Flynn, 1962) and the ventral tegmental area in the mesencephalon (Hunsperger, 1956). Finally, electrical stimulation of the lateral hypothalamic area has been shown to evoke an attack response that is considered to be predatory attack behavior (Wasman and Flynn, 1962). It is of interest that this reactive region in the lateral hypothalamic area overlaps other functional areas like the "feeding center". However, since electrical stimulation methods have been used to define these functional regions, as we will see later in this chapter, uncertainty exists over whether the cell bodies mediating these responses really lie in this region and if the hypothalamus per se is the critical site generating this activity. Although the hypothalamus has been thought to be the major site for initiation and integration of these behaviors, this view has not been substantiated with more contemporary methods (Bandler, 1982; Hilton and Redfern, 1986).

Many of the earlier studies documenting the importance of the hypothalamus in aggressive behavior were carried out in decorticate or high decerebrate cats (in which the hypothalamus is left intact). In these animals, rage behavior was easily evoked by mild stimuli such as stroking the skin (Goltz, 1892). This stereotyped pattern of response included lowering of the head, arching of the back, hissing, growling, retraction of the ears, piloerection, pupillary dilation, and retraction of the nictitating membranes. Cannon and Britton (1925) termed this pattern *sham rage* to denote the lack of higher brain involvement. Animals with this type of lesion appear to lack true perception of their environment and seem to respond inappropriately to innocuous stimuli. Bard (1928) showed that the caudal hypothalamus is critical for the production of sham rage; removal of all tissue rostral and lateral to this area leaves the response intact. These studies implied that the activity of the caudal hypothalamus is inhibited by forebrain areas such as the cerebral cortex or amygdala. These higher centers keep the rage initiating region in check. This is not to deny, as some investigators appear to do, that rostral regions can also facilitate aggressive forms of behavior. More restrictive ablations demonstrated that widespread removal of the cerebral cortex resulted in a behaviorally placid animal whose threshold to aggression was markedly increased (Bard and Mountcastle, 1948). Furthermore, electrical stimulation of cortical and limbic regions can elicit behavioral responses similar to those evoked from the hypothalamus (see Siegel and Edinger, 1981 for review).

The amygdala has often been implicated as another site regulating behavior. In unanesthetized cats, stimulation of this area with low levels of electrical current elicits attentive behavior. With prolonged stimulation, the response progresses to either flight or anger depending on the area of stimulation (Ursin and Kaada, 1960). Fernandez de Molina and Hunsperger (1959, 1962) showed that the region from which defensive behavior could be elicited extended as a continuum from the amygdala through the level of the caudal hypothalamus. This reactive zone coincided with the efferent pathways emanating from the amygdala. In fact, in subsequent investigations, this pathway was traced further caudally in the brain stem where it coincides with the amygdalofugal pathway arising from the central nucleus of the amygdala (Price and Amaral, 1981).

Although it is clear that the behaviors evoked from the amygdala and hypothalamus are similar, they differ in several important respects. One characteristic of the amgydaloid response is the manner in which it gradually builds up during the stimulus and its persistence after the stimulus ceases (MacLean and Delgado, 1953; Hilton and Zbrozyna,

1963). This contrasts with the rapid onset and stimulus locking of the hypothalamically evoked response. In addition, unlike reactions evoked from the hypothalamus or central gray matter, directed attack is not evoked from the amygdala.

The results of electrical stimulation of amygdaloid structures must be questioned, since such stimulation is frequently followed by after-discharges, which spread throughout the tissue and complicate any question of localization of function. More importantly, since the amygdala is reciprocally connected with the cerebral cortex, forebrain, hypothalamus, and brain stem (see Price et al., 1987 for review), electrical stimulation of any site in this nuclear complex will simultaneously antidromically and orthodromically activate multiple CNS areas. In fact, it may be these extra-amygdaloid sites that control behavioral or autonomic responses. However, the contribution of the amygdala to emotion behavior has also been demonstrated by studies that show that ablation of the amygdala results in a reduction of escape behavior (Downer, 1961; Ursin, 1965) and more recent investigations by LeDoux and his associates (see below) also support its role in affective responses.

In addition to the amygdala, other forebrain areas such as the cingulate gyrus and septum have been studied, however, the results from these areas are more equivocal (see Siegel and Edinger, 1981 for review).

NEURAL SITES MEDIATING AUTONOMIC RESPONSES

The studies considered so far have been concerned with somatic and autonomic responses. There is also a wealth of data concerning the effects of studies of electrical stimulation on other specific autonomic responses including blood pressure, heart rate, sympathetic nerve activity, regional blood flow, gastrointestinal motility, and adrenal catecholamine secretion. The discussion here will be restricted to the midbrain, the hypothalamus, and the amygdala.

Before these studies are summarized, the reader should be aware of the limitations of their methodology. Electrical stimulation activates both cell bodies and fibers of passage. Thus, studies of this nature do not provide definitive evidence that a response is due to activation of either the cells at a particular locus, fibers traveling to, or through it. In addition, they cannot be used to determine whether a response is due to orthodromic or antidromic activation of fibers. However, these studies serve as a useful if rather general guide to central autonomic pathways; they are the first systematic studies aimed specifically at providing a functional neuroanatomy of central autonomic circuits. Electrical stimulation of a large zone stretching from the anterior to the posterior hypothalamus elicits marked pressor responses due to vasoconstriction of mesenteric, renal, and cutaneous vascular beds, tachycardia, and increased ventricular contraction. These changes result from increased sympathetic nervous discharges to the heart and resistance vessels. However, in addition to these sympathoexcitatory effects, stimulation at a restricted range of sites rostral to the anterior hypothalamus evokes depressor responses, bradycardia, and vasodilation in many vascular beds. These responses are primarily due to inhibition of sympathetic activity but the heart rate response includes augmentation of parasympathetic drive to the heart. These results have led to the idea of a functional division within the hypothalamus of a posterior sympathoexcitatory region and a rostral sympathoinhibitory/parasympathoexcitatory region. However, this interpretation must be viewed as premature and needs confirmation with chemical microinjection techniques.

Stimulation within the pressor/sympathoexcitatory region evokes a marked vasodilation of resistance vessels in skeletal muscle of cats (Eliasson et al., 1951). In certain species such as the cat, activation of this specialized sympathetic cholinergic vasodilatory system results in a marked increase in blood flow to limb skeletal muscle. This pathway is thought to utilize acetylcholine at the vascular smooth muscle junction because the response can be blocked by the cholinergic antagonist atropine. However, even in those species that do not exhibit this cholinergic vasodilation, increased muscle blood flow is still observed when the hypothalamic sympathoexcitatory region is stimulated. In these cases, vasodilation could result from combinations of inhibition of sympathetic vasoconstrictor fibers, the activation of vasodilator fibers with a noncholinergic mediator, and increased secretion of adrenaline from the adrenal medulla.

In addition to these wide-ranging effects on the cardiovascular system, other autonomic effects can be demonstrated after hypothalamic stimulation such as pupillary dilation, retraction of the nictitating membrane, piloerection, increased sudomotor activity, and a wide range of alterations in gastric and intestinal motility (see Mancia and Zanchetti, 1981 for review).

A variety of autonomic responses can also be elicited by electrical stimulation of the amygdala (Kapp et al., 1983 for review). For example, Ursin and Kaada (1960) described a range of autonomic and somatomotor responses evoked from different amygdaloid nuclei. These included piloerection, pupillary dilation, micturition, defecation, salivation, licking, and a range of respiratory responses.

Whether these are due to activation of efferent or afferent systems remains unknown.

THE BRAIN AS A MEDIATOR OF INTEGRATED BEHAVIOR AND AUTONOMIC ACTIVITY

There are two major concerns with the experiments described so far: (1) the extent to which they relate to real life situations and (2) the accuracy of experimental findings based in large part on electrical stimulation methods. Both of these issues will be discussed in this section.

Although the electrical stimulation mapping studies described above have considered individual autonomic or behavioral variables, it is now clear that the stimulation sites that alter cardiovascular function also modify activity of other autonomic, endocrine, and behavioral functions. This concept developed as a result of studies in which multiple recordings of a range of autonomic and somatomotor activities were made in animals. The responses were studied in free-moving awake cats, which allowed for a correlation with the somatomotor, autonomic, and behavioral responses elicited by the same stimuli (see Mancia and Zanchetti, 1981 for review). The experiments demonstrated that on electrical stimulation, the hypothalamus was capable of producing complex integrated patterns of behavioral, somatomotor and autonomic responses that mirrored the physiological patterns of visceral activity seen in freely moving animals undergoing a variety of motivational behaviors. It is important to stress that although these results do not prove that the response is due to neurons originating within the hypothalamus, they illustrate that the neural system(s) that regulate these physiological patterns of visceral activity are present in conscious animals. Although this concept has now been extended to explain a variety of patterns of activity seen during feeding, drinking, thermoregulation, and exercise, its development was initiated by studies of defense behavior and the autonomic responses accompanying it. Since the concept itself is so clearly applicable to other areas of autonomic control, it is useful to consider in detail its development and standing in relation to our current understanding of autonomic control.

In 1943, Hess and Brugger used electrical stimulation methods in conscious cats to delineate the hypothalamic regions from which a coordinated behavior pattern could be evoked. This response was initially one of alerting, but culminated, if the electrical stimulation was intense, in flight or attack. The response could not be distinguished from those evoked by natural aversive environmental stimuli

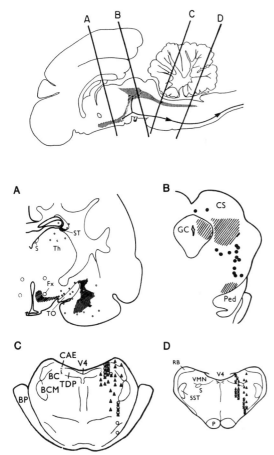

Figure 19-1 Top: A schematic diagram of a parasagittal section of a cat's brain. The diagonal shaded areas represent regions in the hypothalamus, mesencephalon, pons, and medulla oblongata, which integrate defense reactions; the solid line indicates the location of the efferent pathway for the cardiovascular pattern of response and other visceral components. Coronal sections taken at the planes indicated A–D are shown below as indicated. Four representative transverse sections of the cat brain illustrating reactive sites in which electrical stimulation elicits the defense reaction. (A) The reactive zone included the perifornical hypothalamic area (diagonal screening) and the amygdala (cross-hatching). (Reproduced from Hilton and Zbrozyna, 1963, with permission of the authors and publisher.) (B) Regions in the mesencephalon from which active muscle vasodilation is obtained on stimulation. Hatching indicates areas from which vasodilation was regularly obtained; the dots indicate sites of large responses in individual experiments. (Reproduced from Abrahams et al., 1960, with permission of the authors and publisher). (C) Regions in the pons from which increases in blood pressure were obtained, with (open circles) and without (triangles) muscle vasodilation. (Reproduced from Coote et al., 1973, with permission.) (D) Regions in the medulla oblongata from which increases in blood pressure were obtained, with (open circles) and without (triangles) muscle vasodilation. (Reproduced from Coote et al., 1973, with permission.) BC, brachium conjunctivum; BCM, parabrachial nucleus (nucleus of brachium conjunctivum); BP, brachium pontis; CAE, locus coeruleus; CS, superior colliculus; GC, central gray matter; FX, fornix; P, pyramidal tract; Ped, cerebral peduncle; RB, restiform body; S, solitary tract; ST,

and was termed the *defense reaction (Abwehrreaktion)*. It was most eadily evoked from the perifornical hypothalamic area (Figure 19-1A). Stimulation of this region in anesthetized cats evokes an atropine-sensitive vasodilation in skeletal muscle accompanied by sympathetically mediated vasoconstriction in cutaneous and intestinal vascular beds and a rise in arterial blood pressure (Eliasson et al., 1951; Abrahams et al., 1960), renal vasoconstriction (Feigl et al., 1964), increased heart rate and cardiac contractility (Rosen, 1961), and a rise in cardiac output (Kylstra and Lisander, 1970). In addition, pupillary dilation, retraction of the nictitating membrane, piloerection, and rapid, shallow breathing are features of this response (Abrahams et al., 1960). This same coordinated pattern of response can be evoked from a series of sites extending caudally from the hypothalamus into the midbrain (Figure 19-1B) (Abrahams et al., 1960). In particular, an excitable region is found in the dorsolateral part of the central gray matter (Figure 19-1B). Further laterally in the tegmentum and underlying the superior colliculus, similar responses are obtained, except that the pressor response is particularly large and associated with bradycardia. Finally, electrical stimulation of a small area in the mesencephalon dorsal to the cerebral peduncle produces only hindlimb vasodilation. Small lesions of this most ventral region abolish hypothalamically evoked vasodilation, whereas lesions of much of the midbrain, including the central gray matter and the appropriate region of the tegmentum, have little effect. Thus, this ventral region may be part of an efferent pathway controlling muscle vasodilation.

If any site along the pathway from the amygdala to medulla oblongata mediating muscle vasodilation was stimulated in unanesthetized cats (except the area dorsal to the cerebral peduncule), it produced a fairly constant pattern of behavior (Abrahams et al., 1960). A threshold stimulus evoked an alerting reaction. The animal would raise its head to look about and dilate its pupils. With stronger stimulation, the animal would show increased pupillary dilation, piloerection, stand, hiss, or growl, retract its ears, and unsheath its claws. This culminates in attack behavior. With electrodes implanted in either the hypothalamus, central gray matter, or midbrain tegmental area, the behavioral and cardiovascular patterns of response were always evoked in concert. This coordinated response was thought to be due to activation of common regions that subserve integrative cell groups or pathways from which all components of the defense reaction were produced. How-

stria terminalis; TDP, dorsal tegmental nucleus; Th, thalamus; TO, optic tract; VMN, medial vestibular nucleus; V4, 4th ventricle; 5ST, spinal trigeminal tract.

ever, the correlation between the autonomic and behavioral responses elicited from the hypothalamus may be due to the inability of the electrical stimulation technique to discretely stimulate separate populations of neurons or fiber systems controlling these different functional components. The chemical stimulation experiments also have the same problem of spatial resolution. Thus, the brain stem defense region extends from the amygdala complex into the lower brain stem.

Electrical stimulation of the amygdala in unanesthetized cats causes behavioral and autonomic responses qualitatively identical to those evoked by hypothalamic stimulation (Hilton and Zbrozyna, 1963). The area of the amygdala producing defense responses includes part of the anterior amygdala, the magnocellular component of the basal nucleus, and medial part of the central nucleus (Figure 19-1A). However, unlike the responses elicited from the hypothalamus, stimulation within the amygdala produces the entire pattern of response only in awake, or very lightly anesthetized animals (Stock et al., 1978). In addition, Timms (1981) has demonstrated the useful properties of the steroid anesthetic, alphaxalone/alphadolone (Althesin), which is thought not to interfere with the integrative activities of the forebrain in the same way as conventional anesthetics. In Althesin-anesthetized cats, the visceral changes characteristic of a defense reaction can be evoked by stimulation of the amygdala or even reflexly by stimulation of afferent inputs (see Marshall, 1987 for review). Thus, these results clearly show the marked effects anesthetics have on these responses—a factor that has been largely ignored in this area of research.

Stimulation of two regions of the rostral part of the rhombencephalon yields complete patterns of behavioral and autonomic response similar to those seen on hypothalamic stimulation (Figure 19-1C and D). The first area lies in the dorsolateral central gray matter just medial to the parabrachial nucleus. When stimulated in awake or anesthetized animals, it evokes both the behavioral and visceral components of the defense response (Coote et al., 1973). This region may represent the caudal trajectory of the active region identified in the lateral tegmental area of the midbrain. Only two differences are apparent between the responses evoked by stimulation at this site, and those evoked from the hypothalamus or by natural stimuli. First, the brain stem-evoked response is less well integrated and, second, the muscle vasodilation is the result of a reduction in sympathetic vasoconstrictor activity. The second area lies in the ventrolateral tegmentum near the region of the ventral nucleus of the lateral lemniscus.

Electrical stimulation of the medulla oblongata at several loci elicit rises in arterial pressure along with muscle vasodilation (Figure 19-1D). These areas include the dorsal medial medulla (medial vestibular nucleus), the dorsal reticular formation, and the ventral medulla. Only the last area has been studied in detail. Electrical stimulation of the ventral medulla elicits the characteristic cardiovascular patterns of defense response (Hilton et al., 1983). In cats, this narrow pathway runs as a strip about 3 mm lateral to the pyramidal tract. At more caudal medullary levels, the pathway lies ventral to the facial nucleus, very close to the surface of the medulla and coincides with the "rostral ventrolateral medulla." This is considered one of the key autonomic regulatory regions in the brain. It recieves inputs from the hypothalamus, central gray matter, and nucleus tractus solitarius and gives rise to a major projection to the intermediolateral cell column (for review see Ciriello et al., 1986). Bilateral disruption of synaptic transmission in this area totally abolishes the cardiovascular, respiratory, and pupillary responses evoked by stimulation within the defense areas of the amygdala, hypothalamus, or midbrain (Hilton et al., 1983) or by peripheral nerve stimulation (Marshall, 1986).

Neurons in this region are important in the maintenance of vasomotor tone (see Chapters 8 and 9). In a 1986 review, Hilton hypothesized that ongoing activity in the brain stem defense regions is responsible for the tonic activity of the rostral ventrolateral medullary neurons, and, hence, ultimately responsible for vasomotor tone. In contrast, however, Guyenet (Chapter 9) argues that this tonic activity is more likely to be the result of intrinsic pacemaker properties of the neurons themselves. However, the actual neural mechanism(s) responsible for generating vasomotor is still not resolved.

Although electrical stimulation throughout a large continuum of neural tissue can evoke the complex integrated pattern of activity now considered characteristic of affective behavior, the question of which site(s) is important in coordinating and initiating such a response remains unanswered. The hypothalamus, or sites caudal to it have been implicated as the neural centers mediating this behavior because peripheral stimuli can reflexly initiate an almost entire repertoire of responses in the high decerebrate animal. Since the response was produced most reliably by electrical stimulation of the perifornical region of the hypothalamus, the idea arose that this region was of prime importance. However, studies using microinjections of excitatory amino acids that activate only nerve cell bodies and dendrites have cast serious doubt on the accuracy of this hypothesis.

In anesthetized or awake cats and rats, chemical stimulation of midbrain central gray matter can evoke both the behavioral and the cardiovascular patterns of the defense response (Figure 19-2); com-

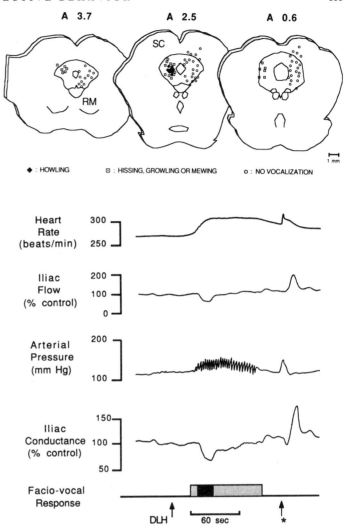

Figure 19-2 Top: Three representative transverse sections of the midbrain of the cat to show location of D,L-homocysteic acid injection sites that elicited vocal reactions (left side). Sites from which no vocal reaction was produced are plotted on the right side. RM, red nucleus (magnocellular division); SC, superior colliculus. Bottom: Example of the cardiovascular changes that accompany vocal reactions after excitatory amino acid injections in the central gray matter. The period of intense vocal reaction is indicated by the dark shading. This was preceded and followed by periods during which the animal exhibited a moderate vocal reaction (indicated by the lighter shading). Note that only the intense reaction was accompanied by a marked decrease in iliac conductance. The first arrow indicates the point at which a microinjection of D,L-homocysteic acid (0.2 μl of 0.2 M solution) was made. The second arrow, marked by an asterisk, indicates the point at which the hindlimb of the animal showed a spontaneous movement. (Reproduced from Carrive et al., 1987, with permission of the authors and publisher.)

parable injections into the hypothalamus and midbrain tegmentum are ineffective (Bandler, 1982; McDougall et al., 1985; Carrive et al., 1987; Hilton, 1986; Bandler and Carrive, 1988; Hilton and Redfern, 1986). This suggests that it is neurons within the midbrain central gray matter that are responsible for coordinating and initiating the responses seen during affective behavior. However, any chemical stimulus must activate a pool of neurons large enough to evoke a measurable peripheral response. Since it is possible that the particular neural architecture of the central gray matter makes it easier for such a pool of functionally homogeneous neurons to be activated by chemical stimuli, even these results must be considered with care.

The midbrain central gray matter (also called the periaqueductal gray matter) receives afferent inputs from the central nucleus of the amygdala, zona incerta, lateral hypothalamic area, substantia nigra, as well as numerous other sites, including the nucleus tractus solitarius and rostral ventrolateral medulla (see Figure 19-3; rat: Beitz, 1982; Luiten et al., 1987; rabbit: Meller and Dennis, 1986; cat: Bandler and McCulloch, 1984; Bandler et al., 1985). These inputs may subserve autonomic, somatomotor, and sensory functions. For example, the afferents from the central nucleus of the amygdala, the lateral hypothalamic area, and the zona incerta may mediate changes in cardiovascular function, since stimulation of each of these areas produces cardiovascular response (Stock et al., 1978; Spencer et al., 1988, 1989) and each connects with autonomic centers of the brain stem and/or spinal cord. The inputs from the substantia nigra may regulate somatomotor functions.

This region of the central gray matter from which defense reactions may be evoked provides descending projections to both medullary and spinal cord

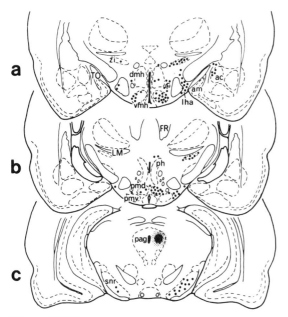

Figure 19-3 The central gray matter receives afferent projections from a variety of forebrain nuclei. Following an injection of the retrograde cell body marker horseradish peroxidase in the midbrain central gray matter of a rat (c), retrogradely labeled cell bodies are found in the central nucleus of the amygdala (ac), zona incerta (zi), lateral hypothalamic area (lha), and a number of other hypothalamic nuclei (a and b). In addition to the substantia nigra, the pars reticulata (snr) also contains retrogradely labeled cells (c). am, medial amygdaloid nucleus; dmh, dorsomedial hypothalamic nucleus; F, fornix; FR, fasciculus retroflexus; LM, medial lemniscus; pag, periaqueductal gray matter; ph, posterior hypothalamic area; pmd, dorsal premammillary nucleus; pmv, ventral premammillary nucleus; vmh, ventromedial hypothalamic nucleus. (Reproduced from Luiten et al., 1987, with permission of the authors and publisher.)

nuclei involved in both autonomic and somatic motor functions (Figures 19-4 and 19-5). It projects to the ventrolateral medulla and the caudal raphe nuclei (Luiten et al., 1987); these two latter areas project to the spinal nuclei containing sympathetic preganglionic neurons and somatic motor neurons (Loewy et al., 1981; Loewy, 1981). However, these projections are considerably less dense than the projection to the rostral ventrolateral medulla (Figure 19-4), so it is likely that the central gray matter projection to the ventral medulla is of prime importance. Thus, this system may influence both sympathetic and somatic responses via direct and indirect pathways.

If the effects of electrical stimulation within the hypothalamus are due to activation of axons arising elsewhere, the origin of these fibers remains to be determined. Numerous neuronal systems project to and through this defense hypothalamic zone. One possibility is the amygdala. However, when this area is stimulated with the excitatory amino acid D,L-homocysteic acid in conscious rats, none of the behavioral or cardiovascular changes seen under anesthesia is observed (Gelsema et al., 1987). Another possibility is the prefrontal and insular regions of the cerebral cortex, which is known to play a role in control of autonomic function. However, functional studies in conscious animals have not yet been reported. Additional sites that provide inputs to the hypothalamus may be involved as well, but the search for the cell group controlling this response will require systematic mapping studies using excitatory amino acids combined with lesions to pinpoint the critical loci.

AFFECTIVE BEHAVIOR AND AUTONOMIC RESPONSES TO NATURAL STIMULI

So far, consideration of the defense reaction has been restricted to those responses that could be elicited by electrical or chemical stimulation of neural tissue. Although this has been productive in providing a conceptual framework, we must now look at how such patterns of response compare to those exhibited by awake animals when confronted with stimuli that would evoke such affective behavior.

When cats are chronically instrumented to measure a range of cardiovascular and motor variables and then studied during confrontation of an aggressor, they display a variety of emotional behavior and cardiovascular responses (Mancia and Zanchetti, 1981). When the aggressor cat was allowed to attack, the instrumented cat would engage in a bout of fighting in which all four limbs were involved. This was termed supportive fighting (as opposed to nonsupportive fighting, which occurred if the subject was initially lying). In this latter case, the subject tended to fight using only the forelimbs to strike out. When the aggressor approached without attacking, the cat was immobile, vocalized, and showed signs of pupillary dilation. During supportive fighting, the pattern of cardiovascular response was similar to that evoked by hypothalamic stimulation. This included tachycardia, a small increase in arterial blood pressure, marked decreases in mesenteric and renal blood flows, and an increased iliac blood flow (Figure 19-6). The vasoconstriction in the mesenteric and renal beds was primarily the result of increased sympathetic vasoconstrictor activity and, indeed, a similar sympathetic vasoconstriction in the iliac bed was occasionally seen at the onset of the response. However, this was overridden at the onset of the muscle movement by vasodilation, which was a consequence of local metabolic factors and activation of sympathetic cholinergic fibers.

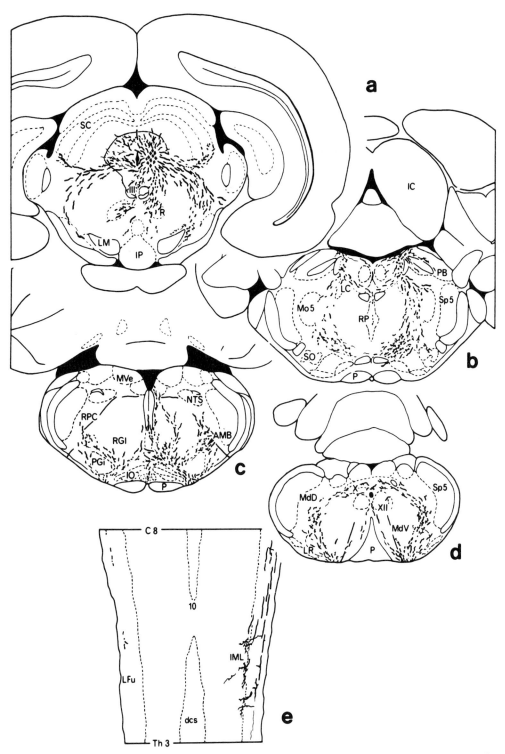

Figure 19-4 The central gray matter sends efferent projections to a number of sites in the brain stem and the spinal cord. After an injection of the anterograde axonal marker *Phaseolus vulgaris* leucoagglutinin (PHA-L) in the central gray matter of a rat (a), labeled axons and terminals can be traced to autonomic centers of the lower brain stem (b–d), including the parabrachial nucleus, the ventral medulla, and the caudal raphe nuclei. The latter two areas project to the intermediolateral cell column (e). Fibers can also be traced to the intermediolateral cell column (IML) in the upper thoracic spinal cord. AMB, ambiguus nucleus; IC, internal capsule; IP, interpeduncular nucleus; IML, intermediolateral cell column; LC, locus coeruleus; LFu, lateral funiculus; MdV, ventral reticular nucleus; MVe, medial vestibular nucleus; NTS, solitary tract nucleus; P, pyramidal tract; PB, parabrachial nucleus; PGI, paragigantocellular reticular formation; RGI, gigantocellular reticular formation; RP, raphe pontis nucleus; RPC, parvocellular reticular formation; SC, superior colliculus; SO, superior olivary nucleus; XII, hypoglossal nucleus. (Reproduced from Luiten et al., 1987, with permission of the authors and publisher.)

A

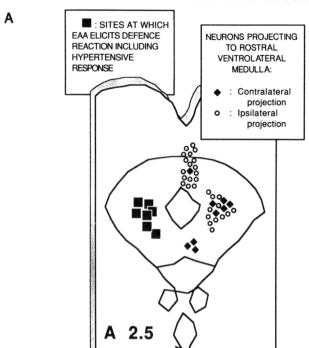

B

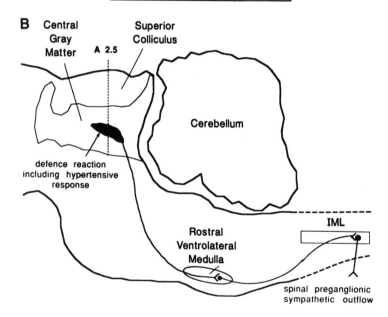

Figure 19-5 (A) Transverse section of the central gray matter showing that the area from which the defense reaction can be elicited with microinjections of excitatory amino acids (EAA) overlaps the same area that projects to the rostral ventrolateral medulla. (Reproduced from Carrive et al., 1988, with permission of the authors and publisher.) (B) Schematic diagram of the postulated pathway that mediates the cardiovascular response component of the defense reaction. IML, intermediolateral cell column.

During nonsupportive fighting, small increases in heart rate and blood pressure were noted. In addition, mesenteric and renal vasoconstriction occurred (Figure 19-6). Since there was no hindlimb muscle movement, vasoconstriction was also prominent in the iliac bed (see also Figure 19-2). This was also the case during immobile confrontation, but in this situation small decreases in blood pressure and heart rate were usual.

Clearly then, during naturally evoked affective behavior, the pattern of evoked response can very depending on how the stimulus is presented, only one of the patterns mirroring that evoked by electrical stimulation of the hypothalamus. Comparing the natural and hypothalamic evoked responses shows some similarities but also some major discrepancies. First, during immobile confrontation, the heart rate and cardiac output often fall. Second, blood pressure responses are never as large during natural responses as during hypothalamic-evoked responses. This may be due to less intense increases in cardiac output and vasoconstrictor activity being evoked during natural

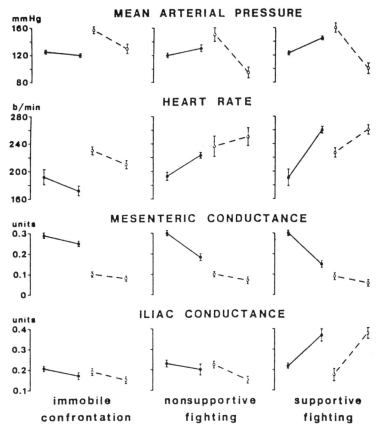

Figure 19-6 The cardiovascular changes recorded during emotional behavior before (filled circles and solid lines) and after (open circles and dashed lines) bilateral sinoaortic deafferentation. Circles on the left of each line indicate values immediately before the onset of emotional behavior; circles on the right indicate maximum changes during emotional behavior. Each panel refers to the type of behavior indicated at the bottom of the figure. Data are shown as means and standard errors of the mean of six trials of each behavior in one cat. (Reproduced with permission from Baccelli et al., 1976.)

confrontation. Third, it may also result from the fact that the baroreceptor reflex remains functional during natural stimulation (see Mancia and Zanchetti, 1981 for review). Finally, the most contentious issue concerns the observation that during natural stimulation active muscle vasodilation occurs only when muscle movements participate in the response. This is clearly different from hypothalamically evoked responses in which muscle vasodilation is so often present that it was considered a feature characteristic of the defense reaction.

Hilton (1982), in his review, has argued that results discussed by Mancia and Zanchetti (1981) can be explained in the following ways: (1) there was selection of subjects on the basis that they showed strong behavioral responses to the stimuli used; and (2) since multiple tests were carried out in each animal, the experiments could be criticized because the subjects were not naive to the stimuli, and the confrontations were not associated with actual noxious stimulation or physical attack. These are important issues since when a cat is confronted by a dog, a threatening reaction is elicited in which the cat remains in the sitting position with its hindlimbs immobile (Martin et al., 1976). During this response, only small changes in blood pressure and heart rate are seen, accompanied by vasoconstriction in the

iliac bed. However, this response occurs only after multiple confrontations, the earlier, naive confrontations being associated with hindlimb vasodilation, and larger increases in blood pressure and heart rate. These responses become habituated on repeated stimulation, the hindlimb vasodilation being most easily extinguished. Although this may, in fact, explain the discrepancies between the two sets of data, it is important to consider that in the natural environment in which we live, by far the majority of aversive or alerting stimuli with which we are confronted are not novel but have been the subject of many previous experiences. Indeed, as attested by the large array of conditioning paradigms studied (see below), the alerting response evoked by a novel tone soon habituates so that the tone can then be employed as a conditioned stimulus.

CONDITIONING OF AFFECTIVE BEHAVIOR

The studies considered so far have suggested a role for the hypothalamus–midbrain axis in the integration of the behavioral and autonomic responses to alerting and defense. However, these experiments have not discounted the possibility that two, or more, anatomically adjacent pathways may separately mediate behavioral and/or autonomic effects and that during electrical or chemical stimulation these pathways are simultaneously activated.

An answer to this problem has been forthcoming in a wide range of species where the combination of autonomic and behavioral responses typical of fear or defense has been conditioned to occur in response to the presentation of a previously unrelated, non-aversive, and emotionally insignificant stimulus such as an acoustic tone or a particular colored light. In particular, Smith and his colleagues have investigated the hypothesis that the hypothalamus influences a variety of different behaviors and that specific cardiovascular responses accompany them (see reviews by Smith et al., 1980, 1986). Using awake baboons that have been chronically instrumented to monitor a range of cardiovascular variables, the effects of various interventions have been studied on a range of behaviors and accompanying autonomic responses. The instrumented animals are trained by operant (reinforcement) techniques to response to colored lights by either performing mild leg exercise or by pressing a lever, a successful performance being rewarded by applesauce. After a stable performance has been reached a classical conditioning series is carried out to develop what Smith terms the *conditioned emotional response,* which is an electric shock to the abdominal skin. During data collection sessions the animal would be signaled to exercise, lever press, or feed, or the conditioned stimulus would be applied during a period of lever pressing. During the conditioned emotional response, a rapid response initiates a neurally mediated renal vasoconstriction and pressor response, followed by secondary increases mediated by adrenal catecholamine secretion. In addition, this mediates the tachycardia, and increased aortic blood flow, that probably represents a hindlimb vasodilation (Figure 19-7).

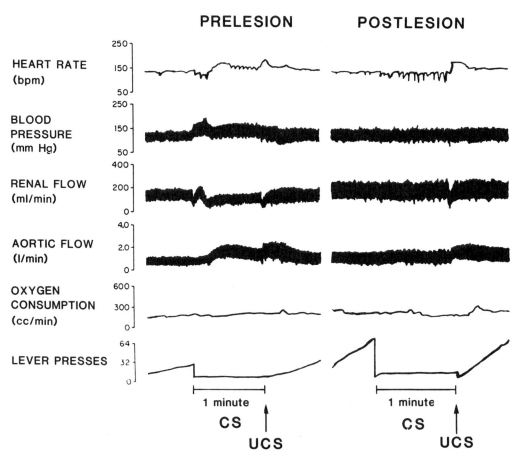

Figure 19-7 The cardiovascular pattern recorded from a chronically instrumented baboon during a conditioned emotional response evoked by presentation of a conditioned stimulus (CS). The panels show the pattern of response evoked before (prelesion) and after (postlesion) destruction of the perifornical region of the hypothalamus. Note that the lesion abolishes the changes evoked by the CS, but not those evoked by the unconditioned stimulus (UCS). (Reproduced with slight modification from Smith et al., 1982, with permission of the authors and publisher.)

Associated with this response, there was inevitably a behavioral suppression of the ongoing lever pressing. When the conditioned emotional response was repeated following localized bilateral lesions of the perifornical hypothalamic region, the cardiovascular response was totally abolished or severely attenuated, even though baseline cardiovascular variables were unaltered. However, these small hypothalamic lesions had no effect on the behavioral suppression of lever pressing (Figure 19-7).

These studies led to the conclusion that this definable area of the hypothalamus controls the whole pattern of cardiovascular response specifically associated with emotional behavior, since animals were still able to evoke the appropriate cardiovascular responses during exercise, feeding, and lever pressing. Although a similar effect may have been expected had the animal simply lost its ability to assess the significance of the conditioned stimulus, this is clearly not the case since behavioral suppression of lever pressing was still effective after the lesions (Figure 19-7).

These studies of chronically instrumented animals have been extended by recording the autonomic response patterns in response to normal environmental stimuli (Smith et al., 1986 for review). Results from studies of a social group of baboons, in which a representative blood pressure recording was taken from a submissive male who was eating, is shown in Figure 19-8. As he was briefly approached by a dom-

inant female, he was placed in a situation of conflict between leaving the area and his desire to remain and continue eating. Although his somatic activity during this encounter was minimal, the emotionally evoked cardiovascular responses were marked. Although this is a preliminary report, the results that may be expected to emanate from extensions of this study should be of immense importance in understanding cardiovascular control during normal behavioral activities.

NEURAL PATHWAYS MEDIATING CONDITIONED RESPONSES

Although it is now well known that aversive conditioning to a variety of auditory or visual stimuli can be easily performed, the neural pathways underlying such a procedure are only now being uncovered. One major question arises at this point—at which neural locus is the emotional significance applied to an otherwise insignificant tone or light? A discussion of how the emotional significance of any particular stimulus is encoded, the factors that determine it, and the neural regions required for its implementation forms a major part of the review on emotion by Le Doux (1987). Only a summary of the main points will be included here.

With regard to visual stimuli, the search for an answer goes back to ablation experiments performed by Kluver and Bucy (1937). They demonstrated that temporal lobe lesions endowed monkeys with what has been termed "psychic blindness" (the Kluver–Bucy syndrome); although able to see, the monkeys were unable to recognize objects (visual agnosia) and were passive or unresponsive to external stimuli. Although these lesions clearly involved the amygdala, subsequent studies in monkeys with more restricted lesions limited to the amygdala have implicated this nuclear complex in emotional processing. If the amygdala is destroyed on one side after sectioning the cerebral commissures then visual stimuli evoke normal emotional reactions. If the optic chiasm is subsequently sectioned, then the monkeys show normal emotional responses if the stimulus is presented to the eye ipsilateral to the intact amygdala, but are "tamed" if the stimulus is applied only to the opposite eye (Downer, 1961).

The pathways mediating the conditioned response to auditory stimuli in rats have been reviewed by Le Doux (1986, 1987). Such emotional responses are unaffected by large ablations of the auditory cortex. However, using microinjections of ibotenic acid (which destroys neuronal cell bodies but not axons) they have demonstrated that emotional responses are disrupted by localized destruction of neurons of the auditory pathway. Lesions of the inferior collic-

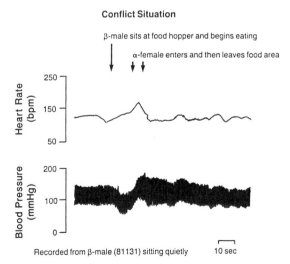

Figure 19-8 Heart rate and blood pressure records from a chronically instrumented submissive male baboon living in a family situation with four other baboons. Heart rate and blood pressure decrease while sitting and eating. When a dominant female walks toward him, there is an increase in blood pressure and heart rate. (Reproduced with slight modification from Smith et al., 1986, with permission of the authors and publisher).

ulus or in the medial geniculate nucleus blocked the response.

Medial geniculate nucleus lesions were specific for the conditioned response to auditory stimulation, but unconditioned responses to auditory stimuli or footshock were unaffected. In addition, the lesioned animals can still learn to associate visual stimuli with footshocks (Le Doux et al., 1986). This implies that the medial part of the medial geniculate nucleus is part of the afferent pathway for learning the emotional significance of auditory stimuli. The ascending pathway from the medial geniculate nucleus projects to several regions in the brain of which the pathway to insular cortex and central nucleus of the amygdala may be of importance in the current context. In addition, the outflow from the central nucleus of the amygdala seems important in this response. Ibotenic acid lesions of the dorsal part of the central nucleus of the amygdala abolish both the behavioral and blood pressure responses to auditory conditioned stimuli, whereas lesions of the lateral central nucleus or medial part of the lateral nucleus of the amygdala disrupt only the behavioral responses. The neurons in the central nucleus of the amygdala project to the bed nucleus of the stria terminalis, lateral hypothalamic area, midbrain central gray matter, and possibly directly to brain stem nuclei. Ibotenic acid lesions of the bed nucleus of the stria terminalis have no effect on blood pressure or somatomotor activity elicited by classical conditioning of fear to an acoustic stimulus, whereas lateral hypothalamic area lesions affect the blood pressure response and central gray matter lesions disrupt the behavioral response (Le Doux et al., 1988). This sug-

gests that the lateral hypothalamic region, which overlaps with a region of neurons projecting to the intermediolateral cell columns, forms part of the efferent pathway, mediating the cardiovascular response (Figure 19-9), whereas the pathways for the behavioral response are controlled separately by the central gray matter. However, if this is the case, it does not resolve the question of the role of the direct pathways from the amygdala to many brain stem nuclei. In addition, although the efferent pathway for the behavioral response may well pass via the midbrain central gray matter, it is known that chemical stimulation of this site also evoked the autonomic components of defensive behavior (Bandler and Carrive, 1988; Carrive et al., 1987; McDougall et al., 1985).

Conditioning of the emotional responses to auditory stimuli appears to be mediated by a direct thalamic–limbic pathway that bypasses the auditory cortex (Figure 19-9). However, this does not necessarily mean that corticolimbic pathways cannot, or do not, normally influence such conditioned responses. Indeed, it is possible that the direct subcortical pathways may provide for conditioned responses to primitive sensory stimuli, whereas thalamocorticolimbic pathways may mediate responses requiring perceptual discrimination between stimuli (Le Doux, 1987). If this is indeed the case, even within the subcortical pathway, neurons must exist that are able to assign affective significance to different stimuli.

Neurons within both the medial geniculate nucleus and the central nucleus of the amygdala receive convergent input from both conditioned and uncon-

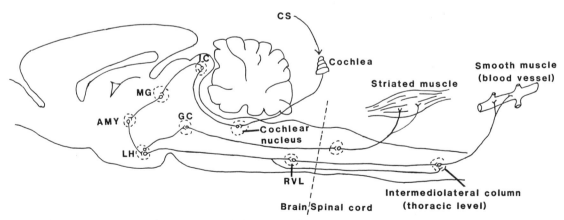

Figure 19-9 Thalamoamygdaloid pathways mediating learned fear responses in the rat. A schematic drawing of sections through the rat brain illustrating the pathways essential for autonomic activity and emotional behavior. The two pathways overlap through the auditory system and the amygdala but different efferent pathways mediate the effects from the amygdala. AMY, amygdala; CS, conditional stimulus; GC, central gray; IC, inferior colliculus; LH, lateral hypothalamus; MG, medial geniculate; RVL, rostral ventrolateral medulla. (Adapted and reproduced from LeDoux, 1987, with permission of the author and publishers.)

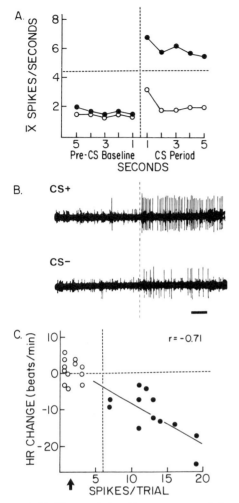

Figure 19-10 Characteristics of a neuron recorded extra-cellularly in the central nucleus of the amygdala of an un-anesthetized rabbit during Pavlovian fear conditioning. The positive conditioning stimulus (CS+) involved pre-sentation of a two-tone stimuli followed by an electrical shock to the eyelid (unconditioned stimulus). The negative conditioned stimulus (CS−) situation also involved a two-tone stimulus, without electrical shock. (A) Cumulative records of the activity of 13 of these neurons during the course of 114 presentations of each of the CS+ (closed circles) and CS− (open circles). Shown are the mean spike counts during CS and pre-CS periods. The dashed horizontal line indicates the level above which unit activity is significantly elevated above pre-CS baseline rates. (B) Oscilloscope traces showing the response of a neuron to presentations of each CS (at the dashed line). Calibration bar = 1 sec. (C) The relationship between the heart rate change and the activity of an amygdala neuron during the course of 12 presentations of each of the CS+ (closed circles) and CS− (open circles). The dashed vertical line indicates the point above which the activity is significantly elevated over the spontaneous firing rate of the neuron (shown by the arrow). (Reproduced with slight modification from Pascoe and Kapp, 1985, with permission of the authors and publisher.)

ditioned stimuli. Some neurons in the amygdala can respond differently to stimuli signifying food and shock, and others can distinguish between edible and inedible objects (Ono et al., 1983; Sanghera et al., 1979). In addition, neurons in both the cat medial geniculate nucleus (Ryugo and Weinberger, 1978) and rabbit central nucleus of the amygdala (Pascoe and Kapp, 1985) (Figure 19-10) change their ongoing activity during the development of fear conditioning. Of course, because any neuron in the efferent pathway of a conditioned response would be expected to demonstrate such differential responses, the question still remains of whether the amygdala complex is simply an outflow pathway or is integrally involved in the development of the emotional significance of stimuli.

PLAYING DEAD: A FURTHER BEHAVIORAL AND AUTONOMIC PARADIGM?

During the development of fear conditioning, rabbits, unlike cats, show a marked bradycardic response. This has been used as a model to describe the contribution of the central nucleus of the amygdala in the acquisition of conditioned response in this species (see review by Kapp et al., 1983). Such a role was proposed since the bradycardic response is attenuated by lesions in the central nucleus of the amygdala, or by injection of opiate agonists or β-adrenoceptor antagonists into this region. In addition, electrical stimulation of the central nucleus of the amygdala evokes a marked, vagally mediated bradycardia.

Although the major part of this chapter has discussed experimental paradigms in which tachycardia and other sympathoexcitatory responses served as a marker of affective behavior, the reader may be puzzled about the use of bradycardia as a functional indicator of this behavior. The reason for this is the observation that electrical stimulation of the central nucleus of the amygdala in awake rabbits evokes an arrest of ongoing behavior, pupillary dilation, rapid shallow breathing, and bradycardia (Applegate et al., 1983), which in the anesthetized animals is associated with a fall in blood pressure and a hindlimb vasodilation (Cox et al., 1987). This pattern of behavior and autonomic responses is considered to be typical of that seen during what has been termed "playing dead." This is often encountered when animals are faced with a threat outside their own territory. They freeze, crouch, and remain immobile. Although this is commonly seen in rabbits, they too can show aggressive behavior in response to some stimuli. Stimulation of regions of the hypothalamus and midbrain in unanesthetized rabbits can evoke flight or escape type behavior. When these animals are anesthetized, the same stimulus then evoked pupillary dilation, exothalamus, hyperventilation, a pressor response, tachycardia, hindlimb vasodilation, and renal vasoconstriction (see Azevedo, 1987 for review).

These results define another pattern of matched autonomic and behavioral responses appropriate to the context of the stimulus. An important question still unanswered is whether in every individual there are always two or more different preprogrammed patterns of behavior and associated autonomic responses that can be switched in and out at will depending on the environmental cues presented? An alternative explanation is that the different patterns of response all rely on one basic efferent outflow pattern that can be modified to suit the particular stimulus. Only a more detailed analysis of the individual components of the neural networks involved will allow this to be answered.

SUMMARY

The autonomic nervous system plays a full and coordinated part in providing an appropriate pattern of activity to complement somatic alterations associated with evoked behavioral patterns. The most widely studied activity, affective attack (defense response), has been used as a model on which general concepts of behavioral–autonomic integration have been based.

The defense response is evoked in a wide range of species when presented with threatening or aversive stimuli. In cats, the animal retracts its head and ears, crouches, vocalizes, and is generally alert. The stereotyped pattern of autonomic activity that accompanies this behavior mediates dilation of the pupils, piloerection of the back and tail, increases in blood pressure and heart rate, and vasoconstriction in renal, mesenteric, and skin beds with increased blood flow to hindlimb muscles.

These behavioral and autonomic patterns of activity can both be evoked by electrical, and sometimes, chemical stimulation of the same parts of a longitudinal continuum of brain tissue stretching from at least the level of the amygdala, through the hypothalamus and midbrain to the medulla. A unified site—probably the midbrain central gray matter—organizes and integrates both the behavior and the autonomic outflow appropriate for that behavior, and this general phenomenon could be extended to other behavior patterns such as feeding, temperature regulation, or exercise.

An output similar to the defense response is evoked in awake animals presented with threatening stimuli, and it can also be conditioned to occur on presentation of a previously nonsignificant stimulus.

The neural networks underlying the conditioning of such affective responses include both cortical and subcortical pathways. In the latter case, the amygdala nuclei seem to be of importance as a site for assessing the emotional significance of the stimuli.

In rabbits, the "playing dead" reaction is a common response to an aggressor. This involves arrest of ongoing locomotor activity, pupillary dilation, rapid shallow breathing, decreases in heart rate and blood pressure, and increased hindlimb muscle blood flow. However, in certain situations, rabbits can also exhibit the classical defense response as described in the cat. It is suggested that in all animals there are always several different preprogrammed patterns of behavior and their associated autonomic responses and that these can be switched in and out at will, depending on the environmental cues provided.

REFERENCES

Reviews

Azevedo, A. D. (1987). The defense reaction in different animal species. In: *Neuroscience and Behaviour,* M. L. Brandao (ed.), Grafica de UFES, Vittoria, Brazil, pp. 263–296.

Bard, P., and Macht, M. B. (1958). The behavior of chronically decerebrate cats. In: *Ciba Foundation Symposium on the Neurological Basis of Behavior,* G. E. W. Wolsteinholme and C. M. O'Connor (eds.), Little, Brown, Boston, pp. 55–75.

Ciriello, J., Caverson, M. M., and Polosa, C. (1986). Function of the ventrolateral medulla in the control of the circulation. *Brain Research Reviews* 11, 359–391.

Hilton, S. M. (1982). The defence-arousal system and its relevance for circulatory and respiratory control. *Journal of Experimental Biology* 100, 159–174.

Hilton, S. M. (1986). The central nervous contribution to vasomotor tone. In: *Central and Peripheral Mechanisms of Cardiovascular Regulation,* A. Magro, W. Osswald, D. J. Reis, and P. Vanhoutte (eds.), Plenum, London, pp. 465–486.

Kaada, B. (1967). Brain mechanisms related to aggressive behaviour. In: *Aggression and Defense,* C. D. Clemente and D. B. Lindsey (eds.), University of California Press, Los Angeles, pp. 95–133.

Kapp, B. S., Pascoe, J. P., and Bixler, M. A. (1983). The amygdala: A neuroanatomical systems approach to its contribution to aversive conditioning. In: *The Neuropsychology of Memory,* N. Butters and L. R. Squire (eds.), Guilford Press, New York, pp. 473–488.

LeDoux, J. E. (1986). Sensory systems and emotion: A model of affective processing. *Integrative Psychology* 4, 237–248.

LeDoux, J. E. (1987). Emotion. In: *Handbook of Physiology—The Nervous System V,* F. Plum (ed.), American Physiological Society, Bethesda, MD, pp. 419–459.

Luiten, P. G. M., ter Horst, G. J., and Steffens, A. B. (1987). The hypothalamus, intrinsic connections and outflow pathways to the endocrine system in relation to the control of feeding and metabolism. *Progress in Neurobiology* 28, 1–54.

Mancia, G., and Zanchetti, A. (1981). Hypothalamic control of autonomic functions. In: *Handbook of the Hypothalamus*, Vol. 3B, P. J. Morgane and J. Panksepp (eds.), Dekker, New York, pp. 147–202.

Marshall, J. M. (1987). Contribution to overall cardiovascular control made by the chemoreceptor-induced alerting/defense response. In: *Neurobiology of the Cardiorespiratory System*, E. W. Taylor (ed.), Manchester University Press, Manchester, pp. 222–240.

Price, J. L., Russchen, F. T., and Amaral, D. G. (1987). The limbic system. II. The amygdaloid complex. In: *Handbook of Chemical Neuroanatomy*, Vol. 5, *Integrated Systems in the CNS. Part I*, A. Bjorklund, T. Hokfelt, and L. W. Swangon (eds.), Elsevier, Amsterdam, pp. 279–388.

Siegel, A., and Edinger, H. (1981). Neural control of aggression and rage behaviour. In: *Handbook of the Hypothalamus*, Vol. 3B, P. J. Morgane and J. Panksepp (eds.), Dekker, New York, pp. 203–240.

Smith O. A., Astley, C. A., DeVito, J. L., Stein, J. M., and Walsh, K. E. (1980). Functional analysis of the hypothalamic control of the cardiovsacular responses accompanying emotional behavior. *Federation Proceedings* 39, 2487–2494.

Smith, O. A., DeVito, J. L., and Astley, C. A. (1982). The hypothalamus in emotional behaviour and associated cardiovascular correlates. In: *Changing Concepts of the Nervous System*, A. R. Morrison and P. L. Strick (eds.), Academic Press, New York, pp. 569–584.

Smith, O. A., Astley, C. A., Chesney, M. A., Taylor, D. J., and Spelman, F. A. (1986). Personality, stress and cardiovascular disease: Human and non-human primates. In: *Neural Mechanisms and Cardiovascular Disease*, B. Lown, A. Malliani, and M. Prosdocimi (eds.), Livianna Press, Padua, Italy, pp. 471–484.

Research Papers

Abrahams, V. C., Hilton, S. M., and Zbrozyna, A. (1960). Active muscle vasodilation produced by stimulation of the brain stem; its significance in the defence reaction. *Journal of Physiology (London)* 154, 491–513.

Applegate, C. D., Kapp, B. S., Underwood, M. D., and McNall, C. L. (1983). Autonomic and somatomotor effects of amygdala central nucleus stimulation in awake rabbits. *Physiology and Behavior* 31, 353–360.

Baccelli, G., Albertini, R., Mancia, G., and Zanchetti, A. (1976). Interactions between sino-aortic reflexes and cardiovascular effects of sleep and emotional behaviour in the cat. *Circulation Research* 38, Suppl. 2, 30–34.

Bandler, R. (1982). Induction of 'rage' following microinjections of glutamate into midbrain but not hypothalamus of cats. *Neuroscience Letters* 30, 183–188.

Bandler, R., and Carrive, P. (1988). Integrated defence reaction elicited by excitatory amino acid microinjection in the midbrain periaqueductal gray region of the unrestrained cat. *Brain Research* 439, 95–106.

Bandler, R., and McCulloch, T. (1984). Afferents to a midbrain periaqueductal grey region involved in the 'defense-reaction' in the cat is revealed by horseradish peroxidase. II. The diencephalon. *Behavioural Brain Research* 13, 279–285.

Bandler, R., McCulloch, T., and Dreher, B. (1985). Afferents to a midbrain periaqueductal grey region involved in the 'defence reaction' in the cat as revealed by horseradish peroxidase. I. The telencephalon. *Brain Research* 330, 109–119.

Bard, P. (1928). A diencephalic mechanism for the expression of rage with special reference to the sympathetic nervous system. *American Journal of Physiology* 84, 490–515.

Bard, P., and Mountcastle, V. B. (1948). Some forebrain mechanisms involved in expression of rage with special reference to suppression of angry behaviour. *Research Publications of the Association for Nervous and Mental Diseases* 27, 362–404.

Beitz, A. J. (1982). The organization of afferent projections to the midbrain periaqueductal gray of the rat. *Neuroscience* 7, 133–159.

Cannon, W. B., and Britton, S. W. (1925). Studies on the conditions of activity in endocrine glands. XV. Pseudoaffective medulliadrenal secretion. *American Journal of Physiology* 72, 283–294.

Carrive, P., Dampney, R. A. L., and Bandler, R. (1987). Excitation of neurones in a restricted portion of the midbrain periaqueductal grey elicits both behavioural and cardiovascular components of the defence reaction in the unanesthetized decerebrate cat. *Neuroscience Letters* 81, 273–278.

Carrive, P., Bandler, R., and Campney, R. A. L. (1988). Anatomical evidence that hypertension associated with the defence reaction in the cat is mediated by a direct projection from a restricted portion of the midbrain periaqueductal gray to the subretrofacial nucleus of the medulla. *Brain Research,* 460, 339–345.

Coote, J. H., Hilton, S. M., and Zbrozyna, A. W. (1973). The ponto-medullary area integrating the defence reaction in the cat and its influence on muscle blood flow. *Journal of Physiology (London)* 229, 257–274.

Cox, G. E., Jordan, D., Paton, J. F. R., Spyer, K. M., and Wood, L. M. (1987). Cardiovascular and phrenic nerve responses to stimulation of the amygdala central nucleus in the anesthetized rabbit. *Journal of Physiology (London)* 389, 541–556.

Downer, J. L. deC. (1961). Changes in visual gnostic functions and emotional behaviour following unilateral temporal pole damage in the 'split-brain' monkey. *Nature* 191, 50–51.

Eliasson, S., Folkow, B., Lindgren, P., and Uvnas, B. (1951). Activation of sympathetic vasodilator nerves to the skeletal muscles in the cat by hypothalamic stimulation. *Acta Physiologica Scandinavica* 23, 333–351.

Feigl, E., Johansson, B., and Lofving, B. (1964). Renal vasoconstriction and the 'defence reaction'. *Acta Physiologica Scandinavica* 62, 429–435.

Fernandez de Molina, A., and Hunsperger, R. W. (1959). Central representation of affective reactions in forebrain and brain stem: Electrical stimulation of amygdala, stria terminalis and adjacent structures. *Journal of Physiology (London)* 145, 251–265.

Fernandex de Molina, A., and Hunsperger, R. W. (1962). Organization of the subcortical system governing defence and flight reactions in the cat. *Journal of Physiology (London)* 160, 200–213.

Gelsema, A. J., McKitrick, D. J., and Calaresu, F. R.

(1987). Cardiovascular responses to chemical and electrical stimulation of amygdala in rats. *American Journal of Physiology* 253, R712–R718.

Glusman, M. (1974). The hypothalamic 'savage' syndrome. *Research Publications of the Association for Nervous and Mental Diseases* 52, 52–92.

Goltz, F. (1892). Der Hund ohne Grosshirn. *Pflugers Archiv* 51, 570–614.

Hess, W. R., and Brugger, M. (1943). Das subkorticale Zentrum der affektiven-Abwehrreaktion. *Helvetica Physiological Acta* 1, 33–52.

Hilton, S. M., and Zbrozyna, A. W. (1963). Amgydaloid region for defence reactions and its efferent pathway to the brain stem. *Journal of Physiology (London)* 165, 160–173.

Hilton, S. M., and Redfern, W. S. (1986). A search for brain stem cell groups integrating the defence reaction in the rat. *Journal of Physiology (London)* 378, 213–228.

Hilton, S. M., Marshall, J. M., and Timms, R. J. (1983). Ventral medullary relay neurones in the pathway from the defence areas of the cat and their effect on blood pressure. *Journal of Physiology (London)* 345, 149–166.

Hunsperger, R. W. (1956). Affektreaktionen auf elektrische Reizung im Hirnstamn der Katze. *Helvetical Physiologica Pharmacologica Acta* 14, 70–92.

Kluver, H., and Bucy, P. C. (1937). "Psychic blindness" and other symptoms following temporal lobectomy in rhesus monkeys. *American Journal of Physiology* 119, 352–353.

Kylstra, P. H., and Lisander, B. (1970). Differentiated interaction between the hypothalamic defence reaction and baroreceptor reflexes. II. Effects on aortic blood flow as related to work load on the left ventricle. *Acta Physiologica Scandinavica* 78, 386–392.

LeDoux, J. E., Iwata, J., Cicchetti, P., and Reis, D. J. (1988). Different projections of the central amygdala and nucleus mediate autonomic and behavioral correlates of conditioned fear. *Journal of Neuroscience* 8, 2517–2529.

LeDoux, J. E., Iwata, J., Pearl, D., and Reis, D. J. (1986). Disruption of auditory but not visual learning by destruction of intrinsic neurons in the medial geniculate body of the rat. *Brain Research* 371, 395–399.

Loewy, A. D. (1981). Raphe pallidus and raphe obscurus projections to the intermediolateral cell column in the rat. *Brain Research* 222, 129–133.

Loewy, A. D., Wallach, J. H., and McKellar, S. (1981). Efferent connections of the ventral medulla oblongata in the rat. *Brain Research Reviews* 3, 63–80.

MacLean, P. D., and Delgado, J. M. R. (1953). Electrical and chemical stimulation of the frontotemporal portion of limbic system in waking animal. *Electroencephalography and Clinical Neurophysiology* 5, 91–100.

Marshall, J. M. (1986). The role of the glycine sensitive area of the ventral medulla in cardiovascular responses to carotid chemoreceptor and peripheral nerve stimulation. *Pflugers Archiv* 406, 225–231.

Martin, J., Sutherland, C. J., and Zbrozyna, A. W. (1976). Habituation and conditioning of the defence reactions and their cardiovascular components in cats and dogs. *Pflugers Archiv* 365, 37–47.

McDougall, A., Dampney, R., and Bandler, R. (1985). Cardiovascular components of the defence reaction evoked by excitation of neuronal cell bodies in the midbrain periaqueductal grey of the cat. *Neuroscience Letters* 60, 69–75.

Meller, S. T., and Dennis, B. J. (1986). Afferent projections to the periaqueductal gray in the rabbit. *Neuroscience* 19, 927–964.

Nakao, H. (1958). Emotional behaviour produced by hypothalamic stimulation. *American Journal of Physiology* 194, 411–418.

Ono, T., Fukuda, M., Nishino, H., Sasaki, K., and Muramoto, K. (1983). Amygdaloid neuronal responses to complex visual stimuli in an operant feeding situation in the monkey. *Brain Research Bulletin* 11, 515–58.

Pascoe, J. P., and Kapp, B. S. (1985). Electrophysiological characteristics of amygdaloid central nucleus neurons during Pavlovian fear conditioning in the rabbit. *Behavioral Brain Research* 16, 117–133.

Price, J. L., and Amaral, D. G. (1981). An autoradiographic study of the projections of the central nucleus of the monkey amygdala. *Journal of Neuroscience* 1, 1242–1259.

Romaniuk, A. (1965). Representation of aggression and flight reactions in the hypothalamus of the cat. *Acta Biologiae Experimentalis* 25, 177–186.

Rosen, A. (1961). Augmented cardiac contraction, heart rate acceleration and skeletal muscle vasodilation produced by hypothalamic stimulation in cats. *Acta Physiologica Scandinavica* 52, 291–308.

Ryugo, D. K., and Weinberger, N. M. (1978). Differential plasticity of morphologically distinct neuron populations in the medial geniculate body of the cat during classical conditioning. *Behavioral Biology* 22, 275–301.

Sanghera, M. K., Rolls, E. T., and Roper-Hall, A. (1979). Visual responses of neurones in dorsolateral amygdala of the alert monkey. *Experimental Neurology* 63, 610–626.

Spencer, S. E., Sawyer, W. B., and Loewy, A. D. (1988). L-Glutamate stimulation of the zona incerta in the rat decreases heart rate and blood pressure. *Brain Research* 458, 72–81.

Spencer, S. E., Sawyer, W. B., and Loewy, A. D. (1989). Cardiovascular effects produced by L-glutamate stimulation of the lateral hypothalamic area. *American Journal of Physiology* 257, H540–H552.

Stock, G., Schlor, K.-H, Heidt, H., and Buss, J. (1978). Psychomotor behaviour and cardiovascular patterns during stimulation of the amygdala. *Pflugers Archiv* 376, 177–184.

Timms, R. J. (1981). A study of the amygdaloid defence reaction showing the value of althesin anaesthesia in studies of the function of the fore-brain in cats. *Pflugers Archiv* 391, 49–56.

Ursin, H. (1965). The effect of amygdaloid lesions on flight and defense behaviour in cats. *Experimental Neurology* 11, 61–79.

Ursin, H., and Kaada, B. (1960). Functional localization within the amygdaloid complex in the cat. *Electroencephalography and Clinical Neurophysiology* 12, 1–20.

Wasman, M., and Flynn, J. P. (1962). Directed attack from the hypothalamus. *Archives of Neurology* 6, 220–227.

Woodworth, R. S., and Sherrington, C. S. (1904). A pseudoaffective reflex and its spinal path. *Journal of Physiology (London)* 31, 234–243.

20

Alterations in Autonomic Functions During Sleep

P. L. PARMEGGIANI AND A. R. MORRISON

Dramatic changes in autonomic function occur in sleep. To the untutored, sleep is a period of quiescence, rest and stability, when little variation in autonomic control is expected. Yet, in one phase of sleep called rapid eye movement (REM) sleep (also referred to as desynchronized, paradoxical, or active sleep), a series of changes occurs in the autonomic outflows through a central disruption of those neural mechanisms controlling homeostasis. REM sleep is characterized by muscle atonia, rapid eye movements, and a low-voltage, fast-wave electroencephalogram (EEG). In terms of control theory, autonomic regulation during REM sleep operates mostly in an open-loop mode (i.e., lacking feedback), in contrast to the closed-loop mode of control (i.e., with feedback) that occurs during other sleep stages and wakefulness (see Parmeggiani, 1985 for review). At present, the specific neural pathways that mediate autonomic control required for homeostatic regulation have not been resolved. Indeed, the functions of sleep are not known, although several obvious possibilities exist, such as neuronal, as well as general body restoration and conservation of energy.

Knowledge of the factors controlling autonomic regulation in sleep is important for a complete understanding of normal and abnormal mammalian physiology. Studies of a variety of autonomic functions during sleep in freely behaving animals have given important insight into control mechanisms that the usual experimental preparations, such as anesthetized or decerebrate animals, could have never revealed. Furthermore, a number of sleep disorders in humans affect autonomic functions, making it essential to obtain a basic knowledge of the neural mechanisms to provide rational treatments. For example, respiratory dysfunction in sleep, most commonly sleep apnea, is not rare and is assuming a significant place in the list of possible causes of arterial hypertension (Lugaresi et al., 1980). Similarly, the study of penile erection in REM sleep, a normal occurrence, can assist in distinguishing organic ver-

sus psychogenic causes of impotence (see Karacan et al., 1978 for review). Moreover, alterations in gastroesophageal function during sleep appear to be an important cause in the pathogenesis of esophagitis (see Orr and Stahl, 1980 for review).

This chapter will focus on the alterations in autonomic activity that occur in sleep. Several examples of these changes will be discussed. Detailed examination of all the work of the past 35 years would be impossible here; the interested reader should consult monographs edited by Orem and Barnes (1980) and Saunders and Sullivan (1984) as well as the review by Phillipson and Bowes (1986) on respiration. There are also compendia of autonomic functions in sleep by Orem and Keeling (1980) and Parmeggiani et al. (1985) that provide very useful overviews.

GENERAL CHARACTERISTICS OF SLEEP

Until quite recently, sleep was generally viewed as a passive process. It was though that sleep depended the withdrawal of sensory inputs to eliminate wakefulness, although evidence from experimental and pathological telencephalic lesions as well as electrical stimulation studies clearly had suggested an involvement of active neuronal processes. Recognition of a "new" phase of sleep, REM sleep, in the 1950s gave rise to the concept that there must be intricate neuronal processes actively involved in sleep and that sleep could not be a unitary process.

In 1953, Aserinsky and Kleitman reported periods during sleep with bursts of rapid eye movements associated with a pattern of desynchronized activity in the EEG (Figure 20-1). Dreaming was reported during these episodes. REM sleep has been observed in a variety of animals as well (Dement, 1958; Jouvet, 1962; Zepelin and Rechtschaffen, 1974). In addition to an EEG pattern that is surprisingly similar to that of wakefulness, REM sleep is also characterized by

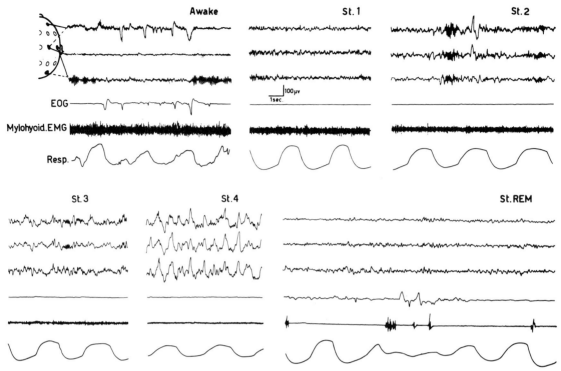

Figure 20-1 Polygraphic records showing the electroencephalogram (EEG) pattern recorded from several pairs of surface electrodes placed at standard positions on the scalp during wakefulness and sleep in humans. A dorsal view of the right scalp is in the upper left. The electroculogram (EOG), the electromyogram of an antigravity muscle (Mylohyoid EMG), and the thoracic pneumogram (Resp.) are illustrated. Non-REM sleep is divided into four stages (st. 1, st. 2, st. 3, and st. 4) based on the frequencies and amplitudes of the waves in the EEG. During REM sleep (st. REM), there are bursts of rapid eye movements, muscle atonia, myoclonic twitches, and irregular respiration all recorded via surface electrodes. (Reproduced from Lugaresi et al., 1978, with permission of the authors and publisher.)

skeletal muscle atonia, which is punctuated with intermittent muscular twitches. This atonia is caused by a central inhibition of the motor neurons (Glenn et al., 1978; Nakamura et al., 1978). During REM sleep, neuronal activity of most cells in the brain exhibit firing patterns similar to those seen in wakefulness with two notable exceptions: serotonergic neurons in the dorsal raphe nucleus and noradrenergic neurons in the locus coeruleus are completely inactive (see reviews by McGinty et al., 1974; Jacobs, 1987). This period is also characterized by a decrease in sympathetic tone (Iwamura et al., 1966; Baust et al., 1968; Reiner, 1986) coupled with a general increase in parasympathetic activity (Berlucchi et al., 1964; Baust and Bohnert, 1969).

Another important feature of REM sleep is its irregularity; phasic features are irregularly superimposed on the tonic components that last the duration of an episode. Tonic REM sleep is characterized by a continuously desynchronized EEG and paralysis of skeletal muscles. Phasic interruptions occur in the form of rapid eye movements and irregular twitches of the skeletal muscles; the eye movements,

of course, result from twitches of the extraocular muscles. Also at these times, respiration and heart rate become irregular, the pupils briefly dilate, and there are bursts of sympathetic activity (see reviews by Orem and Keeling, 1980 and Parmeggiani et al., 1985). The exact source of the bursts of excitatory neural discharges is unknown. Electrolytic lesions of the vestibular nuclei eliminate phasic motor twitches, heart rate irregularities, and episodic pupillary dilation (Morrison and Pompeiano, 1970), but the nonspecificity of this technique does not allow for an accurate determination of the CNS source controlling these phasic alterations (see review of methodologies used in sleep research by Parmeggiani et al., 1985). Nevertheless, these findings reveal two fundamental processes in operation during REM sleep: skeletal muscle atonia and intermittent bursts affecting the autonomic and somatic motor nervous systems. The changes occurring in a variety of autonomic functions will be summarized in this chapter.

Homeostatic controls are dramatically depressed in REM sleep. These REM sleep state-dependent effects are most obvious in certain functions, such as thermoregulation, which are controlled predominantly by higher brain levels. For example, hypothalamic thermosensitive neurons largely lose their sensitivity to thermal stimuli. Other neural systems, such as those controlling vascular baroreceptor and lung inflation reflexes, are depressed. This disruption in control will be discussed in greater depth in the sections that follow concerning circulation, respiration, and thermoregulation.

Changes in motor and secretory activities of the gastrointestinal tract are also observed during sleep (see Orr and Stahl, 1980 for review), but they cannot be simply explained on the basis of sleep state-dependent changes in autonomic outflow. This is due to the fact that the gastrointestinal tract is regulated by the enteric nervous system. The latter provides an intrinsic control that is autonomous in nature.

Sleep as it was classically known before the discovery of REM sleep is now called non-REM sleep. It is characterized by bodily quiescence and high-amplitude, low-frequency EEG waves. Other terms for this state are synchronized, slow-wave, or quiet sleep. In humans, four different stages of non-REM sleep may be distinguished on the basis of the EEG pattern (Figure 20-1); at least two non-REM sleep stages can be discerned in the carnivore EEG as well (see Ursin and Sterman, 1981 for review). During non-REM sleep, muscle tone is reduced and many CNS neurons reach their lowest firing frequency at this time, although some neurons in the limbic system discharge at their highest rate (see McGinty et al., 1974 for review). Homeostasis is maintained, although it is set at a lower level, consistent with a lower level of activity and lower metabolic demands. Furthermore, this period is marked by a great regularity in respiration and heart rate.

These two basic states of sleep (REM and non-REM sleep) alternate periodically in an irregular way. Under normal conditions, non-REM sleep is always the first step of the cycle. The length of a sleep cycle—the beginning of the non-REM sleep stage to the end of the subsequent REM sleep period—varies among species; it is ~10 minutes in rats, ~25 minutes in cats, ~90 minutes in humans, and ~120 minutes in elephants (Zepelin and Rechtschaffen, 1974). While the length of the sleep cycle of humans averages about 90 minutes, the variation has a large standard deviation. In particular, the duration of stage 4 sleep decreases and the length of each REM sleep phase increases as the night progresses, so that REM sleep comprises much of the sleep in the early morning hours (Figure 20-2). REM sleep occupies approximately 25% of total sleep time after early infancy; it dominates sleep in the newborn.

To summarize, sleep is an active and complex process, not a period of passive withdrawal. It con-

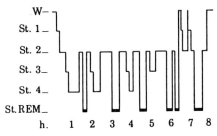

Figure 20-2 Schematic histogram of a night's sleep in a normal adult human. Non-REM sleep and REM sleep alternate regularly five to six times. Slow wave sleep (non-REM sleep stages 3 and 4) peaks during the first part of the night, while REM sleep prevails during the second. (Reproduced from Lugaresi, Coccagna and Mantovani 1978, with permission of the authors and publisher.)

sists of two basic phases, non-REM sleep and REM sleep, that alternate throughout the sleeping period. REM sleep is of particular interest due to the depression of homeostasis that occurs throughout its course.

NEURAL MECHANISMS REGULATING SLEEP

Description of the behavioral and EEG characteristics of sleep is rather straightforward and noncontroversial; the same cannot be said about the sleep regulatory centers and the mechanisms responsible for sleep.

The first studies directed at trying to elucidate the neural centers controlling sleep focused on the diencephalon. Von Economo observed that inflammatory lesions in humans resulting from encephalitis lethargica induced two syndromes that could be correlated with damage in two different brain areas: somnolence resulted from lesions in the wall of the caudal part of the third ventricle, and insomnia followed inflammation associated with the rostral hypothalamus (Von Economo, 1917, 1930; see review by Sterman and Shouse, 1985). Nauta (1946) later found that damage of the posterior hypothalamic area in rats produced a state of hypersomnolence, whereas more rostral hypothalamic lesions led to an insomnia that terminated in death. More recent studies using excitotoxins to produce cell body lesions support the idea that the posterior hypothalamus is involved in waking mechanisms (Leach et al., 1980; Sallanon et al., 1988).

Although these studies suggested that the hypothalamus was the major site in the brain regulating sleep, emphasis began to shift toward the more caudal brain stem with Moruzzi and Magoun's (1949) discovery of the arousal effects obtained with stimulation of the midbrain reticular formation. Two additional findings in the early 1960s led workers to focus almost exclusively on the lower brain stem: (1) Jouvet (1962) demonstrated that some of the features of REM sleep—atonia, muscle twitches, characteristic pontine neuronal discharges—still occurred following midbrain transection, and (2) anatomical techniques revealed that certain groups of serotonergic and noradrenergic neurons in the rostral pons and mesencephalon projected widely throughout the brain, making them good candidates for the regulators of the sweeping changes in neural activity that must accompany shifts in behavioral states (see Jouvet, 1972 for review). Guided by the results of a variety of lesion and pharmacological experiments, Jouvet (1972) proposed that these two types of monoamine-containing neurons were responsible for regulating the onset of sleep and alternation between its two phases. According to this hypothesis, serotonin-containing neurons in the midbrain and pontine raphe nuclei promote non-REM sleep and "prime" the occurrence of REM sleep, whereas noradrenergic neurons of the locus coeruleus control initiation and maintenance of REM sleep.

Neither of these two cell groups has the physiological properties of sleep-generating centers though. For example, several studies have since demonstrated that both raphe dorsalis and locus coeruleus neurons become progressively less active the moment a cat enters non-REM sleep, and become totally silent during REM sleep. Therefore, they cannot function as the main neuronal generators of sleep. The locus coeruleus may play a permissive role in REM sleep generation, wherein the inactivity of the noradrenergic neurons may permit REM sleep to occur (Chu and Bloom, 1974; Hobson et al., 1975; Reiner, 1986). The raphe system may subserve some type of somatic sensation filtering system that is critical for the induction of sleep (Hobson et al., 1975; McGinty and Harper, 1976; Trulson and Jacobs, 1978). Insomnia created by depletion of serotonin via raphe lesions or pharmacologic manipulations has been interpreted to be a consequence of an animal's inability to ignore sensory stimuli in wakefulness after such manipulations (McGinty and Harper, 1976).

Other neuronal cell groups in the brain stem are also involved. Giant reticular neurons of the pontine tegmentum, thought to be specifically active in REM sleep, have been proposed to promote REM sleep actively by inhibiting the noradrenergic neurons (Hobson et al., 1975), but the former are active during specific movements in wakefulness, too (Siegel and McGinty, 1977; Vertes, 1979), so that their prolonged, high activity in REM sleep may be correlative only with that state. In fact, activity of cholinergic neurons lying in the pedunculopontine and laterodorsal tegmental nuclei may be the caudal

brain stem initiators of the process (Mitani et al., 1988). They project to a region of the pontine tegmentum that many have demonstrated to be the site of cholinergic activation of REM sleep (cf., Amatruda et al., 1975).

What induces these cholinergic neurons to initiate REM sleep? The search for these elements need not be limited to the caudal brain stem. In fact, evidence generally overlooked, or not recognized as significant, points to the rostral brain; and the feature of REM sleep that will be a focus of discussion in this chapter, suppressed homeostasis, provides an important clue. Although decerebrate cats exhibit all the peripheral signs of REM sleep (Jouvet, 1962; Villablanca, 1966), their REM sleep-like state has a strikingly abnormal feature that has been generally ignored—a variety of normal non-sleep-promoting stimuli, such as pinching of the ear, passing a stomach tube, or passively moving the limbs, will induce these REM episodes (Jouvet, 1964). This suggests that the caudal brain stem is unusually primed to enter REM sleep abruptly without the normal preparatory period of non-REM sleep. Since the decerebrate cat is not in a well-regulated, homeostatic state, could it be that midbrain transection releases the caudal brain stem from the influence of higher integrative levels that control the transition, non-REM sleep, in intact animals from the homeostatic state of wakefulness to the nonhomeostatic state of REM sleep? This suggestion would lead to the conclusion that the initiation of normal REM sleep requires changes in the forebrain neurons in the latter part of non-REM sleep at least. These ideas are developed more fully in reviews by Parmeggiani (1985) and Morrison and Reiner (1985).

One of the forebrain sites thought to be involved in sleep regulation is the thalamus. This idea dates back to experiments performed by Hess (1944), who demonstrated that electrical stimulation in the ventromedial thalamus of cats would induce the normal sequence of behaviors associated with preparation for sleep and then sleep itself. This work was later extended by numerous investigators who revealed that additional forebrain areas could be stimulated to produce behavioral inhibition and then sleep (Parmeggiani, 1962; Sterman and Clemente, 1962). Although the electrical stimulation does not permit definitive CNS localization, it has directed attention to what appear to be key areas involved in sleep induction. More recent experiments have now revealed neurons in the basal forebrain that are selectively activated before sleep onset (Szymusiak and McGinty, 1986).

The sleep–wakefulness cycle as described so far is clearly an endogenous cyclic phenomenon, but it is likely that the pattern of its occurrence is determined at least in part by cues that result from the changing environmental light intensity. Entrainment is not

dependent on activity generated in the primary visual pathway by light but, rather, involves the action of a more direct bilaterally represented retinohypothalamic pathway that innervates the suprachiasmatic nucleus (see Swanson, 1987 for review). Destruction of this nucleus results in the loss of many features of normal circadian behavior and, strikingly, a loss of the normal distribution of sleep in the light–dark cycle of rodents, but without reducing the normal daily amount of sleep (Ibuka and Kawamura, 1975). Therefore, the suprachiasmatic nucleus is not critical for sleep generation, only its timing. Indeed, as Moore-Ede et al. (1982) state, evidence from primates and rodents indicates that some structure outside the suprachiasmatic nucleus modulates the circadian timing of REM sleep. A circadian rhythm of this sleep stage still remains, even after destruction of the nucleus. The suprachiasmatic nucleus, by virtue of its efferent projection to the parvocellular component of the paraventricular hypothalamic nucleus, may have important consequences for autonomic function as they relate to sleep. Detailed information on connectivity of the suprachiasmatic nucleus and its role in sleep–wake mechanisms may be found in reviews by Swanson (1987) and Moore-Ede et al. (1982), respectively.

Although the actual neural mechanisms that induce sleep are unknown, the idea that neurons release sleep-promoting substance(s) has attracted interest. Although a number of chemicals have been hypothesized to function as putative sleep factors, controversy surrounds the efficacies of these substances individually and the notion that a single compound "turns on" sleep (see Mendelson et al., 1983 for review). However, the idea that over time sleep factors might accumulate that would trigger the brain to enter a particular sleep mode is eminently reasonable. Krueger et al. (1990) reviewed evidence indicating that a variety of chemicals affect various aspects of the sleep cycle and proposed models of how they might influence, or modulate, neuronal elements at various junctures in the sleep–wakefulness continuum.

In summary, many brain structures participate in the regulation of sleep, although their mode of action is not yet fully understood. The mechanisms described here are more extensively covered in reviews by McGinty and Beahm (1984) and Morrison and Reiner (1985).

AUTONOMIC OUTFLOW DURING SLEEP

Most of our information regarding alterations in autonomic function that occur during sleep has resulted from end organ measurements rather than direct recordings of autonomic nerve activity. This is due to the fact that sympathetic nerves are extremely fragile, and it is technically difficult to maintain recordings from these structures in freely behaving animals. For descriptive purposes, different patterns of autonomic functions that occur during sleep will be illustrated. Since most of these observations involve the cardiovascular system, this discussion will extend into the next section on circulation.

The iris is innervated by both the parasympathetic and sympathetic nervous systems. In both normal and blinded cats, Berlucchi et al. (1964) demonstrated that during non-REM sleep pupilloconstriction occurs. Also, during REM sleep the pupil is constricted, although phasic dilations accompany the rapid eye movements. Since this dilation persists after sympathectomy, it is due to a central inhibition of the parasympathetic outflow to the iris. Thus, pupilloconstriction is maintained during sleep as a result of a tonic parasympathetic drive (see Chapter 14 for a discussion of pupillary pathways).

The heart is controlled by both divisions of the autonomic nervous system. The changes occurring in heart rate that are associated with the different stages of sleep are good indicators of such innervation. Baust and Bohnert (1969) observed that the decrease in heart rate that occurs with the change from wakefulness to non-REM sleep is mainly caused by a tonic increase in parasympathetic activity because sympathectomy alone had little effect. The further decrease in heart rate during REM sleep is the result of a tonically reduced sympathetic discharge. Moreover, phasic changes in heart rate associated with rapid eye movements are elicited by short-lasting changes in both parasympathetic and sympathetic activity controlled by phasic alterations in brain stem neural activity (Gassel et al., 1964a).

The pattern of sympathetic nerve activity has been studied in cats during sleep (Baust et al., 1968; Iwamura et al., 1969; Reiner, 1986). Recordings from renal and cervical sympathetic nerves indicate activity is either unchanged or slightly decreased during non-REM sleep. However, during REM sleep, a large decrease in firing rate occurs with intermittant phasic bursts associated with rapid eye movements. During REM sleep-like states, midbrain transected, vagotomized, and sinoaortic denervated cats show an increased activity of sympathetic fibers innervating the hindlimb skeletal muscles and a decrease in neural activity in the sympathetic fibers innervating the kidney, the gastrointestinal tract, and the pelvic viscera (Futuro-Neto and Coote, 1982a). Futuro-Neto and Coote (1982b) found that electrical stimulation of the nucleus raphe obscurus produced similar sympathetic nerve discharge patterns. This indicates that either the raphe obscurus or some neural pathway projecting to or through it is involved in this patterned response.

In summary, a shift to a predominantly "parasympathetic" form of activity occurs in sleep. A dramatic decrease in sympathetic tone occurs in REM sleep, although phasic increases appear coincidentally with rapid eye movements.

CIRCULATION

Sleep-related alterations in autonomic neural activity produce widespread effects on the cardiovascular system. In non-REM sleep, cardiac output of cats is only slightly reduced with respect to the awake state as a result of the moderate decrease in heart rate with no significant change in stroke volume (Mancia and Zanchetti, 1980; Baust and Bohnert, 1969). Arterial pressure decreases as a consequence of this decrease in cardiac output as well as an accompanying fall in peripheral vascular resistance. Small increases in skin, mesenteric, iliac, and renal vascular conductances occur. In REM sleep, there is a more pronounced bradycardia and blood pressure falls as a result of a marked decrease in peripheral vascular resistance, especially due to vasodilation of gastrointestinal vascular beds (Mancia and Zanchetti, 1980). During bursts of rapid eye movements and myoclonic twitches, blood pressure is unstable in animals (Gassel et al., 1964a; Guazzi and Zanchetti, 1965) and humans (Lugaresi et al., 1978) because of phasic periods of vagal inhibition and sympathetic activation. These two factors induce variability in heart rate, and the tonic change in sympathetic activity produces a decrease in vascular resistance in certain vascular beds (Figure 20-3).

In REM sleep, the vasodilation resulting from reduced sympathetic activity is not global. For example, vasoconstrictor activity occurs in the vascular beds supplying the hindlimb musculature even during atonia. This vasomotor tone in flaccid muscles reduces reflexively the hypotension that occurs in this sleep stage (Baccelli et al., 1974). This activity depends on a spinal reflex triggered from muscle afferents. In cats with intact lumbar sympathetic trunks, tonic vasoconstriction can be reversed into vasodilation after dorsal rhizotomies or spinal cord transection caudal to the emergence of the sympathetic fibers. Sinoaortic denervation overrides the reflex by removal of the buffering action of those nerves on the brain stem inhibitory mechanisms controlling the sympathetic outflow (Baccelli et al., 1978). In contrast, Futuro-Neto and Coote (1982a) found in the decerebrate, sinoaortic-vagotomized cat that the increase of sympathetic vasoconstrictor outflow to the hindlimbs depends only on a central mechanism. The high level of activity in the limb vasoconstrictor fibers seen after dorsal rhizotomy, however, may result from the decerebration itself, because somatic reflexes seen during REM sleep can be facilitated or inhibited depending on the midbrain level of transection (Sterman et al., 1974). The specific CNS area modulating these sympathetic responses is unknown.

In REM sleep, a redistribution of blood flow occurs in various vascular beds (Reis et al., 1968). It was reported that blood flow to red muscle (slow twitch) decreases, whereas blood flow to white muscle (fast twitch) is unchanged (Reis et al., 1969). In contrast, Lenzi et al. (1989) were unable to confirm this result since in white muscle they found an increase in blood flow during REM sleep. This latter result is compatible with the principle of blood flow–muscle activity coupling. Flow to red muscles, which sustain postural tonus, should decrease in association with REM sleep atonia. On the other hand, white fibers that are inactive in non-REM sleep

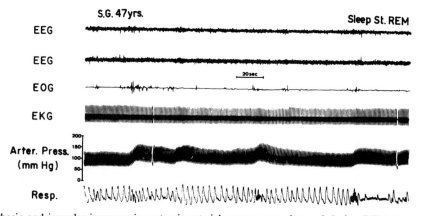

Figure 20-3 Phasic and irregular increases in systemic arterial pressure are observed during REM sleep. Such pressure increases often coincide with the bursts of rapid eye movements and with respiratory irregularities. EEG, electroencephalograms; EOG, electroculogram; EKG, electrocardiogram; Arter. Press., arterial pressure; Resp., thoracic pneumogram. (Reproduced from Lugaresi et al., 1978, with permission.)

twitch in REM sleep, which would account for the increase in blood flow seen by Lenzi et al. (1989). Red muscles twitch as well (Gassel et al., 1964b), but this seems to be quantitatively less significant than the loss of their tonic postural activity.

The decrease in blood pressure that occurs during REM sleep could be disastrous were it not for the buffering action of peripheral reflexes (Guazzi and Zanchetti, 1965). In particular, after sectioning of the aortic and carotid sinus nerves in cats, blood pressure increases mildly during wakefulness, decreases little more than usual during non-REM sleep, but falls precipitously during REM sleep (Figure 20-4). Heart rate diminishes more in both sleep states, although the change is less dramatic than in the case of blood pressure. Sinoaortic denervation induces a greater vasodilation in the splanchnic vascular bed and a reversal of the constriction in the limbs to vasodilation. In a small percentage of debuffered animals, blood pressure drops sufficiently to

cause cerebral ischemia, flattening of the EEG, and arousal. Thus, the sinoaortic afferents temper the usual brain stem-generated changes in REM sleep. Selective removal of either baroreceptor or chemoreceptor afferents demonstrates that the effects are largely due to eliminating the latter. In conclusion, the hypotension of REM sleep is buffered in the cat by chemoreceptor reflexes, whereas baroreceptor reflexes are depressed (Mancia and Zanchetti, 1980; Knuepfer et al., 1986).

However, in other species, such as the rat, the baroreceptor reflexes are more important in the genesis of REM sleep cardiovascular phenomena. In this species, arterial pressure increases during REM sleep as a result of a higher sensitivity of the baroreceptor reflex, whereas in baroreceptor-denervated rats a severe reduction in pressure occurs as in the cat (Junqueira and Krieger, 1976; Lacombe et al., 1988; Meunier et al., 1988). Circulation is affected during REM sleep by the same central influences

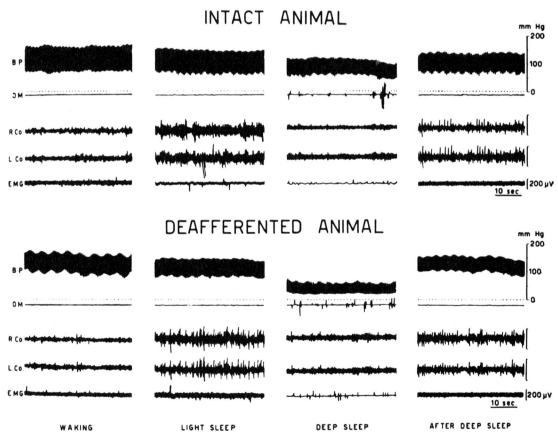

Figure 20-4 Systemic arterial pressure during various stages of the wakefulness–sleep cycle before and after sinoaortic deafferentation in a cat. Recordings of both upper and lower halves of the figure are taken from the same animal. Note that the pressure fall during REM sleep is larger after deafferentation than before it. BP, femoral arterial pressure; OM, electrooculogram; RCo and LCo, electroencephalograms of right and left cerebral cortex; EMG, neck muscle electromyogram; LIGHT SLEEP, non-REM sleep; DEEP SLEEP, REM sleep. (Reproduced from Guazzi and Zanchetti, 1965, with permission.)

that operate in the cat, the prevalence of either baro-receptor (rat) or chemoreceptor (cat) reflexes determining largely the pattern of the cardiovascular response. In humans, the changes in autonomic outflow during non-REM sleep are probably similar to those occurring in the cat (Coccagna et al., 1971; also Jones et al., 1980 for review). Therefore, the tonic decrease in arterial pressure during all stages of non-REM sleep may be explained on the basis of similar changes in heart rate, cardiac output, and peripheral vascular resistance. In contrast to the situation in the cat, heart rate and arterial pressure may not fall further or may even increase in REM sleep in humans, which has been hypothesized by Mancia and Zanchetti (1980) to be the result of a greater incidence of phasic events with accompanying pulses of sympathetic activity (Iwamura et al., 1966; Baust et al., 1968; Reiner, 1986) and a higher sensitivity of baroreceptor reflexes than in the cat.

To summarize, non-REM sleep is characterized by regularity of cardiovascular function at a reduced rate of cardiac contraction and REM sleep by a distinguishable irregularity and a depression of reflexes that are species specific. Further discussion may be found in reviews by Jones et al. (1980), Mancia and Zanchetti (1980), and Coote (1982).

RESPIRATION

Striking changes occur in the control of breathing during different behavioral states. These involve re-adjustments in the various controls, both automatic and voluntary, that operate to drive breathing and to maintain a given rate and depth of respiration (tidal volume) (see Phillipson and Bowes, 1986 for review). Unlike the cardiovascular system, important components of the respiratory system are, of course, somatic, but must be considered along with changes in autonomic functions to present an integrated picture.

Respiratory mechanisms are closely linked to the CNS sleep–wakefulness mechanisms. Certain respiratory neurons in the pons and medulla oblongata decrease their activity with the changes from wakefulness to non-REM sleep and then to REM sleep (Lydic and Orem, 1979; Orem et al., 1974). This is independent of sensory input, as demonstrated by extensive deafferentations (Netick and Foutz, 1980). Other respiratory neurons fire in conjunction with the phasic bursts of activity, such as pontogeniculooccipital (PGO) waves and rapid eye movements, that characterize REM sleep (Orem, 1980; Sieck and Harper, 1980).

The net effect on respiration of these changes in neuronal activity as an animal passes from wakefulness through the various phases of sleep has been suggested to occur as follows: deactivation of neurons in the reticular formation occurs with onset of non-REM sleep and this results in the loss of the so-called "wakefulness stimulus" with a slowing and regularization of respiration and an overall decrease in ventilation, in non-REM sleep stage 4 (Figure 20-5) (Fink, 1961). The neural substrate of the wake-

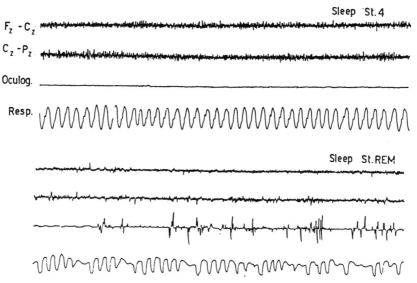

Figure 20-5 Aspects of respiration during sleep in the normal human individual. During stage 4 of non-REM sleep, respiration becomes very regular. During REM sleep, frequency and depth of respiration are irregular and at times short episodes of apnea appear. Respiratory irregularities coincide with bursts of rapid eye movements. F_z–C_z and C_z–P_z, standard electrode placements for human electroencephalograms; Oculog., electrooculogram; Resp., thoracic pneumogram. (Reproduced from Lugaresi et al., 1978, with permission.)

fulness stimulus is not known; however, it is certain from lesion work that there is no simple linkage with the reticular activating system (see Orem, 1984 for review). During REM sleep, respiration becomes irregular in rate and depth, depending on the particular patterns of phasic activations that occur.

Respiratory muscle activity changes with sleep onset (Dick et al., 1982). The most profound alterations appear during REM sleep as is the case with purely postural and locomotor musculature. Many workers report little change in tonic intercostal activity during non-REM sleep and an increase in phasic contractions, leading to an increase in the depth of respiration (Phillipson and Bowes, 1986 for review). On entering REM sleep, though, tone of the intercostal muscles essentially disappears, and phasic respiratory activity in several of these muscles is also markedly reduced or even temporarily suppressed (e.g., see Duron and Marlot, 1980) (Figure 20-6), although they are active in temporal relation to the general muscular twitches (Wurtz and O'Flaherty, 1967; Orem et al., 1977b). During REM sleep, phasic activity of the diaphragm continues almost unchanged in all species studied, or, of course, respiration would cease. Tonic activity of the diaphragmatic musculature, which is present only in humans during non-REM sleep (Muller et al., 1979), not cats (Parmeggiani and Sabattini, 1972), diminishes dramatically.

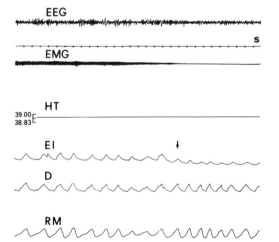

Figure 20-6 Activity of respiratory muscles during sleep in the cat. At the onset of REM sleep tonic postural activity (EMG) disappears and phasic respiratory activity decreases in the external intercostal muscle (EI) recording (arrow). The phasic respiratory activity of the diaphragm persists almost unchanged. Note also the increase in respiratory frequency. D, integrated electromyogram of diaphragm; EEG, electroencephalogram; EI, integrated electromyogram of an external intercostal muscle; EMG, neck muscle electromyogram; HT, hypothalamic temperature; RM, thoracic pneumogram; s, seconds. (Reproduced from Parmeggiani et al., 1973, with permission.)

The tone of the upper airway muscles changes in sleep. These are important determinants of obstructive apneas during sleep (see Phillipson and Bowes, 1986 for review). Tonic tongue (Sauerland and Harper, 1976), pharyngeal (Sauerland et al., 1981), and laryngeal (Orem and Lydic, 1978; Sherry and Megirian, 1980) musculature activity associated with upper airway dilation decreases in non-REM sleep and essentially vanishes in REM sleep. Overall, there are increases in upper airway resistance in sleep that are highest in REM sleep due to partial collapse of the airway and reduction or absence of phasic inspiratory activity of the muscles (Orem et al., 1977a, b).

The transition from wakefulness to non-REM sleep consists of the progressive inactivation of the voluntary control mechanism and release of the automatic control mechanism (see Figure 20-7). Regular breathing begins with stages 3 and 4 of non-REM sleep. At this point, breathing is driven by the automatic control mechanism. Ventilation decreases according to the metabolic rate. Various manipulations—vagotomy (Remmers et al., 1976), spinal cord transection (Foutz et al., 1979), and pontine lesions in the pneumotaxic area (Baker et al., 1981)—do not interfere with the slower, deeper pattern of breathing, suggesting that sleep alters several mechanisms involved in pattern generation and reduces the drive of medullary respiratory neurons (see Phillipson and Bowes, 1986 for review). A concomitant increase in both alveolar and arterial CO_2 partial pressures associated with a decrease in alveolar arterial O_2 partial pressures has been observed (e.g., Guazzi and Freis, 1969). These changes in respiratory variables are appropriate for a state of rest with minimum energy expenditure such as non-REM sleep.

Although the operation of the automatic control mechanism appears to be tuned to a lower activity level in non-REM sleep, all the normal physiological compensatory mechanisms are maintained. The sensitivity to CO_2 and O_2 changes is only moderately reduced (see Phillipson and Bowes, 1986 for review). Pulmonary inflation and deflation reflexes remain effective during non-REM sleep in both infants (Finer et al., 1976) and animals (Farber and Marlow, 1976; Phillipson et al., 1976a,b).

Older experimental evidence obtained via electrical stimulation in the hypothalamus of cats points to the existence of hypothalamic influences on brain stem regulatory mechanism and to the probability that these are operable in wakefulness and non-REM sleep but not in REM sleep (see Parmeggiani, 1979 for review). Hypothalamic stimulation will elicit lung inflation- or deflation-like effects in the first two states but not in REM sleep (Parmeggiani et al., 1981). Vagal stimulation is still effective in

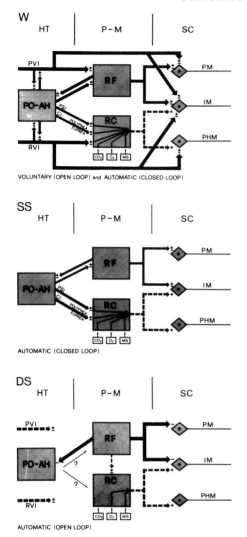

Figure 20-7 Voluntary and automatic control mechanisms of breathing during the wake–sleep cycle. W, voluntary (cortical) and automatic control mechanisms of breathing during wakefulness; SS, automatic control mechanism of breathing during non-REM sleep (synchronized sleep); DS, automatic control mechanism of breathing during REM sleep (desynchronized sleep). Solid lines indicate tonic influences; dashed lines indicate phasic influences; + and −, excitatory and inhibitory net influences, respectively, regardless of the specific synaptic organization. CI, chronotropic influences; CO_2, capnoreceptive inputs; HT, hypothalamus; IM, intercostal motoneurons; MS, mechanoreceptive inputs; O_2, oxyreceptive inputs; P–M, pons and medulla; PHM, phrenic motoneurons; PM, postural motoneurons; PO–AH, preoptic region and anterior hypothalamus; PSI, phase switching influences; PVI, postural voluntary influences; RC, respiratory centers; RF, reticular formation; RVI, respiratory voluntary influences; SC, spinal cord. The simplified scheme shows functional relationships among voluntary and automatic control mechanisms of both breathing and posture in the different behavioral states. Note the slight depression of capnoreceptive respiratory responses in non-REM sleep (SS) and the strong depression of the same responses during phasic activity (rapid eye movements, myoclonic twitches) in REM sleep (DS).

REM sleep, though indicating that the state-related changes are occurring rostral to the lower brain stem. The fact that the central effects are state related strongly supports the conclusion that integrative structures within the hypothalamus, not fibers of passage alone, are being stimulated. Thus, there is justification in including hypothalamic structures in the autonomic control mechanism of respiration in non-REM sleep to explain not only full homeostatic regulation, but also complete integration of all input variables influencing respiration in normal conditions [Figure 20-7, SS(NREM sleep)]. A general reorganization within the forebrain must be considered as well, however, for the effects of orbital cortex stimulation on respiratory cycle timing in cats are also suppressed during REM sleep (Marks et al., 1987) [Figure 20-7, DS(REM sleep)].

During REM sleep, a profound alteration in respiratory rhythmogenesis occurs (see Figure 20-7). Note that potential cortical influences have been reintroduced into the scheme because of the similarity of EEG and single neuronal activity patterns when compared with wakefulness (see McGinty et al., 1974, for review). The respiratory rhythm in humans and animals is very irregular (Aserinsky and Kleitman, 1953; Snyder et al., 1964; Duron and Marlot, 1980), the average frequency being increased or decreased with respect to the rate attained during non-REM sleep in eupnea or polypnea, respectively (Parmeggiani and Sabattini, 1972). Alveolar ventilation may be variable too as shown by either a decrease or no change in alveolar CO_2 partial pressure. It is important to stress that such disturbances are of central origin as they persist after vagotomy (Remmers et al., 1976), section of the spinal cord at T1–T2 (Thach et al., 1977), afferent denervation of the midthoracic chest wall (Phillipson et al., 1977), denervation of carotid and aortic chemo- and baroreceptors (Guazzi and Freis, 1969), hypercapnia (Phillipson et al., 1977), and hypoxia (Phillipson et al., 1978). Respiratory responses to hypercapnia are depressed whereas those to hypoxia are unchanged (Figure 20-8) (Bryan et al., 1976; Phillipson et al., 1977; Bolton and Herman, 1974; Phillipson et al., 1978). The inflation reflex is practically abolished during REM sleep in dogs and human infants (Phillipson et al., 1976a,b; Finer et al., 1976). The arousal threshold is increased in REM sleep as compared to non-REM sleep (see Phillipson and Bowes, 1986 for review).

From these results, it may be surmised that the changes in chemoreceptive and mechanoreceptive

---

Also some mechanoreceptive responses (e.g., lung inflation) are depressed in this stage of sleep. (Reproduced from Parmeggiani, 1979, with permission.)

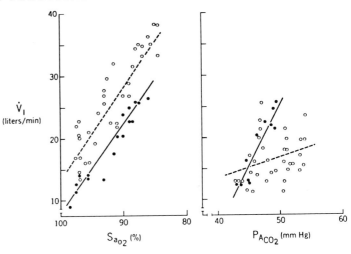

Figure 20-8 Breath-by-breath response of minute volume ventilation ($\dot{V}_I$) response to decreasing arterial O_2 saturation (S_{aO_2}) and to increasing alveolar partial pressure of CO_2 (P_{ACO_2}) in a sleeping dog. Filled circles, non-REM sleep slow wave sleep; open circles, REM sleep. Note scatter of data points around calculated linear regression lines during REM sleep and marked decrease in $\dot{V}_I$ response to increasing P_{ACO_2}. (Reproduced from Phillipson, 1977, with permission.)

respiratory reflexes during REM sleep are different, depending on the degree of their normal subordination to higher levels of integration in various species. In this regard, it is particularly interesting that during REM sleep oxyreceptive inputs maintain their influence not only on breathing (Bolton and Herman, 1974; Fagenholz et al., 1976; Phillipson et al., 1978), but also on blood pressure in cats since baroreceptive, but not chemoreceptive, reflexes are strongly depressed in that species (Mancia and Zanchetti, 1980; Guazzi et al., 1968).

To summarize, the combination of behavioral and metabolic controls of respiration during wakefulness is replaced by purely metabolic control in non-REM sleep. Hypotonia of respiratory muscles places an added burden on the system in REM sleep as well. For more extensive reviews of respiration in sleep, see reviews by Phillipson and Bowes (1986), Orem (1984), Mathew and Remmers (1984), and Sullivan (1980).

THERMOREGULATION

Changes in thermoregulation during sleep provide a very clear example of the effects of behavioral state on physiological functions and autonomic activity. In non-REM sleep, both brain and body temperatures decrease independently of ambient temperature. This phenomenon is consistent with a regulated state of body quiescence. In REM sleep, however, brain temperature increases within a relatively wide range of ambient temperature, whereas body temperature is affected as in poikilothermic animals (Parmeggiani et al., 1971). Only at relatively low ambient temperatures, the absolute value depending on the size of the animal, does brain temperature decrease during REM sleep (Van Twyver

and Allison, 1974; Walker et al., 1983; Parmeggiani et al., 1984). Moreover, the external thermal environment plays a role in determining the appearance of sleep, for at extremes of temperature, both the amount and quality of sleep are significantly changed in animals and humans (e.g., Parmeggiani and Rabini, 1970; Schmidek et al., 1972; Palca et al., 1986). In fact, maximal REM sleep time defines a narrower thermoneutral zone than does minimal metabolic rate (Szymusiak and Satinoff, 1981).

Thermoregulatory responses to thermal loads may be classified as behavioral (posture, motor activity related to the search for thermal comfort) and autonomic or physiological (vasomotion, piloerection, shivering, metabolic heat production, panting, sweating). Here the latter will be considered, but it should be noted that full expression of behavioral thermoregulation—changing of the sleep posture in different ambient temperatures—will occur in non-REM sleep. REM sleep, in contrast, is characterized by a stereotyped skeletal muscle atonia, which is unrelated to the thermal load.

During non-REM sleep, core temperature is regulated at a lower level than in wakefulness, due to the general decrease of energy expenditure typical of this stage of sleep. This could result from a simple resetting of the threshold temperatures of the different thermoregulatory responses, but work in rats (Glotzbach and Heller, 1976), cats (Parmeggiani and Sabattini, 1972), and humans (Sagot et al., 1987) suggests that the gains of the different thermoregulatory mechanisms may be affected during non-REM sleep. As Figure 20-9 illustrates, cooling the hypothalamus with a thermode elicits an increase in metabolic activity as measured by oxygen consumption. This change occurs at a lower hypothalamic temperature in non-REM sleep than in wakefulness, but also has a markedly reduced slope in non-REM

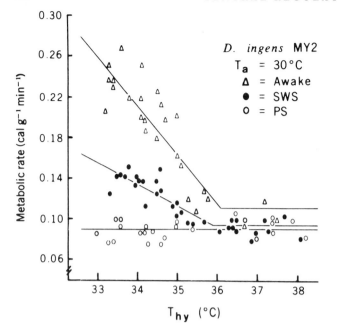

Figure 20-9 Relationship between metabolic rate and hypothalamic temperature in a kangaroo rat during wakefulness, SWS (non-REM sleep), and PS (REM sleep) at 30°C ambient temperature. Note the decrease in the response slope from wakefulness to non-REM sleep and the lack of metabolic response during REM sleep. T_a, ambient temperature; T_{hy}, hypothalamic temperature; MR, metabolic rate. (Reproduced from Glotzbach and Heller, 1976, with permission. Copyright 1976 by the American Association for the Advancement of Science.)

sleep (Glotzbach and Heller, 1976). Although these effects might also involve the impairment of fibers of passage, the presence of a concentration of thermosensitive cells in the hypothalamus that are affected by the behavioral state changes (see below) suggests that the hypothalamus itself is a key structure in this effect. This sleep-dependent depression of metabolic heat production, or nonshivering thermogenesis, is associated with an enhancement of other thermoregulatory responses. For example, both shivering and panting increase in intensity during non-REM sleep with respect to wakefulness in cats (Parmeggiani and Sabattini, 1972).

Temperature regulation is essentially suspended during REM sleep in small, furred animals (see Parmeggiani, 1980; Heller and Glotzbach, 1985 for reviews). It is uncertain whether the same occurs in humans (Parmeggiani, 1987). Thermoregulatory responses to environmental heating and cooling, such as shivering and panting, are suppressed (Parmeggiani and Rabini, 1970) (Figure 20-10). Panting will occur only at unpredictable times during REM sleep when cats have been kept at ambient temperatures over 30°C for several hours, and in situations where the panting rate prior to entering REM sleep is more than 100/minute (Amini-Sereshki and Morrison, 1988). This result may be attributed to activation of extrahypothalamic thermoregulatory mechanisms (see Satinoff, 1978 for review).

Disappearance of shivering in REM sleep is not due to concomitant muscle atonia. Small lesions of the dorsolateral pontine tegmentum eliminate skeletal muscle atonia and allow complex behaviors

(Hendricks et al., 1982), leaving other aspects of REM sleep intact (Jouvet and Delorme, 1965; Henley and Morrison, 1974). In such preparations during "REM sleep without atonia," shivering, although even violent in wakefulness and non-REM sleep, vanishes in REM sleep (Hendricks, 1982). This observation is made even more dramatic by the fact that during wakefulness cats with such lesions both shiver and pant at thresholds lower than normal (Amini-Sereshki and Morrison, 1986).

The decreased sympathetic activity in REM sleep is mirrored in other altered thermoregulatory phenomena. Piloerection in the cold disappears when a cat enters REM sleep (Hendricks, 1982) and thermal sweating in humans is depressed (e.g., Sagot et al., 1987).

Changes in ear skin temperature in response to variations in ambient temperature depend on blood flow, and demonstrate the absence of thermoregulatory vasomotor control during REM sleep in cats (Parmeggiani et al., 1977) and rabbits (Franzini et al., 1982). At a temperature below thermoneutrality, the skin warms on entrance into REM sleep as a consequence of vasodilation following the fall in sympathetic vasoconstrictor activity. At temperatures above or at thermoneutrality, skin temperature drops due to the lowering of blood pressure and accompanying passive vasoconstriction that results from the decrease in transmural pressure.

Thermoregulatory responses to direct thermal stimulation of the hypothalamus are also depressed during REM sleep. There is no metabolic response (Figure 20-9) to cooling the hypothalamus of the

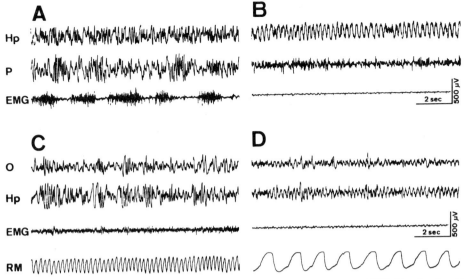

Figure 20-10 Shivering and panting during sleep in the cat. At low ambient temperature (6°C) shivering is evident in the neck muscle electromyogram during non-REM sleep (A) but absent during REM sleep (B). At high ambient temperature (36.5°C) tachypnea is evident during non-REM sleep (C) and disappears during REM sleep (D). P and O, parietal and occipital electroencephalograms; Hp, hippocampogram; EMG, electromyogram of neck muscle; RM, thoracic pneumogram. (Reproduced from Parmeggiani and Rabini, 1970, with permission.)

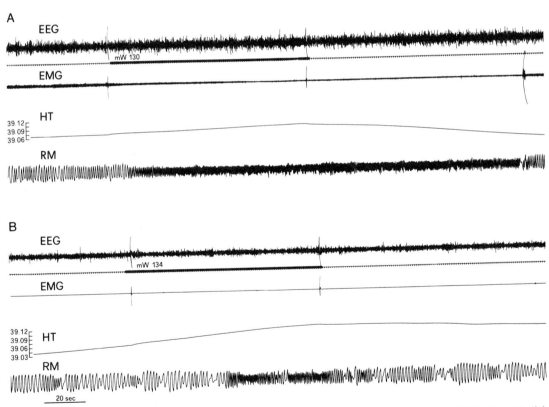

Figure 20-11 Respiratory responses to preoptic warming during sleep. Preoptic warming during non-REM sleep (A) elicits a long-lasting and high-frequency tachypnea in spite of an increase in hypothalamic temperature that is smaller than that eliciting only a short-lasting and irregular tachypnea during REM sleep (B). Note that in the latter case the effect of preoptic warming on hypothalamic temperature is superimposed on its spontaneous increase during REM sleep. EEG, electroencephalogram; EMG, electromyogram of neck muscle; HT, hypothalamic temperature (recorded 5 mm behind the warming electrodes); RM, thoracic pneumogram; mW, milliwatt (diathermy). (Reproduced from Parmeggiani et al., 1973, with permission.)

kangaroo rat in REM sleep (Glotzbach and Heller, 1976). Similarly, warming the hypothalamus in cats (Parmeggiani et al., 1973, 1976) does not induce panting in REM sleep, although it will in non-REM sleep at a specific threshold temperature. Even strong heating elicits a weak tachypneic response during REM sleep, an effect that is in no way comparable to that observed during non-REM sleep under the same experimental conditions (Figure 20-11). Moreover, in cats (Parmeggiani et al., 1977), hypothalamic warming elicits ear skin vasodilation in non-REM sleep, but no such effect in REM sleep (Figure 20-12).

An inactivation during REM sleep of the hypothalamic temperature regulator may be inferred from these changes in thermoregulatory responses to both peripheral and central thermal stimulation. However, a crucial answer to this question awaited study of specific hypothalamic preoptic neurons during the wake–sleep cycle. Studies on thermosensitive neurons in two species, the cat (Parmeggiani et al., 1983) and the kangaroo rat (Glotzbach and Heller, 1984), show consistent changes in neuronal thermosensitivity that are state dependent. Using short-lasting thermal stimuli, it has also been possible in

cats to study the temporal relationship of hypothalamic–preoptic neuronal thermosensitivity changes with EEG patterns and thermoregulatory effector activity (Parmeggiani et al., 1986). Cold- or warm-sensitive neurons respond inversely with either an increase or a decrease in firing rate during wakefulness and non-REM sleep depending on the direction of the temperature change (cooling or warming) induced by thermodes placed in the hypothalamic-preoptic region, but the majority lose their sensitivity to such stimulation during REM sleep (Figure 20-13). Essentially this amounts to an open feedback loop at the hypothalamic preoptic level of the temperature regulator. A more recent study in the cat (Parmeggiani et al., 1987) examined state-specific activity patterns of the population of thermosensitive neurons. Similarly shaped frequency distributions of neuronal thermosensitivity characterize wakefulness and non-REM sleep, but the frequency distribution of neuronal thermosensitivity is modified in REM sleep with respect to the other two states. A drop in the responsiveness to thermal stimulation of a majority of neurons is associated with a reversal in the sensitivity to cooling and warming of a minority of neurons. Such changes in REM sleep

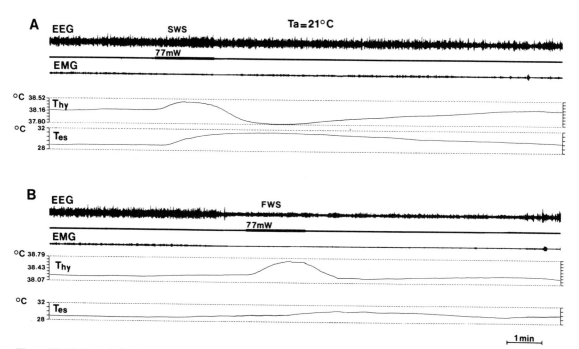

Figure 20-12 Hypothalamic and ear skin temperature changes elicited by preoptic warming during sleep at an ambient temperature slightly below thermal neutrality. (A) Preoptic warming during non-REM sleep elicits a steep increase in ear skin temperature (thermoregulatory heat-loss response). (B) The same preoptic warming during REM sleep does not affect the spontaneous increment of ear skin temperature occurring during this stage of sleep as a result of the decrease in sympathetic vasoconstrictor outflow. EEG, electroencephalogram; EMG, electromyogram of neck muscle; SWS, non-REM sleep; FWS, REM sleep; T_{hy}, hypothalamic temperature (recorded 3 mm behind the warming electrodes); T_{es}, ear skin temperature; T_a ambient temperature; mW, milliwatt (diathermy). (Reproduced from Parmeggiani et al., 1977, with permission.)

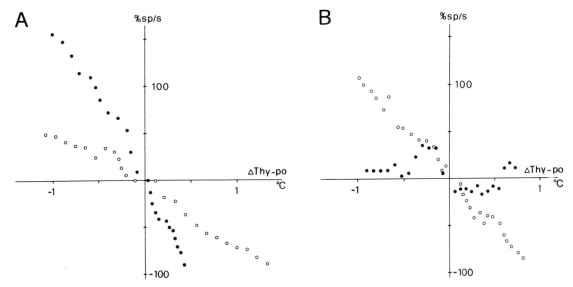

Figure 20-13 Relative changes in firing rate (percentage spikes/second) of thermosensitive neurons as a function of anterior hypothalamic–preoptic temperature changes (filled triangle, Thy-po in degree Celsius) elicited by water-perfused thermodes during the waking–sleeping cycle. (A) The responsiveness of a cold-sensitive neuron is greater in wakefulness (filled circles) than in non-REM sleep (open circles). (B) A cold-sensitive neuron during non-REM sleep (open circles) is thermally insensitive during REM sleep (filled circles). (Data from Parmeggiani et al., 1983, with permission.)

decrease or abolish the hypothalamic preoptic drive on thermoregulatory effectors. A residual thermoregulatory capability may be maintained by the release of subordinate extrahypothalamic brain stem mechanisms (Satinoff, 1978).

To summarize, the thermal environment greatly influences sleep, but the sleep state, in turn, has a profound effect on thermoregulation, most notably in REM sleep when furred animals become essentially poikilothermic. The data and concepts presented in this section are reviewed in more detail by Parmeggiani (1980) and Heller and Glotzbach (1985).

CONCLUDING REMARKS

The chapter has centered on mammalian sleep, although bird sleep has similar properties. Whether other vertebrate classes exhibit REM sleep remains controversial. A key point may be that mammals and birds are endotherms, their highly efficient central thermoregulatory systems enabling them to perform at a high level of activity throughout a wide range of environmental conditions, whereas many other animals cannot. What purpose could be served, then, by surrendering tight homeostatic control while already vulnerable because of reduced sensory responsiveness no less? The answer is not self-evident, in large measure because we simply do not know what purpose(s) REM sleep serves. It could be

that tight regulation is suspended in REM sleep because certain neurons critical for control rest during these periods. Siegel and Rogawski (1988) have reviewed substantial evidence suggesting that REM sleep, with its attendant silence of noradrenergic locus coeruleus neurons, serves an important function in up-regulating or preventing the down-regulation of noradrenergic receptors as a result of the continual waking activity of these neurons. In any event, homeostatic regulation is held in abeyance because for some as-yet-uncertain reason the state of REM sleep seems to take precedence (within certain environmental limits as discussed above). This would not be without precedent; for an interruption of regulation can be accomplished voluntarily for some functions in wakefulness by cortical influences acting on the brain stem, for example, suspension of respiration during speech; but it can also occur without conscious effort, for example, a cessation of shivering with intense arousal to a stimulus. Whatever the reasons might be, though, recognition that changes in the physiology of the body can be quite profound during REM sleep forces one to a broader view of the activity of the autonomic nervous system and the meaning of the phrase, "normal function."

SUMMARY

Sleep is an active, complex state that depends on the engagement of a number of neuronal groups throughout the brain. Two different phases, non-REM sleep and REM sleep, alternate in a predictable way throughout a sleeping period. REM sleep is of particular interest from the standpoint of the autonomic nervous system because regulation of homeostasis is grossly depressed. The reason for this remains a mystery.

Non-REM sleep is characterized by a tonic increase in parasympathetic activity, which is also maintained throughout REM sleep. There is no or only slight attenuation in sympathetic discharge during non-REM sleep, depending on the effect to the organ considered. Deep non-REM sleep (slow-wave sleep) shows the greatest stability of autonomic regulation, a feature common to all mammalian species. A tonic decrease in sympathetic activity characterizes REM sleep in several species. However, irregular episodes of sympathetic activation and parasympathetic deactivation, related to somatic phasic events (rapid eye movements and muscle twitches), underlie the great instability of autonomic functions during REM sleep episodes. REM sleep is characterized by the variety and variability of functional events within and among species.

Cardiovascular changes during non-REM sleep represent a homeostatic response to behavioral quiescence. The stereotype of cardiovascular activity in non-REM sleep across mammalian species is based on the development of efficient automatic regulatory mechanisms, which is a peculiar physiological feature of mammals. In contrast, the variety and variability of functional events within and among species during REM sleep are the result of the interaction between central mechanisms and species-specific reflex mechanisms released from the homeostatic control of hypothalamic structures.

As in the case of circulation, respiration is characterized by a regulation consistent with the decrease in metabolic rate in non-REM sleep and then a removal of CNS modulation of various reflexes and activation of state-specific brain stem neural activity during REM sleep. An added feature for this system is a shift from a combination of behavioral and metabolic controls during wakefulness to purely metabolic regulation involving the hypothalamus and related areas during non-REM sleep, particularly deep non-REM sleep once the wakefulness stimulus is completely withdrawn. Less regular, at times erratic, respiratory movements and decreased responsiveness to a variety of stimuli result from the loss of control by the hypothalamus in REM sleep.

The thermal environment greatly affects both the quality and quantity of sleep. In turn, sleep modifies the nature of thermoregulation. All thermoregulatory responses, both behavioral and physiological, are observed during non-REM sleep. Changes in threshold and gain of the major putative regulator,

the hypothalamus, occur in the transition from wakefulness to non-REM sleep that are specifically related to sleep processes. Most remarkable during REM sleep, besides the lack of behavioral thermoregulation as a consequence of muscle atonia, is the disappearance or depression of the physiological responses such as shivering, panting, vasomotion, piloerection, and sweating to peripheral and central thermal stimuli.

ACKNOWLEDGMENTS

This work was prepared with the support of a grant from the North Atlantic Treaty Organization to the authors and NIMH grant MH 42903 to Dr. Morrison.

REFERENCES

Reviews

Coote, J. H. (1982). Respiratory and circulatory control during sleep. *Journal of Experimental Biology* 100, 223–239.

Heller, H. C., and Glotzbach, S. F. (1985). Thermoregulation and sleep. In: *Heat Transfer in Biological Systems: Analysis and Application,* R. C. Eberhardt and A. Shitzer (eds.), Plenum, New York, pp. 107–134.

Jacobs, B. (1987). Brain monoaminergic unit activity in behaving animals. In: *Progress in Psychobiology and Physiological Psychology,* Vol. 12, A. N. Epstein and A. R. Morrison (eds.), Academic Press, New York, pp. 171–206.

Jones, J. V., Sleight, P., and Smyth, H. S. (1980). Haemodynamic changes during sleep in man. In: *Sleep. Current Topics in Endocrinology,* Vol.3, D. Ganten and D. Pfaff (eds.), Academic Press, New York, pp. 213–272.

Jouvet, M. (1972). The role of monoamines and acetylcholine-containing neurons in the regulation of the sleep-waking cycle. *Ergebnisse der Physiologie* 64, 166–307.

Karacan, I., Salis, P. J., and Williams, R. L. (1978). The role of the sleep laboratory in diagnosis and treatment of impotence. In: *Sleep Disorders, Diagnosis and Treatment,* R. L. Williams and I. Karacan (eds.), Wiley, New York, pp. 353–382.

Krueger, J. M., Obal, F., Jr., Opp, M., Cady, A. B., Johannsen, L., Toth, L., and Majde, J. (1990). Putative sleep neuromodulators. In: *Sleep and Biological Rhythms,* J. Montplaisir (ed.), Oxford University Press, New York, in press.

Lugaresi, E., Coccagna, G., and Mantovani, M. (1978). *Hypersomnia with Periodic Apneas: Advances in Sleep Research.* Spectrum Books, New York.

Mancia, G., and Zanchetti, A. (1980). Cardiovascular regulation during sleep. In: *Physiology in Sleep,* J. Orem and C. D. Barnes (eds.), Academic Press, New York, pp. 1–55.

Mathew, O. P., and and Remmers, J. E. (1984). Respiratory function of the upper airway. In: *Sleep and Breathing,* N. A. Saunders and C. E. Sullivan (eds.), Dekker, New York, pp. 163–200.

McGinty, D. J., Harper, R. M., and and Fairbanks, M. K. (1974). Neuronal unit activity and the control of sleep states. In: *Advances in Sleep Research,* Vol. 1, E. Weitzman (ed.), Spectrum Books, New York, pp. 173–216.

McGinty, D. J., and Beahm, E. K. (1984). Neurobiology of sleep. In: *Sleep and Breathing,* N. A. Saunders and C. E. Sullivan (eds.), Dekker, New York, pp. 1–89.

Mendelson, W. B., Wyatt, R. J., and Gillin, J. C. (1983). Whither the sleep factors? In: *Sleep Disorders, Basic and Clinical Research,* M. H. Chase and E. D. Weitzman (eds.), Spectrum Books, New York, pp. 281–306.

Moore-Ede, M. E., Sulyman, F. M., and Fuller, C. A. (1982). *The Clocks That Time Us.* Harvard University Press, Cambridge.

Morrison, A. R., and Reiner, P. B. (1985). A dissection of paradoxical sleep. In: *Brain Mechanisms of Sleep,* D. J. McGinty, R. Drucker-Colin, A. R. Morrison, and P. L. Parmeggiani (eds.), Raven, New York, pp. 97–110.

Orem, J. (1984). Central neural interactions between sleep and breathing. In: *Sleep and Breathing,* N. A. Saunders and C. E. Sullivan (eds.), Dekker, New York, pp. 91–135.

Orem, J., and Barnes, C. D. (1980). *Physiology in Sleep.* Academic Press, New York.

Orem, J., and Keeling, J. (1980). Appendix: A compendium of physiology in sleep. In: *Physiology in Sleep,* J. Orem and C. D. Barnes (eds.), Academic Press, New York, pp. 315–335.

Orr, W. D., and Stahl, M. L (1980). Alimentary function during sleep. In: *Physiology in Sleep,* J. Orem and C. D. Barnes (eds.), Academic Press, New York, pp. 203–212.

Parmeggiani, P. L. (1979). Integrative aspects of hypothalamic influences on respiratory brainstem mechanisms during wakefulness and sleep. In: *Central Nervous Control Mechanisms,* C. Von Euler and H. Lagercrantz (eds.), Pergamon, Oxford, pp. 53–68.

Parmeggiani, P. L. (1980). Temperature regulation during sleep: A study in homeostasis. In: *Physiology in Sleep,* J. Orem and C. D. Barnes (eds.), Academic Press, New York, pp. 97–143.

Parmeggiani, P. L. (1985). Homeostatic regulation during sleep: Facts and hypotheses. In: *Brain Mechanisms of Sleep,* D. J. McGinty, R. Drucker-Colin, A. R. Morrison, and P. L. Parmeggiani (eds.), Raven, New York, pp. 385–397.

Parmeggiani, P. L. (1987). Interaction between sleep and thermoregulation: An aspect of the control of behavioral states. *Sleep* 10, 426–435.

Parmeggiani, P. L., Morrison, A. R., Drucker-Colin, R., and McGinty, D. J. (1985). Brain mechanisms of sleep: An overview of methodological issues. In: *Brain Mechanisms of Sleep,* D. J. McGinty, R. Drucker-Colin, A. R., Morrison, and P. L. Parmeggiani (eds.), Raven, New York, pp. 1–34.

Phillipson, E. A. (1977). Regulation of breathing during sleep. *American Review of Respiratory Diseases* 115, Suppl., 217–224.

Phillipson, E. A., and Bowes, G. (1986). Control of breathing during sleep. In: *Handbook of Physiology Section III, The Respiratory System,* Vol. II, N. S. Cherniack and J. G. Widdicombe (eds.), American Physiological Society, Bethesda, MD, pp. 642–689.

Satinoff, E. (1978). Neural organization and evolution of thermal regulation in mammals. *Science* 201, 16–22.

Saunders, N. A., and Sullivan, C. E. (1984). *Sleep and Breathing.* Dekker, New York.

Siegel, J. M., and Rogawski, M. A. (1988). A function for REM sleep: Regulation of noradrenergic receptor sensitivity. *Brain Research Reviews* 13, 213–233.

Sterman, M. B., and Shouse, M. N. (1985). Sleep "centers" in the brain: The preoptic basal forebrain area revisited. In: *Brain Mechanisms of Sleep,* (eds.), D. J. McGinty, R. Drucker-Colin, A. Morrison, and P. L. Parmeggiani (eds.), Raven, New York, pp. 277–299.

Sullivan, C. E. (1980). Breathing in sleep. In: *Physiology in Sleep,* J. Orem and C. D. Barnes (eds.), Academic Press, New York, pp. 213–272.

Swanson, L. W. (1987). The hypothalamus. In: *Handbook of Chemical Neuroanatomy. Vol. 5, Integrated Systems of the CNS,* Part I. A. Bjorklund, T. Hökfelt, and L. W. Swanson (eds.), Elsevier, Amsterdam, pp. 1–124.

Ursin, R., and Sterman, M. B. (1981). *A Manual for Standardized Scoring of Sleep and Waking States in the Adult Cat,* University of California, Los Angeles.

Research Articles

Amatruda, T. T., Black, D. A., McKenna, T. M., McCarley, R. W., and Hobson, J. A. (1975). Sleep cycle control and cholinergic mechanisms: Differential effects of carbachol at pontine brainstem sites. *Brain Research* 98, 501–575.

Amini-Sereshki, L., and Morrison, A. R. (1986). Effects of pontine tegmental lesions that induce paradoxical sleep without atonia on thermoregulation in cats during wakefulness. *Brain Research* 384, 23–28.

Amini-Sereshki, L., and Morrison, A. R. (1988). Release of heat-loss responses in paradoxical sleep by thermal loads and by pontine tegmental lesions in cats. *Brain Research* 450, 9–17.

Aserinsky, E., and Kleitman, N. (1953). Regularly occurring periods of eye motility, and concomitant phenomena during sleep. *Science* 118, 273–274.

Baccelli, G., Guazzi, M., Mancia, G., and Zanchetti, A. (1974). Central and reflex regulation of sympathetic vasoconstrictor activity of limb muscle during desynchronized sleep in the cat. *Circulation Research* 35, 625–635.

Baccelli, G., Albertini, R., Mancia, G., and Zanchetti, A. (1978). Control of regional circulation by the sino-aortic reflexes during desynchronized sleep in the cat. *Cardiovascular Research* 12, 523–528.

Baker, T. L., Netick, A., and Dement, W. C. (1981). Sleep-related apneic and apneustic breathing following pneumotaxic lesion and vagotomy. *Respiratory Physiology* 46, 271–294.

Baust, W., and Bohnert, B. (1969). The regulation of heart rate during sleep. *Experimental Brain Research* 7, 169–180.

Baust, W., Weidinger, H., and Kirchner, F. (1968). Sympathetic activity during natural sleep and arousal. *Archives Italiennes de Biologie* 106, 379–390.

Berlucchi, G., Moruzzi, G., Salvi, G., and Strata, P. (1964). Pupil behavior and ocular movement during synchronized and desynchronized sleep. *Archives Italiennes de Biologie* 102, 230–244.

Bolton, D. P. G., and Herman, S. (1974). Ventilation and sleep state in the newborn. *Journal of Physiology (London)* 240, 67–77.

Bryan, H. M., Hagan, R., Gulston, G., and Bryan, A. C. (1976). Co₂ response and sleep state infants. *Clinical Research* 24, A689.

Chu, N. S., and Bloom, F. E. (1974). Activity patterns of catecholamine-containing pontine neurons in the dorsolateral tegmentum of unrestrained cats. *Journal of Neurobiology* 5, 527–544.

Coccagna, G., Mantovani, M., and Lugaresi, E. (1971). Arterial pressure changes during spontaneous sleep in man. *Electroencephalography and Clinical Neurophysiology* 31, 277–281.

Dement, W. C. (1958). The occurrence of low voltage, fast electroencephalogram patterns during behavioral sleep in the cat. *Electroencephalography and Clinical Neurophysiology* 10, 291–296.

Dick, T. E., Parmeggiani, P. L., and Orem, J. (1982). Intercostal muscle activity during sleep in the cat: An augmentation of expiratory activity. *Respiration Physiology* 50, 255–265.

Duron, B., and Marlot, D. (1980). Intercostal and diaphragmatic electrical activity during wakefulness and sleep in normal unrestrained adult cats. *Sleep* 3, 269–280.

Fagenholz, S. A., O'Connell, K., and Shannon, D. C. (1976). Chemoreceptor function and sleep state in apnea. *Pediatrics* 58, 31–36.

Farber, J. P., and Marlow, T. A. (1976). Pulmonary reflexes and breathing pattern during sleep in the opossum. *Respiratory Physiology* 27, 73–86.

Finer, N. N., Abroms, I. F., and Taeusch, H. W. Jr. (1976). Ventilation and sleep states in new born infants. *Journal of Pediatrics* 89, 100–108.

Fink, B. R. (1961). Influences of cerebral activity in wakefulness on regulation of breathing. *Journal of Applied Physiology* 16, 15–20.

Foutz, A. S., Netick, A., and Dement, W. C. (1979). Sleep state effects on breathing after spinal cord transection and vagotomy in the cat. *Respiratory Physiology* 37, 89–100.

Franzini, C., Cianci, T., Lenzi, P. L., and Guidalotti, P. L. (1982). Neural control of vasomotion in rabbit ear is impaired during desynchronized sleep. *American Journal of Physiology* 243, R142–R146.

Futuro-Neto, H. A., and Coote, J. H. (1982a). Changes in synaptic activity to heart and blood vessels during desynchronized sleep. *Brain Research* 252, 259–268.

Futuro-Neto, H. A., and Coote, J. H. (1982b). Desynchronized sleep-like pattern of sympathetic activity elicited by electrical stimulation of sites in the brainstem. *Brain Research* 252, 269–276.

Gassel, M. M., Ghelarducci, B., Marchiafava, P. L., and Pompeiano, O. (1964a). Phasic changes in blood pressure and heart rate during the rapid eye movement episodes of desynchronized sleep in unrestrained cats. *Archives Italiennes de Biologie* 102, 530–544.

Gassel, M. M., Marchiafava, P. L., and Pompeiano, O. (1964b). Phasic changes in muscular activity during de-

synchronized sleep in unrestrained cats. *Archives Italiennes de Biologie* 102, 449–470.

Glenn, L. L., Foutz, A. S., and Dement, W. C. (1978). Membrane potential of spinal motoneurons during sleep in cats. *Sleep* 1, 199–204.

Glotzbach, S. F., and Heller, H. C. (1976). Central nervous regulation of body temperature during sleep. *Science* 194, 537–539.

Glotzbach, S. F., and Heller, H. C. (1984). Changes in the thermal characteristics of hypothalamic neurons during sleep and wakefulness. *Brain Research* 309, 17–26.

Guazzi, M., and Freis, E. D. (1969). Sinoaortic reflexes and arterial pH, PO₂ and PCO₂ in wakefulness and sleep. *American Journal of Physiology* 217, 1623–1627.

Guazzi, M., and Zanchetti, A. (1965). Blood pressure and heart rate during natural sleep of the cat and their regulation by carotid sinus and aortic reflexes. *Archives Italiennes de Biologie* 103, 789–817.

Guazzi, M., Baccelli, G., and Zanchetti, A. (1968). Reflex chemoceptive regulation of arterial pressure during natural sleep in the cat. *American Journal of Physiology* 214, 969–978.

Hendricks, J. C. (1982). Absence of shivering in the cat during paradoxical sleep without atonia. *Experimental Neurology* 75, 700–710.

Hendricks, J. C., Morrison, A. R., and Mann, G. L. (1982). Different behaviors during paradoxical sleep without atonia depend on pontine lesion site. *Brain Research* 239, 81–105.

Henley, K., and Morrison, A. R. (1974). A re-evaluation of the effects of lesions of the pontine tegmentum and locus coeruleus on phenomena of paradoxical sleep in the cat. *Acta Neurobiologiae Experimentalis* 34, 215–232.

Hess, W. R. (1944). Das Schlafsyndrom als Folge dienzephaler Reizung. *Helvetica Physiologica Pharmacologica Acta* 2, 305–344.

Hobson, J. A., McCarley, R. W., and Wyzinski, P. W. (1975). Sleep cycle oscillation: Reciprocal discharge by two brainstem neuronal groups. *Science* 189, 55–58.

Ibuka, N., and Kawamura, H. (1975). Loss of circadian rhythm in sleep-wakefulness cycle in the rat by suprachiasmatic nucleus lesions. *Brain Research* 96, 76–81.

Iwamura, Y., Uchino, Y., Ozawa, S., and Torii, S. (1966). Sympathetic nerve activity and paradoxical sleep in the decerebrate cat. *Proceedings of Japan Academy of Science* 42, 837–840.

Iwamura, Y., Uchino, Y., Ozawa, S., and Torii, S. (1969). Spontaneous and reflex discharge of a sympathetic nerve during "para" sleep in decerebrate cat. *Brain Research* 16, 359–367.

Jouvet, M. (1962). Recherches sur les structures nerveuses et les mécanismes responsables des différentes phases du sommeil physiologique. *Archives Italiennes de Biologie* 100, 125–206.

Jouvet, M. (1964). Cataplexie et sommeil paradoxal réflexes chez le Chat pontique. *Comptes Rendus des Seances de La Societe de Biologie et de Ses Filiales* 159, 383–387.

Jouvet, M., and Delorme, F. (1965). Locus coeruleus et sommeil paradoxal. *Comptes Rendus des Seances de La Societe de Biologie et de Ses Filiales* 159, 895–899.

Junqueira, L. F., Jr., and Krieger, E. M. (1976). Blood pressure and sleep in the rat in normotension and in neurogenic hypertension. *Journal of Physiology* 259, 725–735.

Knuepfer, M. M., Stumpf, H., and Stock, G. (1986). Baroreceptor sensitivity during desynchronized sleep. *Experimental Neurology* 92, 323–334.

Lacombe, J., Nosjean, A., Meunier, J. M., and Laguzzi, R. (1988). Computer analysis of cardiovascular changes during sleep-wake cycle in Sprague-Dawley rats. *American Journal of Physiology* 254, H217–H222.

Leach, L., Whishaw, I. Q., and Kolb, B. (1980). Effect of kainic acid lesions in the lateral hypothalamus on behavior and hippocampal and neocortical electroencephalograph (EEG) activity in the rat brain. *Behavioral Brain Research* 1, 411–431.

Lenzi, P., Cianci, T., Leonardi, G. S., Martinelli, A., and Franzini, C. (1989). Muscle blood flow changes during sleep as a function of fibre type composition. *Experimental Brain Research,* 74, 549–554.

Lugaresi, E., Cirignotta, F., Coccagna, G., and Piana, C. (1980). Some epidemiologic data on snoring and cardiocirculatory disturbances. *Sleep* 3, 221–224.

Lydic, R., and Orem, J. (1979). Respiratory neurons of the pneumotaxic center during sleep and wakefulness. *Neuroscience Letters* 15, 187–192.

Marks, J. D., Frysinger, R. C., and Harper, R. M. (1987). State dependent respiratory depression elicited by stimulation of the orbital frontal cortex. *Experimental Neurology* 95, 714–729.

McGinty, D. J., and Harper, R. M. (1976). Dorsal raphe neurons: Depression of firing during sleep in cats. *Brain Research* 101, 569–575.

Meunier, J. M., Nosjean, A., Lacombe, J., and Laguzzi, R. (1988). Cardiovascular changes during the sleep-wake cycle in spontaneous hypertensive rats and in their genetically normotensive precursors. *Pflugers Archiv* 411, 195–199.

Mitani, A., Ito, K., Hallanger, A. E., Wainer, B. H., Kataoka, K., and McCarley, R. W. (1988). Cholinergic projections from the laterodorsal and peduculopontine tegmental nuclei to the pontine gigantocellular tegmental field in the cat. *Brain Research* 451, 397–402.

Morrison, A. R., and Pompeiano, O. (1970). Vestibular influences during sleep. VI. Vestibular control of autonomic functions during the rapid eye movements of desynchronized sleep. *Archives Italiennes de Biologie* 108, 154–180.

Moruzzi, G., and Magoun, H. W. (1949). Brainstem reticular formation and activation of the EEG. *Electroencephalography and Clinical Neurophysiology* 1, 455–473.

Muller, N. L., Volgyesi, G., Becker, L., Bryan, M. H., and Bryan, A. C. (1979). Diaphragmatic muscle tone. *Journal of Applied Physiology* 47, 279–284.

Nakamura, Y., Goldberg, L. J., Chandler, S. H., and Chase, M. H. (1978). Intracellular analysis of trigeminal motoneuron activity during sleep in the cat. *Science* 199, 204–207.

Nauta, W. J. H. (1946). Hypothalamic regulation of sleep in rats. Experimental study. *Journal of Neurophysiology* 9, 285–316.

Netick, A., and Foutz, A. S. (1980). Respiratory activity and sleep-wakefulness in the deafferented, paralyzed cat. *Sleep* 3, 1–12.

Orem, J. (1980). Neuronal mechanisms of respiration in REM sleep. *Sleep* 3, 251–267.

Orem, J., and Lydic, R. (1978). Upper airway function during sleep and wakefulness: Experimental studies on normal and anesthetized cats. *Sleep* 1, 49–68.

Orem, J., Montplaisir, J., and Dement, W. C. (1974). Changes in the activity of respiratory neurons during sleep. *Brain Research* 82, 309–315.

Orem, J., Netick, A., and Dement, W. C. (1977a). Increased upper airway resistance to breathing during sleep in the cat. *Electroencephalography and Clinical Neurophysiology* 43, 14–22.

Orem, J., Netick, A., and Dement, W. C. (1977b). Breathing during sleep and wakefulness in the cat. *Respiration Physiology* 30, 265–289.

Palca, J. W., Walker, J. M., and Berger, R. J. (1986). Thermoregulation, metabolism, and stages of sleep in cold-exposed men. *Journal of Applied Physiology* 61, 940–947.

Parmeggiani, P. L. (1962). Sleep behavior elicited by electrical stimulation of cortical and subcortical structures in the cat. *Helvetica Physiologica Pharmacologica Acta* 20, 347–367.

Parmeggiani, P. L., and Rabini, C. (1970). Sleep and environmental temperature. *Archives Italiennes de Biologie* 108, 369–387.

Parmeggiani, P. L., and Sabattini, L. (1972). Electromyographic aspects of postural, respiratory and thermoregulatory mechanisms in sleeping cats. *Electroencephalography and Clinical Neurophysiology* 33, 1–13.

Parmeggiani, P. L., Franzini, C., Lenzi, P., and Cianci, T. (1971). Inguinal subcutaneous temperature changes in cats sleeping at different environmental temperatures. *Brain Research* 33, 397–404.

Parmeggiani, P. L., Franzini, C., Lenzi, P. L., and Zamboni, G. (1973). Threshold of respiratory responses to preoptic heating during sleep in freely moving cats. *Brain Research* 52, 189–201.

Parmeggiani, P. L., Franzini, C., and Lenzi, P. L. (1976). Respiratory frequency as a function of preoptic temperature during sleep. *Brain Research* 111, 253–260.

Parmeggiani, P. L., Zamboni, G., Cianci, T., and Calasso, M. (1977). Absence of thermoregulatory vasomotor responses during fast wave sleep in cats. *Electroencephalography and Clinical Neurophysiology* 42, 372–380.

Parmeggiani, P. L., Calasso, M., and Cianci, T. (1981). Respiratory effects of preoptic-anterior hypothalamic electrical stimulation during sleep in cats. *Sleep* 4, 71–82.

Parmeggiani, P. L., Azzaroni, A., Cevolani, D., and Ferrari, G. (1983). Responses of anterior hypothalamic preoptic neurons to direct thermal stimulation during wakefulness and sleep. *Brain Research* 269, 382–385.

Parmeggiani, P. L., Zamboni, G., Perez, E., and Lenzi, P. (1984). Hypothalamic temperature during desynchronized sleep. *Experimental Brain Research* 54, 315–320.

Parmeggiani, P. L., Azzaroni, A., Cevolani, D., and Ferrari, G. (1986). Polygraphic study of anterior hypothalamic-preoptic neuron thermosensitivity during sleep. *Electro-*

encephalography and Clinical Neurophysiology 63, 289–295.

Parmeggiani, P. L., Cevolani, D., Azzaroni, A., and Ferrari, G. (1987). Thermosensitivity of anterior hypothalmic-preoptic neurons during the waking-sleeping cycle: A study in brain functional states. *Brain Research* 415, 79–89.

Phillipson, E. A., Kozar, L. F., and Murphy, E. (1976a). Respiratory load compensation in awake and sleeping dogs. *Journal of Applied Physiology* 40, 895–902.

Phillipson, E. A., Murphy, E., and Kozar, L. F. (1976b). Regulation of respiration in sleeping dogs. *Journal of Applied Physiology* 40, 688–693.

Phillipson, E. A., Kozar, L. F., Rebuc, A. S., and Murphy, E. (1977). Ventilatory and waking responses to CO_2 in sleeping dogs. *American Review of Respiratory Diseases* 115, 251–259.

Phillipson, E. A., Sullivan, C. E., Read, D. J. C., Murphy, E., and Kozar, L. F. (1978). Ventilatory and waking responses to hypoxia in sleeping dogs. *Journal of Applied Physiology* 44, 512–520.

Reiner, P. (1986). Correlational analysis of central noradrenergic neuronal activity and sympathetic tone in behaving cats. *Brain Research* 378, 86–96.

Reis, D. J., Moorehead, D., and Wooten, G. F. (1968). Redistribution of visceral and cerebral blood flow in the REM sleep phase of sleep. *Neurology* 18, 282.

Reis, D. J., Moorhead, D., and Wooten, G. F. (1969). Differential regulation of blood flow to red and white muscle in sleep and defense behavior. *American Journal of Physiology* 217, 541–546.

Remmers, J. E., Barlett, D., Jr., and Putnam, M. D. (1976). Changes in the respiratory cycle associated with sleep. *Respiratory Physiology* 28, 227–238.

Sagot, J. C., Amoros, C., Candas, V., and Libert, J. P. (1987). Sweating responses and body temperatures during nocturnal sleep in humans. *American Journal of Physiology (Regulatory, Integrative, Comparative Physiology)* 21) 252, R462–R470.

Sallanon, M., Sakai, K., Buda, C., Puymartin, M., and Jouvet, M. (1988). Increase of paradoxical sleep—induced by microinjections of ibotenic acid into the ventrolateral part of the posterior hypothalamus in the cat. *Archives Italiennes de Biologie* 126, 87–97.

Sauerland, E. K., and Harper, R. M. (1976). The human tongue during sleep: Electromyographic activity of the genioglossus muscle. *Experimental Neurology* 51, 160–170.

Sauerland, E. K., Orr, W. C., and Hairston, L. E. (1981). EMG activity of oropharyngeal muscles during respiration in wakefulness and sleep. *Electromyography and Clinical Neurophysiology* 21, 307–316.

Schmidek, W. R., Hoshino, K., Schmidek, M., and Timo-Iaria, C. (1972). Influence of environmental temperature on the sleep-wakefulness cycle in the rat. *Physiology and Behavior* 8, 363–371.

Sherry, J. H., and Megirian, D. (1980). Respiratory EMG activity of the posterior cricoarytenoid, cricothyroid and diaphragm muscles during sleep. *Respiration Physiology* 39, 355–365.

Sieck, G. D., and Harper, R. M. (1980). Pneumotaxic area neuronal discharge during sleep-waking states in the cat. *Experimental Neurology* 67, 79–102.

Siegel, J. M., and McGinty, D. J. (1977). Pontine reticular formation neurons: Relationship of discharge to motor activity. *Science* 196, 678–680.

Snyder, F., Hobson, J. A., Morrison, D. F., and Goldfrank, F. (1964). Changes in respiration, heart rate, and systolic blood pressure in human sleep. *Journal of Applied Physiology* 19, 417–422.

Sterman, M. B., and Clemente, C. D. (1962). Forebrain inhibitory mechanisms: Sleep patterns induced by basal forebrain stimulation in the behaving cat. *Experimental Neurology* 6, 103–117.

Sterman, M. B., McGinty, D. J., and Iwamura, Y. (1974). Modulation of trigeminal reflexes during the REM sleep state in brain transected cats. *Archives Italiennes de Biologie* 112, 278–297.

Szymusiak, R., and McGinty, D. J. (1986). Sleep-related neuronal discharge in the basal forebrain of cats. *Brain Research* 370, 82–92.

Szymusiak, R., and Satinoff, E. (1981). Maximal REM sleep time defines a narrower thermoneutral zone than does minimal metabolic rate. *Physiology and Behavior* 26, 687–690.

Thach, B. T., Abrams, I. F., Frantz, I. D., Sotrel, A., Bruce, E. N., and Goldman, M. D. (1977). REM sleep breathing pattern without intercostal muscle influence. *Federation Proceedings* 36, Section 917, 445.

Trulson, M. E., and Jacobs, B. L. (1978). Raphe unit activity in freely moving cats: Correlation with level of behavioral arousal. *Brain Research* 163, 135–150.

Van Twyver, H., and Allison, T. (1974). Sleep in the armadillo Dasypus novemcinctus at moderate and low ambient temperatures. *Brain, Behavior and Evolution* 9, 107–120.

Vertes, R. P. (1979). Selective firing of rat pontine gigantocellular neurons during movement and REM sleep. *Brain Research* 128, 146–152.

Villablanca, J. (1966). Behavioral and polygraphic study of "sleep" and "wakefulness" in chronic decerebrate cats. *Electroencephalography and Clinical Neurophysiology* 21, 562–577.

Von Economo, C. (1917). Encephalitis lethargica. *Wiener Klinische Wochenschrift* 30, 581–585.

Von Economo, C. (1930). Sleep as a problem of localization. *The Journal of Nervous and Mental Disease* 71, 249–259.

Walker, J. M., Walker, L. E., Harris, D. V., and Berger, R. J. (1983). Cessation of thermoregulation during REM sleep in the pocket mouse. *American Journal of Physiology* 244, R114–R118.

Wurtz, R. H., and O'Flaherty, J. J. (1967). Physiological correlates of steady potential shifts during sleep and wakefulness. 1. Sensitivity of the steady potential to alterations in carbon dioxide. *Electroencephalography and Clinical Neurophysiology* 22, 30–42.

Zepelin, H., and Rechtschaffen, A. (1974). Mammalian sleep, longevity and energy metabolism. *Brain, Behavior and Evolution* 10, 425–470.

Index